FUNDAMENTALS
OF VETERINARY
OPHTHALMOLOGY

FUNDAMENTALS OF VETERINARY OPHTHALMOLOGY

SECOND EDITION

Douglas Slatter, B.V.Sc., M.S., Ph.D., F.R.C.V.S.

Diplomate, American College of Veterinary Ophthalmologists
Diplomate, American College of Veterinary Surgeons

Animal Eye and Surgical Clinic
La Habra, California

Animal Eye Clinics
Reno, Nevada
Riverside, California

1990
W.B. SAUNDERS COMPANY
Harcourt Brace Jovanovich, Inc.
Philadelphia London Toronto Montreal Sydney Tokyo

W. B. SAUNDERS COMPANY
Harcourt Brace Jovanovich, Inc.

The Curtis Center
Independence Square West
Philadelphia, PA 19106

Library of Congress Cataloging-in-Publication Data

Slatter, Douglas
Fundamentals of veterinary ophthalmology / Douglas Slatter.—2nd ed.

p. cm.

ISBN 0–7216–2463–4

1. Veterinary ophthalmology.   I. Title.
[DNLM: 1. Eye Diseases—veterinary.   SF 891 S631f]

SF891.S53   1990
636.089'77—dc20
DNLM/DLC   89–70312

Editor: Linda Mills
Designer: Dorothy Chattin
Production Manager: Linda R. Turner
Manuscript Editor: Mimi McGinnis
Illustration Coordinator: Peg Shaw
Indexer: Roger Wall
Cover Designer: Joanne Carroll

Fundamentals of Veterinary Ophthalmology, Second Edition   ISBN 0–7216–2463–4

Printed in the United States of America.

Last digit is the print number: 9   8   7   6   5   4   3   2   1

To
Christine and Diane

Preface

Fundamentals of Veterinary Ophthalmology is a companion for the clinician and student. Its composition has taken into consideration the increasing sophistication of veterinary ophthalmology and the difficulty of adequately covering many newer topics. These topics in detail are relevant to practicing ophthalmologists, and a general knowledge of them is important to veterinarians in general practice who treat the patient first. Many details of less common ocular disorders have been deliberately omitted. For more details, comprehensive reference atlases and texts are available. Constructive suggestions by teachers and users of the text are appreciated.

The passing, after a long, outstanding, and productive professional life, of Dame Ida Mann, who wrote the Foreword to the first edition, is recorded with sadness.

Acknowledgments

I am again indebted to the many colleagues who have contributed the knowledge that makes up this work. Deserving of special mention for their efforts in reviewing and commenting on the text and providing figures and tables are Drs. Peter Bedford, Roy Bellhorn, Rowan Blogg, Jeanette daSilva Curiel, Joan Dziezyc, Lorraine Karpinsky, Tom Kern, Claire Latimer, William Miller, Malcolm and Kim Nairn, Ron Riis, Jeff Smith, Robin Stanley, Ardene Vestre, Ralph Vierheller, and Dan Wolfe. Co-authors Drs. Elizabeth Chambers and Alexander deLahunta assisted in their respective chapters. I thank also the numerous veterinarians and students whose encouraging comments stimulated the continuing process of producing this edition. In attempting to distill and collate the relevant information, I hope that no important contributions have been omitted or misinterpreted. Contributing authors to the literature are encouraged to make available information relevant to the aims of this book for future inclusion.

The staff of the W. B. Saunders Company have again been most helpful, and Linda Mills, Darlene Pedersen, Julie Lawley, and Connie Vrato have earned special mention. Lorie Biederman assisted with many new illustrations.

To my clients whose love for their animals, and whose persistence in the face of both success and disappointment, make the advancement of our specialty possible, I give my sincere thanks.

DOUGLAS SLATTER

Contents

Appendix II

Notice

Extraordinary efforts have been made by the author and publisher of this book to ensure that dosage recommendations are precise and in agreement with standards officially accepted at the time of publication.

However, dosage schedules are changed from time to time in the light of accumulating clinical experience and continuing laboratory studies. This is most likely to occur in the case of recently introduced products. It is urged, therefore, that you check the manufacturer's recommendations for dosage, especially if the drug to be administered or prescribed is one that you use only infrequently or have not used for some time.

In addition, some drugs mentioned have been used as experimental drugs. Others have been used after official clearance for use in one species but not in others described here. This is particularly true for rare and exotic species. In these cases, readers are urged to view the recommendations with discretion and precaution.

PLATE I

A, Entropion. Note the blepharospasm and overflow of tears.
B, Adenoma of the tarsal gland. Note tumor involvement of the tarsal gland deep within the lid.

C, Chalazion. chronic obstruction of the duct of a tarsal gland. (From Muller GH, Kirk RW: Small Animal Dermatology, 4th ed. WB Saunders Co, Philadelphia, 1989.)
D, Chronic staphylococcal blepharitis. Note numerous masses in the palpebral conjunctiva. (Courtesy of Dr. E. S. Chambers.)

E, Equine habronemiasis. Local injection of fenthion caused complete remission.
F, Pemphigus vulgaris. Ulceration and dermatitis were present in the mucocutaneous junction of eyelids, mouth, anus, and prepuce in a 5-year-old greyhound.

G, Canine inhalant dermatitis/conjunctivitis syndrome (atopic disease). Face rubbing causes erythema, whereas eye and nasal discharges caused rust-colored discoloration of hair. (From Muller GH, Kirk RW: Small Animal Dermatology, 4th ed. WB Saunders Co, Philadelphia, 1989.)
H, Chronic pyogenic demodicosis in a dachshund. (From Muller GH, Kirk RW: Small Animal Dermatology, 4th ed. WB Saunders Co, Philadelphia, 1989.)

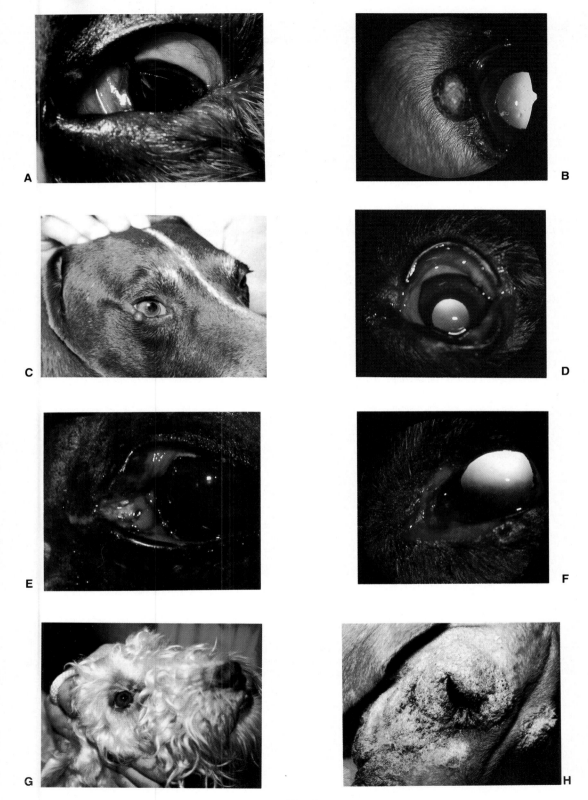

Plate I

PLATE II

A, *Mucopurulent conjunctivitis in a cat with calicivirus infection.*

B, *Conjunctival pallor in a dog with aplastic anemia (packed cell volume 9%).*

C, *Follicle formation in the inferior conjunctival fornix and on the anterior surface of the third eyelid.*

D, *Normal unpigmented third eyelid with hyperemia of the bulbar conjunctiva.*

E, *Descemetocele and corneal ulcer after a minor corneal wound in which subconjunctival corticosteroids were administered. Pseudomonas spp infection occurred, the ulcer progressed to a descemetocele that ruptured, and the eye was lost.*

F, *Corneal edema.*

G, *Intraocular canine lens for placement after cataract removal. (Courtesy of Dr. J. Gaiddon.)*

H, *An intraocular lens implanted in a dog after cataract removal. The pupil has been dilated. Margins of the lens are not normally visible in the undilated resting pupil. (Courtesy of Dr. J. Gaiddon.)*

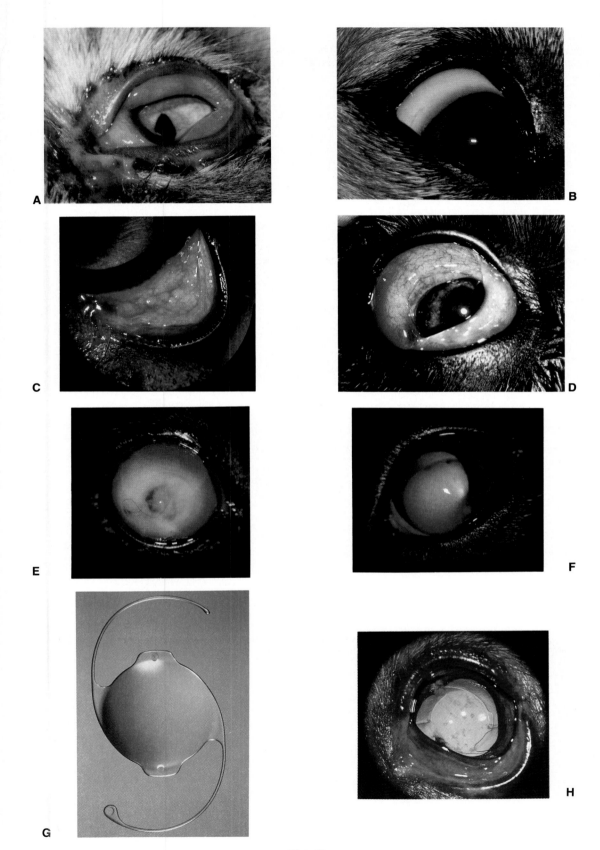

Plate II

PLATE III

A, *Superficial corneal vascularization in a dog. (Courtesy of Dr. G. A. Severin.)*
B, *Deep corneal vascularization and limbal injection in a horse.*

C, *Lipid deposition in the area of an old corneal scar.*
D, *Chorioretinal dysplasia temporal to the optic disc in a collie with scleral ectasia syndrome.*

E, *Scleral coloboma at the posterior pole in a collie with scleral ectasia syndrome.*
F, *Superficial corneal erosion in a corgi.*

G, *Advanced vascularization and pigmentation in chronic immune-mediated keratoconjunctivitis syndrome (Uberreiter's).*
H, *Feline corneal necrosis syndrome (sequestration or mummification) in a 12-month-old Persian cat.*

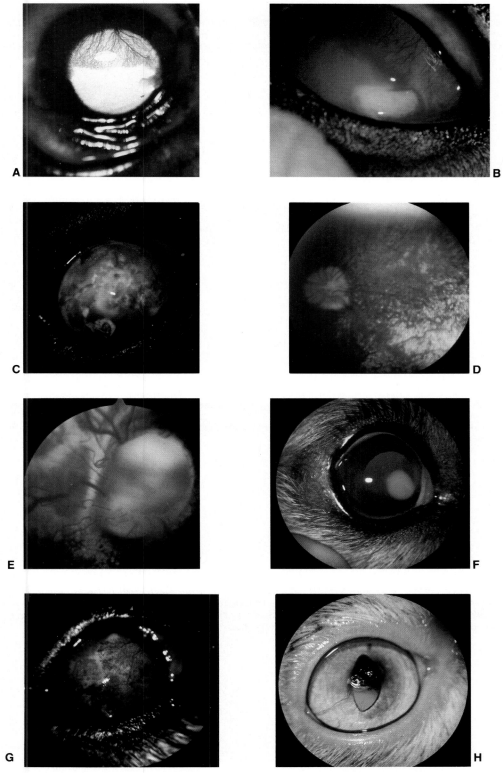

Plate III

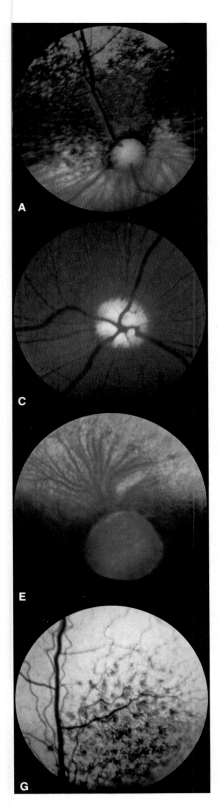

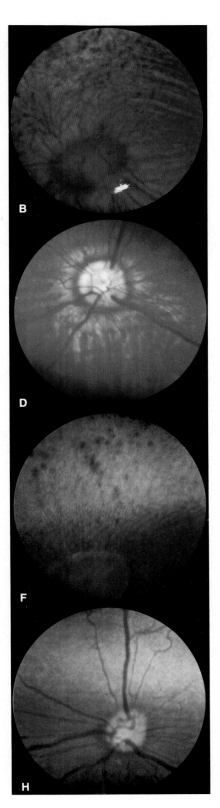

Plate IV

PLATE V

A, *Foci of retinal dysplasia in a 7-month-old American cocker spaniel. Areas overlying the tapetum appear as dark streaks surrounded by a narrow zone of hyperreflectivity. (Courtesy of Dr. A. MacMillan.)*

B, *Early retinal degeneration in a poodle.*

C, *Early vascular attenuation in a poodle with progressive retinal degeneration (PRD) type I. Visual deficits were present by this time.*

D, *Multiple discrete foci of pigmentation over the central tapetum in a 5-year-old Labrador retriever with PRD type II.*

E, *Retinal detachment. The detached retina is white. Note the optic disk visible through folds of detached retina.*

F, *Bright blindness in a sheep. Note increased tapetal reflectivity and vascular attenuation. (Courtesy of Dr. K. Barnett.)*

G, *Peripheral retina of a cow with active retinitis. Pigmentation is evident dorsally, with several areas of active retinitis surrounded by pale edema and cellular infiltration. A hyperreflective margin (yellow) is present around the upper lesion. (Courtesy of Dr. L. Klein.)*

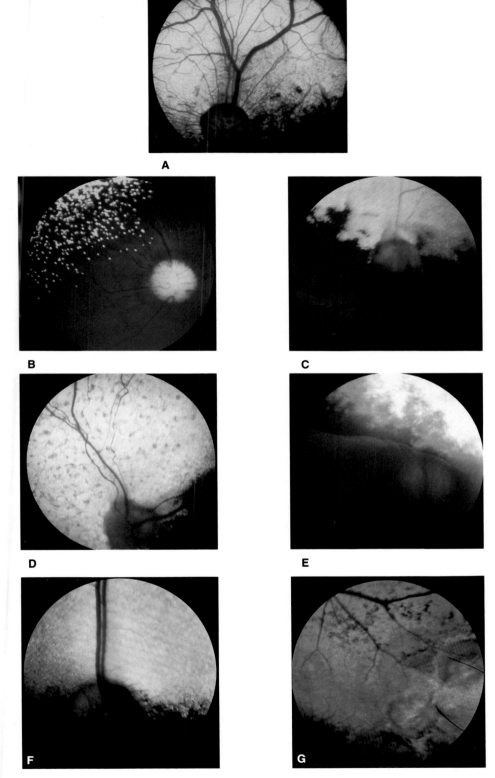

Plate V

Structure and Function of the Eye

VISION AND REFRACTIVE ERRORS	**GENERAL PATTERN OF VASCULAR ANATOMY AND PERIPHERAL NEUROANATOMY**	**OCULAR REFLEXES PHYSIOLOGY OF THE AQUEOUS**
MECHANISMS OF ACCOMMODATION		
CENTRAL VISUAL PATHWAYS		

The visual system collects light and focuses it onto photoreceptors—transducers that convert it to electrical impulses for passage to the visual cortex where the sensation of vision occurs (Figs. 1–1 and 1–2). Homeostatic and anatomical mechanisms that refine and protect the system vary among species depending on functional requirements.

In nonpredatory animals, the eyes are placed with diverging visual axes, so the total visual field approaches 360°. The BINOCULAR FIELD (the area from which light falls onto both retinas from a single object) is relatively small, about 65° (Fig. 1–3). The visual axes in predatory animals are closer to parallel, the eyes are more frontal, the binocular field is larger (85°+) and there is a larger blind zone posteriorly (Fig. 1–4). The greater binocular field gives more accurate depth perception and greater coordination with body movements.

VISION AND REFRACTIVE ERRORS

The principal refracting surfaces of the eye are the cornea and the lens, their refracting powers being determined by their radii of curvature and the refractive index of the air or aqueous in which they are bathed. As the surface curvature increases (the radius of curvature is decreasing), the refractive power increases. If the focal length of the cornea-lens mechanism does not equal the length of the eye, there is a refractive error (Fig. 1–5). AMETROPIA means that no refractive error

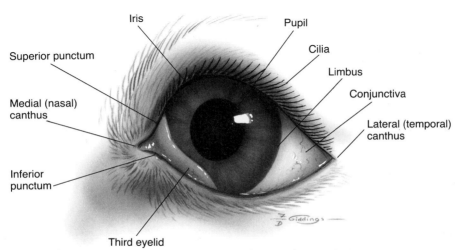

FIGURE 1–1. *Frontal view of the external structures of the canine eye.*

Labels: Iris, Pupil, Superior punctum, Cilia, Limbus, Conjunctiva, Medial (nasal) canthus, Lateral (temporal) canthus, Inferior punctum, Third eyelid

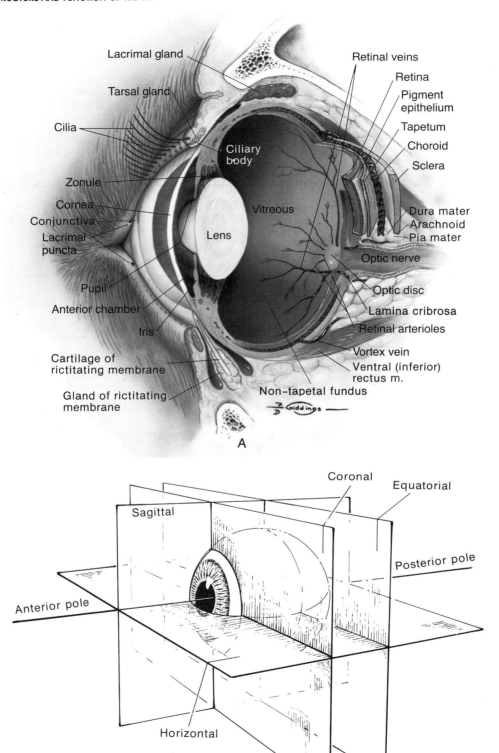

FIGURE 1–2. *Internal structures of the canine eye* (A). *Also shown are the standard reference planes* (B).

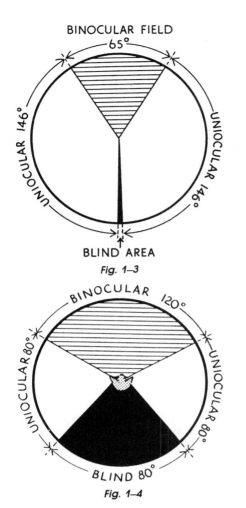

Fig. 1–3

Fig. 1–4

FIGURE 1–3. *The visual field of the horse (a nonpredator), showing a small binocular field (65°), large panoramic uniocular areas (146°), and a minute blind area (3°). (Reproduced by permission from Duke-Elder, Sir Stewart, editor: System of Ophthalmology. Vol I. The Eye in Evolution. St Louis, 1958, The CV Mosby Co.)*

FIGURE 1–4. *The visual field of the cat (a predator), showing a large anterior binocular area (85° +), a large posterior blind area (80°), with relatively small uniocular area. (80°). (Reproduced by permission from Duke-Elder, Sir Stewart, editor: System of Ophthalmology. Vol I. The Eye in Evolution. St Louis, 1958, The CV Mosby Co.)*

is present. Refractive errors can be caused by a change in either the optical power or the axial length of the eye. Refractive errors can be estimated with a **DIRECT OPHTHALMOSCOPE** or measured more accurately with a **RETINOSCOPE**.

In general, dogs have several diopters of myopia, but considerable variation occurs. In clinical practice a detailed knowledge of the refractive state is rarely important, but an understanding is required in order to answer owners' questions and to relate them to their own eyes, and to explain **APHAKIC** vision (without a lens) after cataract surgery.

MECHANISMS OF ACCOMMODATION

In the normal **EMMETROPIC** eye, parallel rays of light from a distant object are focused onto the photoreceptor layer of the retina. Accommodation is the ability of the eye to increase its optical power and bring rays of light from a near object to a focal point on the retina as the object comes closer to the eye. When the eye is adjusted for far vision it is relaxed, and for near vision it is accommodated (Fig. 1–6).

The accommodative power of domestic animal eyes is less than that of the human eye. The normal dog or cat has about 1–2 diopters (D) of accommodation, whereas the young adult human eye has about 10 D. Ungulates have little, if any, accommodation. The mechanisms for varying optical power differ with species. For domestic animals, optical power is varied by altering the power of the lens, by varying its curvature.

The young lens is pliable and soft, and it is molded to a circular shape by its tough elastic capsule. The tendency for the lens to become circular (with maximal optical power) is opposed by the tension of the lens zonules on the capsule. This tension flattens the lens and reduces its optical power. Tension of the zonules is apparently controlled by the ciliary muscle. As the ciliary muscle contracts, the choroid is pulled forward, the zonular tension *decreases,* and the optical power increases as the lens tends to return to its circular shape. When the ciliary muscle relaxes, the zonular

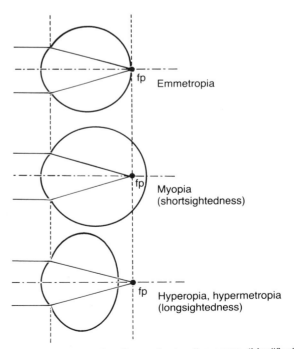

FIGURE 1–5. *Normal optics and refractive errors. (Modified from Magrane WG: Canine Ophthalmology, 3rd ed. Lea & Febiger, Philadelphia, 1977.)*

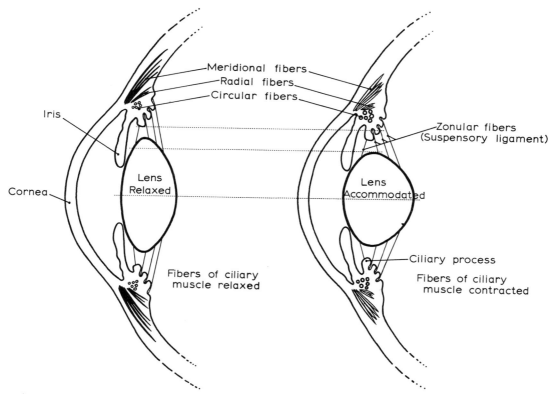

FIGURE 1–6. *Left, Position of the lens and relaxed ciliary muscle fibers when the eye is accommodated for distant vision. Right, Position of the lens and the contracted ciliary muscle fibers when the eye is accommodated for near objects. (From Getty R: Sisson and Grossman's The Anatomy of the Domestic Animals, 5th ed. WB Saunders Co, Philadelphia, 1975.)*

tension is *increased,* the lens is flattened, and its optical power is less (see Fig. 1–6).

> When the ciliary muscle is in the contracted state, the lens zonules are relaxed, the lens has its greatest optical power, and the eye is accommodated for near vision. When the ciliary muscle is relaxed, tension on the zonules is maximal, the lens is flattened anteroposteriorly, the optical power is least, and the eye is relaxed for distant vision.

The mechanism of accommodation in the equine eye is controversial. The "ramp retina" of the horse, in which the distance of the retina from the posterior lens surface varies in different parts of the globe, may contribute to accommodation, and this may explain movements of the equine head.

Form, movement, and brightness are more significant for domestic animals than is fine visual discrimination. Herbivores are assumed to have little if any color vision, but the evidence is contradictory in dogs, where im-

pulses of differing velocities have been recorded in the optic nerve after stimulation of the retina with light of different wavelengths. All domestic species have rods and cones.

CENTRAL VISUAL PATHWAYS

The eye is a small part of the visual system (Fig. 1–7). Fibers originating in the NERVE FIBER LAYER of the retina converge at the OPTIC DISC, turn posteriorly, gain a myelin sheath, and pass through the sieve-like opening in the sclera—the LAMINA CRIBROSA. The fibers pass via the OPTIC NERVE to the OPTIC CHIASM (Fig. 1–8). Fibers coming from different parts of the retina maintain definite positions within the optic nerve and throughout the path to the visual cortex. Fibers from both optic nerves enter the optic chiasm.

Partial DECUSSATION or "crossing over" of fibers from one side to another occurs in the chiasm. Fibers carrying impulses from nasal parts of the respective retinas cross to the opposite side. Thus, impulses caused by an object in one VISUAL FIELD travel to the same part of the visual cortex, even though that object caused

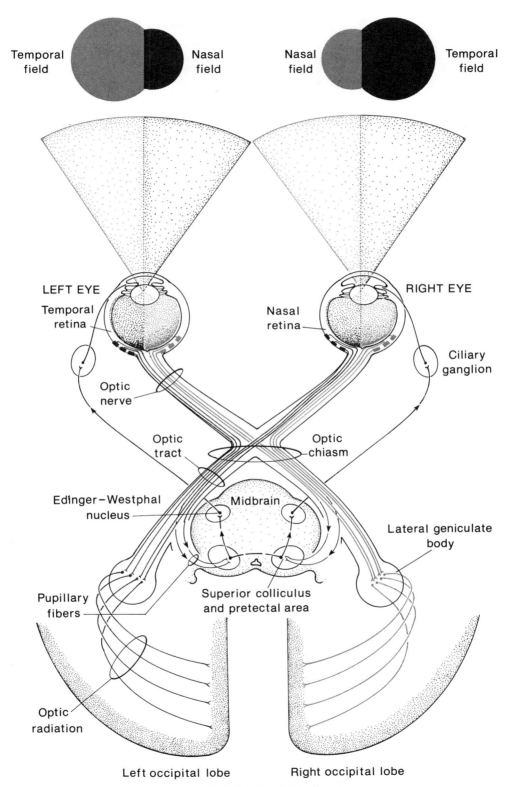

FIGURE 1–7. The visual pathway.

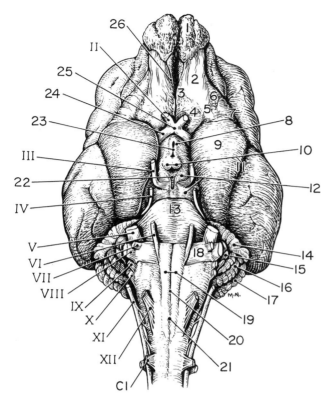

1. Olfactory bulb
2. Olfactory peduncle
3. Medial olfactory tract
4. Rostral perforated substance
5. Lateral olfactory tract
6. Lateral olfactory gyrus
7. Rostral part of lateral rhinal sulcus
8. Tuber cinereum
9. Piriform lobe
10. Mamillary bodies
11. Caudal part of lateral rhinal sulcus
12. Crus cerebri
13. Transverse fibers of pons
14. Ventral paraflocculus
15. Flocculus
16. Dorsal paraflocculus
17. Ansiform lobule
18. Trapezoid body
19. Pyramids
20. Median fissure
21. Decussation of pyramids
22. Caudal perforated substance in intercrural fossa
23. Infundibulum
24. Optic tract
25. Optic chiasm
26. Medial rhinal sulcus

II.	Optic nerve	VIII.	Vestibulocochlear nerve
III.	Oculomotor nerve	IX.	Glossopharyngeal nerve
IV.	Trochlear nerve	X.	Vagus nerve
V.	Trigeminal nerve	XI.	Accessory nerve
VI.	Abducent nerve	XII.	Hypoglossal nerve
VII.	Facial nerve	CI.	First cervical nerve

FIGURE 1–8. Ventral view of the brain and cranial nerves in the dog. (From Evans HE, Christensen GC: Miller's Anatomy of the Dog, 2nd ed. WB Saunders Co, Philadelphia, 1979. © Cornell University 1964.)

impulses in both eyes (see Fig. 1–7). For example, an object in an animal's right visual field (on its right side) falls on the nasal area of the right retina and the temporal area of the left retina. After decussation in the chiasm, all the fibers carrying this information from the right visual field proceed to the left visual cortex.

Objects on one side of an animal are not "seen" solely by the eye on that side but by both eyes. A dog or a cat with binocular vision does not necessarily bump into objects on the side of a blind eye. In cattle and horses with more decussation at the optic chiasm, and less binocular vision, blindness in one eye has a greater effect on vision on that side. The distinctions and differences among species are important when explaining to owners the effects of a blind eye on an animal's behavior.

The proportion of optic nerve fibers that decussate in the chiasm is related to the relative lateral positioning of the orbits and eyes in the skull. In horses and cattle, with laterally directed eyes, the proportion of decussating fibers is high (83%); in dogs and cats with more rostrally placed eyes it is about 75%; and in humans, about 50%. The primitive vertebrate pattern is total decussation. In animals with laterally directed eyes, the majority of visual information from an object falls on the retina on the same side. As the eyes become more

rostrally placed, the information is more equally shared between the two eyes, and the need for decussation to the opposite side diminishes.

The optic chiasm receives the optic nerves as they enter the cranial vault via the OPTIC FORAMEN and CANALS (Fig. 1–9). The chiasm lies at the base of the brain, adjacent and anterior to the HYPOPHYSIS, which sits in the PITUITARY FOSSA of the POSTSPHENOID BONE. This relationship between the pituitary and the chiasm and optic tracts is important in considering the potential effect of space-occupying masses of the pituitary on vision.

From the optic chiasm, fibers enter the LEFT and RIGHT OPTIC TRACTS, which then pass laterally from the chiasm, anterior to the hypophysis, and beneath the ventral surface of the CEREBRAL PEDUNCLE. The tracts then curve dorsally and posteriorly, between the cerebral peduncle to which they are attached laterally, and the PYRIFORM LOBE. The tracts thus pass to the LATERAL GENICULATE BODY. Before reaching the lateral geniculate body, some 20–30% of the fibers leave the tracts and enter the PRETECTAL AREA. Some of these fibers enter the SUPERIOR COLLICULUS directly, and others pass via the tracts and lateral geniculate body to the colliculus indirectly. The majority of fibers entering the lateral geniculate body synapse here with

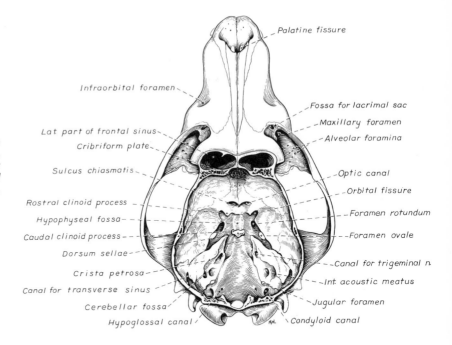

FIGURE 1–9. Skull of the dog with calvaria removed dorsal aspect. (From Evans HE, Christensen GC: Miller's Anatomy of the Dog, 2nd ed. WB Saunders Co, Philadelphia, 1979. © Cornell University 1964.)

Labels on figure: Palatine fissure; Infraorbital foramen; Fossa for lacrimal sac; Maxillary foramen; Alveolar foramina; Lat part of frontal sinus; Cribriform plate; Optic canal; Sulcus chiasmatis; Orbital fissure; Foramen rotundum; Rostral clinoid process; Foramen ovale; Hypophyseal fossa; Caudal clinoid process; Canal for trigeminal n.; Dorsum sellae; Int. acoustic meatus; Crista petrosa; Canal for transverse sinus; Jugular foramen; Cerebellar fossa; Hypoglossal canal; Condyloid canal

the third ascending neuron in the visual system, which passes without further synapse to the visual cortex. The first two synapses are the photoreceptor-bipolar and bipolar–ganglion cell interfaces.

Those fibers that leave the optic tracts before entering the lateral geniculate body pass to the pretectal area, carrying afferent impulses of the PUPILLARY LIGHT REFLEX. In the pretectal area much decussation occurs, and the fibers pass to the midline EDINGER-WESTPHAL NUCLEI of the OCULOMOTOR NERVE (III) (see Fig. 1–8). Efferent impulses pass from these nuclei to the PUPILLARY SPHINCTER MUSCLE in each iris.

A positive pupillary light reflex does not mean the eye can see. Fibers that mediate the reflex arc leave the optic tracts before the tracts enter the lateral geniculate body.

From the lateral geniculate body, fibers pass forward and lateral to the lateral ventricle as the fan-like OPTIC RADIATION, which enters the OCCIPITAL or VISUAL CORTEX where interpretation of some visual stimuli occurs in domestic animals (Fig. 1–10). An increase in intraventricular pressure (HYDROCEPHALUS) can affect the visual pathway at this point.

In dogs and cats the visual cortex is not the sole center of interpretation of visual stimuli. If the cortex is removed, light perception and discrimination of light intensity are retained, but familiarity of surroundings is lost. Subcortical integration is believed to occur in the superior colliculus.

GENERAL PATTERN OF VASCULAR ANATOMY AND PERIPHERAL NEUROANATOMY

Further details of orbital anatomy may be found in Chapter 18.

Arterial Supply

The major arterial supply of the eye is from the EXTERNAL OPHTHALMIC ARTERY, a branch of the INTERNAL MAXILLARY ARTERY that arises from the EXTERNAL CAROTID ARTERY (Fig. 1–11). The contribution from the internal carotid artery is small, unlike the situation in primates, and is via an INTERNAL OPHTHALMIC ARTERY that arises from the CIRCLE OF WILLIS. The internal ophthalmic artery enters the orbit through the optic canal with the optic nerve. From the external ophthalmic artery, numerous SHORT POSTERIOR CILIARY ARTERIES arise (Fig. 1–12) and penetrate the sclera around the optic nerve head. These arteries supply the retina and choroid.

There is no central retinal artery in domestic species. Single MEDIAL and LATERAL LONG POSTERIOR CILIARY ARTERIES pass around the globe horizontally, within the sclera, to supply the ciliary body. Muscular branches of the orbital artery, which supplies the extraocular muscles, also enter the globe near the insertions of these muscles. These ANTERIOR CILIARY ARTERIES anastomose with the long posterior ciliary arteries to form the ciliary arterial supply. When the globe is

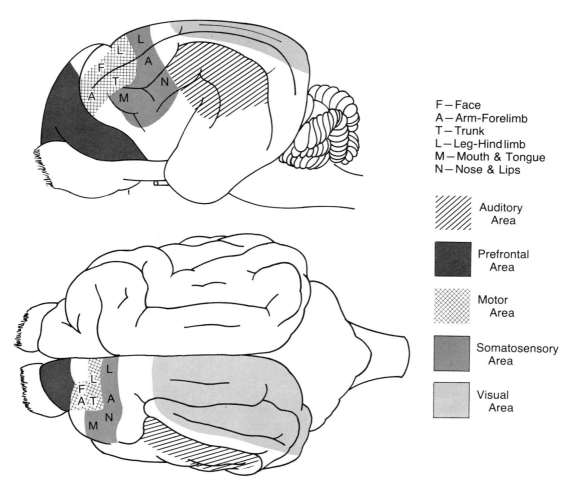

F—Face
A—Arm-Forelimb
T—Trunk
L—Leg-Hindlimb
M—Mouth & Tongue
N—Nose & Lips

Auditory Area

Prefrontal Area

Motor Area

Somatosensory Area

Visual Area

FIGURE 1–10. Motor and sensory areas of the cerebral cortex of the dog. (From Hoerlein BF: Canine Neurology, 3rd ed. WB Saunders Co, Philadelphia, 1978.)

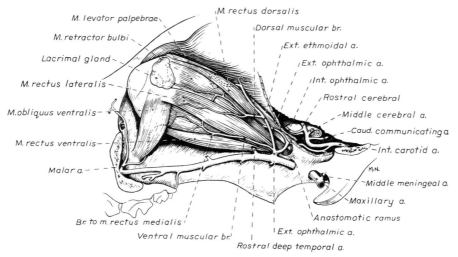

M. levator palpebrae
M. retractor bulbi
Lacrimal gland
M. rectus lateralis
M. obliquus ventralis
M. rectus ventralis
Malar a.
Br. to m. rectus medialis
Ventral muscular br.
Rostral deep temporal a.
Ext. ophthalmic a.
Anastomotic ramus
Maxillary a.
Middle meningeal a.
Int. carotid a.
Caud. communicating a
Middle cerebral a.
Rostral cerebral
Int. ophthalmic a.
Ext. ophthalmic a.
Ext. ethmoidal a.
Dorsal muscular br.
M. rectus dorsalis

FIGURE 1–11. Arteries of the orbit and extrinsic ocular muscles in the dog. Lateral aspect. (From Evans HE, Christensen GC: Miller's Anatomy of the Dog, 2nd ed. WB Saunders Co, Philadelphia, 1979. © Cornell University 1964.)

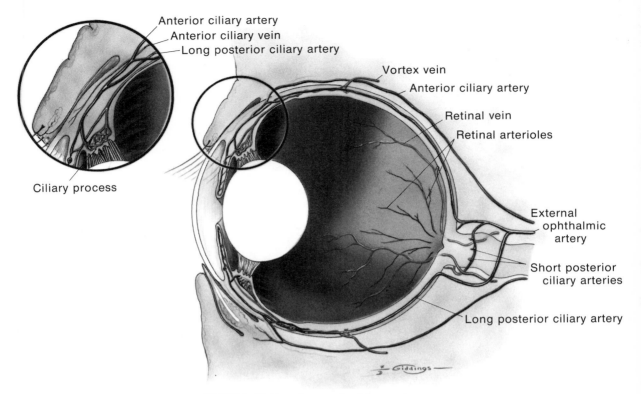

FIGURE 1–12. *Vascular supply of the canine eye.*

prolapsed, these muscular branches may be destroyed, decreasing the available supply to the anterior segment of the eye. Branches from the ciliary arterial network form the **MAJOR ARTERIAL CIRCLE OF THE IRIS**. The deep conjunctival arterioles at the limbus anastomose with the anterior ciliary arteries before they enter the sclera and also with arterioles in the ciliary body. Vascular events of clinical importance, e.g., inflammation, in one area of this network of anastomosing vessels can often be seen in other parts, and their origin must be distinguished (Fig. 1–12).

The eyelids are supplied by the **SUPERFICIAL TEMPORAL ARTERY**, a branch of the **EXTERNAL CAROTID ARTERY**, and by the **MALAR ARTERY**, a branch of the **INFRAORBITAL ARTERY** (Fig. 1–13).

Venous Drainage
(Fig. 1–14; see also Fig. 1–12)

The retina is drained by the retinal veins and venules, which run from the peripheral retina toward the optic nerve head. The venous circle they form at the optic disc may be complete or incomplete in the dog. The venous circle drains posteriorly through the sclera via the **POSTERIOR CILIARY VEINS** to a dilation in the orbital vein—the **SUPERIOR (DORSAL) OPHTHALMIC VEIN**.

The choroid is drained by approximately four **VORTEX VEINS**, which leave the globe near the equator and join the **SUPERIOR** and **INFERIOR OPHTHALMIC VEINS**. The ciliary body is drained by the anterior ciliary veins to the same superior and inferior ophthalmic veins that drain to the **ORBITAL VENOUS PLEXUS** at the apex of the orbit. This plexus drains to the cavernous venous sinus within the cranial vault. The cavernous sinus drains via the **VERTEBRAL SINUSES**, **EXTERNAL JUGULAR VEIN**, and **INTERNAL MAXILLARY VEIN**. Venous blood thus passes posteriorly from the orbit via this route. It may also pass anteriorly via anastomoses between the ophthalmic veins and the **MALAR**, **ANGULARIS OCULI**, and **FACIAL VEINS** to the **EXTERNAL MAXILLARY** and **EXTERNAL JUGULAR VEINS**. Considerable species variation exists in the vascular supply and drainage of the eye and orbit.

Nerve Supply of the Eye and Adnexa

The general plan of nerve supply to the eye is shown in Figure 1–15. For further details see Chapter 17.

Optic Nerve (Cranial Nerve II)

The **OPTIC NERVE** and meninges pass from the globe, through the cone formed by the **RETRACTOR BULBI**

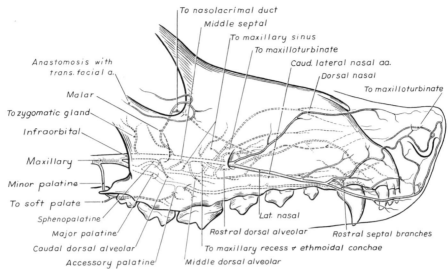

FIGURE 1–13. Scheme of the terminal branches of the maxillary artery in the dog. Lateral aspect. (From Evans HE, Christensen GC: Miller's Anatomy of the Dog, 2nd ed. WB Saunders Co, Philadelphia, 1979. © Cornell University 1964.)

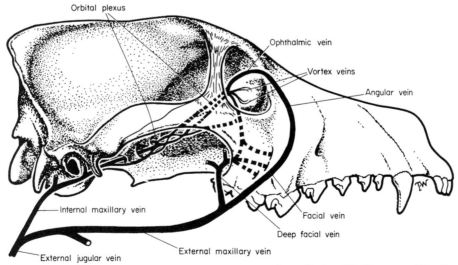

FIGURE 1–14. The venous drainage of the eye and orbit of the dog. (From Startup FG: Diseases of the Canine Eye. © by Williams & Wilkins, 1969.)

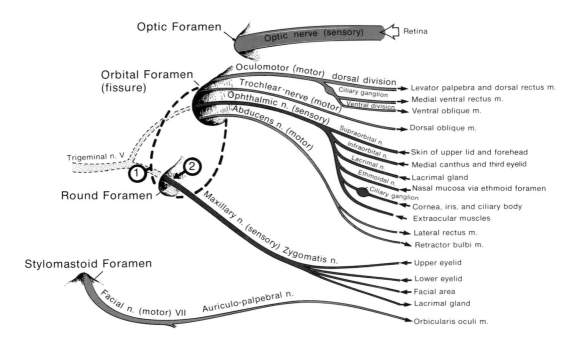

① Round and orbital foramina fuse in the pig and ruminants, forming the <u>foramen orbitorotundum</u>

② Only orbital branches shown here

FIGURE 1–15. *Nerve supply to the eye.*

MUSCLES, via the OPTIC CANAL to the OPTIC CHIASM. The dura covering the nerve is continuous with the outer layers of the sclera. The optic nerve consists of ganglion cells whose cell bodies lie in the ganglion cell layer of the retina. It is a tract of the central nervous system and not a peripheral nerve.

Oculomotor Nerve (Cranial Nerve III)

The nucleus of the oculomotor nerve lies in the brain stem and has several components serving different extraocular muscles—VENTRAL RECTUS, DORSAL RECTUS, MEDIAL RECTUS, INFERIOR OBLIQUE, and LEVATOR PALPEBRAE SUPERIORIS MUSCLES. The nerve also carries parasympathetic fibers originating from the Edinger-Westphal nucleus that lies near the other nuclei of the oculomotor nerve and serves the DILATOR and SPHINCTER PUPILLAE MUSCLES and the CILIARY MUSCLE. The oculomotor nerve thus contains efferent motor fibers to the striated extraocular muscles of mesodermal origin and parasympathetic fibers to the smooth muscles of the iris and ciliary body of neuroectodermal origin.

The oculomotor nerve leaves the brainstem on its ventromedial surface (see Fig. 1–8), passes ventral to the optic tracts through the cavernous sinus, and enters the orbit via the ORBITAL FISSURE (FORAMEN ORBITOROTUNDUM in cattle, sheep, and pigs). In the orbit the nerve divides into dorsal and ventral rami. A branch from the ventral ramus passes to the CILIARY GANGLION, where the preganglionic parasympathetic fibers synapse. For more details of the fibers leaving the ciliary ganglion, see page 14.

Trochlear Nerve (Cranial Nerve IV)

The trochlear nerve leaves the brain stem on the dorsal surface and runs lateral to the tentorium cerebelli to the orbital fissure. It passes through the fissure with the oculomotor nerve and the ophthalmic branch of the trigeminal nerve. The trochlear nerve innervates the DORSAL OBLIQUE MUSCLE only.

Trigeminal Nerve (Cranial Nerve V)

The sensory branches of the trigeminal nerve receive the majority of the input from the orbit and periocular area. The nerve has both motor and sensory roots (see Fig. 1–8), which pass in a common sheath through the PETROUS TEMPORAL BONE to the TRIGEMINAL GANGLION. The three branches of the nerve—OPHTHALMIC, MAXILLARY, and MANDIBULAR—arise from the TRIGEMINAL GANGLION. The ophthalmic nerve leaves the cranial cavity via the orbital fissure, and the maxillary leaves via the round foramen (see Fig. 1–15).

Once in the orbit, the ophthalmic nerve divides into the SUPRAORBITAL, LACRIMAL, and NASOCILIARY NERVES. The supraorbital nerve is sensory to the middle of the upper eyelid and adjacent skin (Fig. 1–16). In horses, cattle, sheep, and pigs it reaches the upper lid via the SUPRAORBITAL FORAMEN, but in dogs and cats it passes beneath the orbital ligament.

The LACRIMAL NERVE supplies the LACRIMAL GLAND. The nasociliary nerve is the major continuation of the ophthalmic nerve in the orbit, and it gives rise to the ETHMOIDAL and INTRATROCHLEAR NERVES. The ethmoidal nerve passes through the ETHMOIDAL FORAMEN to supply the mucous membranes of the nasal cavity. The infratrochlear nerve passes beneath the trochlear, penetrates the SEPTUM ORBITALE (see Fig. 18–13), and innervates the medial canthus, third eyelid, and adjacent lacrimal system (see Fig. 1–16). Within the orbit the nasociliary nerve gives off the LONG CILIARY NERVE that enters the globe near the optic nerve to provide sensory innervation to the globe itself.

The MAXILLARY NERVE passes through the round foramen and passes via the ALAR CANAL to the PTERYGOPALATINE FOSSA. It gives rise to the ZYGOMATIC NERVE, which divides into ZYGOMATICOTEMPORAL and ZYGOMATICOFACIAL branches within the orbit. The zygomaticotemporal supplies sensory innervation to the lateral upper lid and rostral temporal area. The zygomaticofacial emerges from the periorbita ventral to the lateral canthus and supplies the lateral lower lid and surrounding skin. Postganglionic sympathetic fibers from the CRANIAL CERVICAL GANGLION may also be distributed to the orbit via the branches of the maxillary nerve, which has no other branches of ophthalmic significance.

Abducent Nerve (Cranial Nerve VI)

The abducent nerve leaves the ventral surface of the medulla oblongata (see Fig. 1–8) and passes through the wall of the cavernous sinus, forward via the orbital fissure (see Fig. 1–15) to enter the orbit and supply the RETRACTOR BULBI and LATERAL RECTUS MUSCLCES.

Facial Nerve (Cranial Nerve VII)

The mixed facial nerve contains somatic motor and parasympathetic fibers, innervating the ORBICULARIS OCULI and RETRACTOR ANGULI MUSCLES and the LAC-

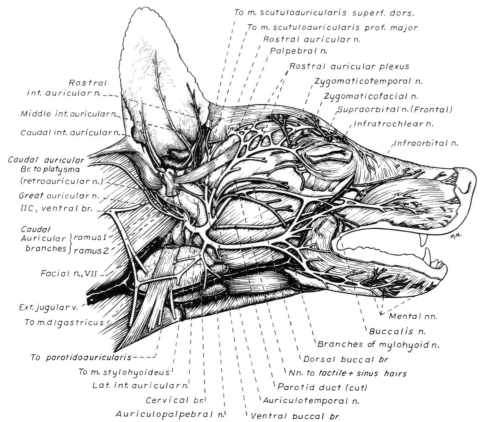

FIGURE 1–16. Superficial branches of the facial and trigeminal nerves in the dog. Lateral aspect. (From Evans HE, Christensen GC: Miller's Anatomy of the Dog, 2nd ed. WB Saunders Co, Philadelphia, 1979. © Cornell University 1964.)

RIMAL GLAND. Cell bodies of the motor fibers are found in the FACIAL NUCLEUS in the medulla oblongata. The parasympathetic cell bodies are located in the ROSTRAL SALIVATORY NUCLEUS in the medulla. The nerve leaves the brainstem lateral to the origin of the abducent nerve (see Fig. 1–8) and, with the VESTIBULOCOCHLEAR NERVE, enters the PETROUS TEMPORAL BONE near the acoustic meatus (Fig. 1–17)—a point of clinical significance to be discussed later under hemifacial spasm (see Chap. 17). The facial nerve enters the facial canal of the temporal bone, where the GENICULATE GANGLION is situated.

From the ganglion arises the MAJOR PETROSAL NERVE. Joined by the DEEP PETROSAL (SYMPATHETIC) NERVE, the NERVE OF THE PTERYGOID CANAL is formed, and it passes via the PTERYGOID CANAL to the PTERYGOPALATINE FOSSA, ending as the PTERYGOPALATINE GANGLION. The parasympathetic fibers synapse here, and some pass to the lacrimal gland.

From the geniculate ganglion, the facial nerve emerges from the STYLOMASTOID FORAMEN to give numerous branches. The facial trunk terminates as the AURICULOPALPEBRAL NERVE, which crosses the temporal region and ZYGOMATIC ARCH (see Fig. 1–16). The PALPEBRAL BRANCH supplies the ORBICULARIS OCULI and RETRACTOR ANGULI OCULI MUSCLES.

Actions of the Ocular Muscles with Autonomic Innervation

m. dilator pupillae	sympathetic
Müller's muscle	sympathetic
m. sphincter pupillae	parasympathetic
ciliary muscle	parasympathetic

The PUPILLARY DILATOR and SPHINCTER MUSCLES are antagonistic to each other and control the size of the pupil. For either to act, the other must relax. If either muscle fails to function, the effects of the remaining muscles predominate; e.g., paralysis of the dilator alone results in a small pupil (MIOSIS) because of the unbalanced action of the sphincter muscle.

The CILIARY MUSCLE controls tension in the lens zonules, which control the curvature and refractive power of the lens. MÜLLER'S MUSCLE together with the LEVATOR PALPEBRAE SUPERIORIS MUSCLE elevates the upper eyelid. If either of these muscles is defective, the upper eyelid is not held up, and it droops (PTOSIS).

Autonomic Innervation
(Figs. 1–18 and 1–19)

PARASYMPATHETIC SUPPLY

Parasympathetic fibers arise from the Edinger-Westphal nucleus of the oculomotor nerve and pass via the nerve to synapse in the ciliary ganglion.

Other fibers that pass into the ciliary ganglion but do not synapse in it include: (1) Postganglionic sympathetic fibers from the cranial cervical ganglion. (2) Sensory fibers from the ophthalmic branch of the trigeminal nerve (V).

SYMPATHETIC SUPPLY

Sympathetic fibers from the brain pass down the cervical spinal cord and leave via spinal nerves of segments T_1 and T_2. The fibers leave the nerves, pass to the sympathetic trunk, and pass cranially with it in its common sheath with the vagus nerve. The sympathetic trunk terminates cranially at the CRANIAL CERVICAL GANGLION, where many of the fibers synapse. Postganglionic fibers pass via a variety of pathways to the pupillary dilator muscle and to Müller's muscle.

OCULAR REFLEXES[1]

Integration of the various sensory and motor functions into protective reflexes of clinical significance are now discussed.

Pupillary Light Reflex
(Fig. 1–20; see also Fig. 1–7)

Nerves: Optic (II) and oculomotor (III).
Stimulus: Light stimulating the photoreceptors of one eye.
Effect: Constriction of both pupils.
Pathway: Impulses pass from the retina to the optic nerve, optic chiasm, both optic tracts, superior colliculus and pretectal area, Edinger-Westphal nuclei of the oculomotor nerve, oculomotor nerves, ciliary ganglia, short ciliary nerves, and pupillary sphincter muscles. Pupillary constriction results.

Constriction of the pupil on the same (IPSILATERAL) side as the stimulus is termed the DIRECT PUPILLARY REFLEX; on the opposite (CONTRALATERAL) side it is called the CONSENSUAL LIGHT REFLEX. The reflexes are elicited with a bright penlight or transilluminator. Both reflexes are present in normal animals, although considerable differences exist in the speed of the reflexes between small and large animal species. The reflexes are of considerable value in localizing lesions within the visual system.

Corneal Reflex

Nerves: Trigeminal (V) and facial (VII).
Stimulus: Painful stimulus to the cornea, e.g., an object or disease process.

1. Modified from Jenkins, 1978. See also Chap 16.

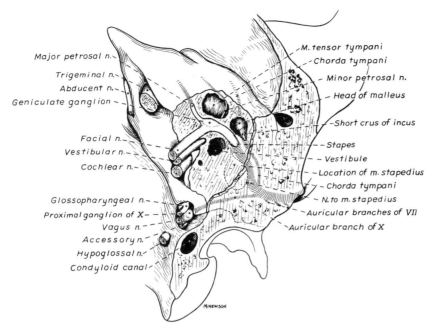

Major petrosal n.
Trigeminal n.
Abducent n.
Geniculate ganglion

Facial n.
Vestibular n.
Cochlear n.

Glossopharyngeal n.
Proximal ganglion of X
Vagus n.
Accessory n.
Hypoglossal n.
Condyloid canal

M. tensor tympani
Chorda tympani
Minor petrosal n.
Head of malleus
Short crus of incus
Stapes
Vestibule
Location of m. stapedius
Chorda tympani
N. to m. stapedius
Auricular branches of VII
Auricular branch of X

M. NEWSON

FIGURE 1–17. *The canine petrous temporal bone, sculptured to show the path of the facial nerve. Dorsal aspect. (From Evans HE, Christensen GC: Miller's Anatomy of the Dog, 2nd ed. WB Saunders Co, Philadelphia, 1979. © Cornell University 1964.)*

AUTONOMIC INNERVATION

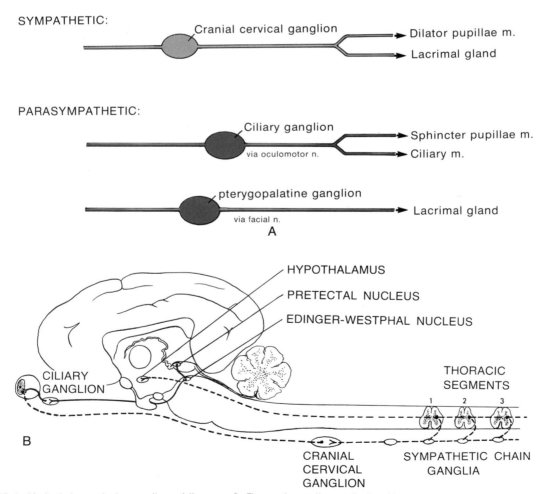

SYMPATHETIC:

Cranial cervical ganglion → Dilator pupillae m.
→ Lacrimal gland

PARASYMPATHETIC:

Ciliary ganglion → Sphincter pupillae m.
via oculomotor n. → Ciliary m.

pterygopalatine ganglion → Lacrimal gland
via facial n.

A

HYPOTHALAMUS
PRETECTAL NUCLEUS
EDINGER-WESTPHAL NUCLEUS

CILIARY
GANGLION

THORACIC
SEGMENTS
1 2 3

B

CRANIAL
CERVICAL
GANGLION

SYMPATHETIC CHAIN
GANGLIA

FIGURE 1–18. *A, Autonomic innervation of the eye. B, The motor pathways to the iris: parasympathetic constrictor and sympathetic dilator. (B from Hoerlein BF: Canine Neurology, 3rd ed. WB Saunders Co, Philadelphia, 1978.)*

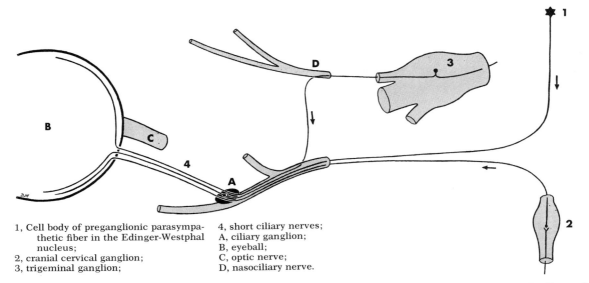

1, Cell body of preganglionic parasympa-
    thetic fiber in the Edinger-Westphal
    nucleus;
2, cranial cervical ganglion;
3, trigeminal ganglion;

4, short ciliary nerves;
A, ciliary ganglion;
B, eyeball;
C, optic nerve;
D, nasociliary nerve.

FIGURE 1–19. Autonomic innervation of the eye. (From Getty R: Sisson and Grossman's The Anatomy of the Domestic Animals, 5th ed. WB Saunders Co, Philadelphia, 1975.)

Effect: Closure of the lids.

Pathway: Impulses arising from the numerous fine sensory **CORNEAL BRANCHES** of the trigeminal nerve pass via the **OPHTHALMIC BRANCH** to the **SEMILUNAR GANGLION** to the upper medulla and **NUCLEI OF THE FACIAL NERVE** on both sides. This nucleus innervates the facial nerve and the **ORBICULARIS OCULI MUSCLE**, which closes the palpebral aperture.

This reflex is important to the protection of the eye; interference with it often results in severe ocular damage, e.g., facial paralysis, trigeminal palsy, local anesthesia. The reflex is used diagnostically to test the function of the two nerves involved. Closure of the lids of the stimulated eye is referred to as the **DIRECT CORNEAL REFLEX**, and closure of the contralateral lids as the **CONSENSUAL CORNEAL REFLEX**. When the stimulus is applied to the lids, the reflex is termed the **PALPEBRAL REFLEX**.

Menace Reflex

Synonym: Blink reflex.

Nerves: Optic (II) and facial (VII).

Stimulus: A sudden visual stimulus, e.g., a hand movement. The stimulus may be applied behind a sheet of glass or plastic in order to prevent air currents from stimulating the corneal reflex and causing a false-positive result. Such false-positive and false-negative results are often misinterpreted by owners as evidence of sight or blindness in an animal.

Effect: Closure of the lids.

Pathway: Impulses pass from the retina to the optic nerve, optic chiasm, optic tracts, and rostral colliculi in the midbrain tectum. Descending axons from the cell bodies in the rostral colliculi form the **TECTOBULBAR TRACTS**, which pass to the motor nuclei of the facial nerve to the palpebral nerve and the **ORBICULARIS OCULI MUSCLE**.

The **MENACE REFLEX** is a reaction to a stronger stimulus than that causing the **PALPEBRAL REFLEX**. It results in turning of the head and neck, and often part of the trunk, away from the stimulus. Tectobulbar fibers passing to **ACCESSORY (XI) NUCLEI** and lower motor neurons from these nuclei to brachiocephalic muscles mediate this reflex. Descending fibers of the **TECTOSPINAL TRACT** pass from the rostral colliculi to the spinal cord and lower motor neurons to innervate

Direct   Consensual

FIGURE 1–20. The pupillary light reflex, showing the difference between the direct and the consensual responses.

body muscles used in this reflex. Cerebellar lesions may interrupt the menace reflex as in any condition that causes the CEREBELLAR SYNDROME. It is assumed that the pathway from the rostral colliculi to the facial nuclei must pass through the cerebellum via a CORTICOPON-TOCEREBELLAR TRACT (see also Chap 17).

PHYSIOLOGY OF THE AQUEOUS

Aqueous fills the AQUEOUS COMPARTMENT—the ANTERIOR CHAMBER between the iris and cornea, and the POSTERIOR CHAMBER, between the anterior lens surface and the posterior iris surface. The posterior chamber should not be confused with the vitreous compartment (Fig. 1–21).

Formation and Composition

Aqueous is produced in the CILIARY BODY, by PASSIVE (DIFFUSION and ULTRAFILTRATION) and ACTIVE (selective transport against a concentration gradient) processes. Ultrafiltration refers to passage of fluid under the influence of the hydrostatic pressure supplied by the arterial system in the ciliary vasculature, against an osmotic gradient into the posterior chamber. Fluid from ciliary capillaries passes into the stroma of the CILIARY PROCESSES through the ciliary epithelium and into the posterior chamber. Aqueous then passes through the pupil into the anterior chamber to the TRABECULAR MESHWORK in the DRAINAGE (IRIDO-CORNEAL) ANGLE and via the meshwork to the systemic venous circulation through a plexus of small veins in the sclera—the SCLERAL VENOUS PLEXUS. Fibers of the

ciliary muscle that insert into the trabecular meshwork affect drainage of aqueous from the eye, probably by increasing the size of the spaces in the meshwork through which the aqueous leaves the eye, when the fibers are placed under tension.

An alternative route of drainage—the UVEOSCLERAL ROUTE—exists and accounts for about 25% of aqueous outflow in the dog. Aqueous is thought to diffuse through the ciliary and choroid to the venous system.

The BLOOD-AQUEOUS BARRIER is a functional barrier between blood in the capillaries of the ciliary stroma and aqueous in the posterior chamber. The capillaries have a thin endothelium with many pores and fenestrations enabling larger molecules to pass into the stroma. Most large molecules, including proteins, are unable to pass through or between the cells in the two layers of ciliary epithelium overlying the ciliary processes, because of the tight intercellular junctions between the cells. The exact anatomical location of the barrier is probably different for different substances, e.g., capillary endothelial cells, endothelial basement membrane, intercellular junctions. The blood-aqueous barrier is frequently broken down by disease processes.

The blood-aqueous barrier restricts the entry of many substances, including drugs, into the aqueous.

An ENERGY-DEPENDENT TRANSPORT MECHANISM similar to that in the renal epithelium is present in the ciliary body, and this results in higher concentrations of certain substances, e.g., ascorbic acid, in the aqueous than in the plasma. *Sodium* and *chloride* ions are actively pumped into the aqueous and draw water passively along a concentration gradient. $Na^+–K^+$ *activated adenosine triphosphatase (ATPase)* is present in the inner layer of the unpigmented ciliary epithelium and may be associated with the sodium pump. The sodium pump probably accounts for the majority of actively formed aqueous.

In some species, *bicarbonate ions* are present in higher concentrations in the aqueous. This is related to the presence of *carbonic anhydrase,* which catalyzes the formation of carbonic acid from CO_2 and water. Carbonic acid dissociates, and bicarbonate ions pass to the aqueous. Carbonic anhydrase inhibitors cause decreased bicarbonate to enter the posterior chamber and less water follows, decreasing aqueous production.

$$H_2O + CO_2 \xrightarrow{\text{carbonic anhydrase}} H_2CO_3 \rightleftharpoons H^+ + HCO_3^-$$

Inhibition of carbonic anhydrase by drugs in some species results in decreased aqueous production.

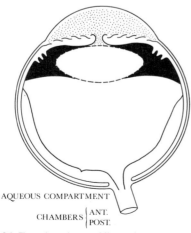

FIGURE 1–21. *The chambers of the aqueous compartment. The aqueous compartment is subdivided into two chambers by the iris diaphragm. The anterior chamber in front of the diaphragm is indicated in stippled black; the posterior chamber behind the iris diaphragm is indicated in solid black. (From Fine S, Yanoff M: Ocular Histology: A Text and Atlas. Harper & Row, New York, 1972.)*

AQUEOUS COMPARTMENT

CHAMBERS | ANT.
| POST.

The concentration of *protein* in aqueous is about 0.5% of the plasma concentration. After damage to the blood-aqueous barrier by inflammation, drugs, or sudden iatrogenic decreases in intraocular pressure by paracentesis, greatly increased amounts of proteins including immunoglobulins and fibrinogen can enter the aqueous. The effect of paracentesis is mediated by prostaglandin release, which affects vessel permeability. As the composition of aqueous approaches that of plasma, it is termed **PLASMOID AQUEOUS**.

Aqueous carries nutrients for the tissues it bathes, e.g., iris, cornea, and it receives constant contributions of waste products of metabolism. Thus the composition of aqueous changes as it passes from the ciliary body to the drainage angle.

Pressure Dynamics

Equilibrium between formation and drainage of aqueous results in a relatively constant **INTRAOCULAR PRESSURE** of 20–30 mmHg that distends the globe to its characteristic form. **DIURNAL VARIATIONS** in pressure occur, and the pressure is also affected by factors such as mean arterial pressure, central venous pressure, and blood osmolality. Several indexes are used to measure features of aqueous production and drainage.

Pressure is defined as force per unit area:

$$P = f/A$$

Fluid flows from areas of high pressure (P_1) to areas of low pressure (P_2) across a **PRESSURE GRADIENT** ($P_1 - P_2$). The rate of flow of a liquid is the volume of liquid transferred in unit time (e.g., milliliters per minute). The rate of flow across a pressure gradient is inversely proportional to the resistance to flow. It is convenient to consider the *ease of flow* of the liquid rather than the resistance; the ease or *facility of outflow (C)* is the reciprocal of the resistance (R).

$$C = 1/R$$

$$F :: P_1 - P_2$$

$$\text{Therefore } F = 1/R(P_1 - P_2)$$

$$\text{Therefore } F = C(P_1 - P_2)$$

where R = resistance
F = flow (microliters per minute)
P_1, P_2 = pressure (millimeters of Hg)
C = facility of outflow (microliters per minute per millimeter of Hg)
$C_{dog} = 0.13 - 0.18$, $C_{cat} = 0.156 - 0.193$

In clinical ophthalmology, C is a measure of the ease with which aqueous passes the trabecular meshwork; P_1 is the **INTRAOCULAR PRESSURE**, and P_2 is the pressure in the venous channels into which the aqueous drains (**EPISCLERAL VENOUS PRESSURE**). As intraocular pressure increases, aqueous production decreases and outflow increases.

REFERENCES

Bill A (1966): Formation and drainage of aqueous humor in cats. Exp Eye Res 5:185.

Braund KG (1986): Clinical Syndromes in Veterinary Neurology. Williams & Wilkins, Baltimore.

de Lahunta A, et al (1967): Neuro-ophthalmologic lesions as a cause of visual deficit in dogs and horses. J Am Vet Med Assoc 150:994.

Duke-Elder S (1958): System of Ophthalmology, Vol 1, The Eye in Evolution. H Kimpton, London.

Duke-Elder S (1968): System of Ophthalmology, Vol 4, Physiology of the Eye and Vision. Kimpton, London.

Evans HE, et al (1979): Miller's Anatomy of the Dog. 2nd ed. WB Saunders Co, Philadelphia.

Hogan MJ, et al (1971): Histology of the Human Eye. WB Saunders Co, Philadelphia.

Jenkins TW (1978): Functional Mammalian Neuroanatomy, 2nd ed. Lea & Febiger, Philadelphia.

Langham ME (1960): Steady-state pressure flow relationships in the living and dead eye of the cat. Am J Ophthalmol 50:950.

Morrin LA, et al (1982): Oval lipid corneal opacities in beagles: Ultrastructure of normal beagle cornea. Am J Vet Res 43:443.

Moses RA (1980): Adler's Physiology of the Eye, 7th ed. CV Mosby, St. Louis.

Neufeld AH, et al (1973): Prostaglandin and eye. Prostaglandins 4:157.

Peiffer RL, et al (1976): Determination of canine facility of outflow, comparing in vivo and in vitro tonographic and constant pressure perfusion techniques. Am J Vet Res 33:1473.

Prince JH, et al (1960): Anatomy and Histology of the Eye and Orbit of Domestic Animals. Charles C Thomas, Springfield, IL.

Schmidt GM, et al (1981): Physiology of the Eye. *In* Gelatt KN (ed): Veterinary Ophthalmology. Lea & Febiger, Philadelphia.

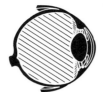

Development and Congenital Abnormalities

DEVELOPMENT	CILIARY BODY AND IRIS	CONGENITAL
FORMATION OF OPTIC PRIMORDIA	SCLERA AND EXTRAOCULAR MUSCLES	ABNORMALITIES
RETINA	CORNEA AND ANTERIOR CHAMBER	DEFINITIONS
OPTIC NERVE	EYELIDS AND THIRD EYELID	ETIOLOGY
VITREOUS	NASOLACRIMAL SYSTEM	ANOPHTHALMOS–MICROPHTHALMOS
LENS		CYCLOPIA–SYNOPHTHALMOS
PRIMITIVE VASCULAR SYSTEM		COLOBOMA

DEVELOPMENT

FORMATION OF OPTIC PRIMORDIA

The PRIMORDIUM of the eye develops from that portion of the embryo that later forms the anterior part of the central nervous system. The process may be divided into three stages:

1. EMBRYOGENESIS—segregation of the primary layers of the developing embryo. This period begins with fertilization and ends with differentiation of the primary germ layers.

2. ORGANOGENESIS—separation into the general pattern of various organs.

3. DIFFERENTIATION—detailed development of the characteristic structure of each organ.

The eye develops from NEUROECTODERM, SURFACE ECTODERM, and MESODERM. Ocular structures are differentiated from the rest of the embryo at the EMBRYONIC PLATE stage. The site of the future eye is indicated by flattened areas on the anterior end of the NEURAL GROOVE. The neural groove becomes deeper, sinks into the mesoderm, and detaches from the overlying surface ectoderm to form the NEURAL TUBE from which the central nervous system develops. Before the anterior end of the neural tube closes, small pits—the OPTIC GROOVES (Figs. 2–1 and 2–2)—form in the neural ectoderm.

The optic grooves invaginate and grow toward the surface ectoderm, forming the OPTIC VESICLES (Fig. 2–3). The forebrain is connected to the optic vesicles by the OPTIC STALK. Surface ectoderm overlying the optic vesicles thickens to form the LENS PLACODE (Fig. 2–4).[1]

The former optic vesicle continues to invaginate to form the double-layered OPTIC CUP (Fig. 2–5). The lens vesicle then lies within the optic cup. A groove called the OPTIC FISSURE forms on the ventral surface of the optic cup and along the optic stalk. Mesoderm enters through this fissure and forms the HYALOID VASCULAR SYSTEM. The optic fissure gradually closes, leaving a small opening at the anterior end of the optic stalk, which the hyaloid artery passes through (Figs. 2–6 and 2–7).

The HYALOID ARTERY supplies the inner layers of the optic cup and associated mesoderm and the developing lens vesicle. Gradually the edges of the optic fissure approximate and fuse, enclosing the hyaloid vessels in the optic nerve (Fig. 2–8). The rostral portions of the hyaloid vessels degenerate at variable times during pre- and postnatal development. In dogs the hyaloid system provides vascular supply to the posterior lens region up to about postnatal day 6, but remnants of the hyaloid system are sometimes visible ophthalmoscopically until 4 months of age; in cattle they may persist visibly until 12 months of age or longer. In beagles, most hyaloid arteries are no longer patent by postpartum day 17. In humans, but not domestic animals, the caudal portion of the hyaloid

---

1. The phenomenon whereby the optic vesicle influences surface ectoderm to thicken and form the lens placode is called *induction*.

18

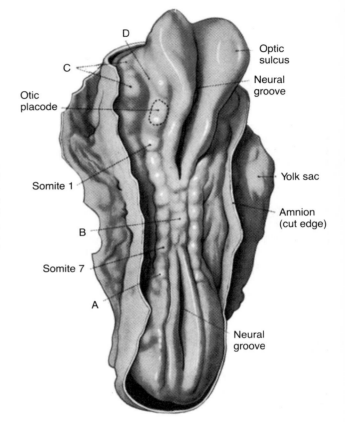

FIGURE 2–1. *Reconstruction of a seven-somite human embryo, showing the dorsal aspect at about the 22nd day. The early optic pit (sulcus) is seen in the prosencephalic region. A, The paraxial mesoderm partially segmented into somites. B, The roof of the neural tube formed in the central area. C, The pericardial area. D, The region of the branchial arches. (From Hamilton, Boyd, Mossman: Human Embryology. W Heffer, Cambridge.)*

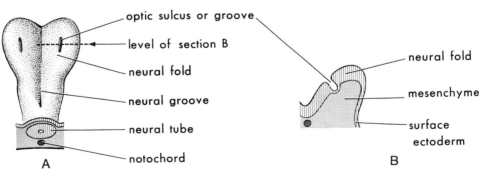

FIGURE 2–2. *Early eye development. A, Dorsal view of the cranial end of 22-day embryo, showing the first indication of eye development. B, Transverse section through an optic sulcus. (From Moore KL: The Developing Human, 4th ed. WB Saunders Co, Philadelphia, 1988.)*

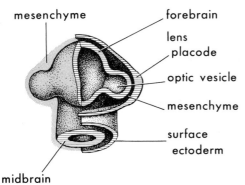

FIGURE 2–3. Schematic drawing of the forebrain, its covering layers of mesoderm and the surface ectoderm from an embryo of about 28 days. (From Moore KL: The Developing Human, 4th ed. WB Saunders Co, Philadelphia, 1988.)

vasculature persists as the central retinal artery and vein.

At this stage of development the general structure of the eye has been determined. Early in gestation, differentiation to adult ocular structures is more rapid in the posterior segment, with the anterior segment developing more rapidly later. The formation of specific structures are now discussed.

RETINA

The outer layer of the optic cup forms the PIGMENT EPITHELIUM OF THE RETINA. The thicker inner layer differentiates to form the NEUROBLASTIC LAYER (Fig. 2–9). The two layers are separated by an INTRARETINAL SPACE. The intraretinal space represents the cavity of the optic vesicle, which is gradually obliterated by invagination of the optic vesicle and thickening of the neuroblastic layer. Retinal detachments in postnatal and adult life occur where this space existed. Nuclei

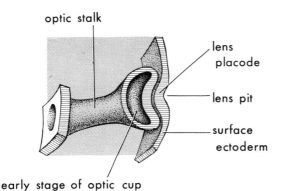

FIGURE 2–4. Schematic section of the developing eye, illustrating early stage in the development of the optic cup. (From Moore KL: The Developing Human, 4th ed. WB Saunders Co, Philadelphia, 1988.)

within the neuroblastic layer migrate into two layers—the inner and outer neuroblastic layers—separated by the fiber layer of Chevitz, which is devoid of nuclei (Fig. 2–10). The cells of the OUTER NEUROBLASTIC LAYER differentiate to form the RODS and CONES, adjacent to the pigment epithelium and the horizontal cells found in the inner nuclear layer. The INNER NEUROBLASTIC LAYER forms the GANGLION, BIPOLAR, AMACRINE, and MÜLLER cells.

The retina is thus inverted, with the rods and cones adjacent to the pigment epithelium. Light must pass through the layers of the retina in order to reach the sensory photoreceptors. The neuroblastic layer of the retina is continuous with the optic stalk. Axons develop from ganglion cells and grow toward the optic stalk, which later becomes the optic nerve.

The stage of development of the retina at birth depends on species. In dogs, the electroretinogram appears during the 1st week of life and reaches adult amplitudes by 5–8 weeks. Microscopically, rod and cone inner and outer segments are observed in the 3rd week of life and further differentiation occurs in weeks 5–8.

OPTIC NERVE

The nerve begins as a single layer of cells with a central lumen. Nerve fibers from ganglion cells in the inner neuroblastic layer grow toward the optic stalk, forming the NERVE FIBER LAYER OF THE RETINA and finally the optic nerve. The fibers later extend posteriorly to form the OPTIC CHIASM and OPTIC TRACTS. Medullation of nerve fibers extends peripherally from the brain toward the lamina cribrosa. As the lips of the optic fissure fuse, the hyaloid system is trapped in the center of the optic nerve.

At a point in the center of the future optic disc, the axons of the retinal GANGLION CELLS pass through the retina to enter the optic nerve. Glial cells are displaced forward at this point to form the sheath of the hyaloid artery. This group of cells may protrude from the OPTIC DISC (OPTIC PAPILLA) throughout adult life as BERGMEISTER'S PAPILLA. Variable atrophy of these cells causes the PHYSIOLOGICAL CUP in the optic disc.[2]

VITREOUS

The vitreous body is formed from the primary, secondary, and tertiary vitreous. PRIMARY VITREOUS consists of mesodermal cells, fibers, and secretions from the neural surface of the retina and the lens, associated with the hyaloid vascular system (Fig. 2–11). It persists

---

2. Normal ophthalmoscopic variations of the optic pit must be distinguished from pathological alterations, e.g., disc ectasia in scleral ectasia syndrome, glaucomatous cupping.

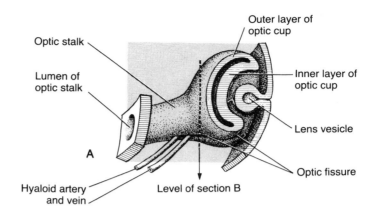

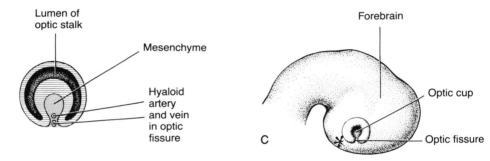

FIGURE 2–5. A, Schematic section of the developing eye, showing stage in the development of the optic cup and lens vesicle. B, Transverse section through the optic stalk, showing the optic fissure and its contents. C, Lateral view of the brain of an embryo at about 32 days, showing the external appearance of the optic cup. (From Moore KL: The Developing Human, 4th ed. WB Saunders Co, Philadelphia, 1988.)

FIGURE 2–6. The invagination of the optic vesicle (A) through the formation of the embryonic fissure (B,C,D) to form the optic cup (E). In E, the hyaloid artery is seen entering the proximal extremity of the fissure. (Reproduced by permission from Duke-Elder, Sir Stewart, editor: System of Ophthalmology. Vol III. Normal and Abnormal Development, Part 1. Embryology [by Duke-Elder, Sir Stewart, and Cook, Charles]. St Louis, 1963, The CV Mosby Co.)

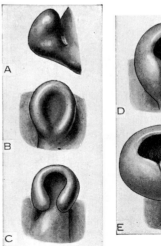

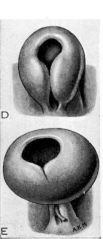

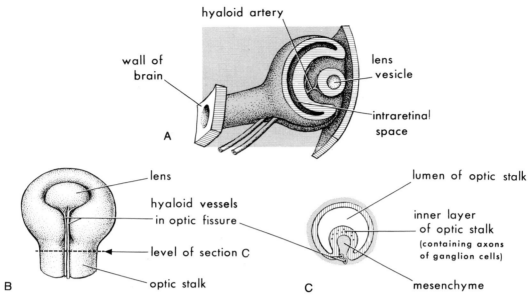

FIGURE 2–7. A, Schematic section of the developing eye, illustrating late stage in the development of the optic cup and lens vesicle. B, View of the inferior surface of the optic cup and stalk, showing early stage in the closure of the optic fissure. C, Transverse section. (From Moore KL: The Developing Human, 4th ed. WB Saunders Co, Philadelphia, 1988.)

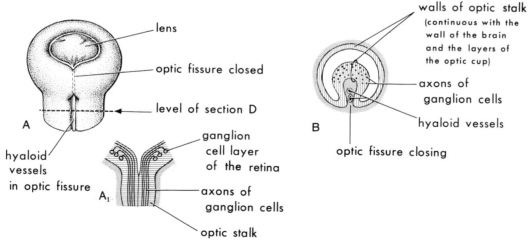

FIGURE 2–8. A, View of inferior surface of optic cup and stalk, showing stage in closure of optic fissure. A₁, Schematic sketch of a longitudinal section of a portion of the optic cup and optic stalk, showing axons of ganglion cells of the retina growing through the optic stalk to the brain. B, Transverse section. (From Moore KL: The Developing Human, 4th ed. WB Saunders Co, Philadelphia, 1988.)

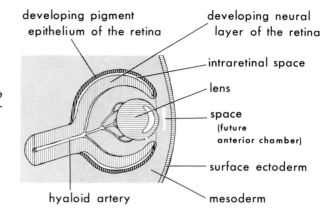

developing pigment epithelium of the retina

developing neural layer of the retina

intraretinal space

lens

space (future anterior chamber)

surface ectoderm

mesoderm

hyaloid artery

FIGURE 2–9. Sagittal section of the eye at 5-week stage of development. (From Moore KL: The Developing Human, 4th ed. WB Saunders Co, Philadelphia, 1988.)

in adults just behind the posterior pole of the lens as the hyaloid canal (Cloquet's canal), which runs to the optic disc. SECONDARY VITREOUS is denser, more homogeneous, and avascular, and it is laid down outside the primary vitreous. It is secreted by the retinal ectoderm, and the vitreous fibrils within it are continuous with Müller's fibers in the retina. TERTIARY VITREOUS is secreted by the ciliary epithelium. Bundles

of vitreous fibrillar condensations extend radially from the future ciliary epithelium to the lens equator, displacing the secondary vitreous. Tertiary vitreous persists in the adult as the LENS ZONULES (suspensory ligament of the lens) (see Fig. 2–11).

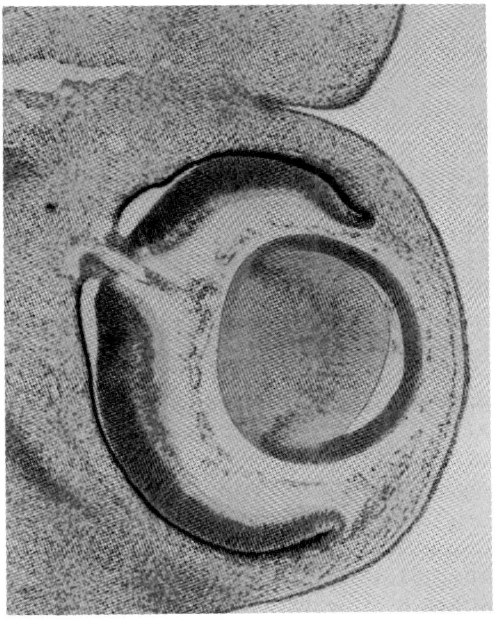

LENS

The surface ectoderm thickens, forming the LENS PLACODE (see Fig. 2–3), which invaginates to become the LENS VESICLE. The apex of these ectodermal cells is directed toward the center of the lens vesicle, whereas the basal portion of the cell is directed outward (see Fig. 2–4). Eventually the lens vesicle is cut off from the parent surface ectoderm. The anterior cells of the optic vesicle remain cuboidal, but the posterior cells elongate, become columnar, and form the PRIMARY LENS FIBERS (Fig. 2–12A, B). These fibers eventually fill the cavity of the lens vesicle when they reach the anterior epithelium (Fig. 2–12C, D). The nuclei of the primary lens fibers gradually fade, but the anterior cuboidal cells remain as the adult LENS EPITHELIUM. The junction of cuboidal and columnar cells is called the EQUATORIAL ZONE OF THE LENS. SECONDARY LENS FIBERS proliferate from this area anteriorly beneath the cuboidal cells and posteriorly beneath the LENS CAPSULE. Secondary lens fibers continue to form during adult life, from the equatorial region, and they are deposited outside the pre-existing fibers like the layers of an onion (Fig. 2–12E). The lens capsule is formed by the cuboidal lens epithelium and primary lens fibers and is the basement membrane of these cells. Secondary lens fibers run from the anterior to the posterior pole of the lens and are thickest in the middle (Fig. 2–12F). Because none of the fibers is quite long enough to reach fully from pole to pole, and because the cells are too thick at the ends for all of them to meet at a single point, they meet in Y-shaped structures known

FIGURE 2–10. Transverse section through a 20-mm embryo fixed in formalin and stained with hematoxylin and eosin. The primary vitreous is well developed, and the hyaloid artery has reached the lens. The corneal epithelium (surface ectoderm) is present, and the corneal stroma (mesenchyma) is developing. The secondary vitreous has begun to form. A nerve fiber layer is in the central aspect of the optic cup, and the future retina has differentiated into an inner and outer neuroblastic layer as far forward as the middle third of the optic cup. (From Bistner SI, Rubin LF, Aguirre G: Development of the bovine eye. Am J Vet Res 34:7, 1973.)

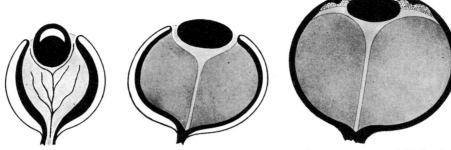

FIGURE 2–11. *Stages in the development of the vitreous body. The primary vitreous is shown in light shading, the secondary is shown in dark shading, and the tertiary is marked by dots. In A, the primary vitreous alone is present; in B, the secondary vitreous occupies the greater part of the picture; and in C, the tertiary vitreous has appeared (after Ida Mann). (Reproduced by permission from Duke-Elder, Sir Stewart, editor: System of Ophthalmology. Vol III. Normal and Abnormal Development, Part 1. Embryology [by Duke-Elder, Sir Stewart, and Cook, Charles]. St Louis, 1963, The CV Mosby Co.)*

as LENS SUTURES.[3] The anterior lens suture is an upright Y, whereas the posterior suture is inverted (Fig. 2–12F, G).

PRIMITIVE VASCULAR SYSTEM[4]

The HYALOID ARTERY, a branch of the ophthalmic artery, enters the optic cup through the optic fissures (see Fig. 2–7). The parent artery continues anteriorly to form an anastomotic ring around the margin of the optic cup, the ANNULAR VESSEL (see Fig. 2–8). The hyaloid vessels form a net (VASA HYALOIDEA PROPRIA) in the developing vitreous, the anterior extension of which envelopes the developing lens (TUNICA VASCULOSA LENTIS). Anastomotic branches extend between the tunica vasculosa lentis and the annular vessel. The outer surface of the optic cup is surrounded by a network of vessels and pigment cells that give rise to the choroid. Within this net the NASAL and TEMPORAL LONG POSTERIOR CILIARY ARTERIES are formed and grow forward in the horizontal plane to supply the future ciliary body. A circular vessel concentric with the annular vessel develops and is connected to it by anastomoses, forming the MAJOR VASCULAR CIRCLE OF THE IRIS. During fetal development, the hyaloid vas-

cular system atrophies, from posterior to anterior. With the exception of variable venous remnants on the surface of the canine optic disc, the remnants that form the central retinal artery and vein in primates do not remain in domestic animals. The retinal circulation of domestic animals is derived from the ciliary circulation around the optic nerve.[5]

CILIARY BODY AND IRIS

The adult CILIARY BODY is lined by two layers of epithelium. The inner layer closest to the vitreous is unpigmented, and the outer layer is pigmented (Fig. 2–13). The pigmented layer is continuous with the PIGMENT EPITHELIUM OF THE RETINA. The unpigmented layer is a forward extension of the inner neuroblastic layer of the retina, but it contains no neural elements. Folds appear in the epithelial layers and are filled by mesoderm at the edge of the optic cup, eventually forming the CILIARY PROCESSES. The CILIARY MUSCLE and stroma of the ciliary body are also derived from mesoderm. The rim of the optic cup, partially covering the lens, forms the iris, which is continuous with the double epithelium of the ciliary body. In the iris both layers are pigmented. The SPHINCTER (M. SPHINCTER PUPILLAE) and DILATOR (M. DILATOR PUPILLAE) MUSCLES are derived from neuroectoderm at the rim of the optic cup, whereas the iris stroma is derived from mesoderm (see Fig. 2–13). A layer of mesoderm, associated with the anterior portion of the tunica vasculosa lentis in front of the lens, stretches over the pupillary opening, forming the pupillary membrane (Fig. 2–14). With further development the pupillary membrane atrophies and disappears, although small strands may remain attached to the anterior surface of the iris or the corneal endothelium (mesothelium). In the basenji, PERSISTENT PUPILLARY MEMBRANES are regarded as a serious congenital ocular defect, inherited as a homozygous recessive.

---

3. Lens sutures are visible in adult life and must be accurately differentiated from pathological lens opacities, especially in young horses.

4. See also p 397.

5. Development of the retinal vasculature of premature human infants is severely disturbed by an elevated PO_2 in the circulation (resulting in the disease known as **retrolental fibroplasia**). Puppies and kittens in the early postparturient period have a retinal circulation similar in stage of development to premature human infants, and they are similarly susceptible to high atmospheric and arterial oxygen concentrations. This susceptibility gradually decreases, disappearing by 21 days. Herbivorous animals (cattle, sheep, and horses) exhibit a later stage of retinal vasculature development at birth and are unaffected. Study of the condition in the kitten retina led to an understanding of the pathogenesis of the human disease, which frequently results in blindness.

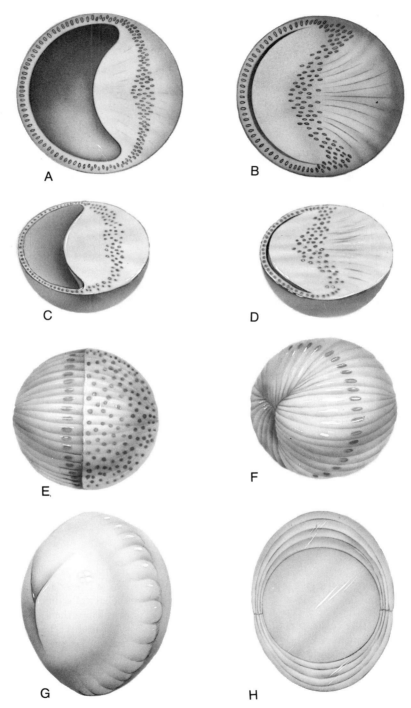

FIGURE 2–12. A, Elongation and anterior growth of posterior cuboidal epithelial cells to form primary lens fibers. (Modified from Severin GA: Veterinary Ophthalmology Notes, 2nd ed. Ft. Collins, 1976.) B, Elongation of primary lens fibers to fill the cavity in the lens vesicle, and formation of the lens bow of cuboidal cell nuclei. C, Secondary lens fibers proliferate from the equatorial region of the lens, covering the primary lens fibers and scattered cuboidal cell nuclei. D, Formation of the anterior Y suture at the junction of the secondary lens fibers. E, The adult lens. F, Successive layers of lens fibers. G, H, New layers of secondary lens fibers are laid down around the central primary lens fibers. Growth continues throughout life.

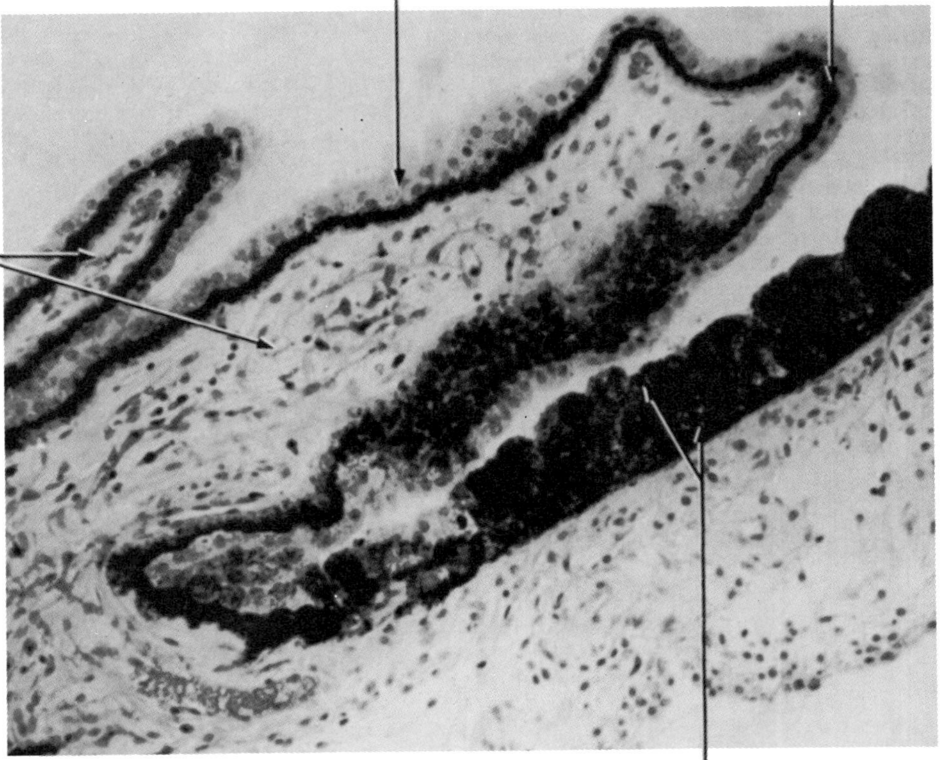

nonpigmented portion of
the ciliary epithelium
(continuous with the
neural layer of the retina)

pigmented portion of
the ciliary epithelium
(continuous with the pigment
epithelium of the retina)

ciliary
processes

double-layered epithelium of the iris
(continuous with the neural and pigmented layers of the retina)

FIGURE 2–13. Photomicrograph of the root of the iris (right) and ciliary processes, showing the ciliary and iridial parts of the retina. (From Leeson TS, Leeson CR: Histology, 2nd ed. WB Saunders Co, Philadelphia, 1970.)

SCLERA AND EXTRAOCULAR MUSCLES

Mesoderm surrounding the optic cup forms two layers, an inner vascular layer (CHOROID) adjacent to the retina and an outer fibrous layer (SCLERA). Condensation of the sclera begins anteriorly near the ciliary body and proceeds posteriorly to the optic nerve, where it is continuous with the DURA MATER of the optic nerve. Extraocular muscles form within the mesoderm of the orbit.

CORNEA AND ANTERIOR CHAMBER

CORNEAL EPITHELIUM is derived from surface ectoderm, but the STROMA, DESCEMET MEMBRANE, and the ENDOTHELIUM (MESOTHELIUM) are mesodermal in origin. Endothelial cells differentiate first and secrete Descemet's membrane (their basement membrane) anteriorly (see Fig. 2–14). Two spaces develop in the mesoderm between the anterior lens capsule and the cornea—the POSTERIOR CHAMBER between the lens and iris and the ANTERIOR CHAMBER between the iris and cornea. The two chambers communicate via the pupil after disappearance of the pupillary membrane. Note that the VITREOUS BODY posterior to the lens should not be confused with the posterior chamber between the lens and the iris. Further ingrowth of mesoderm occurs between the epithelium and the endothelium, forming the CORNEAL STROMA, which is continuous with the sclera.

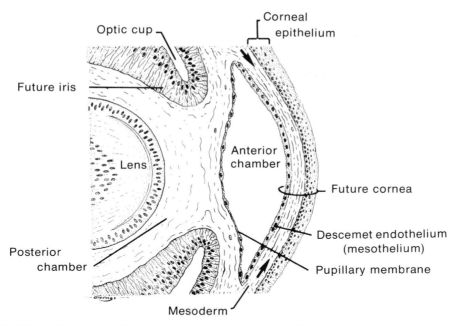

FIGURE 2–14. *Formation of the anterior chamber and cornea. Note the pupillary membrane.*

EYELIDS AND THIRD EYELID

The lower eyelid fold and third eyelid fold are formed by growth of the **MAXILLARY PROCESS** (see Fig. 2–15). The upper eyelid fold is formed from paraxial mesoderm. The folds have an ectodermal surface with cores of mesoderm. During development the upper and lower eyelids are fused, with the time of separation depending on species. In horses, cattle, sheep, and pigs, the lids are open at birth, as a functional eye is required early. In dogs and cats the lids open at 7–10 days postpartum, although visual capabilities are poorly developed before 21 days of age. During formation of the lid folds, the lids and surface of the globe are lined with conjunctiva derived from surface ectoderm. Also formed from the buds of surface ectoderm are the **LACRIMAL** (superotemporal surface of the globe) and **TARSAL** (meibomian) **GLANDS**, the **GLAND OF THE THIRD EYELID**, and the **GLANDS OF ZEIS** (sebaceous) and **MOLL** (sweat).

NASOLACRIMAL SYSTEM

The **NASOLACRIMAL GROOVE** separates the **LATERAL NASAL FOLD** from the **maxillary process.** At the bottom of the groove, a solid cord of ectodermal cells forms and is buried as the maxillary process grows over it to fuse with the lateral nasal fold (Fig. 2–15).

Two additional ectodermal buds grow from the upper end of the buried cord toward the upper and lower lid folds near their nasal ends. These buds develop to form the **SUPERIOR** and **INFERIOR LACRIMAL PUNCTA.** The lower end of the cord enters the rostral portion of the ventral nasal meatus. The entire cord becomes the nasolacrimal duct by a process of **CANALIZATION.** Incomplete canalization is common in domestic animals. The puncta and upper half of the nasolacrimal duct are most commonly affected in dogs and cats. In horses the nasal meatus of the duct may be imperforate.

CONGENITAL ABNORMALITIES

DEFINITIONS

teratology—the branch of embryology that deals with abnormal development and congenital malformations.

developmental abnormalities—those occurring between fertilization of the ovum and the adult stage of development. In this group are included the congenital abnormalities, those present at birth.

anomaly—any deviation from the usual form of a part or organ.

variation—a minor and often fairly common anomaly.

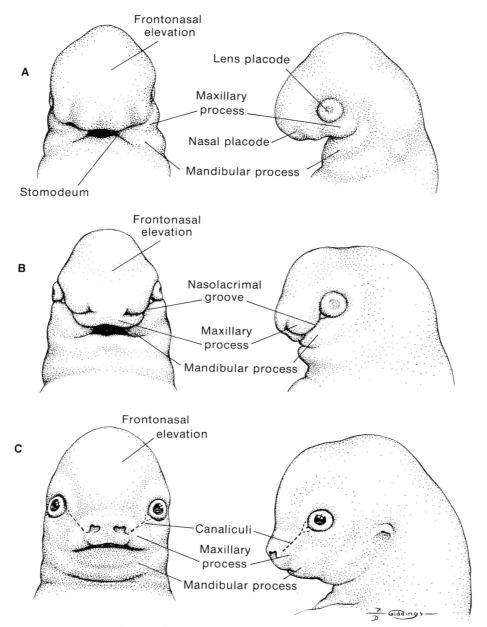

FIGURE 2–15. A–C, Formation of the eyelids and lacrimal drainage system.

atrophy—loss of tissue mass due to diminution in the size of the constituent cells.

degeneration—a broader group of more complex and often irreversible alterations in which metabolism is disturbed. The terms *atrophy, dystrophy,* and *abiotrophy* are often seen in veterinary ophthalmology. In the disease group PROGRESSIVE RETINAL ATROPHY, (PROGRESSIVE RETINAL DEGENERATION), the three terms are often interchanged; for this reason, their definitions are given here. Continuing studies of this disease have shown that abnormalities of the retina may be present very soon after birth, making accurate use of classical definitions more difficult. Dystrophy and abiotrophy have been used interchangeably to such an extent that distinction between them is no longer justifiable.

In this section, common congenital abnormalities of the whole eye of domestic animals are considered. Abnormalities of the individual parts of the eye are discussed in the relevant chapters. Although detailed study of anomalies may seem academic, it is only by such study that etiology and pathogenesis of the lesions are understood and subsequent diagnosis and evaluation simplified.

ETIOLOGY

Some of the causes of ocular abnormalities (modified from Duke-Elder and Cook, 1963, 1964) are

1. Viral infections in utero, e.g., retinal lesions in kittens whose dam was infected with panleukopenia virus during pregnancy, calves with virus diarrhea—mucosal disease virus, lambs with bluetongue virus, and puppies with canine herpes virus.

2. Toxic and chemical agents, e.g., ingestion by the dam of plant toxins that are thought to result in cyclopia in sheep in southwestern Australia and the western United States (*Veratrum californicum*).

3. Genetic factors, e.g., scleral ectasia syndrome (collie eye anomaly), coloboma in charolais, anterior segment dysgenesis with microphthalmia and retina dysplasia in the Doberman pinscher.

4. Inborn errors of metabolism, e.g., mannosidosis in Aberdeen Angus cattle and cats, resulting in retinal lesions in early life, and familial lipodystrophy in English setters.

5. Physical factors, e.g., radiation or low temperature causing ablepharon (lack of lids) in chickens.

6. Mechanical factors, e.g., amniotic bands, intrauterine molding, and abnormal pressure.

7. Nutritional and vitamin deficiencies, e.g., anophthalmia (lack of eyes) and microphthalmia (small eye) in the offspring of vitamin A–deficient sows.

Although many causes have been proposed, actual knowledge of etiological agents of ocular deformities is meager. The most important determining factor of the character of a deformity is the stage of development at which the etiological agent acts. Factors acting during the early period of EMBRYOGENESIS are generally lethal. Those occurring during ORGANOGENESIS result in gross deformities affecting the whole eye (e.g., anophthalmos, microphthalmos, and cyclopia). If the factor acts during the *fetal* period when the most fundamental and active stage has passed, minor defects of individual parts of the eye caused by arrests in development and associated deformities due to aberrant growth may occur.

The stage of development (e.g., embryogenesis, organogenesis, or fetal period) at which a teratogenic factor acts is most important in determining the final effects on the eye.

Surveys indicate that congenital ocular defects affect dogs more frequently than other species. Of these defects affecting the whole eye, microphthalmos-anophthalmos was the most frequent in all species. The following defects, affecting individual parts of the eye, are listed in descending order of frequency: SCLERAL ECTASIA SYNDROME (COLLIE EYE ANOMALY), ENTROPION, ECTROPION, CATARACT, OPACITY OF THE CORNEA, LACRIMAL ANOMALIES, DERMOID CYSTS, and PERSISTENT PUPILLARY MEMBRANE (see later chapters).

ANOPHTHALMOS–MICROPHTHALMOS

These abnormalities occur in association with the development of the PRIMARY OPTIC VESICLE. True anophthalmos, or complete absence of the eye, is very rare, as histological evidence of a rudimentary eye usually can be found. The term CLINICAL ANOPHTHALMOS is applied when no globe can be found on clinical examination. Microphthalmos, or an abnormally small eye, occurs most frequently in pigs and dogs. In pigs, vitamin A deficiency in the dam is the most frequent cause. Administration of griseofulvin to pregnant queens for treatment of dermatomycosis has resulted in anophthalmos, microphthalmos, and cyclopia in cats. In dogs, microphthalmos occurs frequently as part of the scleral ectasia syndrome (see Chap 11), and it is often associated with bilateral convergent strabismus and horizontal nystagmus of fine amplitude and high frequency. In hereditary microphthalmos in white shorthorn cattle, the lids and third eyelid are often present but are too large, and entropion is often the result; microphthalmos may occur in eyes that are otherwise normal, or that show minor or gross abnormalities.

In all species, multiple congenital ocular anomalies are seen and are often thought to be hereditary. The triad of multiple ocular defects, loss of hearing, and partial albinism has been noted in dogs of different breeds.

CONGENITAL NONATTACHMENT OF THE RETINA (due to incomplete involution of the primary optic vesicle, so that the two layers do not come into contact) is frequently seen in microphthalmic eyes. Microphthalmos is often seen with multiple ocular anomalies involving other ocular structures. In Jersey calves, an autosomal recessive condition occurs in which animals are blind at birth and show MICROPHAKIA (small lens), IRIDEREMIA (underdevelopment of the iris), ECTOPIA LENTIS (malposition of the lens), and CATARACT (opacity of the lens). Congenital microphthalmos, ectopia lentis, optic nerve hypoplasia, APHAKIA (absence of the lens), persistent pupillary membrane, colobomata, and nonattachment of the retina were observed in malformed lambs whose dams grazed seleniferous pasture in Wyoming. In Herefords, the ENCEPHALOPATHY-MICROPHTHALMIA syndrome (formerly called congenital hydrocephalus) is inherited as a simple autosomal recessive; it results in a domed skull, degeneration of skeletal muscles, small palpebral fissures and orbits, retinal dysplasia, vitreous liquefaction, malformation of the uvea, microphakia, and bilateral microphthalmos of variable degree. The calves are blind and unable to stand at birth, and they die within a few hours.

CYCLOPIA–SYNOPHTHALMOS

This condition is discussed because of its bizarre nature rather than its frequency. It occurs when elements of the two eyes are either completely fused (cyclopia) or partially fused (synophthalmos) in the midline. The eyes, the anterior part of the brain, and the midline mesodermal structures are involved, and the condition is incompatible with life. Extensive anomalies of the derivatives of the frontonasal process also occur, often resulting in overgrowth and fusion of the maxillary processes in the midline, forming a proboscis dorsal to the eye (Fig. 2–16). The condition occurs in most domestic and laboratory animals. Cyclopia occurs in lambs born to ewes in Idaho and Utah that graze *Veratrum californicum,* containing the teratogenic alkaloid cyclopamine, and to ewes grazing unknown toxic plants in western Australia.

COLOBOMA

A COLOBOMA (pl. colobomata) is a condition in which a portion of the eye is lacking. Most are associated

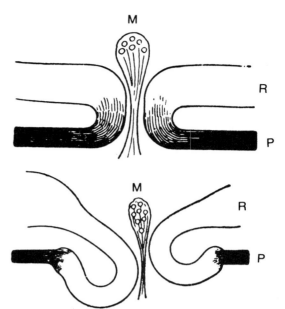

FIGURE 2–17. *The closure of the fetal cleft. R = retina, P = pigment epithelium; M = mesodermal vascular tissue. The margins come together accurately (left), but subsequently an excessive growth of the inner (retinal) layer leads to its eversion (right), a process that occurs normally at the posterior part of the fissure. (Reproduced by permission from Duke-Elder, Sir Stewart, editor: System of Ophthalmology. Vol III. Normal and Abnormal Development, Part 2. Congenital Deformities. St Louis, 1963, The CV Mosby Co.)*

with the embryonic fissure (TYPICAL COLOBOMATA) and are due to incomplete closure of the fissure (Fig. 2–17). ATYPICAL COLOBOMATA are not associated with incomplete closure of the embryonic fissure. TYPICAL COLOBOMATA are usually situated in the inferonasal portion of the ocular structures. They occur between invagination of the optic vesicle and closure of the embryonic fissure. As they may be complete and involve all structures associated with the fissure, or may be incomplete, the term can refer to anything from an extensive series of anomalies involving many ocular structures to a simple lesion such as a notch at the pupillary margin of the iris. Colobomata are most frequently seen in dogs affected with the scleral ectasia syndrome (Chap 11) and basenjis with persistent pupillary membrane, but they are also encountered as a hereditary defect in charolais cattle (Chap 11). Spontaneous ocular colobomata occur in other species of domestic animals and also occur in the eyelids in both dogs and cats (Chap 7).

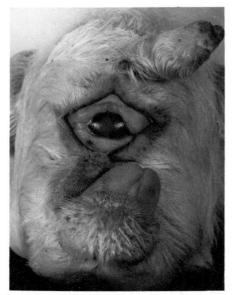

FIGURE 2–16. *Synophthalmos in a lamb whose dam grazed* Veratrum californicum. *(Courtesy of Dr. L.F. James.)*

REFERENCES

Aguirre G, et al (1972): The development of the canine eye. Am J Vet Res 33:2399.

Baker ML, et al (1961): The inheritance of hydrocephalus in cattle. J Hered 52:135.

Barnett KC, Ogden AL (1972): Ocular colobomata in charolais cattle. Vet Rec 91:592.

Bendixen HC (1944): Littery occurrence of anophthalmia or microphthalmia together with other malformations in swine—presumably due to vitamin A deficiency of the maternal diet. Acta Pathol Microbiol Scand Suppl 54:161.

Binns W, et al (1968): Effects of teratogenic agents in range plants. Cancer Res 28:2323.

Bistner SI, et al (1973): Development of the bovine eye. Am J Vet Res 34:7.

Bistner SI, et al (1970): The ocular lesions of bovine viral diarrhea–mucosal disease. Path Vet 7:275.

Duddy JA, et al (1983): Hyaloid artery patency in neonatal beagles. Am J Vet Res 44:2344.

Duke-Elder S, et al (1963, 1964): System of Ophthalmology, Vol 3, Normal and Abnormal Development parts 1 and 2, Embryology. H Kimpton, London.

Gum GG, et al (1984): Maturation of the retina of the canine neonate as determined by electroretinography and histology. Am J Vet Res 45:1166.

Gwin RM, et al (1981): Multiple ocular defects associated with partial albinism and deafness in the dog. J Am Anim Hosp Assoc 17:401.

Jubb KF, Kennedy PC (1984): Pathology of the Domestic Animals, Vol. 2. Academic Press, New York.

Keller RF, Binns W (1966): Teratogenic compounds of *Veratrum californicum* (Durand). II. production of ovine fetal cyclopia by fractions and alkaloid preparations. Canad J Biochem 44:829.

Koppang N (1960): Lipodystrophi i sentral nerve systemet hos hund (Tay-Sachs-lignende sykdom). Nord Med 63:821.

Mann IC (1964): The Development of the Human Eye, 3rd ed. Grune & Stratton, New York.

Moore KL (1988): The Developing Human, 4th ed. WB Saunders Co, Philadelphia.

Pearson AA (1972): The Development of the Eye. Am Acad Ophthalmol Otolaryngol Rochester, Minn.

Peiffer RL, Fischer CA (1983): Microphthalmia, retinal dysplasia and anterior segment dysgenesis in a litter of doberman pinschers. J Am Vet Med Assoc 183:875.

Percy DH, et al (1971): Lesions in puppies surviving infections with canine herpesvirus. Vet Pathol 8:37.

Percy DH, et al (1975): Retinal dysplasia due to feline panleukopenia virus infection. J Am Vet Med Assoc 167:935.

Priester WA (1972): Congenital ocular defects in cattle, horses, dogs and cats. J Am Vet Med Assoc 160:1504.

Scott FW, et al (1974): Teratogenesis in cats associated with griseofulvin therapy. Teratology 11:79.

Silverstein AM, et al (1971): An experimental virus-induced retinal dysplasia in the fetal lamb. Am J Ophthalmol 72:22.

Spencer WH (1985): Ophthalmic Pathology, 3rd ed. WB Saunders Co, Philadelphia.

Urman HK, Grace OD (1964): Hereditary encephalomyopathy. A hydrocephalus syndrome in newborn calves. Cornell Vet 54:230.

3

Ocular Pharmacology and Therapeutics

THERAPEUTIC FORMULATIONS	NONSTEROIDAL ANTI-	TEAR REPLACEMENT AND
ROUTES OF ADMINISTRATION	INFLAMMATORY DRUGS	VISCOUS SOLUTIONS
AUTONOMIC DRUGS	OSMOTIC AGENTS	MISCELLANEOUS THERAPEUTIC
ANTIBIOTICS	CARBONIC ANHYDRASE	AGENTS
ANTIFUNGAL ANTIBIOTICS	INHIBITORS	PHYSICAL THERAPY
ANTIVIRAL DRUGS	LOCAL ANESTHETICS	
CORTICOSTEROIDS	ANTICOLLAGENASE AGENTS	

THERAPEUTIC FORMULATIONS

Drugs are prepared in various ways for ocular administration. The most appropriate choice depends on penetrating characteristics of the drug, required site of drug action within the eye, stability of the drug in the formulation, convenience of application, and duration of action as a function of either its pharmacology or its formulation. Apart from systemic or local parenteral methods of administration, topical DROPS (solution or suspension) and OINTMENTS are most commonly used. The use of powders for ocular treatment is outmoded and may be detrimental to the eye.

Solutions and Suspensions

Tonicity

Drops are formulated with a tonicity similar to human tears (1.4% NaCl). Phosphate buffer is most commonly used to alter tonicity. The eye tolerates some variation in tonicity without great discomfort (e.g., 0.7–2.0% NaCl). Hypertonic solutions are diluted in order to approximate the tonicity of tears.

pH

Most ophthalmic solutions are buffered to the pH range from 3.5 to 10.5. Some unbuffered solutions (e.g., pilocarpine hydrochloride in 2% or higher concentration) are very irritating to the eye and are buffered to about pH 6.8. The pH of a preparation affects the penetrating ability of drugs contained in it. Increasing the pH of alkaloids increases their corneal penetration but decreases solubility and stability.

Stability

TEMPERATURE and pH are the most important factors affecting the stability of drugs in ophthalmic solutions. Alkaloids such as atropine, which are important constituents in many ophthalmic preparations, are more stable at pH 5 than at pH 7. The effect of high pH on decomposition is greatly enhanced by higher storage temperature. Certain ophthalmic preparations (e.g., antibiotics, epinephrine, echothiophate, phenylephrine, and physostigmine) characteristically lose potency with storage.

Sterility

If possible, ophthalmic preparations should be sterile, especially if they enter the interior of the eye. Autoclaving and bacterial filtering are commonly used for sterilization. Preservatives that may be toxic to intraocular tissues (e.g., benzalkonium chloride [Zephiran], chlorobutanol, phenols, and mercurochrome) are often added to multidose containers to prevent bacterial growth. These preservatives may interfere with diagnostic attempts to isolate and grow bacteria from the conjunctival sac. Ophthalmic ointments are prepared aseptically but are not always sterile, although sterile ointments are now becoming available commercially.

Ointments

Drugs do not ionize readily in the common oily ointment bases (paraffin or petrolatum); consequently, pH and tonicity are much less important in their formulation. Although water-soluble bases are available, many drugs (especially antibiotics) rapidly lose their potency when mixed with these bases. Ointments maintain contact of drugs with ocular tissues longer than solutions, resulting in marginally higher tissue concentrations. Ophthalmic ointments are generally more stable than solutions are, but they may interfere with corneal healing more than solutions do. Whether this interference is significant is doubtful. Because oily ointment bases cause severe intraocular inflammation, they are not used after penetrating ocular wounds or prior to or after intraocular surgery until the wound has sealed.

ROUTES OF ADMINISTRATION

Factors governing the choice of the route of administration include
1. Properties of the drug
2. Site of desired action
3. Possible frequency of administration
4. Drug concentration required

Some drugs, because of their properties, are restricted in the routes by which they can be given. For example, polymyxin B cannot be given systemically because of nephrotoxicity nor by subconjunctival injection because of irritation. Drugs required in high concentration in the cornea or conjunctiva are usually administered by TOPICAL APPLICATION or SUBCONJUNCTIVAL INJECTION. If high concentrations are required in the anterior uveal tract (iris, ciliary body), SUBJUNCTIVAL INJECTION, SYSTEMIC ADMINISTRATION (only with drugs that readily pass the blood-aqueous barrier), or FREQUENT TOPICAL APPLICATIONS are used. Drugs that do not pass the blood-aqueous barrier may still reach high concentrations in the anterior and posterior uvea (choroid). If high concentrations are required in the choroid, RETROBULBAR INJECTION or SYSTEMIC ADMINISTRATION is usually used. In inflammation the blood-aqueous barrier is greatly reduced, and drugs that cannot normally enter the aqueous and vitreous may do so.

Some drugs penetrate the eye poorly when placed on the surface of the cornea or conjunctiva. Penetration can be enhanced with a preparation that maintains longer contact with the eye before being washed away by the tears (e.g., an ointment or solution with a viscous vehicle such as polyvinylpyrrolidone or hydroxymethylcellulose). Frequent application of solutions also results in higher local tissue concentrations.

The cornea may be considered a lipid-water-lipid sandwich in which the epithelium and endothelium are lipophilic and hydrophobic, and the stroma is hydrophilic and lipophobic. Lipid-soluble drugs (e.g., chloramphenicol) penetrate more readily, whereas electrolytes and water-soluble drugs (e.g., neomycin, bacitracin, and penicillin) penetrate poorly after topical application. The lipophilic properties of the epithelium may be partially bypassed by subconjunctival injection, provided other properties of the drug are suitable. This

DIFFERENTIAL SOLUBILITY THEORY of drug penetration is illustrated by homatropine, an alkaloid that possesses both lipophilic and hydrophilic properties, depending on pH, and is able to pass both barriers within the cornea (Fig. 3–1).

In this figure, R_3N represents the nonionized fat-soluble (water-insoluble) form of the drug, which is in equilibrium with the ionized water-soluble (fat-insoluble) form, R_3NH^+. The relative proportions of the two forms of the drug depend on the pH. R_3N (being fat-soluble) passes the epithelium and enters the stroma, where it ionizes to R_3NH^+. This hydrophilic form passes the stroma until it is barred by the endothelium. R_3N^+ is then formed and passes the endothelium to enter the aqueous.

Higher or more prolonged drug concentrations and therapeutic effects may be achieved by
1. Increasing the concentration of the drug in the topical preparation (Fig. 3–2); e.g., 3% pilocarpine solution results in higher intraocular concentrations than does a 0.5% solution.
2. Increasing the frequency of application; e.g., 0.5% solution administered at intervals of 10 minutes for an hour results in higher concentrations than does a single application.
3. Slowing down absorption. Drugs released over a long period of time can be used to maintain drug concentrations. For instance, in cattle when frequent medication is inconvenient, subconjunctival injection of benzathine penicillin G (1 million units) may be used to maintain high corneal concentrations for 3–5 days. Other examples include triamcinolone acetonide (7–10 days) and crystalline penicillin G (1 million units) mixed with epinephrine solution (1 ml of 1:1000 solution) by subconjunctival injection. With benzathine penicillin G and triamcinolone acetonide, chemical properties of the drug result in slow absorption, but with penicillin G, absorption is slowed by the vasoconstrictive effect of epinephrine, which lasts about 48 hours.
4. Damaging the lipophilic epithelial layer with a surface-active preservative like benzalkonium chloride. Choice of route is summarized in Figure 3–3. The properties of individual drugs must be considered when choosing a method or group of methods of drug administration.

Ointments

Ointments allow longer contact between the drug and the tissues, less drug enters the lacrimal passages, a soothing effect occurs on instillation, and ointments are a more stable medium for labile antibiotics and drugs. Ointments interfere with corneal healing; they cannot be used after penetrating injuries; and owners tend to overmedicate with them, resulting in loss of medication and increased cost of treatment. Higher

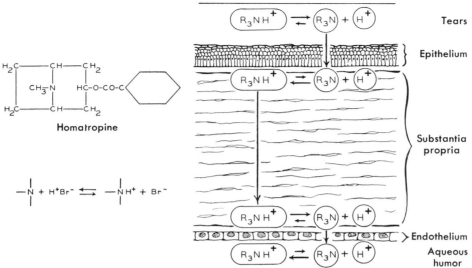

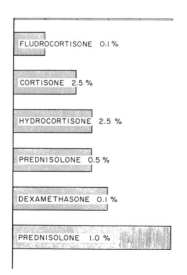

FIGURE 3–1. *Transfer of homatropine through the cornea, according to Kinsey. (Reproduced by permission from Waltman, Stephen R., and Hart, Wm. M., Jr.: The cornea. In Moses, Robert A., and Hart, William M., Jr., editors: Adler's Physiology of the Eye, ed. 8, St. Louis, 1987, The C. V. Mosby Co.)*

drug concentrations can be achieved with solutions than with ointments. Ointments are particularly useful in horses, as a small amount can be placed into the conjunctival sac with the end of a clean finger. Ideally, 1–2 cm of ointment from a fine nozzle is sufficient to medicate an eye. In the horse, the orbicularis oculi is powerful, and it is often impossible to retract the upper eyelid or tilt the head to allow a drop of solution to enter without contaminating the bottle, especially with recurrent treatment of painful eye conditions.

FIGURE 3–2. *Relative anti-inflammatory action of various corticosteroid preparations. (Reproduced by permission from Havener, William H.: Ocular Pharmacology, ed. 5, St. Louis, 1983, The C. V. Mosby Co. Modified from an advertisement by Allergan Pharmaceuticals.)*

Drops

Drops are the most commonly used method of topical treatment. They are easily instilled, especially in dogs and cats; the dosage can be controlled easily and varied; and they interfere less with repair of corneal epithelium. Drops are quickly eliminated from the eye after dilution with tears, and an increased frequency of application or drug concentration may be required. The method for instilling eye drops is shown in Figure 3–4. When properly instructed, clients find the use of drops convenient and economical.

Absorption of drugs from the conjunctival sac may be very rapid, resulting in blood levels comparable with those achieved by parenteral injection (Fig. 3–5). Although ocular penetration studies are frequently extrapolated among species (e.g., from laboratory animals and domestic animals to people), such extrapolation may be inaccurate. Chloramphenicol is commonly supposed to enter the eye readily after topical application, but in the dog it may enter no more rapidly than other drugs (neomycin, polymyxin B) when the corneal epithelium is not intact.

Subconjunctival Injection

Subconjunctival injection bypasses the barrier of the corneal epithelium and allows high drug concentrations in the anterior parts of the eye (see Fig. 3–3). Deeper injections beneath Tenon's capsule allow greater diffusion of drugs through the sclera and into the eye. MYDRIATICS (for pupillary dilation), ANTIBIOTICS, and CORTICOSTEROIDS are the main groups of drugs administered by this route. Some irritating drugs (e.g., polymyxin B) cannot be given subconjunctivally. Potent

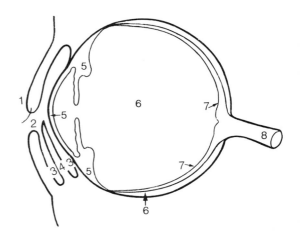

FIGURE 3–3. *Sites of drug administration: 1 and 2, Ointments; 3, Drops; 4, Drops, subconjunctival injection, nasolacrimal lavage; 5, Drops, subconjunctival injection, nasolacrimal lavage; 6, Subconjunctival or deep sub-Tenon's injection, systemic administration; 7, Deep sub-Tenon's or retrobulbar injection, systemic administration; 8, Retrobulbar injection, intra-arterial infusion, systemic administration. (Systemic administration may be by oral route, intramuscular [IM] injection, or intravenous [IV] injection or infusion.)*

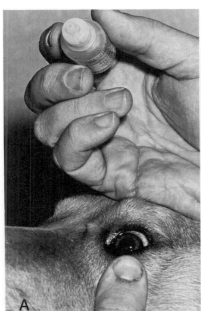

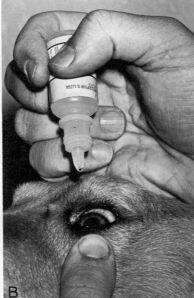

FIGURE 3–4. *A, The lower lid is restrained with the hand holding the head. The upper lid is retracted with the edge of the palm. B, The container is held 2 or 3 cm from the eye, and the dose is instilled.*

FIGURE 3–5. *Blood levels attained with 30 mg of tetracaine by different routes of administration (in dogs). (Reproduced by permission from Havener, William H.: Ocular Pharmacology, ed. 5, St. Louis, 1983, The C. V. Mosby Co. Modified from Adriani J, Campbell D: Fatalities following topical application of local anesthetics to mucous membranes. JAMA 162:1527, 1956.)*

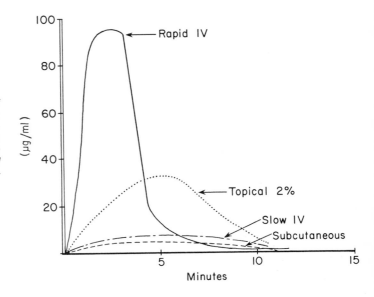

sympathomimetics with vasopressor effects should not be given by this route.

In cooperative patients, the injection is given under topical conjunctival anesthesia. A few drops of a suitable ophthalmic anesthetic (Ophthaine, Ophthetic)[1] are instilled into the conjunctival sac. After 2–3 minutes the application is repeated and the injection is given. Up to 1 ml can be given in separate sites beneath the bulbar conjunctiva, but most injections do not exceed 0.5 ml. The solution is injected through a 25–26-gauge needle with a 1-ml (tuberculin or insulin) syringe (Fig. 3–6), as close as possible to the lesion being treated. The needle is rotated on withdrawal in order to limit leakage through the needle tract. Slight hemorrhage into the injection site occasionally occurs, but this resorbs within 7–10 days. In horses and cattle, tranquilization prior to injection (e.g., xylazine [Rompun] intravenously) is often useful. Hand-held lid retractors are also helpful in all species (Fig. 3–7). Subconjunctival injection results in high drug concentrations in adjacent tissues.

Supplies for Subconjunctival Injection

1-ml syringe (tuberculin or insulin)
25–26-gauge needle
topical anesthetic
injection solution
cotton ball

In addition, for horses and cattle: tranquilizer[2] (e.g., xylazine), hand-held lid retractors, and restraint apparatus—twitch (horses), nose grips (cattle).

---

1. Ophthaine—ER Squibb and Sons, Princeton, NJ; Ophthetic—Allergan Pharmaceuticals, Irvine, CA.

2. Local anesthesia of the palpebral nerve is sometimes used to block motor innervation of the orbicularis oculi. This procedure does not affect pain perception, and topical anesthesia must be used in addition.

Retrobulbar Injection

Local anesthetic may be injected into the muscle cone behind the globe for removal of the bovine eye. Antibiotics are sometimes injected by this route for intraocular infections, retrobulbar cellulitis, or abscesses (note that the sclera does not form a differential barrier to drug penetration as does the cornea). Corticosteroids, usually of the repository kind, are sometimes given by retrobulbar injection. In general, this route of administration is infrequently used except for treatment of disease processes in the orbit or posterior half of the globe.

Intravenous Injection and Infusion

Antibiotics are occasionally given by continuous intravenous (IV) infusion to obtain prolonged high intraocular drug concentrations in severe infections. Unless IV therapy is being used concurrently for another reason, it is more convenient and as effective to give the same total amount of drug by "pulsed" IV injection (Fig. 3–8).

In horses, chloramphenicol must be given frequently (every 3–4 hours) intravenously in order to maintain minimal inhibitory concentrations in plasma. It is unlikely that high intraocular concentrations would be present in the absence of high plasma concentrations. Osmotic agents for reduction of intraocular pressure (IOP) and vitreous volume (e.g., mannitol 20%, urea 30%) are usually given by slow IV infusion.

Oral and Intramuscular Administration

Because continuous treatment is necessary for many ocular disorders, oral drug administration by owners is frequently used. Continuous intramuscular (IM) administration is used less often. Intraocular drug concentra-

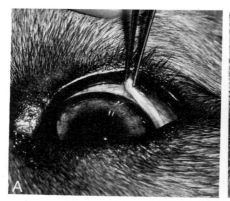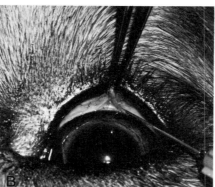

FIGURE 3–6. Subconjunctival injection. A, The mobile conjunctiva is held with fine forceps. B, The needle is inserted, and the solution is injected.

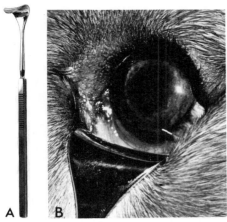

FIGURE 3–7. *Hand-held lid retractor. A, Retractor. B, Retractor in use.*

tions attainable by these routes depend on two important factors:

1. Absorption of the drug from the injection site or gastrointestinal tract, and the plasma concentrations reached.

2. Properties of the drug with respect to the blood-aqueous barrier (in inflamed eyes this barrier is usually much less effective).

Although penicillin is readily absorbed by IM injection, penicillin G is poorly absorbed orally because the low gastric pH destroys it. Also, even when adequate plasma levels are reached, penicillin G penetrates the blood-aqueous barrier poorly. Chloramphenicol is well absorbed by dogs after oral administration (Fig. 3–9), but plasma concentrations after IM injection vary with the preparation used. Chloramphenicol passes the blood-aqueous barrier well. From these examples it follows that the clinician must understand the properties of the individual drugs used in order to predict their applicability for ophthalmic use.

Continuous or Intermittent Lavage

In horses placement of a lavage tube up the nasolacrimal duct, or insertion through the skin of the upper lid into the dorsal conjunctival fornix, allows medications to be conveniently placed into the conjunctival sac (Fig. 3–10). The tube leads back to the shoulder, where it is secured. Drugs are injected into the tube and forced to the eye with a bolus of air from a syringe. Alternatively, by connecting the tube to a gravity-fed bottle or small mechanical infusion pump, a continuous lavage of drug-containing solution may be maintained for 2–3 weeks in valuable animals. Cross tying and supervision may be necessary. This method of therapy

FIGURE 3–8. *Chloramphenicol concentrations in serum and aqueous following continuous IV infusion of 500 mg/kg in rabbits (solid lines) or following administration of the same total amount of chloramphenicol as a 1-minute IV injection (dashed lines). (From Havener WH: Ocular Pharmacology, 7th ed. CV Mosby Co, St Louis, 1987. Modified from Goldman J, et al: Ampicillin, erythromycin and chloramphenicol penetration into rabbit aqueous humor. Ann Ophthalmol 5:147, 1973.)*

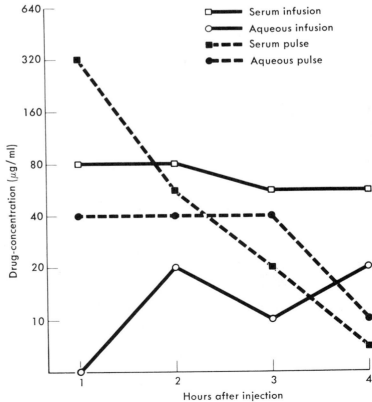

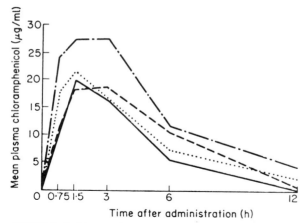

FIGURE 3–9. *Mean plasma chloramphenicol concentrations in three groups of dogs after oral administration of 50 mg/kg in capsule form.* Dashed line, *Greyhounds (mean weight 26.8 kg).* Dotted line, *Same greyhounds after 400 g meal.* Solid line, *Large mongrel dogs (mean weight 24.4 kg).* Dot-and-dash line, *Small mongrel dogs (mean weight 14.1 kg). (From Watson ADJ: Chloramphenicol in the dog: Observations of plasma levels following oral administration. Res Vet Sci 16:147, 1974.)*

is most useful in horses with severe corneal, conjunctival, or uveal disease. High drug concentrations are maintained in the conjunctiva and cornea, and in the anterior chamber if the corneal epithelium is damaged.

Miscellaneous Routes

1. Intra-arterial perfusion. In the dog, a catheter may be passed retrograde up the infraorbital artery into the orbit, and drugs can be injected in high concentration into the external ophthalmic artery and its branches (Fig. 1–12). This method is applicable to radiopaque contrast agents and antimitotic drugs when high concentrations of the drug in tissues other than the target are undesirable.

2. Iontophoresis. The penetration of aqueous solutions of ionized drugs through the cornea may be greatly enhanced by the application of a potential difference (direct current) across the cornea. The technique is rarely used in veterinary ophthalmology.

AUTONOMIC DRUGS

Many of the most important diagnostic and therapeutic drugs used in ophthalmology act on ocular structures with autonomic innervation. The autonomic nervous system is divided into two systems with antagonistic but not necessarily equal actions. Important features of the PARASYMPATHETIC and SYMPATHETIC INNERVATION of the eye, and the sites of action of commonly used drugs, are summarized in Figures 3–

11 and 3–12. In both systems the neurohumoral transmitter at the ganglion is ACETYLCHOLINE, which passes across the synaptic cleft and depolarizes the postsynaptic membrane. This action of acetylcholine is terminated through its cleavage by ACETYLCHOLINESTERASE. In the parasympathetic system the postganglionic transmitter is again ACETYLCHOLINE, but in the sympathetic system it is NOREPINEPHRINE. Norepinephrine also causes depolarization of the muscle cell, but it is not dissipated as simply as acetylcholine in the parasympathetic system. After release by the postganglionic sympathetic terminal, norepinephrine may enter the effector cell, diffuse into the vascular system, undergo enzymatic degradation, or be reabsorbed by the postganglionic terminal (Fig. 3–13). Effector cells that are deprived of transmitter substance become very sensitive to the effects of that transmitter if it is applied after a period of absence. This phenomenon is called DENERVATION HYPERSENSITIVITY and is seen clinically in Horner's syndrome (see p 453).

Drugs may interfere with the passage of a nerve impulse in a number of ways (see Figs. 3–11 and 3–12). The pupillary effects of the autonomic agents commonly used in animals (MYDRIASIS—dilation of the pupil; MIOSIS—constriction of the pupil; CYCLOPLEGIA—relaxation of the ciliary muscle) are tabulated

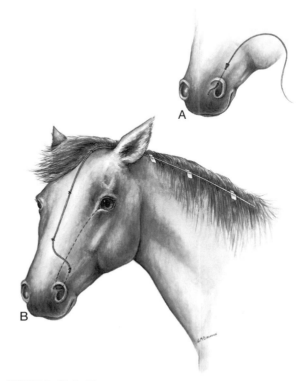

FIGURE 3–10. A, *Placement of the tube (8 French) through the nostril via a large-bore needle under local anesthesia.* B, *Final position of the tube in the nasolacrimal duct, with the opposite end fastened to the skin and mane with sutures and adhesive tape.*

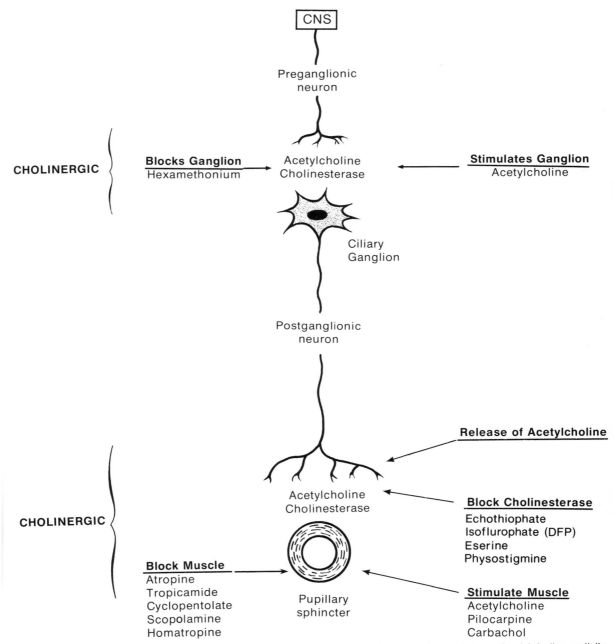

FIGURE 3–11. *Parasympathetic innervation of the eye and sites of action of commonly used drugs. Acetylcholine activity is limited by endogenous acetylcholinesterase.*

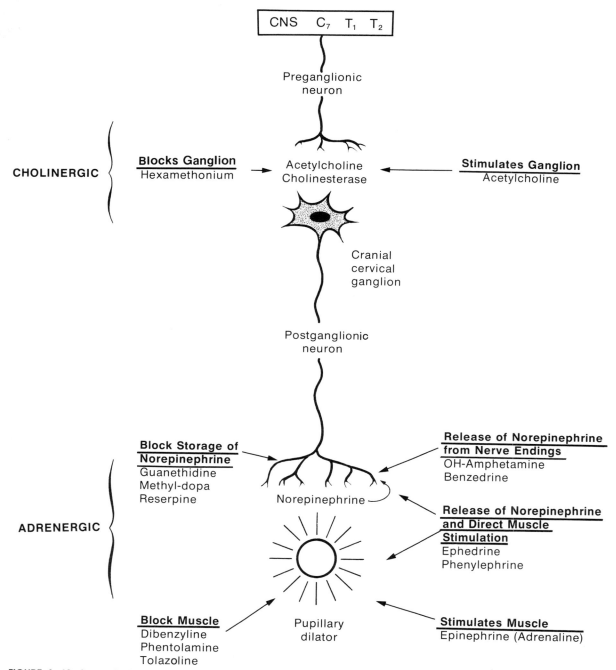

FIGURE 3–12. *Sympathetic innervation of the eye and sites of action of commonly used drugs. Endogenous amine oxidases limit norepinephrine action at the neuromuscular junction. Endogenous catechol-O-methyltransferase limits norepinephrine action within the muscle cell.*

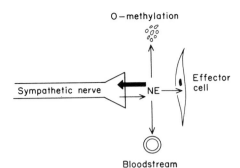

FIGURE 3–13. *Fate of norepinephrine (NE) after release from sympathetic terminal. (Reproduced by permission from Havener, William H.: Ocular Pharmacology, ed. 5, St. Louis, 1983, The C. V. Mosby Co. Modified from Kramer SG, Potts AM: Iris uptake of catecholamines in experimental Horner's syndrome. Am J Ophthalmol 67:705, 1969.)*

in Table 3–1. Note that mydriasis may be caused by paralysis of the sphincter or stimulation of the dilator muscle, whereas miosis may be caused by stimulation of the sphincter or paralysis of the dilator muscle.[3]

Mydriatics and Cycloplegics

PARASYMPATHOLYTIC (ANTICHOLINERGIC) AGENTS

Atropine

Atropine is a parasympatholytic agent used as a mydriatic for examination and preoperative treatment,

---

3. The iris constrictor muscles of some birds are striated, and skeletal muscle relaxants must be used to produce mydriasis because the parasympatholytic agents used in mammals have little or no effect.

TABLE 3–1. Drugs with Autonomic Actions

Adrenergic (Mydriasis and Cycloplegia)	Cholinergic (Miosis)
A. Sympathomimetic (mydriasis)	A. Sympatholytic (miosis)
1. Direct acting	a. Guanethidine
a. Epinephrine	b. Betaxolol
b. Phenylephrine	c. Levobunolol
2. Indirect acting	d. Timolol
a. Hydroxyamphetamine	B. Parasympathomimetic
b. Cocaine	1. Direct acting
c. Ephedrine	a. Acetylcholine
B. Parasympatholytic	b. Carbachol
(cycloplegia)	c. Pilocarpine
a. Atropine	d. Methacholine
b. Homatropine	2. Indirect acting
c. Scopolamine	a. Reversible
d. Tropicamide	i. Eserine
e. Oxyphenonium	ii. Carbachol
	iii. Edrophonium
	b. Irreversible
	i. Isoflurophate
	ii. Echothiophate
	iii. Demecarium

and as a cycloplegic in the treatment of anterior uveitis, iritis, and cyclitis. Paradoxically, atropine solution placed in the oral cavity or reaching it via the nasolacrimal duct acts as a sialagogue (promoter of salivary secretion) because of its bitter taste. This effect, often used to test the patency of a translocated parotid duct, is more noticeable with solution than with ointment and may be especially troublesome in cats. Atropine is infrequently used as a mydriatic for examination because its action may last 24 hours or more (up to 5 days in some dogs and several weeks in horses), and short-acting agents are preferable. Atropine may induce glaucoma in susceptible breeds of dogs (e.g., basset hound, cocker spaniel). Mydriasis induced by atropine may be enhanced by the addition of other belladonna alkaloids (e.g., scopolamine 0.3% drops) or sympathomimetic agents (e.g., phenylephrine 10%).

Note also

1. The cycloplegic effect of atropine relieves the painful spasm of the ciliary muscle caused by anterior uveitis.

2. Sympathomimetic agents do not enhance cycloplegia caused by atropine.

3. Preoperative systemic administration of atropine does not result in increased IOP in glaucomatous eyes controlled with powerful miotics.

4. In rabbits and chickens, the presence of ATROPINE ESTERASE in serum limits the duration of effect and efficacy of atropine.

5. The parasympatholytic properties of atropine decrease tear flow after conjunctival instillation.

6. Atropine (1%) drops and ointment are usually administered therapeutically 2 or 3 times daily. In equine uveitis, more concentrated solutions (4–5%) may be used.

Atropine is *contraindicated* for diagnostic mydriasis in breeds susceptible to glaucoma and in animals affected with lens luxation, glaucoma, and keratoconjunctivitis sicca.

Tropicamide[4]

Tropicamide is a fast-acting parasympatholytic drug of short duration used to induce mydriasis for intraocular examination. When 1% tropicamide is instilled into the conjunctival sac, mydriasis results after 15–20 minutes (or slightly longer in animals with highly pigmented irides). In animals with cataract, lack of mydriasis 20 minutes after one drop of 1% tropicamide indicates MILD UVEITIS may be present. Onset in normal eyes may be hastened by a second drop 5 minutes after the first. Mydriasis and cycloplegia last approximately 2–3 hours (12–18 hours in some dogs and cats), although the drug is insufficiently potent for therapeutic use. There is no evidence that animals dilated with tropicamide suffer retinal damage from

---

4. Mydriacyl—Alcon Laboratories, Fort Worth, TX.

ambient light levels under normal clinical circumstances.

Miscellaneous Anticholinergic Agents

Other parasympatholytic agents are used in selected circumstances:

1. HOMATROPINE (0.5–2%) causes mydriasis and cycloplegia intermediate in duration between atropine and tropicamide, and it is used to dilate the pupil and improve vision when opacities (e.g., nuclear cataract) are present on the visual axis.

2. SCOPOLAMINE (0.3–0.5%) is used before intraocular surgery.

3. *Note:* CYCLOPENTOLATE (Cyclogyl) is a commonly used human diagnostic mydriatic; it is rarely used in animals because its effects last up to 3 days, and it may cause pain and chemosis when administered topically.

SYMPATHOMIMETIC AGENTS

Epinephrine (Adrenalin)

Epinephrine is a sympathomimetic used for vasoconstriction, diagnosis of sympathetic denervation in Horner's syndrome, and mydriasis (without cycloplegia). Epinephrine stimulates contraction of vascular smooth muscle, resulting in vasoconstriction. This effect is used to control conjunctival and scleral hemorrhage by topical application (1:1000) and to retard absorption of drugs (e.g., penicillin, lidocaine) injected with it. It is occasionally used during intraocular surgery (1:10,000) to control hemorrhage, although the danger of causing ventricular fibrillation when halothane is used is significant (the risk is less with methoxyflurane).

Epinephrine stimulates contraction of the pupillary dilator muscle, but it is rarely used alone as a mydriatic, as it penetrates the eye poorly and is quickly destroyed inside the eye. In Horner's syndrome, sympathetic innervation of the eye is interrupted, and denervated structures show DENERVATION HYPERSENSITIVITY. Instillation of a dilute solution of epinephrine into the conjunctival sac results in faster mydriasis than the normal contralateral eye. This phenomenon is occasionally used to help determine the site of interruption in sympathetic supply (see Chap. 17).

Epinephrine decreases aqueous production, and it is used with pilocarpine in the treatment of human glaucoma, but its efficacy for glaucoma in domestic animals is limited. Because of differing vasoconstrictive effects on superficial and deep conjunctival vessels, topical epinephrine may be used to distinguish anterior uveitis from conjunctivitis and in differential diagnosis of protrusion of the third eyelid (haw) in cats, as it is thought to stimulate sympathetic muscles controlling this membrane. Discolored epinephrine solutions should be discarded.

Phenylephrine (Neo-Synephrine)

Phenylephrine is a sympathomimetic agent similar in action to epinephrine. It is used for vasoconstriction (0.125% drops) in differential diagnosis (as for epinephrine) and in the treatment of minor allergic and inflammatory conjunctival disorders. Phenylephrine (10%) is a mydriatic, usually combined with a parasympatholytic agent such as atropine or scopolamine. It is useful as a mydriatic in dogs susceptible to glaucoma, as its action may be reversed with miotics (e.g., pilocarpine 4%, echothiophate 0.25% [Phospholine Iodide], demecarium bromide 0.25% [Humorsol], isoflurophate [diisopropyl flurophosphate—DFP, Floropryl]) if mydriasis results in increased IOP (tropicamide may be similarly reversed). In dogs, phenylephrine causes mydriasis within 1 hour that lasts up to 24 hours. Its effect is additive to other parasympatholytic drugs, but it stings on topical application.

Miotics

All the topical miotics used clinically are parasympathomimetic or sympatholytic agents (see Table 3–1). Miotics are used to treat glaucoma and less frequently to reverse mydriasis after examination. In addition to miosis, miotics may cause painful ciliary spasm in normal patients and those with cyclitis. Careful differential diagnosis will prevent this usage.

DIRECT-ACTING MIOTICS

Pilocarpine

Pilocarpine acts directly on the cells of the pupillary sphincter and is effective even in the denervated eye or after retrobulbar anesthesia when release of acetylcholine at the neuromuscular junction is blocked. Pilocarpine stimulates secretory glands and is used topically and systemically in keratoconjunctivitis sicca. Overdosage, either topical or systemic, may result in salivation, vomiting, and diarrhea, especially in cats. Pilocarpine penetrates the eye after topical instillation (in concentrations ranging from 0.5 to 6.0%); intraocular concentrations depend on frequency of application and concentration of the drops.

In addition to miosis, secretion, and ciliary spasm, pilocarpine and other miotics result in an increased facility of outflow (see p 17) of aqueous in glaucomatous and normal eyes. This effect may be due to stimulation of portions of the ciliary muscle that insert in the area of the iridocorneal angle, resulting in increased drainage via the trabecular meshwork. Contraction of the ciliary muscle may result in larger trabecular spaces through which fluid may exit.

For acute glaucoma, or prophylaxis, 1% and 2% solutions are most frequently used. Use of greater than 2% solution does not enhance reduction of IOP in dogs and increases irritation on instillation. Pilocarpine is less suitable than irreversible indirect-acting miotics for the prolonged prophylaxis of glaucoma in dogs, as it requires more frequent administration (3 or 4 times daily) and may result in pain on application. Therapeutic agents for long-term use must not be painful in order to prevent patient and, ultimately, owner resentment and noncompliance. The relative efficacy of 4% pilocarpine gel has not been determined in dogs.

Acetylcholine

Acetylcholine is destroyed by cholinesterase after topical application and before penetration. It can be used to induce miosis during intraocular surgery, but its action is short-lived.

Carbachol

Carbachol is both a direct- and indirect- (cholinesterase-inhibiting) acting miotic. It has longer action than pilocarpine, requiring administration 2–3 times daily, and frequently causes systemic side effects in dogs. Despite being a more powerful miotic than pilocarpine, carbachol (3%) is less useful in the treatment of glaucoma than are the irreversible cholinesterase inhibitors. Carbachol causes modest decreases in IOP in beagles with inherited open-angle glaucoma.

INDIRECT-ACTING MIOTICS

The indirect-acting miotics are organophosphates, and they are REVERSIBLE and IRREVERSIBLE in nature. They act by inhibition of cholinesterase, causing preservation of acetylcholine, and hence have no effect on denervated structures. Combinations of direct- and indirect-acting miotics do not result in more profound or prolonged miosis, and with some combinations competitive inhibition occurs. The reversible inhibitors (physostigmine [eserine], carbachol, and edrophonium [Tensilon]) are rarely used in the control of glaucoma, because the irreversible agents (echothiophate, isoflurophate, and demecarium) are more effective and require less frequent administration. All drugs of this group may cause severe and even fatal systemic toxicity through incorrect or excessive topical treatment, especially in cats. Signs of systemic toxicity include vomiting, diarrhea, anorexia, and weakness.

Echothiophate (Phospholine Iodide)

Echothiophate is a potent miotic available in a range of concentrations (0.03%, 0.06%, 0.12%, and 0.25%); it requires once or at most twice daily use, penetrates the eye well, and is one of the more effective agents in the medical prophylaxis of canine glaucoma. It has a shelf life of about 2 months after dispensing.

Demecarium (Humorsol)

Demecarium (0.125% and 0.25%) has properties similar to those of echothiophate and isoflurophate. It is indefinitely stable in aqueous solution and is the most toxic of the group. It is usually administered once or twice daily. If treatment with any of the irreversible agents fails, the use of another member of the group is rarely useful. In dogs, demecarium causes ocular irritation more frequently than does echothiophate or isoflurophate.

Isoflurophate (DFP, Floropryl)

The properties and uses of isoflurophate are similar to echothiophate. It is unstable in aqueous solution and is available as an ointment only (0.025%).

The irreversible cholinesterase inhibitors (echothiophate, isoflurophate, and demecarium) are among the most important drugs used in the medical therapy of glaucoma. They are toxic when absorbed systemically, and particular care must be taken to avoid additive effects of these drugs with other organophosphates in fleas collars, washes, and systemic parasitacides.

Sympatholytic Agents

Timolol (Timoptic) and betaxolol (Betoptic) are topical sympatholytic agents used for human glaucoma. They have limited use in glaucoma in dogs and cats, except for ocular hypertension that may be susceptible to medical control. The author's clinical experience indicates that they reduce IOP marginally, if at all. Even in this instance, their efficacy is unproved. Care must be taken in administering these agents to animals with cardiac or respiratory disease.

ANTIBIOTICS

Antibiotics are substances produced by microorganisms that inhibit or destroy other microorganisms. They act by altering cell wall synthesis, protein synthesis, or cell wall permeability in bacteria, but they may also have undesirable effects on the cells of the patient. Antibiotics may be classified as BACTERICIDAL (destroying bacteria) or BACTERISTATIC (inhibiting bacterial growth and reproduction) (Table 3–2). Some antibiotics

TABLE 3–2. Classification of Antibiotics

Bactericidal	Bacteriostatic
Penicillins	Chloramphenicol
Aminoglycosides	Cephalosporins
Polymyxins	Tetracyclines
Bacitracin	Sulfonamides
Vancomycin	

may act in either manner, depending on concentration. Preparations containing both bactericidal and bacteristatic antibiotics are rarely used because antagonism between the agents may result. Combinations of bactericidal drugs (e.g., penicillin with streptomycin) may be synergistic, especially for relatively insensitive organisms, but fixed-dose systemic combinations are not used because of differing properties of the drugs. Combinations of bacteristatic drugs tend to have additive effects, although in some cases the constituents do not influence each other. Bacteristatic combinations are rarely used in ophthalmology.

For resistant infections, combinations of agents with differing mechanisms are sometimes used, e.g., penicillin or a cephalosporin (cell wall synthesis) with an aminoglycoside (intracellular protein synthesis). Combinations of bacteristatic and bactericidal agents and combinations of bacteristatic antibiotics have little justification.

Selection and Administration of Antibiotics[5]

Several factors must be considered in selecting an antibiotic:

1. The offending organism and its sensitivity
2. Location of the organism
3. Penetration, pharmacologic, pharmaceutical, and toxic properties of available antibiotics
4. Spectrum of activity of available drugs

The ideal basis for selection of an ocular antibiotic is an identification of the responsible organism and its antibiotic sensitivity. Often, however, obtaining this information cannot be justified either because of expense or because treatment must be instituted before the results are available. Therefore, a knowledge of the most likely organisms, their sensitivity, and the most likely effective antibiotics is necessary. Treating infections on such an empirical basis, although practical and often unavoidable, does not always lead to a satisfactory result. The use of a Gram-stained smear of either a conjunctival scraping or intraocular material is recommended in severe infections; it is immediately available, and on the basis of staining and morphological characteristics of the organism, a more rational choice of therapeutic agent can be made.

Frequently, simple extraocular infections respond rapidly to treatment. In severe infections or those refractory to initial empirical treatment based on a Gram-stained specimen, culture and sensitivity tests are required. Organisms commonly isolated from the conjunctival sacs of normal and diseased animals, their Gram-staining characteristics, and the antibiotics of choice are given in Tables 3–3 through 3–9.

Samuelson and associates (1984) found fungi common in the conjunctival sac of normal animals in Florida—horses (95%), cows (100%), dogs (22%), and cats (40%). *Aspergillus* spp were also commonly isolated—horses, 56%; cows, 12%; cats, 8%; and dogs, 0%. *Penicillium* spp and *Cladosporium* spp were ubiquitous.

Significant features:

1. The normal conjunctival sac often contains potential pathogens.

2. Geographical differences occur in the organisms present.

3. Because of the variety of organisms present, empirical treatment with standard antibiotics may be unsuccessful.

TABLE 3–3. Normal Flora of the Canine Conjunctival Sac

Area and Flora	Percentage of Cases with Positive Cultures
Western United States*	
Diphtheroids	75.0
Staphylococcus epidermidis	46.0
Staphylococcus aureus	24.0
Bacillus spp	12.0
Gram-negative organisms (*Mima* {*Acinetobacter*} spp, *Neisseria* spp, *Moraxella* spp, *Pseudomonas* spp)	7.0
Streptococcus spp (α-hemolytic)	4.0
Streptococcus spp (β-hemolytic)	2.0
Midwestern United States†	
Staphylococcus epidermidis	55.0
Staphylococcus aureus	45.0
Streptococcus spp (α-hemolytic)	34.0
Diphtheroids	30.0
Neisseria spp	26.0
Pseudomonas spp	14.0
Streptococcus spp (β-hemolytic)	7.3
Eastern Australia‡	
Staphylococcus aureus	39.0
Bacillus spp	29.0
Corynebacterium spp	19.0
Staphylococcus epidermidis	16.0
Yeasts	5.0
Streptococcus spp (α-hemolytic)	3.0
Streptococcus spp (nonhemolytic)	3.0
Micrococcus spp	3.0
Neisseria spp	2.0
Streptococcus spp (β-hemolytic)	1.0
Pseudomonas sp	1.0
Nocardia sp	1.0
Escherichia coli	1.0
Clostridium sp	1.0
Enterobacter sp	1.0
Flavobacterium sp	1.0
Branhamella catarrhalis	1.0

*Data from Bistner SI, et al: Conjunctival bacteria: Clinical appearances can be deceiving. Mod Vet Pract 50:45.
†Data from Urban W, et al: Conjunctival flora of clinically normal dogs. Am J Vet Med Assoc 161:201, 1972.
‡Data from McDonald PJ, Watson ADJ: Microbial flora of normal canine conjunctivae. J Sm Anim Pract 17:809, 1976.

5. Modified from Ellis PP: Handbook of Ocular Therapeutics and Pharmacology, 7th ed. CV Mosby Co, St Louis, 1985.

TABLE 3–4. Flora From Dogs with External Ocular Disease

Area and Flora	Percentage of Cases with Positive Cultures
*The Netherlands**	
Streptococcus canis	20.3
No growth	18.7
Staphylococcus epidermidis	14.0
Staphylococcus aureus	7.8
Other nonpathogenic *Streptococcus* sp	7.8
Nocardia sp	7.8
Absidia ramosa (fungus)	7.8
Pseudomonas aeruginosa	6.1
Corynebacterium sp.	4.6
Other pathogenic *Streptococcus canis* sp—3.1; *Proteus vulgaris*—3.1; *Clostridium perfringens*—1.5; *Candida* sp—1.5	
Colorado†	
Staphylococcus aureus	68.0
Staphylococcus epidermidis	27.0
Streptococcus sp (β-hemolytic)	19.0
Streptococcus sp (α-hemolytic)	17.0
Proteus mirabilis	11.0
Escherichia coli	10.0
Bacillus spp	5.0
Corynebacterium spp—3.0; *Pseudomonas aeruginosa*—2.0; *Klebsiella* spp—1.0	
Illinois‡	
Staphylococcus spp	39.4
Coagulase positive	29.0
Staphylococcus intermedius	17.0
Staphylococcus epidermidus	11.0
Streptococcus spp	25.2
β-hemolytic streptococci	17.0
Pseudomonas spp	9.4

*Data from Verwer MAJ, Gunnick JW: The occurrence of bacteria in chronic purulent eye discharge. J Sm Anim Pract 9:33, 1968.
†Data from Murphy JM, et al: Survey of conjunctival flora in dogs with clinical signs of external eye disease. J Am Vet Med Assoc 172:66, 1978.
‡Data from Gerding PA, et al: Pathogenic bacteria and fungi associated with external ocular diseases in dogs: 131 cases (1981–1986). J Am Vet Med Assoc 193:242, 1988.

TABLE 3–6. Flora from Horses with External Ocular Disease (123 Eyes)

Organism	Percentage of Cases with Positive Cultures
Streptococcus spp (total)	43.9
β-hemolytic	26.0
Other hemolytic	17.9
Staphylococcus sp	24.4
Pseudomonas sp	13.8
Bacillus sp	10.6
Enterobacter sp	6.5
Escherichia coli	4.0
Corynebacterium sp	3.2
Proteus sp	3.2
Aspergillus sp—2.4; *Klebsiella* sp—2.4; *Moraxella* sp—2.4; *Pasteurella* sp—2.4; *Mima*—1.6; *Diplococcus* sp—0.8; *Flavobacterium* sp—0.8; *Fusarium* sp—0.8; *Neisseria* sp—0.8; *Nocardia* sp—0.8; *Penicillium* sp—0.8; *Rhizopus* sp—0.8; *Trichosporon* sp—0.8	

Data from McLaughlin SA, et al: Pathogenic bacteria and fungi associated with extraocular disease in the horse. J Am Vet Med Assoc 182:241, 1983.

4. Moore and coworkers (1986 and 1988) found a high proportion (>95%) of isolates from Wisconsin horses were susceptible to neomycin–bacitracin polymixin combinations and chloramphenicol, conflicting with McLaughlin and colleagues' findings from Ohio (1983). Moore and associates' earlier study from Missouri (1983) did not test antibiotic susceptibility for all of the antibiotics in this combination. Natamycin had a high efficacy for filamentous fungi (97% susceptible), and miconazole was highly efficacious (100%) against *Fusarium* spp and *Aspergillus* spp.

5. Care is advisable in interpreting frequency and sensitivity data from different hospitals and geographical areas.

Gram-stained smears or culture and sensitivity tests are necessary for rational treatment of serious or difficult ocular infections. For suspected bacterial ocular infections, the choice of antibiotic is based on known

TABLE 3–5. Normal Flora of the Feline Conjunctival Sac

Area and Flora	Percentage of Cases with Positive Cultures	
	Conjunctiva	*Lids*
*Western United States**		
Staphylococcus epidermidis	16.3	13.3
Staphylococcus aureus	10.4	8.8
Mycoplasma spp	5	—
Bacillus spp	2.9	1.7
Streptococcus spp (α-hemolytic)	2.5	1.7
Corynebacterium spp	1.3	—
Escherichia coli	—	0.4

*Data from Campbell L: Ocular bacteria and mycoplasma of the clinically normal cat. Feline Pract Nov–Dec:10, 1973.

TABLE 3–7. Fungal Flora from Normal Horses (50 Horses)

Organism	Percentage of Cases with Positive Cultures
Aspergillus spp	36.0
Cladosporium spp	34.0
Positive but no quantitative data given; *Alternaria, Fusarium, Monotospira, Paecilomyces, Phoma, Pullularia, Scopulariopsis, Streptomyces, Trichoderma, Verticillium* spp	

Data from Riis RC: Equine ophthalmology. *In* Gelatt KN (ed): Textbook of Veterinary Ophthalmology. Lea & Febiger, Philadelphia, 1981.

TABLE 3–8. Normal Flora of the Bovine
Conjunctival Sac

Area and Flora	Percentage of Cases with Positive Culture
*Northeastern Australia**	
Unidentified gram-positive cocci	54.4
Corynebacterium spp	27.4
Moraxella nonliquefaciens	26.9
Streptococcus faecalis	20.0
No growth	13.4
Neisseria (Branhamella) catarrhalis (nonhemolytic)	10.5
Unidentified gram-negative rods	8.5
Acinetobacter spp	8.0
Moraxella bovis	6.5
Coliforms	6.5
Staphylococcus aureus	4.1
Moraxella liquefaciens	2.2
Bacillus spp	1.3
Unclassified *Moraxella*	1.0
Actinobacillus spp	0.7
Proteus spp	0.0

*Data from Wilcox G: Bacterial flora of the bovine eye with special reference to Moraxella and Neisseria. Aust Vet J 46:253, 1970.

incidence of pathogens in the locality, and their probable sensitivity (Tables 3–10 and 3–11). Cultures may be necessary in a series of cases to gain this information. Most ocular infections can be controlled with the initial drug treatment.

The use of stained smears for bacterial morphology and conjunctival cytology can assist in reaching a presumptive diagnosis. When using Tables 3–10 and 3–11, remember that previously untreated infections often have a different spectrum of sensitivity than those from hospital populations, e.g., untreated *Staphylococcus* spp is often sensitive to penicillin, but it is frequently resistant if isolated from a hospital population or from a previously treated animal. Also, organisms that are resistant in vitro may be susceptible in vivo to the same antibiotic in suitable concentrations and given by an appropriate route.

Routine use of culture-sensitivity tests in simple,

TABLE 3–9. Normal Flora of the Ovine
Conjunctival Sac

Area and Flora	Percentage of Cases with Positive Culture
*Eastern Australia**	
No growth	60
Neisseria ovis	24.0
Micrococcus spp	NQD†
Streptococcus spp	NQD†
Corynebacterium spp	NQD†
Achromobacter spp	NQD†
Bacillus spp	NQD†
Moraxella spp	NQD†

*Data from Spradbrow P: The bacterial flora of the ovine conjunctival sac. Aust Vet J 44:117, 1968.
†NQD—present in small numbers, but no quantitative data given.

TABLE 3–10. Antibiotics of Choice for Common
Organisms

Gram-positive Cocci	Drug of Choice
Staphylococcus spp	Neomycin
	Bacitracin
	Penicillin
	Cephalosporins
	Erythromycin
	Enrofloxacin
Staphylococcus aureus	Gentamicin
	Oxacillin
	Methicillin
	Cephalosporins
	Enrofloxacin
Staphylococcus epidermidis	Neomycin
	Gentamicin
	Erythromycin
	Enrofloxacin
Streptococcus spp	Penicillin
	Chloramphenicol
	Amoxicillin
	Cephalosporins

Gram-negative Cocci	Drug of Choice
Neisseria spp	Penicillin Tetracycline
	Sulfonamides
	(± trimethoprim)

Gram-positive Rods	Drug of Choice
Corynebacterium spp	Penicillin
	Tetracycline
	Sulfonamides
	(± trimethoprim)

Gram-negative Rods	Drug of Choice
Pseudomonas aeruginosa	Polymixin B
	Gentamicin
	Tobramycin
	Amikacin
Escherichia coli	Chloramphenicol
	Tetracyclines
	Gentamicin
Enterobacter spp	Amoxicillin
	(± streptomycin)
Proteus spp	Gentamicin
	Chloramphenicol
	Tobramycin
	Amikacin
Hemophilus spp	Amoxicillin
	Tetracycline
Moraxella spp	Penicillin
	Sulfonamides
	(± trimethoprim)

previously untreated infections may be helpful for scientific purposes, but it is difficult to justify economically. For topical therapy, combinations of bactericidal drugs infrequently used elsewhere in the body are commonly employed. This allows a wider spectrum of activity than with single drugs, and it reduces the chance of drug resistance. The combination of neomycin, polymixin B, and bacitracin (or gramicidin)[6] is

6. Neosporin Ophthalmic Solution or Ointment—Burroughs Wellcome Co, Research Triangle Park, NC, or its generic equivalents.

TABLE 3–11. Chemotherapeutic Agents for Miscellaneous Organisms

Fungi and Yeasts	Drug of Choice
Fursarium spp	Natamycin
	Thiabendazole
Aspergillus spp	Amphotericin B
	Ketaconazole
	Flucytosine
	Nystatin
Candida spp	Nystatin
	Amphotericin B
	Flucytosine
	Ketaconazole
Cryptococcus spp	Ketaconazole
	Flucytosine
Penicillium spp	Natamycin
Blastomyces and	Ketaconazole
Histoplasma spp	Amphotericin B
Microsporon } spp {	Griseofulvin
Trichophyton	Ketaconazole
Epidermophyton	

Actinomycetes	Drug of Choice
Actinomyces spp	Penicillin
	Tetracycline
Nocardia spp	Chloramphenicol
	(± streptomycin)
	(± isoniazid)

Chlamydia	Drug of Choice
Chlamydia spp	Chloramphenicol
	Tetracyclines
	Sulfonamides

Mycoplasma	Drug of Choice
Mycoplasma spp	Tetracyclines
	Erythromycin
	Chloramphenicol

TABLE 3–12. Steps in the Treatment of Ocular Infections

Diagnostic Level	Therapy
Initial Presentation	
No diagnosis	Neosporin or similar drops every 4–6 hours
Presumptive diagnosis	Specific antibiotic therapy (see Table 3–9)
Diagnosis based on clinical impression or smear	Topical and periocular treatment for local disease Topical, periocular, and systemic treatment if infection is generalized
Bacteriological Diagnosis (Severe or Recurrent Infections)	
No sensitivity available	Use of optimal drug (see Table 3–11)
Sensitivity available	Antibiotic indicated by sensitivity
Clinical Improvement	
Culture positive	Continue use of current treatment if appropriate
Culture negative	Repeat culture; consider diagnostic and culturing techniques for *Mycoplasma, Chlamydia*, and fungi
Culture negative twice	Discontinue treatment

thus useful. In more severe infections (e.g., corneal ulceration or endophthalmitis), the organism should be identified, and a combination of routes of administration, such as topical and subconjunctival injection and systemic administration, are appropriate (Table 3–12). The important properties of the common antibiotics are considered below.

If ocular infection persists despite treatment with the appropriate antibiotic (Table 3–13), the infection may be secondary to an underlying disorder or pathological process.

Penicillin

Penicillin refers to a number of natural and synthetic derivatives of 6-aminopenicillanic acid that vary considerably in stability, solubility, spectrum of activity, ocular penetration, and resistance to beta lactamase.

Sodium and Potassium Penicillin G (Crystalline Penicillin)

Penicillin G is soluble in water, attains high levels in blood, and is excreted in urine in 4–6 hours. It is

suitable for IM, IV, or subconjunctival use; it does not penetrate the intact cornea when applied topically, because of its water solubility. It can be used by nasolacrimal lavage for ulcerative corneal lesions. Penicillin G is most effective against gram-positive organisms, but it is susceptible to beta lactamase. It does

TABLE 3–13. Dose Rates for Subconjunctival Antibiotics

Drug	Dose
Amikacin	75–100 mg
Amphotericin B	2–3 mg
Ampicillin	40–50 mg
Amoxicillin	40–50 mg
Bacitracin	10,000 units
Carbenicillin	100 mg
Cefazolin	50–100 mg
Cephaloridine	50–100 mg
Cephalothin	50–100 mg
Chloramphenicol	40–50 mg
Colistin	15–20 mg
Erythromycin	10–20 mg
Gentamicin	10–20 mg
Kanamycin	10–20 mg
Lincomycin	300 mg
Methicillin	50–100 mg
Miconazole	5 mg daily
Neomycin	100–500 mg
Nystatin	10,000 units
Oxacillin	50–100 mg
Penicillin G'	500,000 units
Polymixin B	5 mg
Streptomycin	40–50 mg
Tobramycin	20–30 mg
Vancomycin	15–25 mg

Reproduced (modified) by permission from Ellis PP: Handbook of Ocular Therapeutics and Pharmacology, 7th ed. St Louis, 1985, The C. V. Mosby Co.

not pass the intact blood-aqueous barrier. Instability at low pH precludes oral administration.

Procaine Penicillin G

This preparation is slowly absorbed after IM injection and maintains blood levels for up to 24 hours. It is unsuitable for IV injection or application to denuded tissue. It is often injected intramuscularly with crystalline penicillin, giving early and prolonged high blood levels.

Benzathine Penicillin G

This preparation, like procaine penicillin G, is irritating when injected intravenously. It is released as penicillin G for 4–5 days after IM injection, although blood levels reached during the first few days are below therapeutic levels. It is usually injected intramuscularly with procaine penicillin and crystalline penicillin, giving immediate and prolonged therapeutic levels. Subconjunctival injections are sometimes used in diseases in which frequent applications of medication are inconvenient (e.g., infectious bovine keratoconjunctivitis). The spectrum of activity and ocular penetration are the same for all types of penicillin G.

Phenoxymethyl and Phenoxyethyl Penicillin

Both of these compounds are more acid-stable than penicillin G is, and are used orally. They, like penicillin G, are most effective against gram-positive cocci, are less effective against gram-negative bacteria, and are susceptible to beta lactamase.

Sodium Methicillin

Methicillin is resistant to beta lactamase and is used by IV infusion for resistant staphylococci. Renal excretion is rapid. Because the drug is unstable in solution, it should be dissolved just before use. Methicillin can be used by nasolacrimal lavage or by subconjunctival injection for corneal infections. Methicillin may be expected to enter the aqueous in therapeutic concentrations when the blood-aqueous barrier is disrupted by inflammation.

Sodium Oxacillin

Oxacillin is resistant to beta lactamase; it is also acid-stable and may be used orally. Unfortunately, much of it is bound to plasma protein in the circulation and cannot enter the aqueous, even in an inflamed eye. It is useful in orbital and adnexal infections when given orally.

Ampicillin and Amoxicillin

Ampicillin is a broad-spectrum penicillin that is often effective against *Escherichia coli* and *Proteus* spp. It penetrates the aqueous, and it may be given orally, intramuscularly, or subconjunctivally. Ampicillin is not the agent of first choice for gram-negative infections because the necessary higher inhibitory concentrations are not always reached in the aqueous. Amoxicillin has a spectrum of activity similar to ampicillin (the manufacturer recommends the same sensitivity test discs), and it is better absorbed from the gastrointestinal tract than ampicillin is. Both ampicillin and amoxicillin are susceptible to beta lactamase. Amoxicillin results in blood levels two to three times higher than ampicillin after oral administration, but both drugs enter the noninflamed eye to about the same degree.

Clavulanic acid (Clavamox) is added to preparations of amoxicillin, because it inhibits beta lactamases specifically. This preparation is frequently useful in the initial treatment of chronic canine staphylococcal blepharitis.

SYSTEMIC DOSAGE OF PENICILLINS

Penicillins are useful for infections of the orbit and lids, and in intraocular infections if the blood-aqueous barrier is reduced by inflammation. In clinical situations, many staphylococci do not produce penicillinase. Diseases (e.g., blepharitis) caused by susceptible bacteria often respond dramatically to penicillin. Systemic dose rates are shown in Table 3–14.

Despite poor intraocular penetration, penicillin is useful for

1. Infections of the lids and orbit
2. Infections of the anterior segment (conjunctiva, cornea, iris), administered by subconjunctival injection
3. After intraocular surgery or injury, by subconjunctival injection of 1 million units of penicillin G, 0.1 ml of 1:1000 epinephrine, and 10 mg of streptomycin followed by systemic therapy (Fig. 3–14)
4. Surface infections of the conjunctiva and cornea, when included in lavage solutions, or by subconjunctival injection
5. Specific infections with susceptible organisms for which efficacy has been previously proved; e.g., combinations of penicillin G by subconjunctival injection in infectious bovine keratoconjunctivitis (see Chap 11).

Chloramphenicol

Chloramphenicol is a broad-spectrum bacteristatic antibiotic, effective against a wide range of gram-positive and gram-negative organisms, Rickettsia, spirochetes, and chlamydia. *Pseudomonas aeruginosa* is often resistant. Because of its lipid solubility, chloramphenicol passes the blood-aqueous, blood-brain and corneal barriers better than most water-soluble antibiotics.

TABLE 3–14. Systemic Penicillin Dosages

Drug	Route*	Dose Rate	Frequency
Penicillin G	PO	40,000 units/kg	every 6 hours
	IV, IM, SC	20,000 units/kg	every 4 hours
Procaine penicillin	IM, SC	20,000 units/kg	every 12–24 hours
Benzathine penicillin	IM	40,000 units/kg	every 5 days
Amoxicillin	PO	25 mg/kg	every 12 hours
Clavamox	PO	15 mg/kg	every 12 hours
Ampicillin	PO	10–20 mg/kg	every 6 hours
	IV, IM, SC	5–10 mg/kg	every 6 hours
Phenoxymethyl penicillin	PO	10 mg/kg	every 8 hours
Phenoxyethyl penicillin	PO	10 mg/kg	every 8 hours
Methicillin	IV, IM	20 mg/kg	every 6 hours
Oxacillin	PO	15–25 mg/kg	every 8 hours
Cloxacillin	PO, IV, IM	10 mg/kg	every 6 hours

*IM = intramuscular; IV = intravenous; PO = per os (by mouth); SC = subcutaneous.

Chloramphenicol may be administered orally, intramuscularly, subcutaneously, intravenously (50 mg/kg every 8 hours in dogs, every 12 hours in cats), subconjunctivally, or by nasolacrimal lavage. Because absorption after oral administration results in high blood levels, this is the route of choice for infections in the posterior globe and orbit. In horses, IV administration 3–4 times daily may be more convenient.

Bone marrow aplasia and hypoplasia seen in humans after systemic and topical therapy with chloramphenicol are not significant in domestic animals. Despite controversial toxicity studies in cats, the drug has undergone prolonged clinical usage with few ill effects except anorexia and occasional pyrexia in some cats after systemic administration, provided administration is not prolonged. Because of its wide spectrum of activity and intraocular penetration, chloramphenicol (1%) ointment and drops are widely used in veterinary practice for superficial injuries and infections before culture results are available. Polymyxin B is often added to aid in control of *Pseudomonas* spp.

In simple disease processes, it is more suitable to use a broad-spectrum bactericidal mixture mentioned earlier, retaining chloramphenicol for use when intraocular penetration is required. For severe intraocular infections a bactericidal antibiotic is more appropriate. The use of mixtures of any antibiotic in the same preparation with a corticosteroid is not recommended, except in special circumstances, and certainly not as "shotgun therapy" in lieu of a rational clinical diagnosis.

Aminoglycosides (Neomycin, Streptomycin, Dihydrostreptomycin, Kanamycin, Framycetin, Gentamicin, Tobramycin, Amikacin)

Neomycin, Framycetin, Kanamycin, and Streptomycin

Neomycin is a particularly useful bactericidal agent for ocular use, and it is active against gram-positive and gram-negative bacteria including *Staphylococcus aureus*. Bacterial resistance develops less readily to neomycin than to streptomycin, and neomycin is more effective against *Proteus vulgaris* than is polymyxin B. Because of nephrotoxicity and ototoxicity, neomycin is administered topically or by subconjunctival injection. Allergic reactions to topical neomycin occasionally develop. Framycetin (neomycin B) has properties similar to neomycin but is more consistently effective against *Pseudomonas* spp and *E. coli*. Kanamycin is similar to

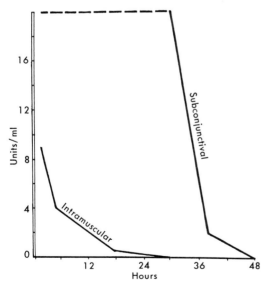

FIGURE 3–14. Penicillin in rabbit aqueous (units/ml) after injection of 1 million units in a 1:1000 solution of epinephrine by subconjunctival and IM routes. (Reproduced by permission from Havener, William H.: Ocular Pharmacology, ed. 5, St. Louis, 1983, The C. V. Mosby Co. Modified from Sorsby A, Ungar J: Distribution of penicillin in eye after injections of 1,000,000 units by subconjunctival, retrobulbar and intramuscular routes. Br J Ophthalmol 32:864, 1948.)

neomycin but is less effective against *Pseudomonas* spp. Because of rapid development of resistance, and ototoxicity, streptomycin is rarely used as an agent of first choice in ocular therapy.

Gentamicin

Gentamicin is effective against many strains of *S. aureus, Pseudomonas* spp, *E. coli, Aerobacter,* and *Klebsiella* spp. *Proteus* spp are frequently susceptible. Topical application does not result in high intraocular concentrations, although subconjunctival and IV injections do penetrate the eye. Long-term systemic therapy is limited by ototoxicity, nephrotoxicity, and cost. Vitreous penetration is poor regardless of route of administration. Gentamicin is mainly useful for infections of the anterior segment with *Pseudomonas* spp and *Staphylococcus* spp. Gentamicin causes cataract and severe retinal degeneration when injected intraocularly.[7] Gentamicin is a valuable drug but should not be used as agent of first choice in routine infections.

Tobramycin

Tobramycin is similar to gentamicin. It is effective against beta lactamase–producing staphylococci and is synergistic with carbenicillin in the treatment of resistant *Pseudomonas* infections. Resistance is less frequent, probably because of its more recent introduction. It is also oto- and nephrotoxic when given systemically. Its use should be restricted to gentamicin-resistant *Pseudomonas* and enterobacterial infections. Tobramicin may be administered topically, by subconjunctival injection, and by nasolacrimal lavage.

Amikacin

Organisms that are resistant to gentamicin, neomycin, and tobramycin are frequently susceptible to amikacin. When other aminoglycosides are effective it has no advantage over them. Amikacin is oto- and nephrotoxic and may be administered topically, by subconjunctival injection, and by nasolacrimal lavage. Its use should be restricted to *Pseudomonas* and other documented gram-negative infections resistant to other aminoglycosides. For *Pseudomonas* infections the order of choice for usage is neomycin, gentamicin, tobramycin, and amikacin.

Bacitracin

Bacitracin is effective against gram-positive organisms and is mainly used topically. It is not inactivated

by inflammatory exudates, and resistance develops rarely. Intraocular penetration after topical application is poor; because of nephrotoxicity, it is not used systemically. Bacitracin is used very frequently in combinations with an agent(s) effective against gram-negative organisms and for surface infections of the lids, conjunctiva, and cornea. It is particularly useful for staphylococcal blepharoconjunctivitis in dogs.

Polymyxin B and Colistin

Polymyxin B and colistin are noteworthy because of their activity against *Pseudomonas*, and they have similar spectra of activity. Both drugs are effective against *E. coli* but not against *Proteus* spp. Neither penetrate intact corneal epithelium significantly, although epithelial defects allow therapeutic concentrations in the stroma. Polymyxin B causes severe chemosis and necrosis after subconjunctival injection, whereas colistin is not irritating by this route.

Pseudomonas may cause infections of the cornea and conjunctiva in dogs, horses, and cats with disastrous effect because of antibiotic resistance and production of collagenase. Polymyxin B, colistin, gentamicin, tobramycin, and amikacin are useful especially when given by frequent topical instillation, or by nasolacrimal lavage in horses, for such infections.

Cephalosporin Derivatives

A range of cephalosporins is available. They are generally similar in mechanism of action and pharmacology to the penicillins but are less susceptible to staphylococcal beta lactamases. Beta lactamases produced by gram-negative organisms may inactivate them. The true place of cephalosporins, if any, in veterinary ophthalmology remains to be determined.

Tetracyclines

Tetracyclines are broad-spectrum bacteristatic antibiotics to which *Staphylococcus, Pseudomonas*, and *Proteus* spp are usually resistant. Ocular penetration is very poor regardless of route of administration. Tetracyclines are useful in the treatment of surface infections with *Chlamydia* and *Mycoplasma* spp. To avoid permanent dental discoloration, tetracyclines must not be administered to young animals with ocular manifestations of systemic diseases, e.g., distemper, infectious tracheobronchitis, *calicivirus* and *herpesvirus felis* infection.

Systemic administration to dogs affected with periocular staining from pigments in the tears results in a decrease in staining while the drug is being administered. This may be due to chemical similarities between tetracyclines and the pigments. Long-acting parenteral tetracycline preparations have been proposed for treatment of *Moraxella bovis* infection in cattle, but convinc-

---

7. All aminoglycosides are toxic to the retina when injected intra-camerally—in order of toxicity from highest to lowest: gentamicin, tobramicin, amikacin, and kanamycin.

ing studies of their significant superiority over existing treatment methods are lacking.

Vancomycin

Vancomycin is rarely used in ophthalmic therapy except for treatment of resistant staphylococcal infections. It may be given topically, subconjunctivally, or intravenously. As ophthalmic solutions are not available, the following may be used: vancomycin, 500 mg sterile water, 10 ml.[8]

Sulfonamides

Sulfonamides are bacteristatic and act by blocking utilization of para-aminobenzoic acid (PABA) by bacteria. All have the same range of therapeutic action and exhibit mutual cross resistance. For any given infection, the appropriate antibiotic is superior to a sulfonamide (Leopold, 1984). Drugs (e.g., procaine, tetracaine) that are esters of PABA, and purulent exudates that contain PABA, interfere with the action of sulfonamides. Sulfonamides have largely been replaced by antibiotics for topical use, but sulfacetamide (10% and 30%) and sulfafurazole (4%) are useful for minor infections. Sulfonamide powders should not be used in the eye. Sulfonamides inhibit many gram-positive and some gram-negative organisms, including *Pseudomonas* sp. The action of gentamicin against *Pseudomonas* sp is inhibited by sulfacetamide.

Because antibiotics are more effective for intraocular infection, systemic sulfonamides are rarely indicated in ophthalmic therapy, with the possible exception of IV treatment of infectious bovine keratoconjunctivitis due to *Moraxella bovis* and treatment of ocular toxoplasmosis. Intravenously administered sulfonamide is excreted in the lacrimal secretions in sufficient quantities to control *Moraxella bovis*, but oral sulfonamides do not reach sufficiently high concentrations in tears for long enough periods to be of therapeutic value. Several sulfonamides are confirmed causes of keratoconjunctivitis sicca in dogs (see Chap 10).

Antibacterials

Antibacterials are substances that inhibit or destroy bacteria but that are not derived from bacteria. The agent with the most potential importance to ophthalmology is enrofloxacin.

Enrofloxacin

Enrofloxacin is a member of the fluorinated 4-quinolones. It is a potent broad-spectrum bactericidal agent,

---

8. Modified from Havener WH: Ocular Pharmacology, 7th ed. CV Mosby Co, St Louis, 1987.

active against the majority of canine bacterial pathogens. It acts by inhibiting DNA gyrase. No plasmids capable of inactivating or preventing quinolone activity are known, reducing the chance of resistance developing.

Enrofloxacin is rapidly absorbed after oral administration, with peak serum concentrations (approximately 1.0 mcg/ml) being reached in 30–60 minutes. Enrofloxacin enters the tears in inhibitory concentrations. It is eliminated by glomerular filtration and biliary secretion. Suggested dosages are 2.5–5.0 mg/kg twice a day per os. Insufficient data are available to recommend its use for intraocular infections, but it appears suitable for staphylococcal infections of the eyelids and orbital area. Enrofloxacin is contraindicated in young dogs of the smaller breeds between 2 and 8 months of age, in large breeds until 12 months, and in giant breeds until 18 months.

Minimal inhibitory concentrations of common organisms are *Staphylococcus* spp—0.125 mcg/ml; *Pseudomonas aeruginosa*—0.5–8.0 mcg/ml; *Escherichia coli*—0.016–0.031 mcg/ml; *Proteus mirabilis*—0.062–0.125 mcg/ml.

ANTIFUNGAL ANTIBIOTICS

Important ophthalmic fungal infections are classified in three groups:

1. Infections of the lids and surrounding skin
2. Intraocular infections (e.g., endophthalmitis associated with systemic infections or penetrating foreign bodies), cryptococcosis, blastomycosis, histoplasmosis, and coccidioidomycosis
3. Mycotic keratitis following corneal injuries by foreign vegetable objects

Group 1 is treated with therapeutic agents for dermatomycosis; groups 2 and 3 are treated with agents discussed briefly here.

Bacterial and viral infections of the cornea are much more common than are fungal infections. Any nonspecific corneal ulcer associated with corneal opacity that does not respond to antibiotic therapy should be scraped, stained, and cultured for possible mycotic involvement, especially in horses. Fungal infections have a much slower onset and course than do bacterial infections, and they may be difficult or impossible to resolve despite therapy. Where antifungal sensitivity tests are available, they should be used, as the agents are usually expensive.

For mycotic keratitis, surgical removal of the infected tissue by superficial keratectomy (see Chap 11) is often as effective as drug therapy and should be combined with it. A 360° conjunctival flap (see Chap 11) may be placed over the lesion for 3–4 weeks during drug treatment. Commonly used antifungal agents are shown in Table 3–11.

Natamycin

Natamycin (pimaricin, Natacyn) is effective against *Candida, Aspergillus, Cephalosporium, Fusarium*, and *Penicillium* spp. Natamycin is available in topical preparations for infections of the lids, conjunctiva, and cornea.

Thiabendazole

Thiabendazole has been documented for the treatment of mycotic keratitis in horses and humans. It is not irritating, penetrates the cornea after topical instillation, and has a broad spectrum of activity. Ophthalmic preparations are not available, but Joyce (1983) used 14.29% TBZ Pig Wormer Paste[9] twice a day in horses for 30 days without sequelae.

Ketaconazole

Ketaconazole (Nizoral) is a member of the imidazole group including clotrimazole, miconazole, and econazole. It is especially useful for the treatment of systemic and ocular *Cryptococcus* spp and *Coccidioides immitis* infection. It is absorbed after oral administration in dogs and cats. In dogs, side effects include inappetence, pruritus, alopecia, and reversible lightening of the hair coat. In cats, anorexia, fever, depression, and diarrhea may occur, and lower doses (50 mg on alternate days) have been used to reduce toxicosis. Long-term therapy, up to 6 months or more, may be necessary, as ketaconazole is fungistatic.

Dosage: dogs—20 mg/kg daily; cats—50 mg daily or 20 mg/kg every 2nd day.

Flucytosine

Flucytosine (Ancobon) has activity against *Cryptococcus, Aspergillus*, and *Candida* spp, and it is useful combined with ketaconazole in the treatment of feline endophthalmitis and meningitis due to *Cryptococcus* spp.

Dosage: Dogs and cats—100 mg/kg every 12 hours orally.

Nystatin

Nystatin is a fungistatic agent used primarily for keratitis and endophthalmitis due to *Candida albicans*. Because of systemic toxicity, it is used topically and subconjunctivally. Ophthalmic preparations are prepared from soluble powder (50,000 units/ml in 1.2% NaCl) and applied every 1–2 hours. Dermatological preparations (e.g., Panalog) containing corticosteroids *must not be used* for treatment of ocular mycotic infections.

Amphotericin B

Amphotericin B may be used topically, subconjunctivally, or systemically. It has a wide range of activity against fungi but is also toxic to host cells. Because of systemic toxicity and the serious nature of lesions for which it is used, amphotericin B should be used only in institutions where complete ophthalmic care and laboratory monitoring are available. Amphotericin is used in the treatment of systemic infections with *Histoplasma, Blastomyces, Cryptococcus*, and *Coccidioides* spp, although treatment with less toxic agents such as ketaconazole should be considered.

In a series of 35 fungal isolates from equine eyes, Moore (1986) found the following susceptibilities—natamycin, 97%; nystatin, 74%; miconazole, 69%; amphotericin, 51%; 5-fluorocytosine, 49%; and ketaconazole, 31%. Such series must be interpreted with caution, as frequency of different organisms shows geographical variation.

ANTIVIRAL DRUGS

The use of antiviral drugs in veterinary ocular therapy is restricted to treatment of keratitis due to *Herpesvirus felis* in cats. Although many viral diseases of domestic animals have secondary ocular manifestations, systemic therapeutic agents are not available.

Idoxuridine

Idoxuridine (IDU) is chemically similar to thymidine, one of the constituents of nucleic acids. IDU replaces thymidine in DNA synthesis and inhibits viral replication. IDU is stored in a refrigerated, dark bottle. Solutions in vehicles other than polyvinyl alcohol are less irritating to feline eyes.

IDU penetrates the eye poorly after topical application, but therapeutic corneal concentrations can be reached with drops every 2 hours or with ointment 5 or 6 times daily. Therapy is continued until the lesion and fluorescein staining disappear. Herpetic keratitis is resistant to cure, and relapses are not uncommon. In susceptible infections, results are often dramatically successful.

IDU is the antiviral of first choice in feline herpetic keratitis because of cost and efficacy. If resistance occurs, particularly in an eye with characteristic lesions, or after immunofluorescent confirmation, trifluridine is the next choice. Vidarabine has the least effect on *herpesvirus felis*, and acyclovir has no effect. None of the agents has activity against feline *calicivirus*.

Trifluorothymidine

Trifluridine (Viroptic) inhibits DNA polymerase and thymidine synthetase and is the most active (and most

---

9. Merck, Sharp & Dohme, Rahway, New Jersey.

expensive) agent for feline *herpesvirus*. Like IDU it is used every 2 hours until re-epithelialization occurs, then every 4 hours for another 7 days. An effect should be seen within 7 days.

Vidarabine

Vidarabine (Vira-A ophthalmic ointment) interferes with viral DNA synthesis, and it is active against feline *herpesvirus*, but less so than trifluorothymidine and IDU. Teratogenic effects have been recorded after topical use in experimental animals.

CORTICOSTEROIDS

Although frequently misused with disastrous results, corticosteroids are among the clinician's most useful and powerful drugs, with specific properties, indications, and contraindications that must be understood.

1. Corticosteroids must not be used topically or subconjunctivally when fluorescein indicates a corneal epithelial defect.

2. Corticosteroids should not be used unless a diagnosis has been made, and a specific immunological or inflammatory response is to be inhibited.

3. Every "red" eye should be stained with fluorescein and have its IOP measured.

4. The cornea should be routinely stained with fluorescein before use of a topical or subconjunctival corticosteroid.

5. Corticosteroids are of no therapeutic value in primary glaucoma.

Properties of Corticosteroids[10]

Corticosteroids decrease cellular and fibrinous exudation and inflammatory tissue infiltration, inhibit degranulation of mast cells with release of inflammatory mediators including prostaglandins, inhibit fibroblastic and collagen-forming activity, retard epithelial and endothelial regeneration and repair, diminish postinflammatory neovascularization, inhibit humoral and cell-mediated immune responses, and tend to restore normal permeability to inflamed capillaries. The degree of response is related to dosage, which must be adjusted to gain the desired effect. Corticosteroids are particularly useful in treating ocular disease when correctly used, because aftereffects of inflammation that would be desirable in other organs and tissues (e.g., fibrous tissue formation and contraction, neovascularization, infiltration with inflammatory cells) may be particularly damaging in the eye if allowed to proceed unchecked. In addition to controlling undesirable side effects of wound-healing processes and nonpyogenic inflamma-

10. Modified from Havener WH: Ocular Pharmacology, 7th ed. CV Mosby Co, St Louis, 1987.

tion, corticosteroids can cause desirable effects in immunologically mediated ocular diseases, e.g., lens-induced uveitis and chronic immune-mediated keratoconjunctivitis syndrome.

Corticosteroids reduce resistance to many microorganisms and should not be used in their presence without effective antibiotic coverage. There is no convincing evidence for the use of corticosteroids in any ocular microbial infection. Accurate differential diagnosis is essential whenever steroids are used. In addition to potentiating microbial infection, corticosteroids increase the activity of collagenases present in corneal ulcers by up to 13 times, often resulting in rapid dissolution of the cornea with prolapse of the ocular contents.

Inhibition of collagen formation and fibroblastic activity by corticosteroids is useful in reducing corneal scarring, but it is detrimental to the healing of surgical wounds. Corticosteroids decrease the strength of healing corneal wounds, and suture removal should be delayed. The inhibition of neovascularization, especially in the cornea, is particularly useful in control of chronic immune-mediated keratoconjunctivitis syndrome (Überreiter's syndrome) in dogs and after corneal injury when fluorescein staining indicates that epithelium has covered the lesion.

Ocular Penetration of Corticosteroids

Dexamethasone, betamethasone, prednisolone, prednisone, triamcinolone, fluorometholone, medrysone, and hydrocortisone are commonly used in ophthalmic therapy. All penetrate the cornea to some extent when applied topically. Factors affecting the penetration and effect of a corticosteroid include:

1. The salt used. Acetates are more lipid-soluble and penetrate the cornea better than succinates or phosphates do.

2. Frequency of application. More frequent application results in higher intraocular levels.

3. Concentration of the drug. Low concentrations of a highly potent steroid may have less anti-inflammatory effect than a high concentration of a less-potent steroid does, e.g., topical 1.0% prednisolone has an anti-inflammatory effect similar to that of 0.1% dexamethasone, although dexamethasone has a relative ocular anti-inflammatory potency greater than prednisolone (see Fig. 3–2).

4. Proximity of the site of administration to the site of inflammation. The route of administration is chosen in relation to the site (see Fig. 3–3). Corneal and conjunctival conditions are usually treated topically, although in severe diseases subconjunctival injection may be used. The latter route is suitable for disorders of the iris and anterior uveal tract; it is often combined with topical treatment if external disease is present, or

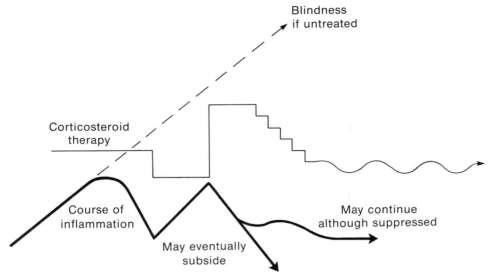

FIGURE 3–15. *Modification of the course of chronic intraocular inflammation by corticosteroid therapy. The diagram illustrates control by treatment, relapse with reduction of treatment, control by higher level treatment, and final quiescence. (Modified from Gordon D: The treatment of chronic uveitis: Preliminary comments on chronic degenerative diseases. Arch Ophthalmol 62:400, 1959. Copyright 1959, American Medical Association.)*

with systemic dosage if posterior uveal involvement is suspected. Retrobulbar and systemic routes are used for disorders of the choroid, retina, optic nerve, and orbit.

5. Affinity for the glucocorticoid receptor. Fluoromethalone has a high affinity for the receptor and more rapid degradation than dexamethasone does, and it is more suitable for external than internal ocular disease.

For most superficial disorders, 0.5% prednisolone or 0.1% dexamethasone is adequate. If the clinical effect is less than desired, it is often better to increase the frequency of dosage rather than to change the concentration of the drug. Severe inflammatory diseases of the eye often result in loss of vision and must be treated vigorously if irreparable damage is to be averted (Fig. 3–15). For long-term inhibition of less serious inflammation, e.g., seasonal and allergic inhalant conjunctivitis (atopy), 0.5% hydrocortisone is suitable.

Most injectable steroids are suitable for subconjunctival use. Several repository forms are available (e.g., methylprednisolone, triamcinolone acetate, dexamethasone disodium phosphate) with periods of activity varying from 7–10 days (triamcinolone, dexamethasone) to 2–4 weeks (methylprednisolone). When given subconjunctivally, methylprednisolone may cause chemosis with severe conjunctival erythema in horses; in dogs, it may leave unsightly white plaques that require surgical removal, as they stimulate local inflammation. Repository corticosteroids have the distinct disadvantage that they cannot be removed if the disease process changes.

Case Report

A 9-year-old collie with proliferative keratoconjunctivitis syndrome was treated successfully with daily topical 0.1% dexamethasone drops. Treatment was changed to monthly subconjunctival injections of methylprednisolone. After 6 months, the dog developed a greenish purulent ocular discharge and pain, which the owner disregarded for 3 days. At presentation, a corneal abscess and endophthalmitis were present. *Pseudomonas* spp were cultured. Despite topical, subconjunctival, and systemic therapy with an antibiotic (gentamicin) indicated by sensitivity testing, the eye was lost.

The hazard of long-term corticosteroid treatment with a repository agent is evident. A topical agent, in contrast, may be withdrawn immediately and appropriate treatment instituted.

Long-Term Therapy

Ocular discharge or *pain* in any patient undergoing long-term corticosteroid treatment requires an immediate and complete ophthalmic examination. Unlike its use in the human eye, long-term (e.g., 7 years) topical corticosteroid therapy in dogs does not predispose the eye to glaucoma or cataract. Occasional statements in veterinary texts that such treatment in dogs results in fungal superinfection (infection with unusual organisms) are incorrect.

Long-term topical usage in dogs causes increases in liver enzymes and mild adrenal suppression, and this should be taken into account in interpretation of laboratory tests and in management of aged patients or patients with suspected endocrine disorders. Serious clinical disturbances due to such treatment are *rare*. The lowest concentration and frequency of dosage that produce the desired clinical effect should be used. In older animals on continuous therapy, regular laboratory evaluation may be considered, e.g., every 6–12 months.

At normal therapeutic dosages, the adrenocortical suppression caused by subconjunctival methylprednisolone (10 mg) in dogs is of no clinical significance (Regnier et al, 1982), and this is consistent with clinical observations with a variety of corticosteroids. Higher doses or patients with adrenocortical abnormalities should be treated with caution.

Long-term use of topical corticosteroids may cause reversible adrenocortical supression. Clinical consequences in otherwise healthy patients are rare.

General Indications for Corticosteroid Usage

1. Immune-mediated ocular disorders (seasonal allergic conjunctivitis, drug and contact allergies, lens-induced uveitis, chronic immune-mediated keratoconjunctivitis syndrome)
2. Traumatic conditions resulting in severe inflammation (prolapse of the globe, contusion with hyphema)
3. Nonpyogenic inflammation (e.g., episcleritis)
4. Postoperative immunosuppression (e.g., corneal transplants, cataract extraction)
5. Reduction of neovascularization and scarring in the cornea (provided it is fluorescein-negative)
6. Reduction of postoperative swelling and inflammation after cryosurgery (e.g., cyclocryotherapy, cryoepilation for distichiasis)

Corticosteroids are often harmful if infectious agents are present. They are of no value as shotgun therapy in old scars, glaucoma, keratoconjunctivitis sicca, and degenerative disorders, although they may have specific indications in certain patients.

Specific Indications for Corticosteroid Usage

Corticosteroids can be used in these conditions:
Seasonal allergic blepharitis and conjunctivitis

Canine allergic inhalant dermatitis syndrome (atopy)
Staphylococcal blepharitis with hypersensitivity
Reduction of corneal scar formation
Reduction of corneal neovascularization and vascularization
Chronic immune-mediated keratoconjunctivitis syndrome (Überreiter's syndrome, chronic superficial keratitis)
Immune reactions in keratoplasty
Scleritis and episcleritis
Proliferative keratoconjunctivitis syndrome in collies
Recurrent equine uveitis
Uveitis (general, nonsuppurative, and traumatic)
Lens-induced uveitis
Chorioretinitis and retinitis
Serous retinal detachment
Optic neuritis
Traumatic proptosis of the globe
Malignant lymphoma
Generalized histiocytoma

NONSTEROIDAL ANTI–INFLAMMATORY DRUGS

Nonsteroidal anti-inflammatory drugs (NSAIDs) are numerous, and they have an important place in ophthalmology, because of their potency and the undesirable side effects of corticosteroids. The most commonly used for ocular disorders in animals are acetylsalicylic acid (aspirin), flunixin meglumine (Banamine),[11] and phenylbutazone. Many more NSAIDs are available for human use, but caution must be used in extrapolating their use to animals because of severe side effects. Topical flurbiprofen (Ocufen) has recently become available, but specific indications for its use have not yet been established. Systemic ibuprofen and naproxen should not be used in dogs.

Mechanism of Action

Prostaglandins are formed from arachidonic acid by the **cyclooxygenase** and **lipoxygenase** pathways. They are released into the eye when it is exposed to irritative stimuli, e.g., trauma, paracentesis, surgery. This release causes miosis, a rise in aqueous protein concentration, vasodilatation of conjunctiva and iris, and a transient rise in IOP. This group of drugs inhibits the cyclooxygenase pathway but not the lipoxygenase path-

---

11. Flunixin is not approved by the FDA for use in dogs, but its use is widespread, apparently without significant undesirable side effects. Ibuprofen is not approved and may have serious side effects, including death, in dogs.

TABLE 3–15. Clinical Use of Nonsteroidal Anti-inflammatory Agents

Drug	Species	Route and Dose	Conditions
Aspirin	Dog	Oral—25 mg/kg twice a day	Uveitis, cataract surgery, cyclocryotherapy and cryoepilation, trauma to globe and lids
	Cat	Oral—10 mg/kg every 48 hours	Trauma, cataract surgery
	Horse	Oral (mixed in food)—30 mg/kg every 24 hours	Acute and chronic equine recurrent uveitis, trauma to globe and lids, cataract surgery
Flunixin	Dog*	IV—1.0 mg/kg daily	Trauma, cyclocryotherapy, cryoepilation, cataract surgery, proptosis of the globe, uveitis
	Cat*	IV—1.1 mg/kg daily	As for the dog
	Horse	IV, IM—1.1 mg/kg twice a day	Acute and subacute equine recurrent uveitis, trauma to globe and lids, cataract surgery, premedicant before *Onchocerca* therapy
Flurbiprofen (Ocufen)	Dog	Topical	Preparation for cataract surgery
Phenylbutazone	Horse	Oral—1–2 gr daily IV—1–2 gr daily	Acute trauma, uveitis, premedicant before *Onchocerca* therapy
	Dog	Oral—22 mg/kg twice a day	As for aspirin
Meclofenamic acid (Arquel)	Horse	Oral—44 mg/kg	As for phenylbutazone
	Dog*	Oral—44 mg/kg	As for aspirin

This information is given *without regard to FDA approval for use in a particular species or otherwise.* It is the individual clinician's responsibility to determine the conditions for appropriate use in a particular patient. Because of the incidence of gastrointestinal and renal side effects with this group of drugs, care is necessary in their use.
*Use not FDA approved.

way. Glucocorticoids induce production of an inhibitor of phospholipase A_2 in both pathways. Cromolyn sodium by definition fits in this group, but it acts by stabilization of mast cells to prevent release of mediators of inflammation including histamine.

Clinical use of NSAIDs is summarized in Table 3–15. When given orally, these drugs concentrate in areas of low pH, e.g., gastric mucosa and renal papillary epithelium, sometimes resulting in gastric ulceration and hemorrhage. This effect is *not* related to hydrochloric acid production per se, and cimetidine (Tagamet) has been proved to have *no protective effect* in dogs. Preoperative use of flunixin meglumine before intraocular surgery in dogs reduces aqueous protein by 22.4%; dexamethasone alone, 45.6%; and dexamethasone and flunixin together, 64.2%.

The supposed association between flunixin and renal failure in dogs and cats is unproved, but caution is advisable. Uncontrolled preliminary reports indicate a *possible* association between flunixin meglumine and methoxyflurane and reversible renal tubular necrosis. Patients in which this combination is used should be well hydrated and have normal renal function.[12]

Cromolyn Sodium (Cromolyn, Opticrom)

Cromolyn sodium is used topically to stabilize mast cells and to prevent release of histamine and other

mediators of inflammation. It is useful for treatment of seasonal allergic conjunctivitis and atopic conjunctivitis in dogs, usually in association with topical corticosteroids.

OSMOTIC AGENTS

An osmotic agent increases the osmotic concentration of blood perfusing the eye. Because of the blood-aqueous and blood-retinal barriers, the osmotic agent enters the aqueous or vitreous only in limited amounts. The osmotic gradient causes withdrawal of water from the eye to the vascular system. This results in

1. Reduction in IOP
2. Reduction in vitreous volume and frequently posterior movement of the lens with disruption of pupillary block (see Chap 13)
3. Clearing of corneal edema (if the drug is applied topically)

Osmotic agents are used for

1. Emergency reduction of IOP in acute glaucoma
2. Reduction of IOP and vitreous volume prior to intraocular surgery
3. Clearing of corneal edema to allow intraocular examination

The routes of administration are summarized in Table 3–16. Mannitol, glycerol (glycerin), and topical NaCl (5%) ointment are most commonly used in veterinary ophthalmology. Mannitol and glycerol should be immediately available for the treatment of glaucoma, as pressure levels of 50–60 mmHg for more than 24–48 hours may result in irreparable visual loss.

---

12. Such uncontrolled reports must be interpreted cautiously—previous, widely disseminated views about methoxyflurane and renal failure in dogs, because of extrapolation of toxicity data from humans, were proved groundless.

Mannitol

Mannitol is a vegetable sugar that is not metabolized and is passed in the urine, causing osmotic diuresis. (The diuresis is *not* the cause of reduced IOP.) Mannitol is not absorbed after oral administration (although it does cause osmotic catharsis). After IV administration, IOP falls in 30–60 minutes and remains low for 5–6 hours. As vitreous volume falls, the iridocorneal angle may open, increasing aqueous outflow facility.

As mannitol increases the serum osmolality, thirst ensues. Water intake must be controlled (by feeding ice cubes) if the ophthalmic effect is to be maintained. Mannitol, unlike urea, does not cause tissue necrosis after extravenous leakage. Mannitol is *not* used for long-term treatment of glaucoma. Dehydrated animals should be rehydrated before using mannitol in order to prevent hypovolemia. Suggestions that mannitol used with methoxyflurane anesthesia cause pulmonary edema in dogs have been disproved.

Method of Use for Acute Glaucoma

1. 2 g/kg IV over 10–15 minutes (10 ml/kg of 20% solution or 12 ml/kg of 16⅔% solution).
2. 500 mg acetazolamide IV. Care must be taken if the patient has had carbonic anhydrase inhibitors previously.
3. Topical pilocarpine (2%) every 5 minutes until pressure begins to fall, or up to 30 minutes, then every 3–4 hours.

Glycerol

Glycerol is less effective than other agents, but it can be administered by an owner during acute relapses of glaucoma until professional evaluation is available. The dosage in dogs is 1–2 ml/kg orally. After oral administration, IOP falls in 20–30 minutes. After repeated administration, emesis may occur. Glycerol is cheap, readily available (as glycerin), nontoxic, can be used orally, and is rapid in action. If administered chilled, 50% in water, emesis is uncommon.

Urea and isosorbide may be used for lowering IOP (see Table 3–16), but mannitol is recommended. Hypertonic osmotic agents are usually used in the treatment of acute glaucoma. Chronic glaucoma is controlled mostly by cyclocryotherapy or intraocular prosthesis insertion, with miotics and carbonic anhydrase inhibitors as adjuncts.

Topical Hyperosmotic Agents

Topical glycerol (after local anesthesia), and 2% or 5% NaCl ointment or drops can be used for temporary clearing of corneal edema for examination. NaCl (2% or 5%) can be used for treatment of bullous keratopathy, superficial corneal erosion, and chronic corneal edema due to endothelial dysfunction, but responses are limited to minor disease states owing to the very short time (about 90 seconds) such applications alter tear osmolality.

TABLE 3–16. Properties of Osmotic Agents

Drug	Dose	Route	Molecular Weight	Advantages	Disadvantages
Mannitol	1.5–3.0 gm/kg	20% solution IV in 20–30 minutes	182	Extracellular Few complications No caloric value No hyperglycemia in diabetics	IV only Large volume required because of molecular weight
Glycerol (glycerine)	1.0–1.5 gm/kg	50–75% solution, oral, ice cold	92	Readily available Little diuresis Penetrates poorly	Very sweet, nauseating High caloric value Slow IOP fall Causes hyperglycemia in diabetics
Isosorbide	1–2 gm/kg	50% solution, oral, cold	146	Extracellular No caloric value No taste	Slower than IV Not yet available
Dextrose	1–2 gm/kg	50% solution, IV	180	Readily available Useful in emergencies	Very short acting Causes hyperglycemia in diabetics
Urea	1–2 gm/kg	30% in invert sugar 10% solution, IV, 60 drops/minute	60	Intra- and extracellular	Solution is unstable Extravascular sloughs Rebound effect because penetrates blood-eye barriers
NaCl	5% ointment	Topical	58	Useful topically	Short acting

CARBONIC ANHYDRASE INHIBITORS

The enzyme carbonic anhydrase is present in the ciliary body and is associated with aqueous production. Inhibition by carbonic anhydrase inhibitors reduces aqueous production by up to 50%, decreasing IOP. These drugs also inhibit carbonic anhydrase in the renal tubular epithelium, causing diuresis. Like the osmotic agents, their effect in reducing IOP is *not* the result of diuresis. Conversely, other diuretics such as furosemide (Lasix) and the benzothiadiazides have no significant effect on aqueous production or IOP.

Any carbonic anhydrase inhibitor may cause undesirable side effects in a particular patient, necessitating a change to a different member of the group. Because of increased urinary loss of potassium with long-term use, oral supplementation (20–30 mg/kg) may be indicated if serum potassium is depressed. Care must be taken when administering them intravenously to patients that have been medicated orally until that time, as *acute severe metabolic acidosis* may occur.

Carbonic anhydrase inhibitors are sometimes used long term in individual patients for glaucoma, but definitive surgical control with cyclocryotherapy, intraocular prosthesis insertion, or removal of a primary luxated lens is preferable.

Acetazolamide

Acetazolamide may be given orally or intravenously. In high doses (50–100 mg/kg) intravenously, it may reduce aqueous production by up to 75% and greatly reduce IOP. Consequently, IV acetazolamide is used in the emergency treatment of acute canine glaucoma. The drug is well absorbed after oral administration, and its action lasts 4–6 hours. More prolonged blood levels and fewer side effects occur when prolonged-release oral preparations are used. In dogs, oral acetazolamide causes vomiting more frequently than other carbonic anhydrase inhibitors do, and long-term use is often unsatisfactory.

Dichlorphenamide, Ethoxzolamide, and Methazolamide

The newer carbonic anhydrase inhibitors are used orally and cause fewer side effects than acetazolamide does. If side effects (see the next heading) occur in a particular patient, another drug of the same group is often more suitable. Occasional patients show disorientation with Daranide.

Dose Rate:

Dichlorphenamide (Daranide) 2 mg/kg daily in 2 or 3 divided doses

Ethoxzolamide (Ethamide) 5 mg/kg daily in 2 or 3 divided doses

Methazolamide (Neptazane) 5 mg/kg daily in 2 or 3 divided doses

Side Effects of Carbonic Anhydrase Inhibitors in Dogs

Clients should be warned of the possible side effects.

1. Disorientation and behavioral changes
2. Vomiting
3. Polyuria (usually decreases after a few weeks)
4. Diarrhea
5. Polydipsia
6. Drowsiness
7. Pruritus of paws
8. Hyperventilation

LOCAL ANESTHETICS

Topical local anesthetics are used for ocular examinations and minor manipulative and surgical procedures but not for therapeutic purposes.

1. All topical anesthetics inhibit corneal epithelialization and are toxic to normal corneal epithelium. They produce minute punctuate ulcerations in normal cornea.

2. Some are extremely toxic systemically (5 ml of 2% tetracaine solution is a fatal human dose) and are rapidly absorbed from the conjunctival sac.

3. Some are antigenic and may cause sensitization.

4. Local anesthetics should *not* be dispensed to owners for any reason.

5. Local anesthetics placed into diseased, painful eyes abolish protective reflexes and increase the chance of further injury (e.g., entropion) as well as causing corneal lesions themselves.

Local anesthetics should not be used therapeutically or included in any therapeutic regimen or preparation.

Within 15–20 seconds of instillation, some degree of corneal anesthesia is present. A second drop after 1–2 minutes enhances anesthesia. After effective anesthesia is achieved, further drops increase the duration of anesthesia. Ophthalmic anesthetics are unsuitable for injection, and great care must be exercised when applying them to diseased corneas—sloughing of the entire corneal epithelium after application of benoxinate to a dog with glaucoma has been reported.

Bacterial samples should be taken before local anesthetics are placed in the eye, because they and the preservatives they contain often kill bacteria in the conjunctival sac and on swabs taken for culture. Local anesthesia reduces Schirmer tear test values by about 50% and should not be used prior to such tests. Of the many agents available—proparacaine, lignocaine (lidocaine), tetracaine, benoxinate, butacaine, cocaine, phenacaine, dibucaine, and piperocaine—0.5% proparacaine[13] is generally the most useful. Brownish solutions of proparacaine are inactivated and should not be used. Tetracaine may cause sensitivity reactions in dogs.

ANTICOLLAGENASE AGENTS

Collagenases are important in the pathogenesis of certain types of corneal ulceration. Collagenases are produced by corneal epithelial cells, stromal fibrocytes, inflammatory cells, and certain bacteria such as *Pseudomonas* spp. Various inhibitors of collagenase and other proteases are used in the treatment of corneal ulceration (Table 3–17). Acetylcysteine is the most frequently used, as it is commercially available. Because of its mucolytic and collagenase-inhibiting properties, it is also used in the treatment of keratoconjunctivitis sicca. Occasional animals may show irritation with acetylcysteine, and the preparation (see Chapter 11) may be diluted appropriately. Acetylcysteine has been demonstrated to have no adverse effect on the healing of corneal epithelial wounds. Penicillamine, in addition to its collagenase-inhibiting action, has anti-inflammatory properties. It has recently been shown in humans and animals that exhaustion of the naturally occurring antiproteases alpha$_2$-macroglobulin and alpha$_1$-antitrypsin is associated with continuing infection in herpetic keratitis (Chesnokova and Maichuk, 1986).

13. Opthetic—Allergan Pharmaceuticals, Irvine, CA; Ophthaine—E. R. Squibb & Sons, Princeton, NJ; Alcaine—Alcon Laboratories, Fort Worth, TX.

TEAR REPLACEMENT AND VISCOUS SOLUTIONS

Aqueous solutions such as normal saline are unsuitable for tear replacement because these hydrophilic solutions do not adhere to the lipophilic corneal epithelium. Viscous agents bind the solution to the epithelium. In the normal precorneal tear film this function is performed by mucopolysaccharide molecules having both hydrophilic and lipophilic ends. Polyvinylpyrrolidone is an artificial mucin used for this purpose. Artificial tear solutions stabilize the precorneal tear film and prevent its breakup, as measured by the tear breakup time. Small cylinders of hydroxypropyl cellulose (Lacrisert) are available for placement beneath the lower lid, but these have not found wide application in veterinary ophthalmology.

Artificial tear solutions are used when tear production is decreased, when loss by evaporation is increased, when corneal treatment with water-soluble drugs is required, or when tear breakup time is abnormal owing to corneal pathology or abnormal precorneal tear film. These solutions are indicated in the following situations:

1. In treatment of keratoconjunctivitis sicca, exposure keratitis (e.g., in facial paralysis), glaucomatous buphthalmos, breed-associated lagophthalmos, and abnormal tear breakup time
2. During prolonged anesthesia, in order to prevent drying
3. As a lubricant and cushioning solution during gonioscopy
4. As an ingredient in ophthalmic drops to increase contact time with the cornea

The most commonly used solutions are:
1. Polyvinylpyrrolidone (1.67%).[14] In this author's

14. Adsorbotear—Alcon Laboratories, Ft Worth, TX.

TABLE 3–17. Anticollagenase Agents for Topical Use

Agent	Concentration Used	Mode of Action	Stability (Room Temperature)	Available Preparations*
N-Acetylcysteine	20% or less (less irritation at 5%)	Chelates Ca^{++}	4–6 weeks (at 4°C)	Mucomyst (20% solution)
Dimethylcysteine (penicillamine)	0.15 M	Chelates Zn^{++} (also anti-inflammatory)	?	Cuprimine (capsules) D-Penamine (capsules)
Autologous serum	Optional	α_2-Macroglobulin inhibits collagenase	Indefinite if frozen	From patient
Na EDTA	0.15 M	Chelates Ca^{++}	Indefinite	From chemical supply houses as generic drug
Cysteine	0.15 M	Chelates Ca^{++}	2–3 days	From chemical supply houses as generic drug
Cystine (in solution)	0.15 M	Chelates Ca^{++}	3 days	From chemical supply houses as generic drug
Cystine (in suspension)	0.15 M	Chelates Ca^{++}	15 days	From chemical supply houses as generic drug

*Mucomyst—Mead Johnson Pharmaceuticals, Evansville, IN; Cuprimine—Merck Sharp & Dohme, West Point PA: D-Penamine—Dista Products, Sydney, Australia.

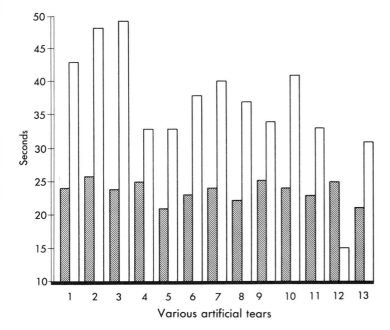

FIGURE 3–16. Duration in seconds of average tear film breakup time following instillation of various artificial tears. Solid bar represents baseline; shaded bar, value with medication. The products evaluated were 1, Adapt; 2, Adapettes; 3, Adsorbotear; 4, Contique; 5, Isopto Tears; 6, Ultra Tears; 7, Liquifilm I; 8, Liquifilm II; 9, Lacril; 10, Pre-Sert; 11, Lyteers; 12, Tearisol; and 13, Tears Naturale. (From Havener WH: Ocular Pharmacology, 5th ed. CV Mosby Co, St Louis, 1983, p 627; modified from Lemp MA, et al: The effect of tear substitutes on tear film break-up time. Invest Ophthalmol 14:255, 1975.) [Author's Note: Some of these products are no longer on the market. Check for equivalent products.]

opinion, the best of the available agents (as Adsorbotear). It has the longest effect on tear breakup time of the commonly available agents (Fig. 3–16).

2. Methylcellulose (0.5–1.0%) (including hydroxyethyl cellulose and hydroxypropyl methylcellulose).

3. Polyvinyl alcohol (1.4%). Polyvinyl alcohol is frequently irritating to dogs and cats.

Manufacturers' claims of prolonged contact time with any of these agents should be viewed with caution.

MISCELLANEOUS THERAPEUTIC AGENTS

Surgical Adhesives

Tissue adhesive (methyl-2-cyanoacrylate) has been advocated for treating leaking and erosive corneal lesions in dogs. It is useful when corneal closure by microsurgical methods is not possible because of tissue destruction or loss, or to supplement surgical closure, but the method is not a substitute for correct surgical repair, and it should be used only by experienced persons. Cyanoacrylate is used on the corneal surface where it results in some inflammatory reaction that may be beneficial in the lesions discussed here, but it must not enter the eye. Large amounts or long-term use results in severe inflammation. Usage is at the clinician's discretion, as surgical tissue adhesives are not approved for ocular application in humans or animals.

Eye Washes (Collyria)

Sterile eye wash is used for removal of purulent exudates, foreign bodies, and irritants from the eyelids and conjunctival sac. Boric acid solution was commonly used, but because of its weak germicidal action and systemic toxicity it is no longer advocated. Commercial formulas (Eye-Stream, Dacriose) are suitable. Eye washes in examination rooms are changed regularly in order to prevent overgrowth with contaminating bacteria.

Germicides

Germicides are used for disinfection of delicate instruments, for preoperative preparation of the lids and conjunctival sac, and as preservatives in eye drops.

Povidone-Iodine

Povidone-iodine is a reliable and nonirritating agent for removal of bacteria from the conjunctival sac prior to surgery. It is mixed as a 1:25 solution in normal saline. Povidone-iodine solution and not surgical scrub solution must be used.

Benzalkonium Chloride (Zephiran)

This drug is commonly used for the three purposes mentioned previously. It is a wetting agent and enhances the corneal penetration of certain drugs (e.g., carbachol) when used as a preservative (1:5000). It is incompatible with nitrates, salicylates, sulfonamides, and fluorescein. Pseudomonas spp. may persist for several days in solutions of 1:5000. A solution of 1:750 is used as an instrument disinfectant, but it will not reliably kill spores, fungi, or viruses. It should not be used on aluminum instruments or with cotton pads, which absorb the drug from the solution. Sodium nitrate (0.5%) is added as a rust inhibitor. For skin preparation, 1:750 solution is used to remove dirt, fat, and superficial bacteria, and 1:5000 may be used to irrigate the conjunctival sac before surgery. Benzalkonium chloride should not be relied upon to sterilize surgical instruments.

Hexachlorophene

The skin preparation pHisoHex contains, in addition to hexachlorophene, a substance that is extremely toxic to the cornea.

Cresol

Cresol is contained in Post's Solution No. 4, used for rapid instrument disinfection:

Saponated cresol compound (NF) 8 ml
Oil of lavender 2 ml
Thymol crystals 2 g
Ethyl alcohol 88 ml

Silver Compounds (Silver Nitrate and Argyrol)

Silver nitrate was once used to kill conjunctival bacteria. It is very irritating, and its use is *contraindicated*. The ophthalmic use of silver nitrate applicator sticks (used for hemostasis after nail trimming in dogs) results in severe keratitis and epithelial sloughing in dogs. Argyrol (10% silver proteinate) was also used for cleaning the conjunctival sac. It has very weak germicidal properties and has been replaced by antibiotics and povidone-iodine. It should not be confused with silver nitrate.

Mercuric Oxide (Golden Eye Ointment)

This is an outmoded agent once used for its antiseptic properties and abrasive action as a mild irritant. Many more effective agents are available, and its use is not recommended.

Ethylene Oxide

Ethylene oxide is a toxic gas that kills bacteria, fungi, viruses, and spores (and humans if it is inhaled). It is widely and effectively used for sterilizing sharp instruments, glass, plastic, rubber, and perishable goods. Sterilized items must be properly aired before use, and a well-ventilated area must be provided for use of the gas in order to avoid toxic effects on humans. Portable bench sterilizers employing ethylene oxide are useful for sterilizing delicate ophthalmic instruments.

Glutaraldehyde

Glutaraldehyde is used as a sterilizing agent for instruments and to preserve tissues for histopathological examination. It is *never* to be placed near the eye! After ethylene oxide, it is one of the more effective chemical sterilizing agents. Stock solutions of glutaraldehyde are acidic; for sterilizing, alkaline solutions (pH 7.5–8.3) must be used. Stock solutions must be changed every 2–4 weeks, as decomposition occurs.

Astringents and Cauterants

Astringents are locally acting protein precipitants, cauterants are severe protein-precipitating agents that cause local tissue destruction. Astringents are occasionally used in inflammation of the conjunctiva, and cauterants are used to remove tissue. In the latter case, surgical removal usually accomplishes the same result and does not leave necrotic debris. The antibacterial action of cauterants gives them a minor place in the treatment of corneal ulcers. They are also useful for sealing minor leaking wounds of the cornea.

Copper Sulfate

Copper sulfate crystals were formerly used for removing lymphoid follicles in chronic follicular conjunctivitis. Such usage is of historical interest only. Surgical methods of follicle removal are just as effective and are only necessary in the rare case when inhibition of the immune reaction to the antigen is unsuccessful.

Trichloroacetic Acid

Trichloroacetic acid (25%) is a powerful cauterant used occasionally to treat leaking corneal fistulae. Its use in corneal ulcer therapy is not recommended.

Phenol (Carbolic Acid)

Phenol is similar in action and properties to trichloroacetic acid. It has the advantage of quickly precipitating protein and turning it opaque, allowing the treated area to be instantly seen. A concentrated solution, made by exposing the hygroscopic crystals to air, is applied carefully with a cotton-tipped applicator or toothpick.

Iodine

Iodine is a milder cauterant used for superficial corneal erosions. Tincture (1–6%), 7% iodine, or alcoholic potassium iodide solution may be used. Iodine has the disadvantage that the treated area is difficult to see. Its use in the treatment of superficial corneal erosion in dogs has been decreased by accurate surgical superficial keratectomy.

Zinc Sulfate

Zinc sulfate solution (0.2% and 0.25%) and ointment (0.5%) have mild astringent and antiseptic properties. Zinc sulfate is used for mild nonspecific conjunctivitis and is often combined with vasoconstrictor and antihistaminic drugs.

Antihistamines

Antihistamines are little used in ocular therapy. Systemic antihistamines are useful in acute allergic conjunctivitis. Antazoline (0.5%) is of marginal use in this condition; when it is combined with zinc sulfate and vasoconstrictors, some therapeutic benefit can be obtained. Contact dermatitis and conjunctivitis, especially of the drug-induced variety, are not histamine-mediated. In almost all ocular disorders for which antihistamines have been advocated, corticosteroid therapy and antiprostaglandin therapy are more effective.

Vitamins

Various vitamins have been advocated for their supposed therapeutic efficacy in the treatment of ocular disorders of animals. In the absence of a specific vitamin deficiency, there is little to be gained from such local therapy. For disorders in which a systemic vitamin deficiency is suspected, multivitamin therapy may be useful. Specific vitamin therapy may be used to prevent progression of disease states caused by vitamin deficiency (e.g., night blindness due to vitamin A deficiency in cattle). Ocular signs of vitamin deficiencies may also assist in diagnosis (e.g., microphthalmia in the offspring of vitamin A–deficient sows). Systemic and ocular signs of warfarin poisoning are treated with vitamin K and its analogues.

Miscellaneous Agents

ANTIPARASITICIDES

Ivermectin

Ivermectins are used for treatment of *Onchocerca* microfilariae in horses (see "Recurrent Equine Uveitis," Chap 12) and equine habronemiasis affecting the lids, third eyelid, and conjunctiva. Toxic reactions have occurred with their use in dogs including blindness, hindlimb ataxia, recumbency, and stupor, and in cats ataxia, blindness, vocalization, and dementia.

Phenothiazine

Orally administered phenothiazine may cause corneal epithelial and stromal edema in cattle when the animals are exposed to sunlight. Phenothiazine is metabolized in the bovine liver to phenothiazine sulphoxide, which enters the aqueous and is responsible for the photosensitization reaction in the cornea. Cattle on a low plane of nutrition may be more susceptible than those on a high plane. If the supplement is removed and the animals are not exposed to bright sunlight, resolution may be expected in 60–90 days.

Rafoxanide

Rafoxanide is a fasciolode used in sheep. At doses of 100 mg/kg, it causes status spongiosis of the central nervous system with blindness.

Immunosuppressants[15]

A complete discussion of immunosuppressants is beyond the scope of this book, and only those currently used for specific ocular disorders in animals are referred to. For a discussion of the chemotherapy of such systemic disorders and feline lymphosarcoma (feline leukemia virus infection), readers are referred elsewhere.

Azathioprine

Azathioprine is an antimetabolite and T-cell suppressor used to treat uncontrolled uveitis in dogs, e.g., Vogt-Koyanagi-Harada–like syndrome (uveodermatological syndrome) in akitas, in which it can be particularly effective if corticosteroids have failed. It is variably useful for nodular granulomatous keratoconjunctivitis syndrome in collies. Azathioprine has a lag phase of 3–5 weeks before its effects become evident. In both disorders, a dosage of 2 mg/kg is used daily for 2 weeks, then 1 mg/kg every 2nd day for 2 weeks, then 1 mg/kg once weekly for 4 weeks. Lower doses and shorter durations may be used if responses are rapid.

Liver enzymes and total white cell and platelet counts are monitored every 2 weeks for the first 8 weeks, then monthly during therapy. Total white cell counts should remain above 4000/cu mm. Elevations of liver enzymes may occur because of corticosteroids used concurrently. Long-term therapy in cats may cause leukopenia.

Cyclophosphamide

Cyclophosphamide is an alkylating agent, used for treatment of ocular and periocular neoplasms, both orally and by injection into extraocular neoplasms, and for multiple histiocytomas of the lids and conjunctiva in dogs. It may be used systemically after removal of neoplasms from the eye and orbit in the treatment of metastases. *Alternate-day therapy* with adequate water intake and urination in the evening to minimize cystic

---

15. See also Chap 7.

mucosal exposure reduces hemorrhagic cystitis due to metabolites of the drug.

Dosage: 50 mg/sq m once daily on alternate days, orally or IV; 6.6 mg/kg orally for 3 days, then 2.2 mg/kg once daily.

Cyclosporine

Cyclosporine is a T-cell inhibitor with an affinity for the cornea and sclera. Cyclosporine affects cell-mediated immunity and possibly humoral immunity by inhibition of helper T cells, but it does not affect epithelial wound healing. Preliminary reports indicate it is effective in inhibiting unspecified immune reactions in these tissues, e.g., graft rejection, autoimmune keratitis in dogs, and possibly in the severe immune reactions seen in some cats to herpetic keratitis.[16] It is potentially useful to reduce corneal opacity in the postoperative treatment of vascularized superficial corneal erosion syndrome in certain breeds.

It is also effective in some cases of canine keratoconjunctivitis sicca, but the mechanism is unknown. The drug is applied as a 2% solution in olive oil, and it is irritating if applied to the skin. Controlled studies on its efficacy are currently lacking.

Immune Globulins

Subconjunctival injection of autologous[17] or allogenic[18] globulin (or even blood) has been advocated for corneal ulceration because serum contains an alpha$_2$-macroglobulin capable of inhibiting collagenase, perhaps accounting for such efficacy. Collection of this plasma from the patient, using ethylenediaminetetraacetic acid (EDTA) as an anticoagulant, adds another collagenase inhibitor to this old remedy.

Immunostimulants

Nonspecific immune stimulants are sometimes used in the therapy of ocular neoplasia with variable results. The most consistently useful has been treatment of periocular equine sarcoid with both live bacille Calmette-Guérin (BCG) vaccine and cell wall extracts (Ribigen,[19] Regressin-Ragland Research), of the same organism. Extracts of other organisms (Immunoregulin-ImmunoVet, which stimulates the reticuloendothelial system) and nonspecific stimulants such as levamisole (2–5 mg/kg orally) may be used in immunosuppressed animals, e.g., cats with chronic herpesvirus infection, chronic canine staphylococcal blepharitis with hypersensitivity. Staphylococcal bacterins are also useful in the latter condition.

Levamisole is useful in the treatment of recurrent stromal herpetic keratitis in cats.

Enzymes

Enzyme preparations are rarely used in veterinary ophthalmology. For a discussion of fibrinolysin, streptokinase, and urokinase, an ophthalmic pharmacology text should be consulted.

Alpha Chymotrypsin

This enzyme is used in human intracapsular cataract extraction to digest lens zonules. It is not used in veterinary ophthalmology, as the zonules are more resistant to enzymatic digestion.

Hyaluronidase

Hyaluronidase depolymerizes hyaluronic acid, an important constituent of connective tissue, allowing faster passage of drugs through tissues (e.g., in retrobulbar local anesthesia). The permeability of tissues returns to normal in 1–2 days. The enzyme is nontoxic, does not cause inflammation or affect capillary permeability, and will not dissolve fibrin or inflammatory exudates. Duration of anesthesia may be increased by addition of epinephrine to the solution. Hyaluronidase is also used to promote dispersion of contrast agents through orbital tissues in radiographic orbitography.

PHYSICAL THERAPY

Heat and Cold

Hot and cold compresses are useful in treating blepharitis because of the prolific eyelid blood supply. Edema, postoperative swelling, and pain may be reduced by frequent application of heat and cold in cooperative patients.

Contact Lenses

Hydrophilic contact lenses have been used and advocated in dogs and horses

1. As a bandage to protect the cornea during healing. The lenses are usually dislodged in less than 5 days in dogs, and they are unsuitable in cats. To assist retention, the use of cyanoacrylate adhesive has been advocated. In general, animal patients are better served by a third eyelid flap, which results in longer coverage and fewer patient management problems for both veterinarian and owner.

---

16. It is *ineffective* in chronic immune-mediated keratoconjunctivitis syndrome (Überreiter's) in German shepherds.
17. Autologous—from the patient.
18. Allogenic—from a genetically dissimilar donor of the same species.
19. Fort Dodge Laboratories, Ft Dodge, IA.

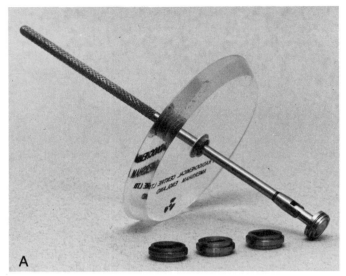

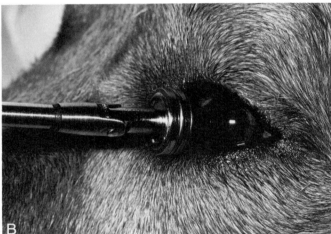

FIGURE 3–17. A, A strontium-90 ophthalmic applicator. B, The applicator in position.

2. As a vehicle for delivery of hydrophilic drugs. The lens is soaked in a concentrated solution of the drug and placed on the eye. In lenses sufficiently large for use in cattle, the center of the lens is too thick and oxygen permeability is too low, causing corneal hypoxia, edema, and ulceration.

Tarsorraphy has been shown experimentally to enhance corneal epithelial wound healing, and therapeutic bandage lenses have been shown to *reduce* the rate of healing.

Radiation

Two forms of radiation—beta and x (or gamma) rays—are used for the treatment of ocular disease. The effects of radiation on rapidly dividing cells, lymphocytes, and vascular endothelium are used in therapy.

Beta Therapy

Beta rays are low-energy electrons that penetrate tissue to a depth of 3–4 mm. They are used to treat superficial lesions only. Beta radiation for ophthalmic use is obtained from a strontium-90 ophthalmic applicator (Fig. 3–17). Because of the dangers inherent in the use of radioactive materials, such applicators are strictly licensed and should be treated with due respect. Beta therapy is used to control corneal neovascularization and pigmentation as in chronic immune-mediated keratitis syndrome (Überreiter's syndrome) in dogs and to treat malignant neoplasms including squamous cell carcinoma of the lids, third eyelid, and conjunctiva in cattle, cats, and horses especially. Because of shallow penetration, beta radiation from an applicator applied

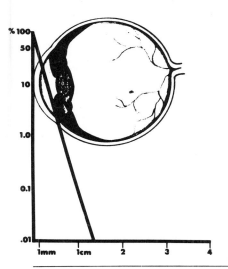

DEPTH—DOSE AS A PERCENTAGE OF SURFACE—
DOSE SHOWN IN RELATION TO EYE STRUCTURE

FIGURE 3–18. This curve indicates the decrease in intensity of beta-radiation emitted from a ⁹⁰Sr ophthalmic applicator as a function of tissue depth. At 1-mm depth the intensity is decreased by 50%. The diagram of the eye is drawn to scale to show the relationship of decreasing intensity to various structures of the eye. (From Gillette EL: Veterinary radiotherapy. J Am Vet Med Assoc 157:1707, 1970.)

to the limbus does not reach the equatorial zone of the lens (Fig. 3–18). The canine cornea can withstand up to 7000 cGy/site.

Gamma and X Radiation

Gamma and x radiation have similar wavelengths, energy, and penetrating properties but differ in origin—gamma radiation emanates from the nucleus and x-radiation from the extranuclear portion of the atom. Both penetrate deeply and are used for infiltrating or inaccessible lesions not suitable for treatment by beta radiation. Sources include superficial (10–125 keV), orthovoltage (125–400 keV), and megavoltage (500–1000 keV) radiotherapy units and cobalt-60 therapy machines, cesium-135 and cobalt-60 needles, and radon and gold implants (*brachytherapy*). Important ophthalmic sequelae of treatment, either of the eye itself or of the adjacent nasal and paranasal sinuses, occur.

Because of safety precautions, licensing, and expense, treatment is performed by trained veterinary radiologists in institutional veterinary hospitals. Referral of cases requiring such therapy is advocated.

Penetrating (x and gamma) radiations may interfere with cell division in the equatorial region of the lens, especially in young animals, resulting in partial or complete **RADIATION CATARACT**. Very high doses of radiation may result in a superficial keratopathy, although the eye of domestic animals appears to be less

sensitive than the human or rabbit eye is at comparable dosage levels. Reported ocular side effects of megavoltage therapy to canine nasal and paranasal sinuses includes severe keratitis (41%), conjunctivitis (mild 34%, severe 28%), cataract (28%), and keratoconjunctivitis sicca including corneal perforation (24%), with 63% of conjunctivitis and keratitis refractory to treatment. The maximal permissible dose to the eye for orthovoltage and megavoltage radiation is approximately 4500–5000 cGy. Ultraviolet radiation also causes painful corneal lesions and photophthalmia in animals exposed to high doses of solar radiation (e.g., snowblindness of cattle and polar bears).

Hyperthermia

Hyperthermia (local induction of heat within a tissue) is used to treat squamous cell carcinoma of the eye and adnexa in horses and cattle (Fig. 3–19). The temperature of the tissue is increased (50° C for 30 sec/sq cm) by the local passage of radiofrequency current through the tissue. In both horses and dogs, corneal lesions produced with hyperthermia resolve with little alteration in structure, indicating that the method may be useful for lesions involving the cornea.

Lasers in Veterinary Ophthalmology

Lasers have not achieved significant clinical use in veterinary ophthalmology because of lack of indications and expense. The neodymium:yttrium-aluminum-garnet laser is sometimes used to remove postoperative

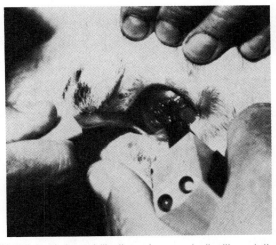

FIGURE 3–19. Immobilization of an eyeball with a slotted retractor during hyperthermic therapy of a squamous cell carcinoma, using the surface probe of a device. (From Kainer RA, et al: Hypothermia for treatment of ocular squamous cell tumors in cattle. J Am Vet Med Assoc 176:356, 1980.)

cyclitic membranes after cataract surgery, but it is not used in the primary lens removal procedure. The CO_2 laser has been used for removal of adnexal lesions, but similar results can be achieved with conventional surgical techniques.

REFERENCES

Ali Z, Insler MS (1986): A comparison of therapeutic bandage lenses, tarsorraphy, and antibiotic and hypertonic saline on corneal epithelial wound healing. Ann Ophthalmol 18:22.

Beale KM (1988): Azathioprine for treatment of immune-mediated diseases of dogs and cats. J Am Vet Med Assoc 192:1316.

Bistner SI, et al (1969): Conjunctival bacteria: Clinical appearances can be deceiving. Mod Vet Pract 50:45.

Bistner SI, et al (1981): Ocular manifestations of low level phenothiazine administration to cattle. Cornell Vet 71:136.

Boulay JP, et al (1986): Effect of cimetidine on aspirin-induced gastric hemorrhage in dogs. Am J Vet Res 47:1744.

Brightman AH, et al (1981): Effect of aspirin on aqueous protein values in the dog. J Am Vet Med Assoc 178:572.

Campbell L (1973): Ocular bacteria and mycoplasma of the clinically normal cat. Feline Pract Nov–Dec:10.

Cattabiani F, et al (1976): Bacterial flora of the conjunctival sac of the horse. (Italian.) Ann Sclavo 18:91.

Chesnokova NB, Maichuk YF (1986): Antiproteases in herpetic keratitis. Metab Pediatr Syst Ophthalmol 9:593.

Clare NT, et al (1947): Identification of the photosensitizing agent in photosensitized keratitis in young cattle following use of phenothiazine as an anthelmintic. Aust Vet J 23:344.

Cross Canada Disease Report (1987): Ivermectin toxicity in small animals. Can Vet J 28:18.

D'Amico DJ, et al (1984): Retinal toxicity of intravitreal gentamicin. An electron microscopic study. Invest Ophthalmol 25:564.

D'Amico DJ, et al (1985): Comparative toxicity of intravitreal aminoglycoside antibiotics. Am J Ophthalmol 100:264.

van Delft JL, et al (1988): Comparison of the effects of corticosteroids and indomethacin on the response of the blood-aqueous barrier to injury. Curr Eye Res 6:419.

Dice PF, Cooley PL (1988): Use of contact lenses to treat corneal diseases in small animals. Semin Vet Med Surg 3:46.

Eichenbaum JD, et al (1988): Effect in large dogs of ophthalmic prednisolone acetate on adrenal gland and hepatic function. J Am Anim Hosp Assoc 24:705.

Ellis PP (1985): Handbook of Ocular Therapeutics and Pharmacology, 7th ed. CV Mosby Co, St Louis.

Faigenbaum SJ, et al (1976): Intraocular penetration of amoxicillin. Am J Ophthalmol 82:598.

Gavin PR, Gillette EL (1978): Interstitial radiation therapy of equine squamous cell carcinomas. J Am Vet Rad Soc 19:138.

George L, et al (1988): Topically applied furazolidone or parentally administered oxytetracycline for the treatment of infectious bovine keratoconjunctivitis. J Am Vet Med Assoc 192:1415.

Gerding PA, et al (1988): Pathogenic bacteria and fungi associated with external ocular diseases in dogs: 131 cases (1981–1986). J Am Vet Med Assoc 193:242.

Gilmour MA, Walshaw R (1987): Naproxen-induced toxicosis in a dog. J Am Vet Med Assoc 191:1431.

Glaze MB, Turk MA (1986): Effects of radiofrequency hyperthermia on the healthy canine cornea. Am J Vet Res 47:913.

Glaze MB, et al (1988): Ophthalmic corticosteroid therapy: Systemic effects in the dog. J Am Vet Med Assoc 192:73.

Greene GE, (ed) (1984): Clinical Microbiology and Infectious Diseases of the Dog and Cat, p 172. WB Saunders Co, Philadephia.

Greer RT, Ryoo JP (1987): Development of ocular inserts for cattle. Scanning Microsc 1:863.

Havener WH (1987): Ocular Pharmacology, 7th ed. CV Mosby Co, St Louis.

Joyce JR (1983): Thiabendazole therapy of mycotic keratitis in horses. Equine Vet J Supp 2:45.

Kainer RA, et al (1980): Hyperthermia for treatment of ocular squamous cell tumors in cattle. J Am Vet Med Assoc 176:356.

Kern TJ, et al (1983): Equine keratomycosis: Current concepts of diagnosis and therapy. Equine Vet J Supp 2:33.

Kinsey VE, cited by Moses RA (1970): Adler's Physiology of the Eye, 5th ed. CV Mosby Co, St Louis.

Koch SA, Rubin LF (1969): Ocular sensitivity of dogs to topical tetracaine HCl. J Am Vet Med Assoc 154:15.

Kray KT, et al (1985): Cromolyn sodium in seasonal allergic conjunctivitis. J Allergy Clin Immunol 76:623.

Krohne SDG, Vestre WA (1987): Effects of flunixin meglumine and dexamethasone on aqueous protein values after intraocular surgery. Am J Vet Res 48:420.

Legendre AM, et al (1982): Treatment of cryptococcosis with ketaconazole. J Am Vet Med Assoc 181:1541.

Legendre AM, et al (1984): Treatment of canine blastomycosis with amphotericin B and ketaconazole. J Am Vet Med Assoc 184:1249.

Leopold IH (1984): Glaucoma. In Sears ML (ed): Pharmacology of the Eye. Springer-Verlag, New York.

Lynch R, Rubin LF (1965): Salivation induced in dogs by conjunctival instillation of atropine. J Am Vet Med Assoc 147:511.

Mathews K, et al (1987): Renal failure in dogs associated with flunixin meglumine and methoxyflurane anesthesia. Vet Surg 16:323.

McDonald PJ, Watson ADJ (1976): Microbial flora of normal canine conjunctivae. J Sm Anim Pract 17:809.

McLaughlin SA, et al (1983): Pathogenic bacteria and fungi associated with extraocular disease in the horse. J Am Vet Med Assoc 182:241.

Moore CP (1986): Ocular microbial isolates from two groups of Southern Wisconsin horses. Proc Am Coll Vet Ophth 17th Ann Mtg, New Orleans, p 366.

Moore CP, et al (1983): Bacterial and fungal isolates from equids with ulcerative keratitis. J Am Vet Med Assoc 182:600.

Moore CP, et al (1983): Keratopathy induced by beta radiation in a horse. Equine Vet J Supp 2:112.

Moore CP, et al (1988) Prevalence of ocular microorganisms in hospitalized and stabled horses. Am J Vet Res 49:773.

Moriello KA (1986): Ketaconazole: Clinical pharmacology and therapeutic recommendations. J Am Vet Med Assoc 188:303.

Murphy JM, et al (1978): Survey of conjunctival flora in dogs with clinical signs of external eye disease. J Am Vet Med Assoc 172:66.

Murphy JM, et al (1979): Immunotherapy in equine sarcoid. J Am Vet Med Assoc 170:202.

Myers-Elliot RH, et al (1988): Effect of cyclosporine A on the corneal inflammatory response in herpes simplex virus keratitis. Exp Eye Res 45:281.

Nasisse MP, et al (1986): In vitro susceptibility of feline herpesvirus to inhibition by idoxuridine, vidarabine, trifluorothymidine, and acyclovir. Proc Am Coll Vet Ophth Proc 17th Ann Mtg, New Orleans, p 234.

Neaderland MH, et al (1987): Healing of experimentally induced corneal ulcers in horses. Am J Vet Res 48:427.

Newton C, et al (1988): Topically applied cyclosporine in azone prolongs corneal allograft survival. Invest Ophthalmol 29:208.

Owen RA, Jagger DW (1987): Clinical observations on the use of BCG cell wall fraction for treatment of periocular and other equine sarcoids. Vet Rec 120:548.

Paulsen ME, et al (1987): Nodular granulomatous episclerokeratitis in dogs: 19 cases (1973–1985). J Am Vet Med Assoc 190:1581.

Pedersen KB (1973): Excretion of some drugs in bovine tears. Acta Pharmacol et Toxicol 32:455.

Petrousos G, et al (1982): Effect of acetylcysteine (Mucomyst) on epithelial wound healing. Ophthalmic Res 14:241.

Prozesky L, et al (1977): Amaurosis in sheep resulting from treatment with rafoxanide. Onderstepoort J Vet Res 44:257.

Punch PI, et al (1985): Investigation of gelatin as a possible biodegradable matrix for sustained delivery of gentamicin to the bovine eye. J Vet Pharmacol Ther 8:335.

Punch PI, et al (1987): The use of plastic rings to determine the dimensions of ocular inserts for insertion into the conjunctival sac of cattle. J Vet Pharmacol Ther 10:85.

Regnier PL, et al (1982): Adrenocortical function and plasma biochemical values in dogs after subconjunctival treatment with methylprednisolone acetate. Res Vet Sci 32:306.

Riis RC (1981): Equine ophthalmology. *In* Gelatt KN (ed): Textbook of Veterinary Ophthalmology. Lea & Febiger, Philadelphia.

Roberts SM, et al (1984): Effect of ophthalmic prednisolone acetate on the canine adrenal gland and hepatic function. Am J Vet Res 45:1711.

Roberts SM, et al (1987): Ophthalmic complications following megavoltage irradiation of the nasal and paranasal cavities in dogs. J Am Vet Med Assoc 190:43.

Rowley RA, Rubin LF (1969): Penetration of penicillin into the aqueous humor of the dog. Am J Vet Res 30:1945.

Rubin LF, Gelatt KN (1967): Corneal epithelial sloughing in dogs with glaucoma. J Am Vet Med Assoc 151:1449.

Samuelson DA, et al (1984): Conjunctival fungal flora in horses, cattle, dogs, and cats. J Am Vet Med Assoc 184:1240.

Semrad SD (1985): Flunixin meglumine given in small doses: Pharmacokinetics and prostaglandin inhibition in healthy horses. Am J Vet Res 46:2474.

Sisodia CS, et al (1975): A pharmacological study of chloramphenicol in horses. Can J Comp Med 39:216.

Slatter DH, Severin GA (1975): Collagenase inhibitors in veterinary ophthalmology. Aust Vet Pract 5:174.

Slatter DH, et al (1982): Ocular inserts for application of drugs to bovine eyes—Effects of hydrophilic contact lenses. Aust Vet J 59:1.

Slatter DH, et al (1983): Ocular sequelae of high dose periocular gamma radiation in a horse. Eq Vet J Supp 2:110.

Slatter DH, et al (1985): Ocular inserts for application of drugs to bovine eyes—In vitro studies on the release of gentamicin from collagen inserts. Aust Vet J 62:79.

Smolin G (1985): Immunotherapy of herpetic infections. Int Ophthalmol Clin 25:165.

Smolin G, et al (1978): Treatment of herpetic keratitis with levamisole. Arch Ophthalmol 96:1078.

Spradbrow P (1968): The bacterial flora of the ovine conjunctival sac. Aust Vet J 44:117.

Urban W, et al (1972): Conjunctival flora of clinically normal dogs. J Am Vet Med Assoc 161:201.

Verwer MAJ, Gunnick JW (1968): The occurrence of bacteria in chronic purulent eye discharge. J Sm Anim Pract 9:33.

Watson ADJ (1974): Chloramphenicol in the dog: Observations of plasma levels following oral administration. Res Vet Sci 16:147.

Wilcox G (1970): Bacterial flora of the bovine eye with special reference to the Moraxella and Neisseria. Aust Vet J 46:253.

Wilson WD, et al (1987): Ormetoprim-sulfadimethoxine in cattle: Pharmacokinetics, bioavailability, distribution to the tears, and in vitro activity against *Moraxella bovis*. Am J Vet Res 48:407.

Yeary RA, Swanson W (1973): Aspirin dosages for the dog. J Am Vet Med Assoc 163:1177.

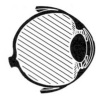

4

Ocular Inflammation and Ophthalmic Pathology

INFLAMMATION	GRANULOMATOUS	SEQUELAE OF INTRAOCULAR
IMMUNE PHENOMENA	INFLAMMATION	INFLAMMATION
NONGRANULOMATOUS		FIXATION
INFLAMMATION		

General principles of ophthalmic pathology are introduced in this chapter. Details of more common ocular diseases are included with clinical discussions in relevant chapters.

INFLAMMATION

Inflammation[1] is the response of tissue to a noxious stimulus. The response varies depending on whether the tissue is predominantly cellular (retina), extracellular products (vitreous, cornea), or a mixture (uvea, conjunctiva). Infection should not be confused with inflammation; although inflammation is often present with *infection,* inflammation may be present without infection. In certain altered immune responses, infection may be present without inflammation. Before summarizing the main features of inflammation, it is well to recall its clinical significance (Fig. 4–1) (Aronson and Elliott, 1972).

Structural alterations of ocular tissues due to inflammation are often the cause of visual loss. Inflammation may be divided into two phases: acute and chronic. Neutrophils and mononuclear phagocytes predominate in the acute phase, lymphocytes and mononuclear phagocytes in the chronic phase.

Although inflammation is a protective response, its consequences, although preserving the physical integrity of the eye, frequently result in complete or partial destruction of ocular function.

Acute Phase

The initial noxious stimulus causes release of many chemical mediators (histamine, serotonin, kinins, plasmin, complement system, prostaglandins, and the slow-reacting substance of anaphylaxis) that results in the cardinal signs of inflammation—heat, pain, swelling, redness, and loss of function. The release of these chemical mediators results in increased vascular permeability and vasoconstriction. Fluid from the vessels passes out between adjacent endothelial cells, leukocytes attach to endothelial walls and emigrate from the vessels, and erythrocytes pass between endothelial cells into the tissue spaces. In the eye, protein gains access to the aqueous (plasmoid aqueous) and is visible as an AQUEOUS "FLARE" when a focal light source illuminates the anterior chamber. If sufficient protein and fibrinogen escape, clots of fibrin may form in the anterior chamber. Release of leukocytes is usually seen clinically in the later stages of inflammation as a collection of yellowish material in the ventral anterior chamber called HYPOPYON (Fig. 4–2). Hypopyon is usually sterile and is a frequent result of inflammation of the anterior uvea (iris and ciliary body). Vasoconstriction gives way to vasodilatation very soon (5 minutes) after the injury, and blood flow to the area increases. Eventually the flow falls below normal because of increased viscosity caused by fluid loss through the vessel walls, which are more permeable than normal. During this acute phase, neutrophils attach to vessel walls (margination) and then move between endothelial cells at their junctions to leave the vessel (emigration). Red blood cells pass out of the vessels (diapedesis).

NEUTROPHILS move to sites of tissue damage by chemotaxis in response to lysozymal enzymes, complement, kinins, and bacterial products, and they remove bacteria and debris by phagocytosis and digestion by lysosomal enzymes. They soon die and release lysosomal

---

1. For further discussion, see Spencer WH: Ophthalmic Pathology, 3rd ed. WB Saunders, Philadelphia, 1985; and Yanoff M, Fine BS: Ocular Pathology, 2nd ed. Harper & Row, Philadelphia, 1982.

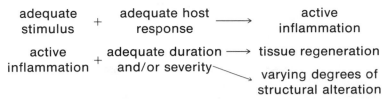

FIGURE 4–1. Features of inflammation.

enzymes, which cause tissue necrosis. Eosinophils and mast cells are also involved in the acute phase of inflammation. EOSINOPHILS increase in allergic states and especially in parasitic infestations. MAST CELLS and BASOPHILS release heparin and histamine in the initiation of hypersensitivity responses. MONONUCLEAR PHAGOCYTES (macrophages or histiocytes) are essential to wound healing, are the hallmarks of granulomatous inflammation, and in contrast to neutrophils, may proliferate in tissues. Macrophages have many functions including phagocytosis, cellular secretion, and antigen processing, and they act as an effector cell in the immune response.

Acute inflammation is characterized by outpourings of fluid and cells from the circulation through openings in the vascular endothelium (exudation). The type of exudate often determines the clinical appearance of the acutely inflamed eye:

1. SEROUS exudate, which is high in protein, causes aqueous flare **in the anterior chamber** (see p 87).

2. FIBRINOUS exudate is high in fibrin, and it is visible as a "plasmoid" (similar to plasma) or "plastic" aqueous.

3. PURULENT exudate contains neutrophils, some lymphocytes, and necrotic products; it is seen as hypopyon or KERATIC PRECIPITATES in the ventral portion of the anterior chamber, and it is usually sterile (Figs. 4–2 and 4–3).

4. SANGUINEOUS exudate is composed of red blood cells and often fibrin; it is visible in the anterior chamber as HYPHEMA.

Chronic Inflammation

Acute inflammation is rapid in onset and has a short duration with pronounced vascular changes. Chronic inflammation starts more slowly, lasts longer, and is both exudative and proliferative.

Two features may be observed: (1) exhaustion of local protective mechanisms, resulting in necrosis, extension of infection, local recurrence, or development of a chronic lesion; (2) restoration of normal structure, with healing and formation of granulation tissue. The degree of structural alteration present varies but frequently has important consequences for ocular function (e.g., a central corneal scar in a well-healed cornea [Fig. 4–4]).

Lysosomal enzymes released by neutrophils at the site of inflammation increase capillary permeability, cause tissue destruction, and activate kinins, which in turn stimulate mast cells to release histamine and induce chemotaxis of mononuclear phagocytes. Collagenases released from neutrophils and mononuclear cells cause digestion of tissues and further structural alterations (e.g., certain corneal ulcers). Bacteria such as *Pseudomonas* also produce collagenases.

In larger injuries that are too extensive for neutrophils and mononuclear cells to resolve, granulation tissue is laid down to repair the structure and limit spread of the disease process. Granulation tissue consists of fibroblasts, proliferating blood vessels, and leukocytes. Inflammation may become chronic because the initial stimulus persists (e.g., dead tissue, foreign body) or because of the presence of an immune or hypersensitivity reaction.

NONGRANULOMATOUS INFLAMMATION

This form of chronic inflammation is the most common, and it is characterized by the presence of lymphocytes and plasma cells, by which humoral and cell-mediated immunity are mediated.

CHRONIC GRANULOMATOUS INFLAMMATION

Granulomatous inflammation is characterized by the presence of EPITHELIOID CELLS and INFLAMMATORY

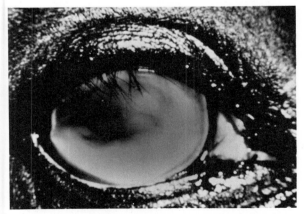

FIGURE 4–2. Sterile hypopyon in the ventral anterior chamber.

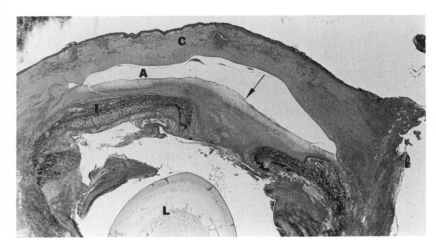

FIGURE 4–3. *Purulent exudate of neutrophils and fibrin (arrow) in the anterior chamber (A). C = cornea, I = iris, L = lens.*

(LANGHANS') GIANT CELLS, which are derived from mononuclear phagocytes. Considerable species variation is seen in the frequency of these cell types in chronic inflammation. The agents that cause granulomas have the following features:

1. Low-grade irritants cause a mononuclear infiltrate.

2. Normal inflammatory cells have difficulty digesting them—particulate materials, lipids (extravasated from sebaceous glands), complex microorganisms such as fungi (e.g., *Coccidioides immitis*), spirochetes, algae (*Geotricha* and *Prototheca* spp), protozoa, and helminths. Obligate intracellular bacteria often produce this reaction—*Mycobacteria* spp, *Listeria monocytogenes*, *Brucella* spp.

The clinical significance of identifying granulomatous inflammation is that it aids in the search for the etiology.

IMMUNE PHENOMENA

The functions of cellular immunity (delayed hypersensitivity) and humoral immunity are summarized in Figures 4–5 to 4–10. Virtually all kinds of cellular and humoral immune reactions may occur in the eye. These reactions are frequently modified by distinctive anatomical, physiological, and biochemical features of the eye (Rahi and Garner, 1976).

Immunoglobulin G (IgG) is the major circulating immunoglobulin active against microorganisms, and its level may remain elevated for long periods. IgM is predominantly an agglutinating and complement-fixing antibody. IgA is found in secretions, e.g., lacrimal, conjunctival, and salivary secretions, and on mucosal surfaces and is a first line of defense in bacterial and viral infections. IgE is an important mediator of hypersensitivity reactions and is found attached to the surface of basophils and mast cells.

Types of Ocular Hypersensitivity Reactions

TYPE I—IMMEDIATE OR ANAPHYLACTIC HYPERSENSITIVITY

The specific antibody, IgE, is located on the surface of mast cells and basophils, and it reacts with the

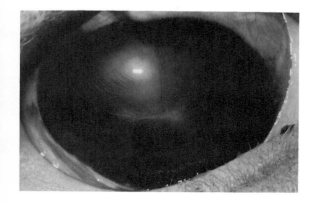

FIGURE 4–4. *A corneal scar. Collagen fibrils are laid down in an irregular manner, restricting the passage of light.*

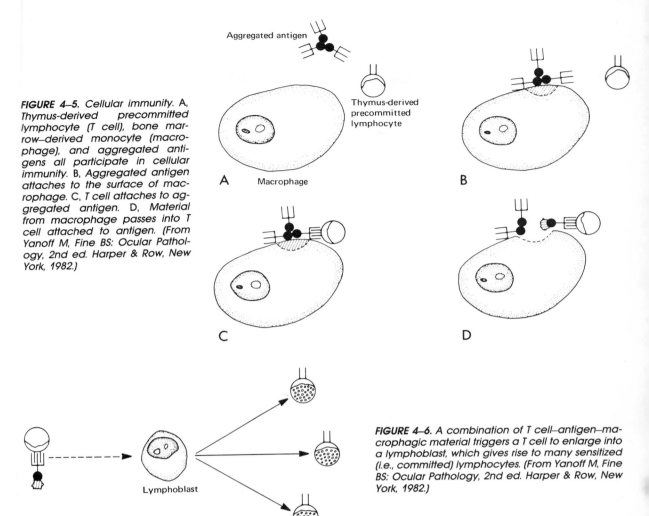

FIGURE 4–5. *Cellular immunity. A, Thymus-derived precommitted lymphocyte (T cell), bone marrow–derived monocyte (macrophage), and aggregated antigens all participate in cellular immunity. B, Aggregated antigen attaches to the surface of macrophage. C, T cell attaches to aggregated antigen. D, Material from macrophage passes into T cell attached to antigen. (From Yanoff M, Fine BS: Ocular Pathology, 2nd ed. Harper & Row, New York, 1982.)*

FIGURE 4–6. *A combination of T cell–antigen–macrophagic material triggers a T cell to enlarge into a lymphoblast, which gives rise to many sensitized (i.e., committed) lymphocytes. (From Yanoff M, Fine BS: Ocular Pathology, 2nd ed. Harper & Row, New York, 1982.)*

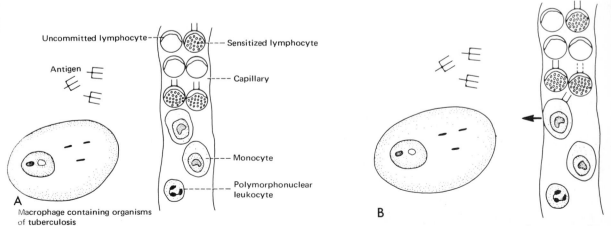

FIGURE 4–7. *Cellular immunity. A, Sensitized lymphocytes (SL) in capillary arrive with other leukocytes, including monocytes, at antigenic site where macrophage contains tubercle bacilli and antigens are present in surrounding tissue. B, Monocytes become sensitized by transfer of cytophilic antibody from SL and leave circulation to migrate toward antigenic stimulus. (From Yanoff M, Fine BS: Ocular Pathology, 2nd ed. Harper & Row, New York, 1982.)*

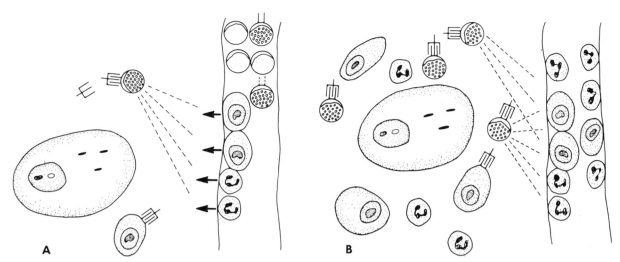

FIGURE 4–8. *A, SL encounter a specific antigen and release biologically active molecules that draw monocytes and other leukocytes to the area. B, When monocytes arrive at the site, they become immobilized by migration inhibition factor (MIF) released by SL. SL also release cytotoxin, which causes tissue necrosis (caseation), and mitogenic factor, which causes proliferation of cells, some of which undergo transformation into epithelioid cells; hence, tuberculoma is formed. (From Yanoff M, Fine BS: Ocular Pathology, 2nd ed. Harper & Row, New York, 1982.)*

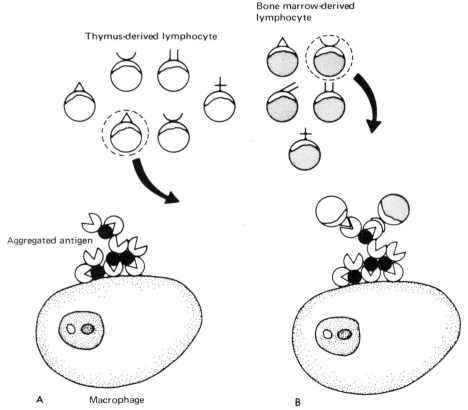

FIGURE 4–9. *Humoral immunoglobulin (anitibody). A and B show four prerequisites for immunoglobulin formation: thymus-derived lymphocyte (T cell); bone marrow–derived lymphocyte (B cell); bone marrow–derived monocyte (macrophage); and aggregated antigens. After aggregated antigens become attached to macrophages, T cell and B cell attach to different determinants on aggregated antigen. (From Yanoff M, Fine BS: Ocular Pathology, 2nd ed. Harper & Row, New York, 1982.)*

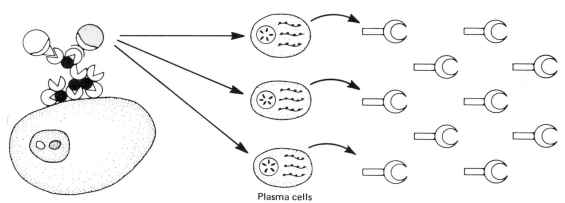

Immunoglobulin (antibody)

Plasma cells

FIGURE 4–10. *Synergistic action between T cell and B cell causes B cell to differentiate and proliferate into plasma cells. (From Yanoff M, Fine BS: Ocular Pathology, 2nd ed. Harper & Row, New York, 1982.)*

antigen, degranulates these cells, and releases mediators such as histamine, prostaglandin, serotonin, slow-reacting substance of anaphylaxis, and eosinophilic chemotactic factor. The reaction may be local, e.g., in the conjunctiva where it may be termed *atopy,* or systemic.

TYPE II—CYTOTOXIC HYPERSENSITIVITY

A cell becomes coated with antibody (IgG or IgM) because of antigens on its surface. The antibody activates the complement system and destroys the cell, or antibody-dependent cell-mediated toxicity destroys the cell. This type of reaction is seen in autoimmune diseases and tumor immunity and when viral antigens occur on cell surfaces.

TYPE III—IMMUNE COMPLEX–MEDIATED HYPERSENSITIVITY

Antigen-antibody complexes form and damage tissue primarily through activation of complement and its associated inflammatory changes. These complexes form either through circulation of soluble antigens combining with antibodies and depositing on blood vessel walls throughout the body or by a combination of soluble antigen with antibody in extracellular spaces.

TYPE IV—CELL-MEDIATED HYPERSENSITIVITY

This type of hypersensitivity is mediated by lymphocytes and macrophages rather than by antibodies, and it is important in allograft rejection, tumor immunity, contact hypersensitivity, microbial hypersensitivity, and some autoimmune diseases. Cell-mediated or delayed hypersensitivity requires 24–72 hours to develop.

TYPE V—STIMULATORY HYPERSENSITIVITY

Circulating antibody causes hyperplasia in target tissues containing a specific antigen, by activating cyclic AMP within the cell and inducing hyperplasia.

Avascularity and Isolation of Cornea and Lens

The healthy cornea is avascular; thus antigens within it, present as a result of exogenous infection, traumatic implantation, or transplantation, can reach lymphoid centers only in low concentration and with difficulty. Humoral antibodies and sensitized lymphocytes have similar difficulty in reaching these antigens. Descemet's membrane in the cornea is a barrier. The avascular lens, which is surrounded by a capsule and suspended in aqueous, is also isolated. Because the lens is isolated from the body by the lens capsule early in fetal development, it is not exposed to the developing immune system and its tissues are immunologically "foreign" in later life. Lens antigens are potent autoantigens in adult animals if released from the lens.

Absence of Ocular Lymphatic Drainage

Intraocular structures and the corneoscleral coat have no lymphatic drainage. Thus, antigens drain directly into the vascular system, rather than into regional lymph nodes, exposing immunologically competent cells in numerous sites throughout the body.

Blood-Aqueous and Blood-Retina Barriers

Under normal conditions, the vascular endothelium and two layers of ciliary epithelium limit passage of

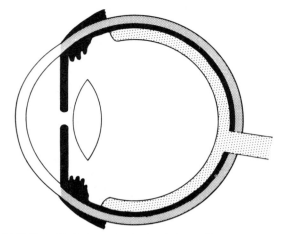

FIGURE 4–11. Immunological privilege. The cornea and lens, being avascular and devoid of lymphatics, enjoy a considerable measure of privilege. The retina also is largely impervious to lymphocytes and immunoglobulins, whereas the uvea and conjunctiva provide the principal centers of lymphoid activity. The sclera is intermediate in its propensity to manifest immunological reactions. (From Rahi AHS, Garner A: Immunopathology of the Eye. Blackwell, Oxford, 1976.)

immunoglobulins and cells into the aqueous (Fig. 4–11). The location of the blood-aqueous barrier varies for different substances, but it is probably due to zonulae occludentes (tight junctions) between the apical ends of nonpigmented ciliary epithelial cells. In inflammation these barriers are broken down, and cells and proteins may enter the aqueous.

The retina is separated from its vascular supply both by tight junctions between endothelial cells in the vessels supplying the inner retinal layers and by junctions between pigment epithelial cells between the retina and the choroid. "In the absence of vascular damage or defective pigment epithelium, immune reactions in the retina probably do not occur" (Rahi and Garner, 1976) (Table 4–1).

Immune Functions of Uvea and Limbus

The eye is not associated with local lymph nodes and, except for the conjunctiva, has no lymphatic drainage. Antigens are processed at distant sites, and sensitized lymphocytes move back to the eye to engage in humoral or cell-mediated immune responses depending on whether they are B or T lymphocytes. The mucopolysaccharide components of ocular basement membranes (Descemet's membrane, lens capsule) and the vitreous accumulate antigens. For this reason and because of vascular supply in these areas, lymphocytes gather in the uvea and limbus.

The majority of antibodies and sensitized lymphocytes produced in response to ocular antigens are produced in ocular tissues rather than in regional lymph nodes or other lymphoid tissues. After an episode of inflammation has subsided, "memory lymphocytes" remain in the uvea and ocular tissues. Further release

TABLE 4–1. Summary of Cellular and Tissue Reactions

Hypertrophy:	Increaase in the normal size of individual cells without an increase in the number of cells (e.g., hypertrophy of pigment epithelium) (Fig. 4–12).
Hyperplasia:	Increase in the number of cells in a tissue. Hypertrophy may occur concurrently. Hyperplasia does not progress indefinitely, and an equilibrium is eventually reached (e.g., hyperplasia of corneal epithelium in an epithelial facet after injury) (Fig. 4–13).
Aplasia:	Lack of development of a tissue during embryonic life.
Hypoplasia:	Arrested development of a tissue during embryonic life (e.g., optic nerve hypoplasia) (Fig. 17–19B).
Metaplasia:	Transformation of one type of tissue into another type.
Atrophy:	Diminution in size or shrinkage of cells, fibers, or tissues that had reached full development (e.g., progressive retinal degeneration or atrophy) (Fig. 4–14).
Dysplasia:	Abnormal growth or development of tissue during embryonic life (e.g., retinal dysplasia) (Fig. 4–15).
Neoplasia:	Unrestricted continuous increase in the number of cells in a tissue above a normal level (e.g., sebaceous adenoma of a tarsal gland) (Fig. 4–16 and Table 4–2).
Degeneration:	A secondary phenomenon resulting from previous disease in an adult tissue (e.g., corneal "mummification") (Fig. 4–17).
Dystrophy:	Primary, bilateral, genetically influenced disorder with distinct clinicopathological findings. The term **abiotrophy** is now used interchangeably with dystrophy.

Modified from Yanoff M, Fine BS: Ocular Pathology, 2nd ed. Harper & Row, New York, 1982.

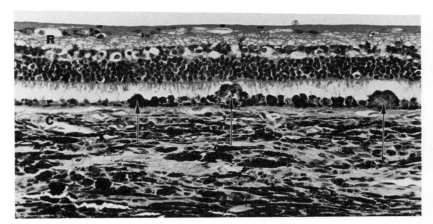

FIGURE 4–12. Hypertrophy of the pigment epithelium (arrows). R = retina, C = choroid.

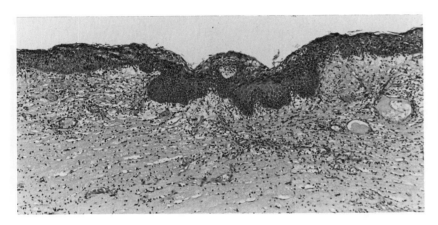

FIGURE 4–13. Epithelial facet with hyperplasia of the corneal epithelium after a superficial injury.

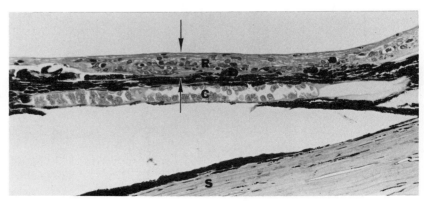

FIGURE 4–14. Progressive retinal degeneration (type I). Most layers are missing (between arrows). R = retina; C = choroid; S = sclera.

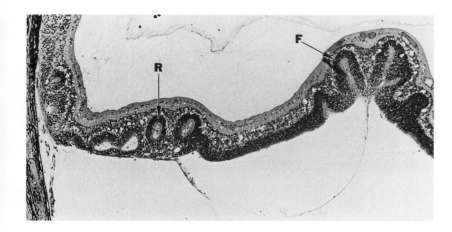

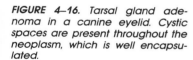

FIGURE 4–15. Retinal dysplasia in a shorthorn calf with cerebellar hypoplasia. R = rosette; F = fold.

FIGURE 4–16. Tarsal gland adenoma in a canine eyelid. Cystic spaces are present throughout the neoplasm, which is well encapsulated.

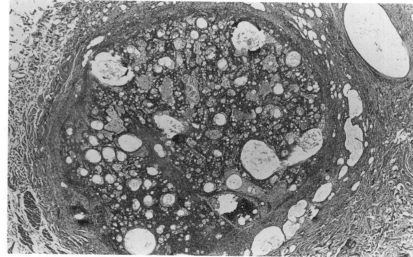

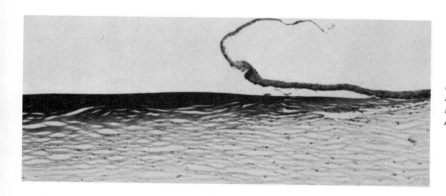

FIGURE 4–17. Feline corneal necrosis syndrome. (From Saunders LZ, Rubin LF: Ophthalmic Pathology of Animals. S Karger, Basel, 1975.)

TABLE 4–2. Differences Between Benign and Malignant Neoplasms

Factor	Benign	Malignant
Growth	Noninvasive; often surrounded by a capsule of compressed or fibrous tissue	Invasive and infiltrating
Spread	Does not metastasize	Has ability to metastasize (form secondary centers of neoplastic growth distant from the primary focus)
Cell appearance	Lack of anaplasia	Exhibits anaplasia (reversion to a primitive cell type with loss of adult characteristics, e.g., secretory activity)
	Nuclei and nucleoli small	Nuclei and nucleoli usually prominent
	Mitotic figures absent	Mitotic figures present
Necrosis	Absent	Often present because growth rate outstrips blood supply
Prognosis	Good	Guarded to poor, depending on biology of specific tumor type, site, and state of metastasis when treated

of antigens, either locally or in distant tissues, readily induces inflammation in the uvea. Thus uveitis is relatively common and may be associated with distant sources of antigen (e.g., prostatitis, pyometra, apical dental abscesses in dogs); its cause often remains undiagnosed.

NONGRANULOMATOUS INFLAMMATION

Nongranulomatous inflammation may be suppurative (pus-producing) or nonsuppurative. In acute suppurative inflammation the neutrophil is the predominant cell; this condition is often associated with bacterial infection or contamination. In acute nonsuppurative inflammation the neutrophil is still the predominant cell, but no purulent exudates are formed. In chronic nonsuppurative inflammation, lymphocytes and plasma cells predominate.

Terminology

Inflammations are named by the tissue(s) or ocular cavities involved:

lids—blepharitis
conjunctiva—conjunctivitis
cornea—keratitis
cornea and conjunctiva—kerato conjunctivitis
iris—iritis
ciliary—cyclitis
iris and ciliary body—iridocyclitis, anterior uveitis
choroid—choroiditis
choroid and ciliary body—posterior uveitis
iris, ciliary body, and choroid—anuveitis
sclera—scleritis
cornea and iris—keratouveitis
retina—retinitis
optic nerve—optic neuritis

If two tissues are involved and the primary site is in one tissue, the inflammation is named after the primary site (e.g., retinochoroiditis in toxoplasmosis, chorioret-

initis in recurrent equine uveitis). ENDOPHTHALMITIS is inflammation of one or more coats of the eye and adjacent cavities. PANOPHTHALMITIS is inflammation of all coats of the eye (fibrous, vascular, neural), often with spread to orbital tissues.

Suppurative Endophthalmitis and Panophthalmitis

These conditions are caused by either exogenous factors (e.g., penetrating foreign bodies) or endogenous factors (e.g., streptococcal or coliform septicemia), which include a variety of agents—retained foreign materials, bacteria, fungi, viruses, and algae. The clinical signs of endophthalmitis and panophthalmitis are similar.

1. Pain (orbital pain on pressure or on opening the mouth is also evident with panophthalmitis)
2. Severe conjunctival congestion
3. Opacity of cornea, anterior chamber, and vitreous
4. Miosis
5. Congestion and edema of lids and conjunctiva

Examples. Bovine malignant catarrhal fever, feline infectious peritonitis, *Aspergillus* endophthalmitis in turkeys, endophthalmitis after penetrating cat claw injuries in dogs, *Listeria* ophthalmitis in cattle and sheep.

Treatment. Treatment depends on the causative agent and is aimed at achieving high concentrations of appropriate antimicrobial drugs in affected tissues by systemic and local administration. The prognosis for endophthalmitis and panophthalmitis is always grave. Infectious processes occasionally progress to meningitis and encephalitis.

Nonsuppurative Endophthalmitis and Uveitis

This type of intraocular inflammation occurs frequently in clinical veterinary ophthalmology. Although the etiology may be endogenous or exogenous and the course may be acute, subacute, or chronic, the exact

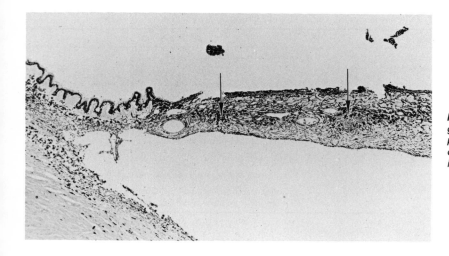

FIGURE 4–18. Nonsuppurative nongranulomatous inflammation after a penetrating injury (arrows). Numerous inflammatory cells are present in the iris stroma.

cause often remains undetermined even after histopathological examination.

The most common causes of acute nonsuppurative inflammation are penetrating and nonpenetrating trauma and inflammation secondary to corneal ulceration and injury. Anterior uveitis is a common sequel to corneal injury and is frequently mistaken clinically for an infectious process requiring radical therapy. This inflammation allows immunoglobulins and inflammatory cells to enter the aqueous and corneal stroma, promoting resolution of the corneal disease. Lympho-

---

Nonsuppurative nongranulomatous anterior uveitis is a frequent sequel to severe corneal disease and is not always detrimental.

---

cytes, plasma cells, monocytes, and occasional neutrophils are present in this form of inflammation.

Examples. Penetrating injuries of the globe (Fig. 4–18); endophthalmitis following traumatic proptosis of the globe; chronic idiopathic uveitis in dogs (Fig. 4–19); optic neuritis, retinitis, and conjunctivitis of canine distemper; uveitis and keratitis in infectious canine hepatitis; optic neuritis and retinitis in hog cholera (swine fever) (Figs. 4–20 and 4–21).

GRANULOMATOUS INFLAMMATION

Chronic granulomatous endophthalmitis and panophthalmitis are usually associated with etiologic agents—including foreign bodies, fungi (Fig. 4–22), resistant bacteria (e.g., tubercle bacilli, (Fig. 4–23), lens mate-

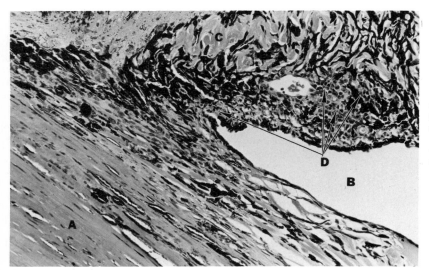

FIGURE 4–19. Nonsuppurative nongranulomatous uveitis (D) in a bassett hound that eventually developed unilateral secondary glaucoma. A = cornea; B = anterior chamber; C = iris.

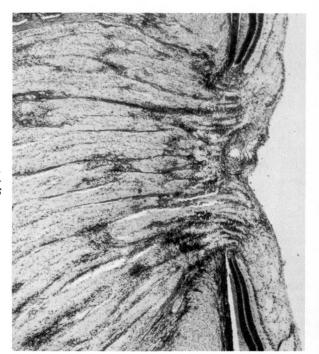

FIGURE 4–20. Optic neuritis, papilitis, and retinitis in a hog. The tissues are heavily infiltrated by glial cells. (From Saunders LZ, Rubin LF: Ophthalmic Pathology of Animals. S Karger AG, Basel, 1975.)

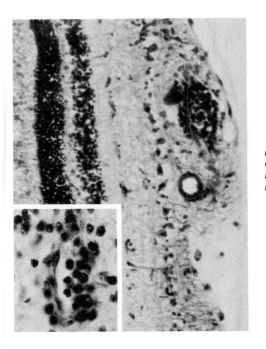

FIGURE 4–21. Retinitis in hog cholera. Perivascular cuffing with lymphocytes extending into a contiguous glial nodule. Inset: Endothelial swelling in a retinal vessel. (From Saunders LZ, Rubin LF: Ophthalmic Pathology in Animals. S Karger AG, Basel, 1975.)

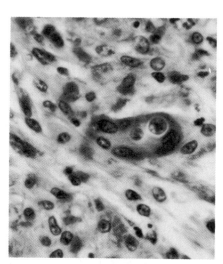

Fig. 4–22

Fig. 4–23

FIGURE 4–22. A giant cell containing a budding blastomycete in the optic nerve of a dog with ocular and systemic blastomycosis. (From Saunders LZ, Rubin LF: Ophthalmic Pathology in Animals. S Karger AG, Basel, 1975.)

FIGURE 4–23. A, Anterior segment from a calf with generalized tuberculosis. The anterior chamber is filled with caseous exudate, some of which has calcified (arrow). The iris and lens have been severely damaged by granulomatous inflammation. B, Higher magnification of A, showing invasion and destruction of the ciliary body. C, Higher magnification of B. The inner two thirds of the cornea are affected by chronic keratitis. Numerous confluent tubercles in the anterior chamber from a granulomatous mass that is diffusely adherent to the cornea. D, Typical Langhans' giant cells in a section of C. (From Saunders LZ, Rubin LF: Ophthalmic Pathology in Animals. S Karger AG, Basel, 1975.)

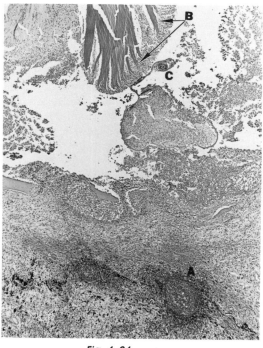

Fig. 4–24

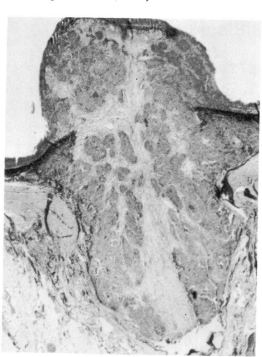

Fig. 4–25

FIGURE 4–24. Severe inflammation (A) associated with lens capsule rupture (phacoanaphylactic endophthalmitis) in a dog. Neutrophils, lymphocytes, and macrophages are dissecting between the lens fibers (B). The ruptured, coiled lens capsule is visible (C).

FIGURE 4–25. Giant cells containing extruded lens substance in a dog with phacoanaphylactic endophthalmitis after lens capsule rupture. (From Saunders LZ, Rubin LF: Ophthalmic Pathology in Animals. S Karger AG, Basel, 1975.)

rial after rupture of the capsule (Figs. 4–24 and 4–25), and algae—that have not been controlled by acute defense mechanisms.

> The epithelioid cell, derived from the macrophage, is the hallmark of granulomatous inflammation.

In addition to epitheloid cells, Langhans', Touton's, and foreign body giant cells may be observed. The reaction induced by lens proteins (lens-induced or phacoanaphylactic uveitis caused by hypersensitivity to the "foreign" proteins formerly sequestered within the lens capsule) is variable, and it is less severe in young animals. In older animals severe reactions are frequent, especially when bacterial contamination occurs with the injury (e.g., trauma by a cat's claw).

Experimentally, strongly antigenic adjuvants (bacterial toxins), when added to lens proteins, greatly enhance the subsequent inflammatory reaction. The reaction to lens proteins that leak out through the capsule (e.g., in spontaneous resorption of cataracts in dogs) is less severe but still very significant. This reaction is particularly significant in relation to post-operative inflammation after cataract surgery in dogs and horses.

> When lens proteins are released, either by lens capsule rupture or by leakage through an intact capsule, severe inflammation usually results.

When all eyes enucleated for endophthalmitis and glaucoma are examined histologically, penetrating injuries, with and without lens capsule rupture, are common in dogs.

SEQUELAE OF INTRAOCULAR INFLAMMATION

IRIS AND CILIARY BODY

The inflamed iris becomes engorged and swollen, and protein-rich fluid and cells enter the aqueous. Ciliary processes become edematous and may contain leukocytes. In the later stages these exudates may organize to form sheets of epithelial cells and fibroblasts stretching from the ciliary processes to the posterior surface of the lens—a CYCLITIC MEMBRANE. The iris may form an adhesion to the lens capsule (POSTERIOR SYNECHIAE) or to the corneal endothelium (ANTERIOR SYNECHIAE) (Fig. 4–26). If the pupil is bound to the lens and is immobile, it is referred to as a SECLUDED PUPIL. If the pupil is adhered around its circumference, aqueous builds up in the posterior chamber and pushes the iris forward (IRIS BOMBÉ), forcing the peripheral part of the iris against the peripheral posterior cornea. Drainage of aqueous to the trabecular meshwork is prevented and chronic secondary narrow-angle glaucoma results. This kind of glaucoma occurs frequently following severe intraocular inflammation in dogs.

In chronic inflammation the iris may atrophy, with loss of the dilator or sphincter muscle and the posterior pigmented epithelium. Contraction of a cyclitic membrane draws in the ciliar processes and may eventually detach the retina from the pigment epithelium at the ora ciliaris retinae. Although the pigment epithelium remains attached, its cells may hypertrophy. Atrophy and detachment of the ciliary body results in *hypotony* lowered intraocular pressure).

CORNEA

Chronic inflammation may damage the corneal endothelium, causing CHRONIC STROMAL EDEMA and a bluish appearance. Eventually, BULLOUS KERATOPATHY with accumulations of fluid may result. NEOVASCULARIZATION (new vessel penetration) and PIGMENTATION of the corneal stroma may also occur (Fig. 4–27). Chronic inflammation may also lead to deposits of

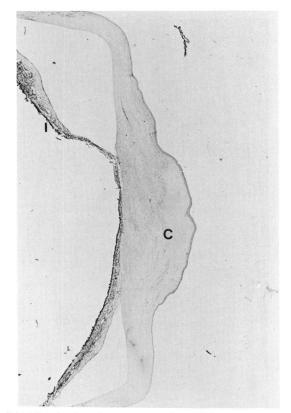

FIGURE 4–26. Anterior synechia with attachment of the iris (I) to the posterior (endothelial) surface of the cornea (C).

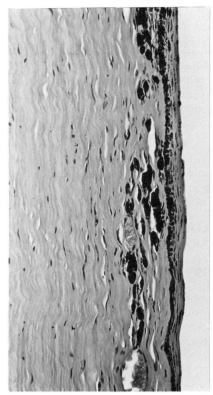

FIGURE 4–27. Neovascularization and pigmentation of the peripheral corneal stroma in a dog.

lipid and, especially in aged animals, calcium. Both lipid and calcium can stimulate further local inflammation. Keratic precipitates (accumulations of lymphocytes and plasma cells) may attach to the corneal endothelium; they are yellow and are frequently associated wtih granulomatous inflammation. Severe suppurative endophthalmitis may lead to corneal stromal abscess formation and rupture, with loss of intraocular contents.

LENS

The most common complication of ocular inflammation is CATARACT (opacity of the lens). The lens capsule is resistant but frequently degenerates in severe intraocular inflammation. Synechiae to the lens capsule may form (see the previous discussion). Deposition of cells, pigment, and fibrin frequently results. Small deposits of pigment are indicators of previous inflammation.

VITREOUS

Inflammatory cells may accumulate in the vitreous, with shrinkage, fibrous membrane formation, organization of the anterior vitreous, and retinal detachment. Large abscesses may form in the vitreous. Chronic inflammation may lead to liquefaction of the vitreous (SYNERESIS) or accumulations of lipid-calcium complexes (ASTEROID HYALOSIS).

CHOROID

Focal or diffuse areas of atrophy and scarring are a frequent sequel to choroiditis. Exudation of fluid or release of inflammatory cells in choroiditis may cause detachment of the overlying retina. The pigment epithelium is frequently destroyed, resulting in fusion of retina and choroid by scar tissue.

RETINA

Retinal perivasculitis and cuffing with lymphocytes occur commonly in intraocular inflammation, even when the inflammation occurs in parts distant from the retina (Fig. 4–28). Retinochoroiditis and chorioretinitis often cause local atrophy and scarring of the retina, usually with some proliferation of the pigment epithelium. Retinal detachment is frequently caused by traction by fibrous membranes in the vitreous or at the ora ciliaris retinae or by exudation of fluid or cells beneath the retina. Detachment occurs *between* the photoreceptor layer and the pigment epithelium and is *intraretinal.*

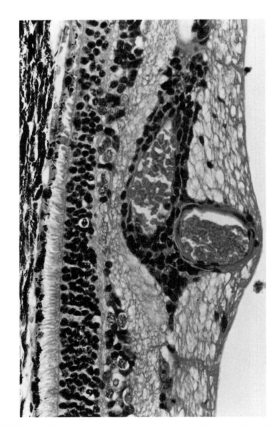

FIGURE 4–28. Retinal perivascular cuffing with lymphocytes.

GLAUCOMA

Glaucoma is characterized by *increased intraocular pressure* and follows inflammation if

1. cells and debris block the drainage angle.
2. peripheral anterior synechiae cause secondary angle closure (Fig. 4–29).
3. posterior synechiae and iris bombé cause angle closure.
4. inflammation and trabeculitis damage the trabecular meshwork in the drainage angle.

For pressure to rise, aqueous drainage must be affected, but the ciliary body must still be able to secrete sufficient aqueous to elevate the intraocular pressure. If the ciliary body is severely damaged, hypotony occurs.

FINAL STAGES OF SEVERE INTRAOCULAR INFLAMMATION

Three final stages may be reached:
1. atrophy without shrinkage
2. atrophy with shrinkage
3. atrophy with shrinkage and disorganization (phthisis bulbi)

In atrophy without shrinkage, the eye is normal in size but many ocular tissues are atrophic (e.g., iris, ciliary body, retina, optic disc). Vision is usually lost. This form is common when secondary glaucoma has been caused by the inflammation. In atrophy with shrinkage, the eye is small and soft, the cornea is frequently pigmented and vascularized, and the internal structure of the eye is well preserved. In atrophy with disorganization (PHTHISIS BULBI) the eye is small, internal structures are severely disorganized, sclera is thickened, cornea is opaque, and much of the ocular contents may be replaced by scar tissue. In severely damaged eyes with chronic atrophy, calcium may be deposited and intraocular ossification rarely occurs.

FIXATION

The method of fixation of globes for pathological examination can significantly affect the quality of sections produced. In order of preference, the fixatives are: glutaraldehyde (2%), Zenker's acetic acid fixative, and buffered neutral formalin (10%). Glutaraldehyde must be refrigerated for storage.

Clients should be advised that enucleated eyes should be submitted for histopathological examination.

REFERENCES

Aronson SB, Elliott JH (1972): Ocular Inflammation. CV Mosby Co, St Louis.
Duke-Elder S (1966): System of Ophthalmology, vol 9, Diseases of the Uveal Tract. H Kimpton, London.
Hogan MJ, Zimmerman LE (1962): Ophthalmic Pathology, 2nd ed. WB Saunders Co, Philadelphia.
Howes EL (1985): Basic mechanisms in pathology. *In* Spencer WHJ (ed): Ophthalmic Pathology, 3rd ed, vol 1. WB Saunders Co, Philadelphia.
Lillie RW (1965): Histopathologic Technic and Practical Histochemistry. McGraw-Hill, New York.
Rahi AHA, Garner A (1976): Immunopathology of the Eye. Blackwell, Oxford.
Saunders LZ, Rubin LF (1975): Ophthalmic Pathology of Animals. S Karger, Basel.
Silverstein AM (1975): Allergic reactions of the eye. *In* Gell PGH (ed): Clinical Aspects of Immunology, 3rd ed. Blackwell, Oxford.
Smolin G, O'Connor CR (1981): Ocular Immunology. Lea & Febiger, Philadelphia.
Yanoff M, Fine BS (1982): Ocular Pathology, 2nd ed. Harper & Row, New York.

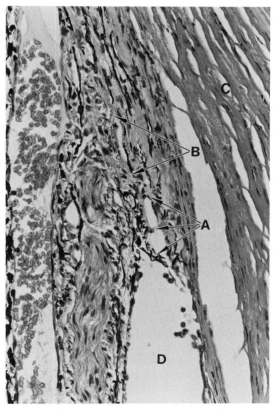

FIGURE 4–29. *Peripheral anterior synechiae* (A) *and secondary angle closure* (B). C = *cornea;* D = *anterior chamber.*

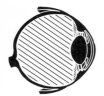

Basic Diagnostic Techniques

"We are constantly misled by the ease with which our minds fall into ruts of one or two experiences."—Sir William Osler

---

HISTORY	COLLECTION OF BACTERIAL	ELECTRORETINOGRAPHY
EXAMINATION PROCEDURE	AND FUNGAL SPECIMENS	ULTRASONOGRAPHY
ANESTHESIA AND RESTRAINT	SCRAPINGS	FLUORESCEIN ANGIOGRAPHY
FOR EXAMINATION	SCHIRMER TEAR TEST	EVALUATION OF VISION
LIGHT SOURCES	TESTS OF LACRIMAL PATENCY	SUMMARY OF TERMS
MAGNIFICATION	TONOMETRY	
VITAL DYES	TONOGRAPHY	OPTICS
OPHTHALMOSCOPY	GONIOSCOPY	NATURE OF LIGHT
THE NORMAL FUNDUS	BIOMICROSCOPY	PRISMS AND LENSES
RETINOSCOPY	RADIOGRAPHIC TECHNIQUES	

The aims of this chapter are to assist the reader in developing a systematic ocular examination procedure, to understand the nomenclature of the more common changes seen, and to understand the range and basic principles of more specialized diagnostic methods. A summary of terms is given in Table 5–5.

A basic eye examination is an essential part of a thorough physical examination and can be performed quickly and efficiently.

HISTORY

To use the problem-oriented approach, the clinician first determines the problems that have caused the owner to present the animal for examination. These problems are noted in the temporary problem list and often suggest further avenues of questioning when obtaining the history from the owner. By obtaining the history after the initial problems have been determined, one saves time and avoids the collection of historical data of little relevance. For instance, a knowledge of an animal's day and night vision over the past 3 months is rarely of significance to the treatment of traumatic proptosis of the globe, but it may be of considerable importance in the differential diagnosis of a chronic progressive visual disorder. A thorough, relevant history

is an important part of the diagnostic process. Although in many cases patients with ocular disorders are presented because of distinct symptoms, important ocular diseases are often detected during routine examination.

Questions that are often helpful include:

1. Is the animal experiencing visual difficulties? Are they worse at night or during the day? In familiar or unfamiliar environments?

2. How long have the visual problems been present? (A condition may be present for a considerable time before being noticed by the owner.) What were the circumstances in which the problem was first noticed (e.g., on return from boarding kennels)? Animals with severe visual deficits, who are adapted to their home environment, may "forget" when taken away, and on return their deficit is obvious. Visual problems may be manifested as colliding with or tripping over objects, reluctance to move, holding the head close to the ground, walking with a high-stepping gait, misjudging the flight of a ball, reluctance to move in the dark, or inability to pass through a gate or over steps.

3. Is the visual problem slowly improving or getting worse?

4. Is the visual deficit worse on one side than on the other?

5. Where does the animal live, and what is its diet?

6. Has the patient had any major diseases or injuries in the past?

7. Have there been any discharges from the eye? If so, what kind?

8. Has the affected eye been painful? If so, for how long and how has it been manifested (e.g., rubbing with a paw or along the ground, painful to touch, blepharospasm, reluctance to open the mouth or to eat, hiding beneath furniture, general malaise and depression, photophobia)?

9. Has the eye appeared more red than normal?

10. Has the eye appeared abnormal in any other way?

11. Has the animal's head or eye been subjected to any trauma recently?

12. Has the animal shown any behavioral or locomotor disturbances recently?

13. Have any of the animal's close relatives been affected with ocular disease? During the examination, heritable conditions present should be recorded (see Appendix I).

14. If the animal has already lost one eye, an attempt should be made to determine the cause of loss. This may be of considerable assistance in diagnosing the current problem and may affect the client's understanding of the disease and his or her reactions to proposed treatment.

EXAMINATION PROCEDURE

BASIC INSTRUMENTS AND SUPPLIES

Focusing penlight
Ocular magnifying loupe
Direct ophthalmoscope
Schirmer tear test strips
Fluorescein test strips
Schiøtz's tonometer
Tropicamide (1%)
Cotton
Eye wash
Sterile applicators for bacterial sampling

Early and correct diagnosis of ocular disorders is essential to a successful clinical result and a satisfied client.

An ophthalmic examination is conducted in subdued light, and preferably in a darkened room, to allow examination of intraocular structures without interference from reflections. Certain tests compromise later parts of the ocular examination; when these tests are indicated, they are performed before systematic examination of the eye.

Schirmer Tear Test. If keratoconjunctivitis sicca is suspected, this test is performed first because parasympatholytic drugs (mydriatics) and local anesthetics reduce values. Manipulative procedures such as conjunctival scrapings, flushing of lacrimal puncta, and fluorescein staining may result in artificially elevated values.

Bacterial Sampling. If indications for sampling are present, samples are taken next, on moistened swabs. Preservatives present in diagnostic drugs (e.g., fluorescein, local anesthetics, and mydriatics) prevent growth of bacteria on samples contaminated by the preservatives.

Direct and Consensual Pupillary Light Reflexes. These reflexes are evaluated before mydriatics or miotics are used.

Systematic Examination (Fig. 5–1)

The eye and periocular region are examined in normal light for gross abnormalities, including discharges, redness, swelling, periocular alopecia, deviations of the visual axes, nasal discharges or dryness, or asymmetry of any kind. During this initial inspection the animal may be spoken to by name and stroked to relieve its apprehension. If necessary, physical and chemical restraint may be applied. Tonic eye reflexes are then examined. As the head is elevated, depressed, and moved laterally, the eye should return to the center of the palpebral fissure.

1. Elevate and depress the head.

2. Move the head to the left and right.

3. Rotate the head clockwise and counterclockwise.

Examination in the dark is commenced with a magnifying loupe and focal light source (e.g., focusing penlight or Finnoff's transilluminator). The ocular structures are examined from anterior to posterior.

EYELID AND MARGINS

Magnification is necessary in order to examine the eyelid margins adequately. Look for

1. Entropion—lacrimal discharge, pain, epiphora, blepharospasm, pale discoloration, or excoriation of epidermis indicating contact with the tear film.

2. Ectropion—discharge, conjunctival erythema, malformation of the lower lid.

3. Epiphora—due to poor drainage or increased production of tears.

4. Disorders of the marginal cilia—epiphora, blepharospasm, pain, corneal ulceration, conjunctival erythema.

5. Ptosis—drooping of the upper lid.

6. Lack of palpebral reflex or asymmetry between palpebral fissures.

7. Blepharitis—discharge, swelling, alopecia, discoloration, erythema.

8. Blepharospasm—caused by local or intraocular pain or stimulation of the palpebral nerve.

THIRD EYELID

The third eyelid is extruded by pressing on the globe through the upper lid. It is everted under topical

OUTLINE OF OPHTHALMIC EXAMINATION PROCEDURE

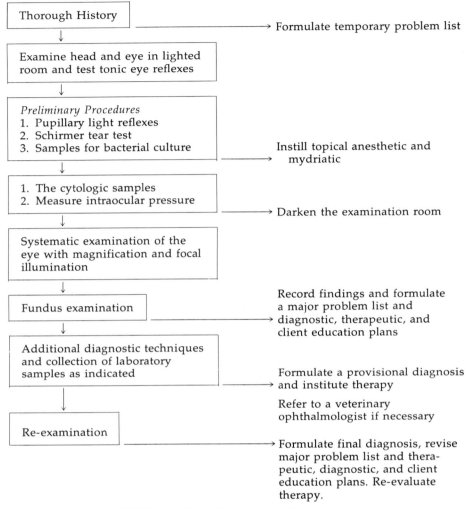

FIGURE 5–1. Ophthalmic examination procedure.

anesthesia with von Graefe's fixation forceps (see Fig. 6–29S). Look for

1. Prominence of the third eyelid—distinguish from lack of pigmentation of the margin.

2. Eversion of the margin.

3. Neoplasms—masses, erythema, irregularities of the margin, erosive lesions, epiphora.

4. Prolapse of the gland of the third eyelid.

5. Prominent follicles on either palpebral or bulbar surface.

6. Foreign bodies on the bulbar surface—epiphora, purulent discharges, blepharospasm, and conjunctival erythema associated with erosive corneal lesions.

7. Microphthalmia—a small globe or enophthalmos often results in apparent prominence of the third eyelid.

CONJUNCTIVA

1. Erythema—engorgement of superficial vessels is common in excited animals. Is the erythema constant or intermittent?

2. Chemosis (edema).

3. Discharges—mucopurulent, mucoid, serous, purulent, or dried exudates. Note whether gas bubbles are grossly visible in the accumulated exudate. Distinguish normal accumulations of mucus (gray) at the medial canthus in dogs with a deep inferior conjunctival fornix—Irish setter, Doberman pinscher—from abnormal discharges. Note any streaking or different colors within accumulated mucus.

4. Thickening of the conjunctiva associated with chronic inflammation.

5. Subconjunctival hemorrhage or emphysema. Resorbing hemorrhages are yellow.

6. Masses and nodules.

7. Hyperplasia of lymphoid follicles.

CORNEA

The normal cornea is transparent and avascular.

1. Loss of transparency may be caused by

a. Disorganized collagen in scar formation—nebula, macula, leukoma.

b. Corneal edema.

c. Pigment.

d. Infiltrates within the corneal stroma (e.g., cholesterol crystals, diffuse lipid droplets, virus particles).

e. Cellular infiltrates.

2. Vascularization is one of two types

a. Superficial—a tree-like or arborizing pattern.

b. Deep—shorter, deeper red, brush-like straight vessels near the limbus.

3. Changes in contour

a. Keratoconus, keratoglobus, cornea plana.

b. Increase in corneal diameter.

c. Depressions in the corneal stroma, giving a pitted appearance (similar to an orange peel), which is covered with epithelium (fluorescein negative).

d. Ulceration—stain all red, painful eyes with fluorescein.

SCLERA

1. Decrease in thickness (ectasia)—the vascular pigmented uveal tract appears blue through a thin sclera. Large nodular protrusions alter the scleral symmetry and shape if large areas are ectatic because of either primary scleral disease or an expanding intraocular lesion. Thinning of the entire sclera (total ectasia) is usually associated with buphthalmos and uncontrolled glaucoma. If stretching involves both the fibrous coat (sclera or cornea) and the underlying uvea, it is termed a STAPHYLOMA.

2. Focal nodules beneath the bulbar conjunctiva.

3. Rupture of the sclera—usually associated with a history of recent trauma. Most ruptures occur near the equator, although limbal ruptures are frequent in horses. Ocular contents (especially iris, lens, and vitreous) may protrude from the rupture.

4. Inflammation and erythema—usually associated with overlying conjunctival disorders.

5. Pigmentation of the sclera (e.g., blue or dark brown)—melanosis, neoplasm; yellow indicates resorbing hemorrhage.

LACRIMAL SYSTEM

1. Epiphora—moistening of the skin next to the eyelid margins or ventrally from the medial canthus.

Chronic epiphora may be associated with brown staining of the hair by pigments in the tears.

2. Negative fluorescein test (see p 95).

3. Occlusion of the puncta (tested by cannulation).

4. Abscessation or purulent dermatitis near the medial canthus.

5. Chronic purulent ocular diseases of any apparent cause.

6. Chronic accumulation of mucus in the conjunctival sac.

7. Corneal vascularization.

8. Corneal pigmentation.

9. Extreme drying, epithelial exfoliation, and keratinization around the external nares (usually unilateral and associated with chronic ipsilateral ocular disease).

10. Lagophthalmos—inability to close the lids completely. Lagophthalmos in brachycephalic breeds results in increased loss of precorneal tear film by evaporation.

ANTERIOR CHAMBER

1. Alterations in depth (distance between the corneal endothelium and the anterior surface of the iris, estimated subjectively in clinical practice)

a. Increased—associated with posterior lens luxation, microphakia (small lens), chronic glaucoma with iris atrophy. In some dog breeds and in the cat, the anterior chamber is naturally deep.

b. Decreased—anterior lens luxation, anterior uveal tumors, iris bombé and narrow-angle glaucoma, chronic anterior uveitis, anterior synechiae, foreign bodies.

2. Abnormal contents

a. Hypopyon—purulent material (usually neutrophils, lymphocytes, macrophages, and plasma cells) in the lower anterior chamber.

Hypopyon should not be "drained."

---

b. Hyphema—blood in the anterior chamber. Note whether it is clotted, free, or associated with fibrin or hypopyon.

c. Fibrin—yellow or brownish.

d. Foreign bodies—gonioscopy may be necessary to find them. If a perforating wound of the cornea or sclera is present, a search for the foreign body is made.

e. Abnormal tissues—iris cysts, tumors, anterior synechiae, persistent pupillary membranes.

f. Keratic precipitates (KPs)—yellowish focal cellular deposits on the corneal endothelium, associated with uveal inflammation.

g. Aqueous flare—cloudiness or turbidity of the aqueous when illuminated with a narrow beam of light, caused by the presence of protein, cells, pigment granules, and crystals. Flare is often visible only with a slit lamp (p 109) and is a valuable sign of inflammation even in the absence of other signs.

    3. Filtration angle

        a. Narrow (or closed) angle.

        b. Open angle.

IRIS AND PUPIL

    1. Congenital conditions of little visual significance

        a. Polycoria—more than one complete pupil.

        b. Coloboma—sector defects in the iris.

        c. Iris cysts—translucent bodies in the anterior chamber.

        d. Heterochromia iridis—the iris may be wholly or partly blue.

        e. Corectopia—eccentric pupil.

    2. Congenital conditions of visual significance

        a. Persistent pupillary membranes.

    3. Size and reactions of the pupil

        a. Mydriasis—dilated.

        b. Miosis—constricted.

        c. Anisocoria—pupils of different sizes.

        d. Hippus—physiological rhythmic constriction and dilatation of the pupil.

        e. Iridodonesis—fluttering of the iris margin in aphakia, lens luxation, or subluxation.

        f. Lack of pupillary light reflexes. The direct pupillary reflex of the cat is the fastest of the domestic animals. When illuminated by a bright penlight, the pupil of the normal dog contracts 2–3 mm; however, this may be inhibited in a frightened dog by epinephrine release. The normal equine pupil in bright sunlight is a horizontal slit that dilates to become almost circular in a darkened room. It constricts slowly in response to a bright light. The pupils of the cow and sheep are similar in shape to those of the horse, but the reflex is more rapid.

        g. Synechiae binding one part of the iris may cause a pupil of elliptical, tear-drop, or irregular shape when the iris dilates or contracts.

    4. Position of the iris

        a. Synechiae.

        b. Occluded pupil—obstruction of the pupil by a pupillary membrane (an acquired membrane across the pupil).

        c. Secluded pupil—annular posterior adhesion resulting from iritis and separating the anterior from the posterior chamber (Fig. 5–2).

        d. Pupillary block—resistance to the passage of aqueous between the pupillary border of the iris and the anterior lens capsule.

    5. Change in appearance

        a. Iris atrophy—iris stroma is more transparent.

        b. Erythema—vessels within the iris stroma may become engorged and impart a pinkish appearance in pale eyes.

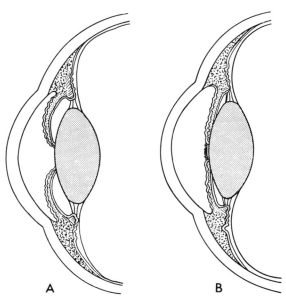

FIGURE 5–2. A, *Secluded pupil with annular synechia causing iris bombé.* B, *Occluded pupil with total posterior synechia. (From Trevor-Roper PD: The Eye and Its Disorders. Blackwell, Oxford, 1974.)*

        c. Neovascularization—growth of small vessels on the surface of the iris (rubeosis iridis).

        d. Decreased light reflectivity—the iris has a "muddy" or dull appearance when inflamed.

        e. Darkening in color of the iris.

        f. Leucocoria—white pupil due to a tissue mass behind the lens.

LENS

    1. Size

        a. Aphakia—lack of lens.

        b. Microphakia—small lens.

        c. Spherophakia—spherical lens.

        d. Lenticonus and lentiglobus—cone-shaped and globoid deformations of the lens capsule.

    2. Position

        a. Luxation—the lens is completely displaced from the hyaloid fossa.

        b. Subluxation—the lens is partially displaced from the hyaloid fossa.

        c. Anterior—the lens may push the iris forward, causing a shallow anterior chamber; or it may luxate completely into the anterior chamber, where it is readily visible.

        d. Posterior—the anterior chamber is deeper, iridodonesis is usually present, and an aphakic crescent may be seen. An aphakic crescent is the portion of fundus visible between the edge of a displaced lens and the pupillary border of the iris (Fig. 5–3)

    3. Cataract—a lens opacity. Cataracts of various types are discussed in Chapter 14. They must be

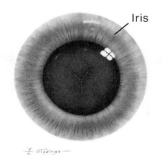

Iris

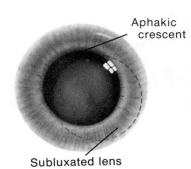

Aphakic crescent

Subluxated lens

FIGURE 5–3. The aphakic crescent seen with lens luxation or subluxation.

distinguished from NUCLEAR SCLEROSIS (p 370), which is a normal aging change.

4. Ruptures and tears of the lens capsule. Opacities within the lens may be localized with a focal light beam shone obliquely into the lens. Presence of the lens can be verified by the PURKIN-SANSON IMAGES, of which three can be usually seen—the corneal, anterior lens capsule, and posterior lens capsule (Fig. 5–4). Parallax and the relative motion of objects when viewed with the light from different oblique angles can be used to localize visible objects with the eye (Fig. 5–5).

VITREOUS

1. Congenital abnormalities
   a. Persistent hyaloid artery or its remnants (p 397).
   b. Persistent hyperplastic primary vitreous (PHPV)—seen as an opacity behind the lens, with blood vessels penetrating the lens (p 397).
   c. Bergmeister's papilla over the optic disc (p 20).
   d. Mittendorf's dot on the posterior lens capsule.
2. Acquired conditions
   a. Asteroid hyalosis—hyperreflective, small dots fixed in position in the vitreous.

b. Synchysis—liquefaction of the vitreous. Often associated with retinal detachment, extensive ocular inflammation, and lens luxation.

c. Synchysis scintilans—small, hyperreflective, mobile opacities (lipid-calcium complexes) in the vitreous, giving a "falling-snow" effect.

d. Inflammatory exudates.

e. Vitreous hemorrhages.

f. Vitreous haze—often found with severe inflammation of the ciliary body, choroid, retina, optic nerve, or vitreous.

g. Traction bands—narrow bands of contracting fibrous tissue within the vitreous, usually attached to the retina.

RETINA

1. Changes in color
   a. Increased tapetal reflectivity (p 417).
   b. Pigmentation over the tapetum.
   c. Loss of pigment or pigmentation in the nontapetal area.
   d. Exudates within the retina.
   e. Hemorrhages within, over, or under the retina (pp 418–419).

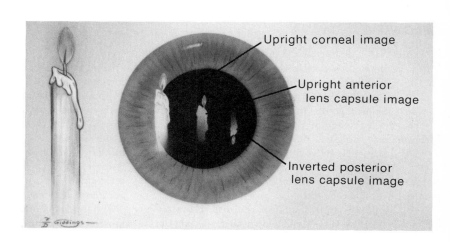

Upright corneal image

Upright anterior lens capsule image

Inverted posterior lens capsule image

FIGURE 5–4. Purkinje's images.

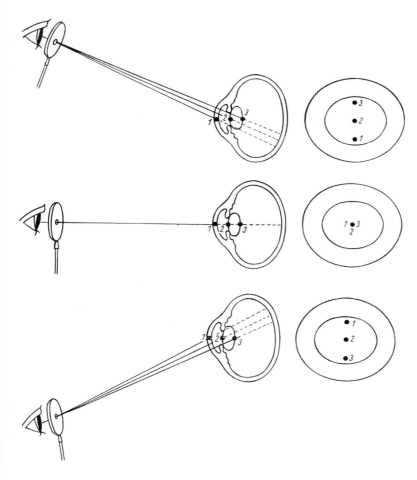

FIGURE 5–5. *The use of parallax to localize intraocular opacities. 1, Corneal opacity. 2, Cataract on anterior lens capsule. 3, Cataract on posterior lens capsule. The pupil is dilated for this examination. (From Komar G, Szutter L: Tierarztliche Augenheilkunde. Paul Parey, Publishers, Berlin, 1968.)*

2. Changes in general appearance
    a. Retinal detachment—complete or partial.
    b. Retinal vessel attenuation.
    c. Retinal tears.

For a more detailed discussion of retinal disorders, many of which have a characteristic appearance, see Chapter 16.

OPTIC NERVE

1. Excavative lesions of the optic disc
    a. Colobomas—optic disc or surrounding tissue.
    b. Glaucomatous cupping of the nerve head.
2. Vascular changes
    a. Hemorrhages on the disc.
    b. Engorgement or proliferation of capillaries in inflammatory disorders.
3. Primary optic nerve alterations
    a. Myelination of the nerve fiber layer of the retina, appearing as an extension of the whitish disc material over adjacent retina.
    b. Swelling (papilledema) of the disc, characterized by a bend as vessels pass down over the edge of the disc onto the adjacent retina.

    c. Atrophy—the disc is smaller and is white or pale gray in color; the disc capillaries are diminished. The lace-like lamina cribrosa may be visible on the surface if atrophy is advanced.

After examination of the anterior segment, mydriatic drops are instilled if ophthalmoscopic examination of the fundus is to be performed. A skilled examiner can often perform this examination through a partly dilated pupil by indirect ophthalmoscopy. Mydriatics take about 20 minutes to dilate the pupil. During this time the lacrimal puncta may be flushed, if indicated by epiphora.

Intraocular pressure (IOP) is determined by Schiøtz tonometry after administering topical local anesthesia. Calibration tables for use with human patients supplied with the instrument are more accurate than are veterinary versions. Breeds predisposed to glaucoma (e.g., basset hound, cocker spaniel) should receive sympathomimetic mydriatics such as phenylephrine 10%, which is reversible with parasympathomimetic miotics (e.g., pilocarpine 4%, echothiophate [Phospholine iodide] 0.25%) if IOP rises.

The fundus is examined systematically with a direct ophthalmoscope, and significant findings are recorded (Fig. 5–6). During the examination, the clinician may

OPHTHALMOLOGY

Date:_____ Clinician:_____
Referring
Veterinarian:_____

Telephone:_____

History:_____
_____
_____
_____

RIGHT EYE	LEFT EYE
Reflexes: ☐ Direct: ☐ Consensual	Reflexes: ☐ Direct: ☐ Consensual
Schirmer 1:____ mm/min Schirmer 2:____ **mm/min**	Schirmer 1:____ mm/min Schirmer 2:____ mm/min
Microbiology ☐ Cytology ☐	Microbiology ☐ Cytology ☐
I.O.P. Schiøtz ____ / ____ / ____	I.O.P. Schiøtz ____ / ____ / ____
reading / wt. / mmHg	reading / wt. / mmHg
Applan._____ mmHg	Applan._____ mmHg

1. Eyelids_____

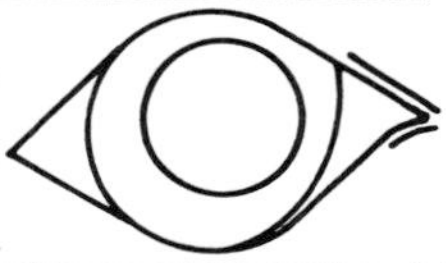

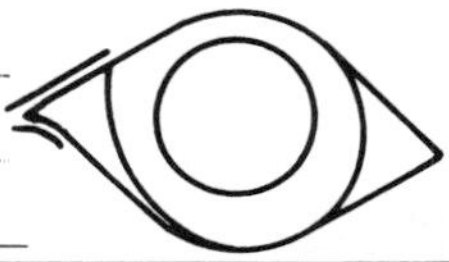

2. Lacrimal_____

3. Conjunctiva_____

4. Cornea_____

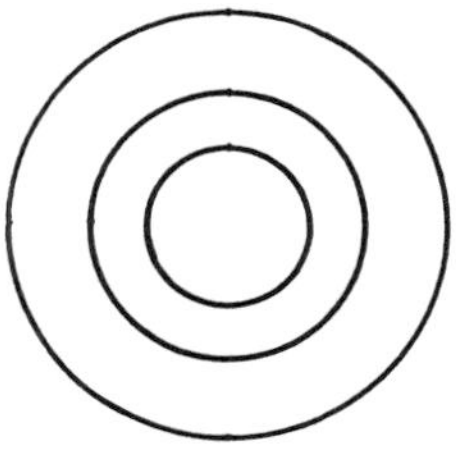

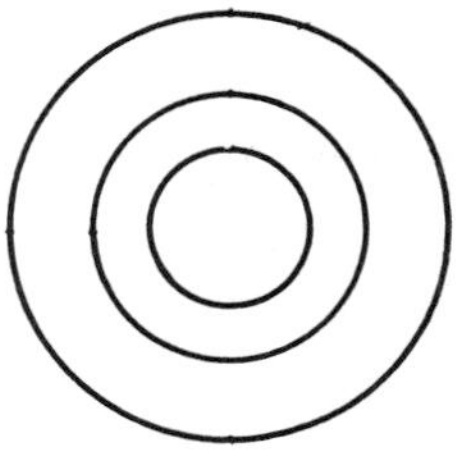

Fluorescein ( ) (±)

Fluorescein ( ) (±)

OPHTHALMOLOGY

FIGURE 5–6. Sample of an ophthalmic examination sheet.

Illustration continued on following page

RIGHT EYE	LEFT EYE

5.   Anterior Chamber and Drainage Angle

_____

_____

(   )   Gonioscopy

5.   Anterior Chamber and Drainage Angle

_____

_____

(   )   Gonioscopy

6.   Pupil and Iris _____

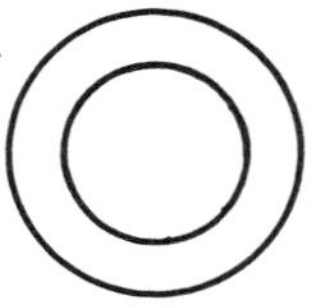

_____

_____

6.   Pupil and Iris _____

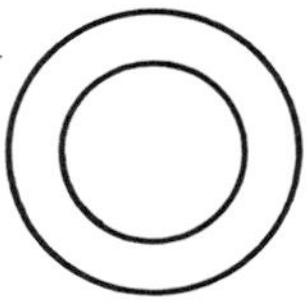

_____

_____

7.   Lens _____

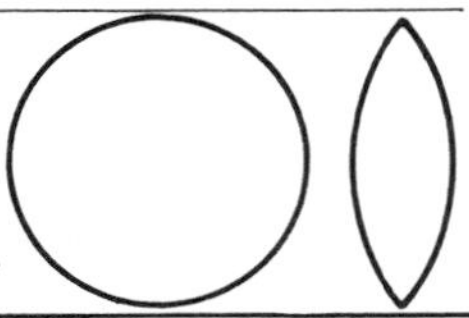

_____

_____

_____

7.   Lens _____

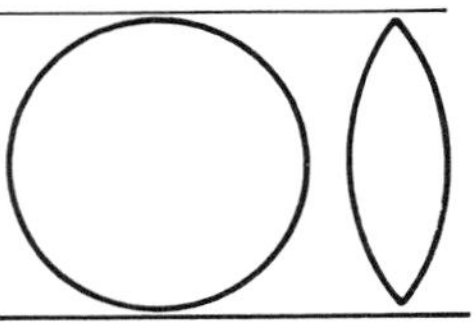

_____

_____

_____

8.   Fundus and Vitreous _____

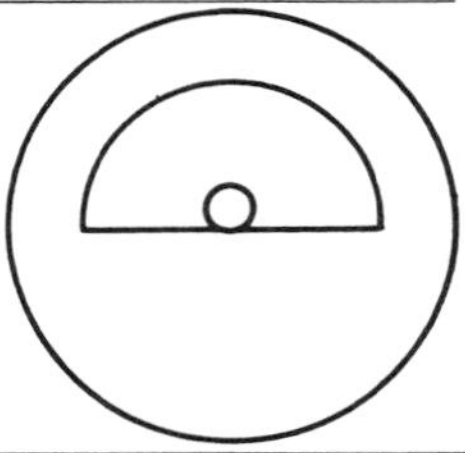

_____

_____

_____

_____

8.   Fundus and Vitreous _____

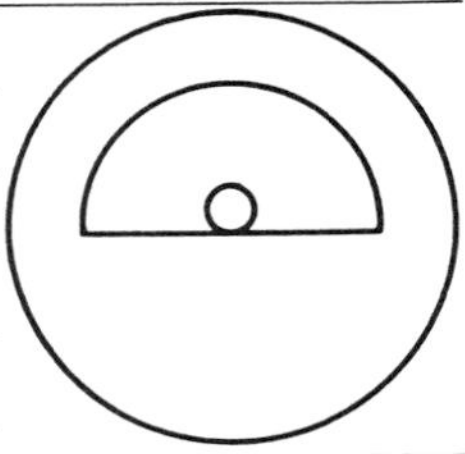

_____

_____

_____

_____

9.   Special Procedures   (   ) ERG   (   ) Photo

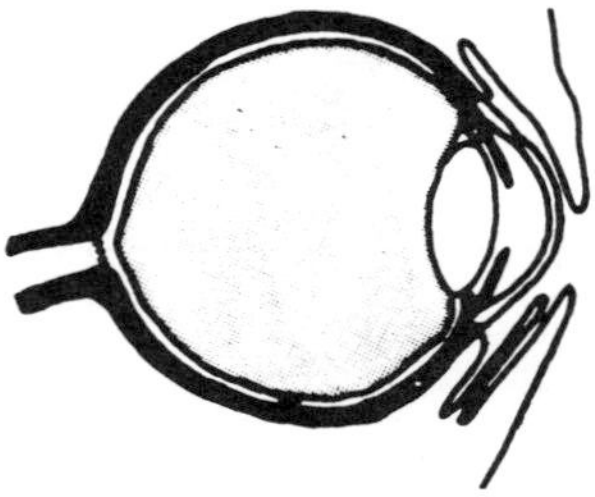

9.   Special Procedures   (   ) ERG   (   ) Photo

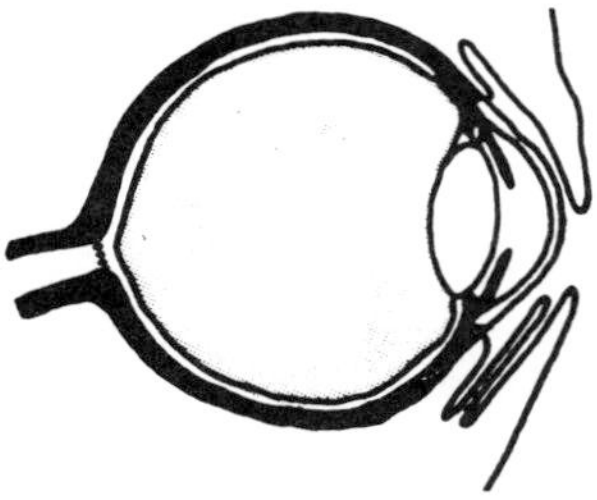

PRELIMINARY PROBLEM LIST	PLANS

1. _____
2. _____
3. _____
4. _____
5. _____

1. _____
2. _____
3. _____
4. _____
5. _____

OPHTHALMOLOGY

FIGURE 5–6 Continued

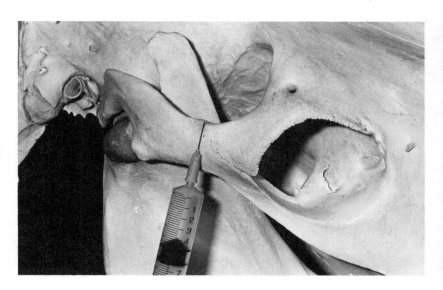

FIGURE 5–7. Injection site for blocking the auriculopalpebral nerve in the horse. Inject 5 ml of lidocaine with epinephrine where the nerve crosses the zygomatic arch.

recall common hereditary or acquired disorders to which the breed of animal is predisposed (see Appendix I). For example, a young Afghan hound presented with unilateral corneal opacity and ocular enlargement (buphthalmos) should prompt further questioning about recent vaccinations, because sight hounds are susceptible to glaucoma secondary to postvaccinal ocular reactions to live hepatitis viruses, both attenuated and virulent.

Indications for more specialized diagnostic techniques performed by a veterinary ophthalmologist (e.g., electroretinography, gonioscopy, slit-lamp biomicroscopy, indirect ophthalmoscopy, fluorescein angiography, and contrast radiography) are noted. If such indications are present, or specialist care is required, the situation must be discussed with the owner.

ANESTHESIA AND RESTRAINT FOR EXAMINATION

Dog

Most dogs may be examined without chemical restraint. In the occasional uncooperative patient, tranquilization with ketamine/diazepam, fentanyl/droperidol, or acepromazine[1] may be useful. With acepromazine, the third eyelid protrudes and may cover the pupil, which inconsistently becomes miotic. Before administration of all tranquilizers, first dilate the pupil with topical atropine 1%. In some animals, general anesthesia, using an ultra–short-acting barbiturate (thiamylal[2] or thiopental[3]), may be necessary, but the eye must be physically mobilized, because under anes-

thesia it is directed ventromedially (the reversed Bell phenomenon). Ketamine/diazepam causes this phenomenon less often than other drugs and is usually preferable. Most tranquilizers and anesthetics decrease IOP and Schirmer tear test readings. Local anesthesia of the auriculopalpebral nerve is rarely used in dogs.

Cat

Although rarely required, intramuscular (IM) ketamine is useful, as are intravenous (IV) ketamine/diazepam and ultra–short-acting barbiturates. Ketamine may elevate IOP by increasing tension in the extraocular muscles, and it is contraindicated when penetrating wounds of the eye are present.

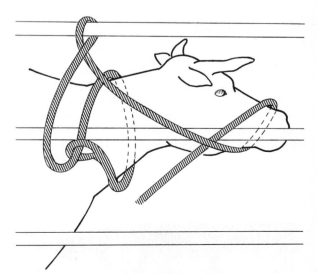

FIGURE 5–8. Method of restraining a cow for ocular examination. (Courtesy of Dr. A. C. Bryant.)

---

1. Acetylpromazine—Ayerst Laboratories, New York, NY.
2. Surital—Parke-Davis, Morris Plains, NJ.
3. Pentothal—Abbott Laboratories, North Chicago, IL.

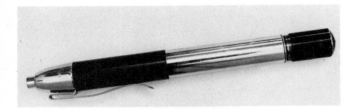

FIGURE 5–9. The Welch Allyn focusing penlight.

Horse

A twitch is frequently indispensable for ocular examination. In intractable animals, xylazine (Rompun; 1 mg/kg IV) quiets the horse and lowers the head and eye. The addition of 5–10 mg of acepromazine to the Rompun enhances tranquilization but causes some horses to lie down. With Rompun, local anesthesia of the auriculopalpebral nerve is less frequently required. It is still useful for preventing spasm of the orbicularis oculi muscle by the patient (Fig. 5–7). (*Note*: Anesthesia of this nerve abolishes motor supply of the muscle, but not ocular sensation.) Lid retractors (Fig. 6–29Z), held by an assistant, are useful in examining the equine eye.

Cattle, Sheep, Goats

Nose tongs and a suitable crush or race or physical restraint method are usually sufficient in cattle (Fig. 5–8). Xylazine (Rompun) is less useful in cattle, as it tends to cause recumbency, but anesthesia of the auriculopalpebral nerve is useful. Chemical restraint is rarely required for ocular examination of sheep and goats.

LIGHT SOURCES

A simple penlight with bright illumination is useful, although a focusing lens is worthwhile (Fig. 5–9). A Finnoff transilluminator attached to an ophthalmoscope handle is useful (Fig. 5–10). A blue filter may be attached to these instruments in order to observe lesions stained with fluorescein. Through the dilated equine pupil, the fundus can be viewed directly with a light source in which the light beam and the observer's visual

axis are parallel (Fig. 5–11). In TRANSILLUMINATION a bright light source is placed on the sclera slightly posterior to the limbus (Fig. 5–12). Light passes through the sclera and outlines the ciliary body and any opaque structures such as ciliary body and iris tumors, foreign bodies, or exudates within the eye. A darkened room is necessary for transillumination.

MAGNIFICATION

Magnification is essential for accurate ophthalmic observation and diagnosis. The most useful instrument for general practice is a simple magnifying loupe with a power of 2× to 4× and a focal length of 15–25 cm (6–10 inches) (Fig. 5–13). Many sophisticated optical instruments combining magnification and illumination (e.g., head-mounted fiberoptic magnifying loupe, slit-lamp biomicroscope) are available if required. For accurate treatment of some ocular disorders such as distichiasis, an operating microscope is essential. These instruments are usually available to specialist veterinary ophthalmologists, skilled and trained in their use.

VITAL DYES

Vital dyes stain living tissues. Fluorescein and rose bengal are the most commonly used.

Fluorescein

Fluorescein is a water-soluble dye that does not stain normal cornea because it does not pass the hydrophobic epithelium. If the epithelium is incomplete, fluorescein

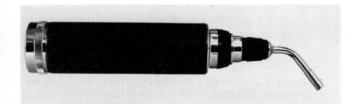

FIGURE 5–10. A Finnoff transilluminator and ophthalmoscope handle.

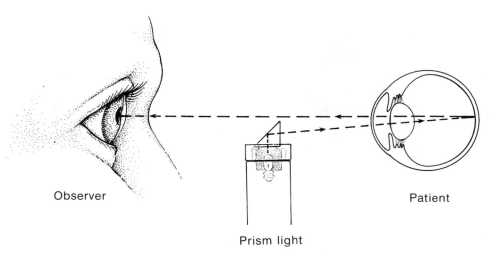

FIGURE 5–11. Examination of the equine fundus with a prism light.

penetrates the hydrophilic corneal stroma and stains it bright green. The green color is best excited with blue light from a cobalt filter attached to a penlight or Finnoff transilluminator. A wood light may also been used. Fluorescein is commonly used in ophthalmic diagnosis for detection of corneal epithelial defects, and it is an essential part of every clinician's armamentarium. All red, inflamed, or painful eyes should be stained with fluorescein routinely. Note that the surface of a vascularized corneal lesion may show diffuse, faint fluorescein staining.

Fluorescein may be applied either as a solution from a multidrop container or on an impregnated paper strip. If a solution is used, care must be taken to prevent contamination of the container. An impregnated paper strip is preferable. The strip is removed from the packet, moistened with a drop of sterile saline solution, and placed into the conjunctival sac. After 60 seconds, excess dye is removed with sterile saline solution, and the eye is examined. Appearance of dye at the nares confirms patency of the nasolacrimal duct on that side (Jones's or fluorescein passage test). The interval required for fluorescein to appear is variable (up to 5–10 minutes in some normal dogs). False-negative results occur owing to drainage from the nasolacrimal duct into the posterior nasal cavity—this test is useful *only* if positive.

Defects in the corneal epithelium appear as bright green areas. In deep corneal lesions, the center of the lesion may fail to take up the stain and appears black, indicating that Descemet's membrane, which does not stain with fluorescein, is protruding into the deeper part of the corneal defect (Fig. 5–14), i.e., a descemetocele is present. If the nonstaining area is large, the descemetocele is large, and immediate surgical intervention is needed (Fig. 5–14).

Fluorescein is also used in fluorescein angiography (see p 113).

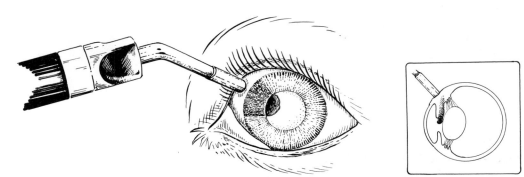

FIGURE 5–12. Transillumination of a mass protruding from the ciliary body into the pupil. The degree of involvement of the ciliary body can be determined.

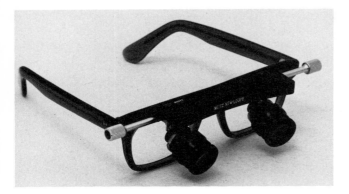

FIGURE 5–13. A simple magnifying loupe (2× or 4×).

All reddened, inflamed, painful, or very moist eyes should be stained with fluorescein. If this test is negative, the IOP should be measured.

Rose Bengal

Rose bengal (0.5% or 1% solution) stains necrotic and devitalized cells and mucus. It confirms the diagnosis of keratoconjunctivitis sicca, where deficiency of precorneal tear film causes necrosis and desquamation of corneal and conjunctival epithelium and retention of mucus in the conjunctival sac.

OPHTHALMOSCOPY

Ophthalmoscopy is the study of the interior of the eye with the ophthalmoscope. When a beam of light enters the eye, some light is reflected back along the same line. If the eye of an observer is positioned on the reflected beam, details of the fundus (the TAPETAL FUNDUS or FUNDUS REFLEX) may be seen. If the observer's eye is off the reflected beam, reflection of the beam on the inner surface of the cornea prevents it from reaching the observer's eye. The DIRECT OPHTHALMO-SCOPE directs a beam of light into the patient's eye and places the observer's eye in the correct position to view the reflected beam and details of the interior of the eye (Fig. 5–15). It is a direct ophthalmoscope because the upright fundus image is viewed directly, rather than an inverted virtual image provided by the indirect ophthalmoscope (see p 97).

Direct Ophthalmoscopy

The direct ophthalmoscope (Fig. 5–16) has a rheostat to control the light intensity, colored filters, a slit beam for viewing the lens and elevations of the retina, an illuminated grid to project onto the fundus in order to measure lesions. It also has a series of lenses on a rotating wheel that adjusts the depth of focus within the eye (Fig. 5–17) in order to examine structures other than the fundus or to measure the height of lesions by changing the focus from the tip of the lesion to the

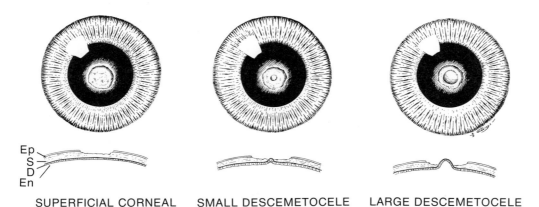

Ep
S
D
En

SUPERFICIAL CORNEAL   SMALL DESCEMETOCELE   LARGE DESCEMETOCELE
LESION

FIGURE 5–14. Staining characteristics of corneal lesion. Ep = epithelium; S = stroma; D = Descemet's membrane; En = endothelium.

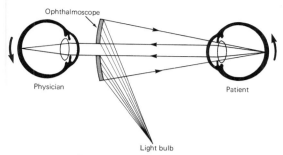

FIGURE 5–15. *Direct ophthalmoscopy. Arrows show orientation of images in examiner's and patient's eyes. (From Vaughan D, Asbury T: General Ophthalmology, 10th ed. Lange Medical Publications, Los Altos, CA, 1983.)*

surrounding retina and determing the dioptric difference (at the posterior pole of the eye, 1 diopter [D] = 0.3 mm). Before fundus examination the pupil is dilated with tropicamide (1%). The observer uses his or her left eye when examining the patient's left eye and vice versa. The examiner's unused eye is left *open*. With the ophthalmoscope set on 0 D, the eye is viewed from approximately 25 cm to locate opacities and alterations of the ocular media outlined against the tapetal reflex. This step is important because lesions, especially in the lens, may be missed during examination at higher magnification.

With the ophthalmoscope still set on 0 D, the observer moves to within 2–3 cm of the patient's eye (Fig. 5–16B), and the optic disc is located. If necessary, adjustment may be made to the lens settings in order to bring the fundus into focus. The fundus is then searched in quadrants. The direct ophthalmoscope is analogous to the high-power lens of a microscope,

resulting in an *upright* image magnified 15–17 times. Thorough examination of the fundus by direct ophthalmoscopy may be time-consuming because the field examined is small and constantly moving.

Constant initial practice is necessary for the beginner to master the techniques of ophthalmoscopy.

Although the direct ophthalmoscope is used predominantly for examination of the fundus, other structures of the eye may be examined at the settings shown in Figure 5–17. The slit beam of the direct ophthalmoscope may be used with a magnifying loupe to determine the positions of opacities within the lens.

Indirect Ophthalmoscopy

In this technique, a convex lens (10–30 D) is placed between the observer's eye and the patient's eye (Fig. 5–18). An inverted real image is formed between the lens and the observer's eye, the magnification depending on the focal length of the lens. With a 20-D lens, the magnification is 4× to 5×; more powerful lenses provide less magnification, but the field of view is larger. In animals, indirect ophthalmoscopy allows examination of more fundus in each field, and it is faster than direct ophthalmoscopy. It is analogous to the low-power setting of a microscope, but it is more expensive and requires considerable practice in order to gain proficiency.

Two kinds of indirect ophthalmoscope are commonly

FIGURE 5–16. A, *A direct ophthalmoscope.* B, *Direct ophthalmoscope in use. Note that the observer's left eye examines the patient's left eye.*

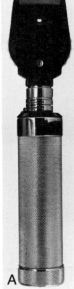

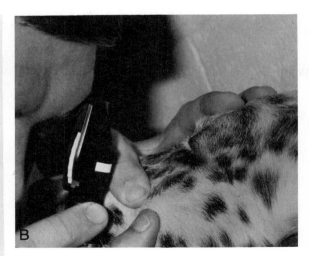

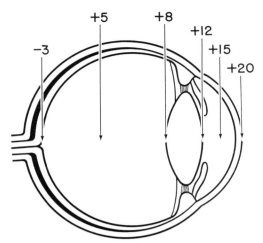

FIGURE 5–17. *Ophthalmoscopic examination of the canine eye. With the ophthalmoscope 2 cm in front of the patient's eye, the structures indicated are in focus with the appropriate lenses on the rotating wheel. (From Magrane WG: Canine Ophthalmology, 3rd ed. Lea & Febiger, Philadelphia, 1977.)*

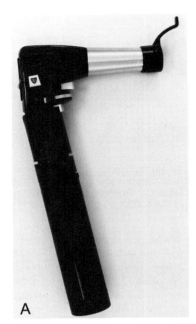

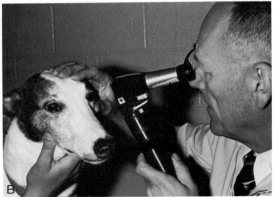

FIGURE 5–19. *A, A monocular indirect ophthalmoscope. B, Monocular indirect ophthalmoscope in use.*

used, monocular[4] (Fig. 5–19A, B) and binocular (Fig. 5–20A, B). The monocular instrument is small and gives an erect image, and it is easier for the beginner and infrequent user to master. The condensing lens is inside the instrument, and it can be used one-handed. Because the observer uses only one eye, there is no depth perception; also, the instrument is relatively expensive. This instrument is ideal for general use in animals.

With the binocular indirect ophthalmoscope (Fig. 5–20) the observer uses both eyes, giving depth perception. A head-mounted light source is used (Fig. 5–20B). The patient's head is positioned at arm's length with one hand, while the other hand is used to position the lens and eyelids. A *magnified inverted image* of the fundus is obtained. Alternatively, indirect ophthalmoscopy may be performed, but less conveniently, with a condensing lens (20 D) and a direct ophthalmoscope (lens setting 0 D) as a light source.

Methods of ophthalmoscopy are summarized in Table 5–1.

---

4. Monocular Indirect Ophthalmoscope—American Optical Co, Buffalo, NY.

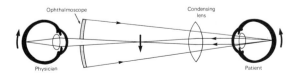

FIGURE 5–18. *Indirect ophthalmoscopy. (From Vaughan D, Asbury T: General Ophthalmology, 10th ed. Lange Medical Publications, Los Altos, CA, 1983.)*

THE NORMAL FUNDUS

The fundus of each domestic species has a characteristic but highly viable appearance, which must be learned by constant practice with a reliable ophthalmoscope. If a veterinary ophthalmologist is not available for consultation, readers are referred to available atlases. The following structures are found in the fundus of all domestic species (Fig. 5–21).

1. Tapetum—a highly reflective structure in the dorsal portion of the fundus. (The pig has no tapetum.)

2. Nontapetal area—the nonreflective ventral portion.

3. Optic disc—the area at the posterior pole where the optic nerve enters the eye.

4. Physiological cup—a small depression of variable size in the center of the optic disc.

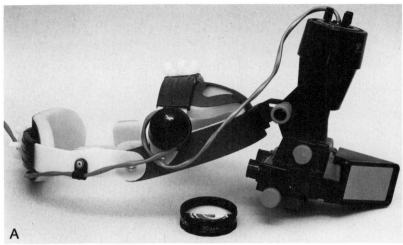

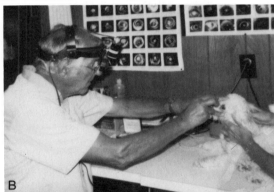

FIGURE 5–20. A, A binocular indirect ophthalmoscope. B, Binocular indirect ophthalmoscope in use.

TABLE 5–1. Comparison of Methods of Ophthalmoscopy

Factor	Direct	Monocular Indirect	Binocular Indirect
Magnification	15–17 ×	3–5 ×	2–4 ×
Stereopsis	No	No	Yes
Image	Inverted	Erect	Inverted
Ease of use	Intermediate–difficult	Simple to master	Requires considerable practice
Speed of examination	Slow, especially if patient uncooperative	Fast	Fast
Portability	Excellent	Excellent	Poor
Area of field examined	2 disc diameters	6–8 disc diameters (approx.)	8–14 disc diameters (approx.)
Cost	Low	High	High

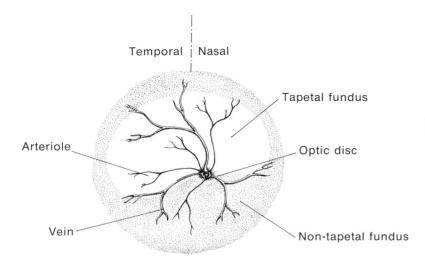

Temporal | Nasal

Tapetal fundus

Arteriole

Optic disc

Vein

Non-tapetal fundus

GENERALIZED
FUNDUS

FIGURE 5–21. Structures in the normal fundus (species differences ignored).

5. Retinal vasculature—considerable species variation occurs in type of vascular patterns (see the following discussion).

6. Retina—transparent and cannot normally be seen in front of the tapetum.

Unlike the human eye, the eyes of domestic animals do not possess a fovea or central retinal artery and vein.

Dog

A tapetum and nontapetal areas are present in the canine fundus (Fig. 5–22A). Tapetal color varies from a golden yellow to bluish green and orange brown. There is a variable association among coat color, iris pigmentation, and tapetal color (e.g., in the golden Labrador the tapetum is usually yellow with greenish margins, in the black cocker spaniel it is yellowish gold, and in liver-colored coats such as the Weimaraner it is a light orange brown). In young dogs, the fundus is grayish soon after the eyes open (7–10 days). A progression occurs through lilac and successively lighter blues to the adult color at 4–4½ months of age.

The tapetum has a fine-beaded appearance, which increases in granularity with age and with distance from the optic disc. The junction between tapetal and nontapetal areas is often irregular. The nontapetal fundus is deep brown, owing to pigment in the pigment epithelium of the retina. The coloration varies from a smooth homogeneous brown to a slightly mottled appearance. Severe mottling must be distinguished from disease processes. In albinotic, subalbinotic, and lightly colored animals, pigment may be reduced or absent from the nontapetal fundus, allowing the larger vessels of the underlying choroid to be seen. Absence of the tapetum is unusual but does occur in dogs.

The OPTIC DISC (papilla) usually lies in the tapetal

area or at its ventral edge, and may have a narrow margin of nontapetal fundus around it. Similarly, the disc may be displaced ventrally into the nontapetal fundus and be surrounded by a narrow margin of tapetum. Small hyperreflective areas immediately adjacent to the margin of the disc (PERIPAPILLARY CONUS) are common in older dogs and in younger dogs of specific breeds, e.g., flat-coated retriever. The disc surface is pink, owing to numerous small capillaries. The PHYSIOLOGICAL CUP is a small gray depression in the center of the optic disc (see Chap 2, p 20). In some animals, a mesh-like pattern can be seen in the disc, owing to to fenestrations in the sclera at the LAMINA CRIBROSA, through which the optic nerve fibers pass. The VENOUS CIRCLE on the surface of the disc may be complete or incomplete. These veins penetrate the lamina cribrosa with the nerve fibers but soon leave the nerve to enter the orbit. RETINAL ARTERIOLES (about 20 in number) emerge from the outer portions and margin of the disc and are considerably smaller than the veins. There are THREE MAJOR RETINAL VEINS (VENULES)—SUPERIOR, INFERONASAL, and INFEROTEMPORAL—although additional veins and variations are common. Over the nontapetal fundus the retinal vessels exhibit a grayish-silver sheen or "reflex" in the center of the vessel, which is not seen over the tapetum.

Cat

The feline fundus is more uniform in appearance than is the canine fundus (Fig. 5–22B). The optic disc is smaller and circular; it is surrounded by a slightly pigmented ring in adult animals and is usually present in the tapetal area. There is no venous circle. There are generally THREE ARTERIOLES—SUPERIOR, INFERO-

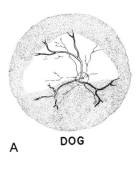

A DOG

area centralis

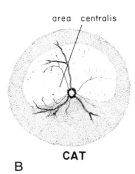

B CAT

stars of Winslow

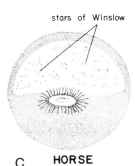

C HORSE

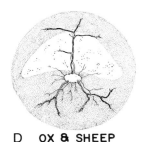

D OX & SHEEP

FIGURE 5–22. Fundi of different species. (Refer to the general diagram shown in Fig. 5–21.) A, Canine fundus. B, Feline fundus. C, Equine fundus. D, Bovine and ovine fundi.

NASAL, and INFEROTEMPORAL—which are ciliary in orgin. The tapetum is more uniformly greenish yellow. Superior and temporal to the optic disc is the AREA CENTRALIS, which is usually devoid of large blood

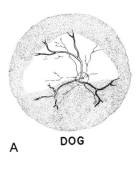

vessels. The nontapetal fundus is frequently unpigmented, especially in Siamese and other blue-eyed or white cats, revealing the larger vessels of the choroid beneath. Complete absence of the tapetum occurs occasionally. The lamina cribrosa is often visible, but a physiological cup usually cannot be seen ophthalmoscopically in the optic disc.

Horse

The equine fundus differs greatly in appearance from canine and feline fundi. The optic disc is a horizontal ellipse and has 30–60 short vessels supplying the surrounding retina (Fig. 5–22C). Arterioles and venules are indistinguishable. The lamina cribrosa is often visible. The optic disc is in the nontapetal area. The junction between tapetal and nontapetal areas is uniform. The tapetum varies in color from bluish purple to green and yellow. The STARS OF WINSLOW—small, uniformly scattered red or dark dots and lines, representing end-on views of capillaries traversing the choriocapillaris—are visible throughout the tapetal area. The nontapetal area is brown and homogeneous. Absence of the tapetum or unpigmented nontapetal areas occur infrequently, allowing the choroidal circulation to be seen. The choroidal circulation is often visible dorsal to the optic disc, where both tapetum and nontapetal pigment may be lacking.

Sheep and Cattle

The fundi of sheep and cattle are similar. Three or four major venules and arterioles radiate from the elliptical optic disc (Fig. 5–22D). The dorsal vein and arteriole often intertwine, and tributaries of the dorsal vessels often appear like the hanging branches of a tree. The tapetum is bluish green in most animals. The nontapetal area is homogeneous brown except in albinotic and subalbinotic animals, in which it may be unpigmented, revealing the choroidal vasculature. Remnants of the hyaloid vascular system persist longer in sheep and cattle than in other species. These remnants may be seen ophthalmoscopically up to 2 or 3 years of age in cattle, sheep, and goats.

RETINOSCOPY

Retinoscopy is a specialized technique for objective evaluation of the refractive state of the eye, and it allows determination of refractive errors, e.g., hyperopia and myopia. It is used in evaluation of refractive errors after cataract extraction and for evaluation of the visual state of animals in which no apparent abnormalities are found on ophthalmoscopy or electroretinography.

COLLECTION OF BACTERIAL AND FUNGAL SPECIMENS

INDICATIONS

1. Severe purulent inflammations at first presentation.

2. Persistent purulent or nonpurulent inflammations in any part of the eye that do not respond to routine antibiotics.

3. Corneal lesions associated with a gelatinous appearance or with an enlarging geographical or focal stromal opacity.

4. Severe ulcerative, seborrheic, or pruritic lesions of the lids or periocular area.

Bacterial specimens are taken on a sterile, moist swab and plated onto suitable media as soon as possible. In addition, collection of the specimen into tubes of thioglycollate broth and cooked meat broth often results in a higher yield and earlier identification. Properly labeled, separate samples are taken from the conjunctiva and eyelid margins of each eye and plated into different portions of the agar plate. Antibiotic sensitivity testing is not performed on mixed cultures. If the samples are to be transported, they must not dry out.

Fungal specimens are usually taken as corneal or skin scrapings (see the next section). Because saprophytic fungi, especially those of plant origin, may cause ocular disease, samples are cultured on both Sabouraud's agar and Sabouraud's agar without inhibitors (the inhibitors may prevent growth of saprophytic fungi). Growth of fungi may take several weeks.

SCRAPINGS

EQUIPMENT

Kimura spatula (Fig. 5–23)
Alcohol lamp
Clean microscope slides
Fixative (either spray or immersion)

Corneal and conjunctival scrapings are collected for cytological and immunocytological examination and Gram's staining. Scrapings are removed from the palpebral conjunctiva after topical anesthesia with 0.5% proparacaine. Examination of the types and numbers of cells present assists with etiologic diagnosis or, if only general changes are noted, in determining the stage of disease process present. The mucus thread in the ventral conjunctival fornix accumulates cells and debris and can be easily removed with a spatula for examination. Giemsa's stain or new methylene blue may be used for cytological examination. Papanicolaou's stain may be used if neoplastic changes are suspected (e.g., in bovine squamous cell carcinoma). Impression smears, stained in the same way as scrapings, are useful in the diagnosis of neoplasia and mycotic and chlamydial infections. For further details of conjunctival cytology, see Chap 8.

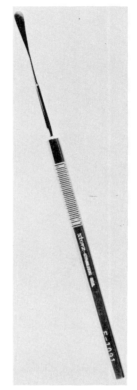

FIGURE 5–23. Kimura spatula.

Special handling may be required for immunocytological examination of scrapings, e.g., for canine distemper and feline herpesvirus diagnoses.

SCHIRMER TEAR TEST

The Schirmer tear test is a semiquantitative method of measuring production of the precorneal tear film. The test is performed with sterile, individually packaged strips of absorbent paper with a notch 5 mm from one end (Fig. 5–24). Each strip is folded at the notch and hooked over the middle of the lower lid for 60 seconds (Fig. 5–25). The distance from the notch to the end of the moistened paper is measured immediately on removal of the strip from the eye. In this method (Schirmer test no. 1), corneal sensation, including stimulation from the test strip, is intact. Normal values are shown in Table 5–2. In the Schirmer test no. 2, corneal sensation is abolished with topical anesthetic, and lower test values result. The local anesthetic desensitizes the cornea, blocks the afferent limb of the reflex path, and prevents reflex secretion by the lacrimal and nictitans glands. The Schirmer test no. 2 has little clinical application in animals. Normal animals without clinical signs may show values below the normal range. Avoid measuring tear production after the administration of drugs—local anesthetics and parasympatholytic

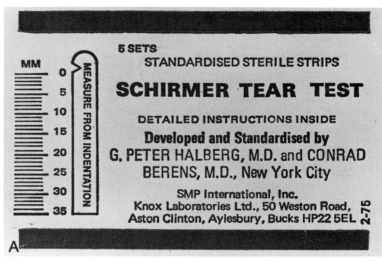

FIGURE 5–24. A, A packet of five sets of Schirmer tests. B, A pair of tear test strips for one patient.

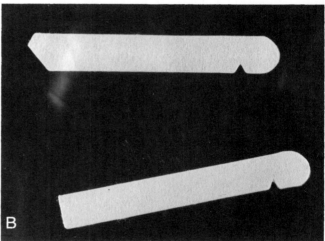

drugs (atropine, tropicamide) lower tear production; parasympathomimetic drugs (pilocarpine, echothiophate, demecarium, isoflurophate) increase tear production. Commercial strips are often unsuitable for horses because of greater tear production, which quickly saturates the entire strip. Larger strips (7.5 mm × 8.0 cm) may be prepared from Whatman's no. 42 filter paper (normal values 12.7 ± 9.5 mm/min). Variations

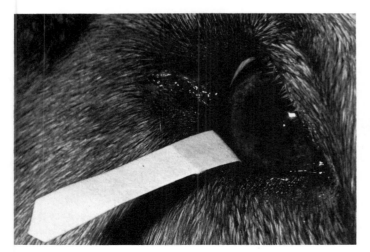

FIGURE 5–25. Schirmer tear test strip in position.

TABLE 5–2. Normal Schirmer Tear Test Values (mm/min)

Animal	No. 1	Low, But Disease Usually Not Present	Abnormal	No. 2
Dog	19.8 ± 5.3	5–8	<5	11.6 ± 6.1
Cat	16.9 ± 5.7	5–8	<5	—
Horse	>15	10–15	<10	—
Cow	>15	10–15	<10	—

between brands of Schirmer tests strips are of little clinical significance but should be noted in experimental situations.

TESTS OF LACRIMAL PATENCY

Blockage of the nasolacrimal ducts causes overflow of tears (EPIPHORA) at the lid margin near the medial canthus, with staining of the surrounding hair. Blockage of the nasolacrimal ducts may be determined by

1. negative fluorescein passage test
2. inability to flush the duct
3. inability to pass a catheter
4. demonstration by dacryocystorhinography

The lacrimal ducts are flushed, under topical anesthesia, by passing a 20- or 22-gauge curved or malleable lacrimal cannula (Fig. 5–26A) through the punctum (the superior punctum is more convenient), occluding the remaining punctum with a finger, and applying pressure to the saline-filled syringe (Fig. 5–26B). The cannula is passed through the canaliculus into the lacrimal sac within the lacrimal bone. So that the cannula can enter the bony portion of the nasolacrimal duct, the medial portion of the upper lid and superior canaliculus is stretched dorsolaterally to straighten the canaliculus. For more detailed examinations of the lacrimal system, see Chapter 10.

The nasolacrimal duct in some dogs opens into the posterior nasal cavity, so that saline solution fails to appear at the external nares when the duct is flushed. These animals may cough slightly as the saline solution runs posteriorly. For this reason, lacrimal flushing is performed with the nose held low to prevent respiratory embarrassment and to allow fluid to pass visibly from the nose. In horses the lacrimal ducts are usually flushed from the nasal end (Fig. 5–27) with a plastic tube such as a flexible plastic tomcat catheter or tubing (PE 90). The tube is passed up the duct 8–10 cm before flushing.

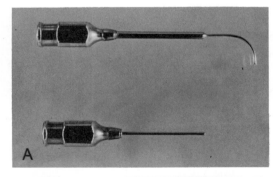
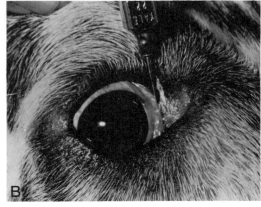

FIGURE 5–26. A, Lacrimal cannulae. B, Flushing of the superior lacrimal punctum.

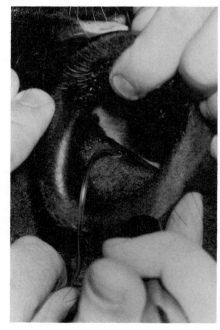

FIGURE 5–27. Flushing of the equine nasolacrimal duct.

TONOMETRY

TONOMETRY is the measurement of IOP, whereas TONOGRAPHY is the study of aqueous outflow facility in response to pressure applied to the eye.

Pressure within the eye results in tension in the cornea and sclera. Various methods employ this tension to estimate the IOP. Cannulation measures pressure directly; it is used experimentally but not clinically. Pressure may be roughly estimated by palpation of the globe through the upper lid during physical examination; however, this method is inadequate for routine ophthalmic use. The accuracy of digital palpation depends on the clinician's experience, IOP range, relative prominence of the globe, and cooperation of the patient. Dependence on this method leads to inaccurate diagnosis and inappropriate ocular therapy, with unfortunate sequelae for veterinary patients.

An instrumental method of IOP measurement is an essential part of a thorough ophthalmic evaluation.

Two basic methods of IOP measurement are useful: INDENTATION and APPLANATION TONOMETRY.

Indentation Tonometry

In indentation tonometry, a standard force is applied to the anesthetized cornea with a metal rod. The distance the rod indents the cornea, which is related to the IOP, is measured. This method is easily understood by considering the eye to be analogous to a water-filled balloon. If the blunt end of a pencil is applied to the balloon with a given force (e.g., the weight of the pencil placed vertically), the pencil indents the surface of the balloon by a certain distance. If the pressure in the balloon is decreased (some of the water is let out), the tension in the rubber wall decreases, and the same pencil resting on the balloon indents it further. Conversely, if the pressure in the balloon is increased, the same pencil indents it less. This is the principle of the SCHIØTZ TONOMETER.

The Schiøtz tonometer (Fig. 5–28) consists of three parts—the plunger (analogous to the pencil), the footplate assembly (a device to measure indentation), and the handle. A further refinement is added—the weight applied to the eye through the rod may be varied by adding or subtracting weights (5.5 g, 7.5 g, 10.0 g, or 15.0 g). The greater the weight applied to the eye at a given IOP, the greater the penetration of the rod (if the pencil is pressed into the balloon with more force, it penetrates further).

PROCEDURE

1. A drop of local anesthetic is placed in each eye. The patient is restrained if necessary, and the lids are

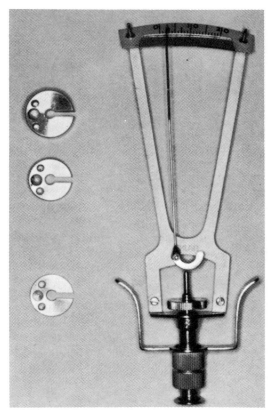

FIGURE 5–28. *Schiøtz's tonometer with extra weights. (From Scheie HG, Albert DM: Textbook of Ophthalmology, 9th ed. WB Saunders Co, Philadelphia, 1977.)*

carefully retracted without placing pressure on the globe. The head is elevated so that the corneal surface is horizontal.

2. The tonometer is placed on the eye, either with no weight in place (the plunger weighs 5.5 g) or with the 7.5-g weight in place. The scale reading is recorded. The *greater* the scale reading, the *lower* the IOP.

3. The calibration table supplied with the instrument is entered with the scale reading, and the appropriate column is selected according to the weight used (5.5 g); this yields the IOP. The data are recorded as scale reading per weight per pressure (e.g., 5.0 units/5.5 g/21 mmHg).

Because of difficulties in head positioning and patient cooperation, Schiøtz's tonometry is unsuitable for large domestic animals; on the basis of disease incidence, it is rarely required. Calibration tables for dogs are available, but more consistent results are obtained with the human tables supplied with the Schiøtz tonometer. Applanation tonometry is suitable for large animals.

OCULAR RIGIDITY

If, under the influence of the Schiøtz plunger, the sclera and cornea stretch because of the slight increase in IOP caused by the indentation, then a higher scale

TABLE 5–3. Normal Intraocular Pressure Values

Species	Values (mmHg)	Reference
Canine	20–25 (20–30)	Magrane, 1971
	14–28	Severin, 1976
	16–30	Startup, 1969
	10–31	Heywood, 1971
Feline	14–26	Severin, 1976
	17.4–19.2	Bill, 1966
Bovine	14–22	Severin, 1976
	16.5 ± 5.5	Woelfel, 1964
Equine	14–22	Severin, 1976
	16.5–32.5	Cohen and Reinke, 1970
	28.6 ± 4.8	McClure et al, 1976

reading and a lower IOP are measured because the ocular rigidity has changed. This ocular rigidity varies considerably in dogs. A quick check to determine the influence of ocular rigidity on the accuracy of the readings may be performed by measuring the pressure with two different tonometer weights (using the lighter weight first). If the pressures obtained are similar, the influence of ocular rigidity is small. If the pressure obtained with the heavier weight is considerably less, the ocular rigidity is low and the walls of the globe are stretching. Applanation tonometry is unaffected by variations in ocular rigidity. Normal values for Schiøtz tonometry are shown in Table 5–3.

FACTORS AFFECTING IOP READINGS

State of the Instrument. The plunger assembly of the Schiøtz tonometer is removed after use, and the plunger, plunger housing, and footplate are cleaned with a pipe cleaner soaked in ether. Deposits of mucus and tears can dry on the surfaces and prevent free movement of the plunger, causing inaccurate results. The instrument may be sterilized with ethylene oxide to prevent transfer of pathogenic microorganisms between patients.

Prior Medication. Most sedatives, tranquilizers, and anesthetic drugs cause lowered IOP. Ketamine causes increased IOP, possibly by inducing spasm in the extraocular muscles.

Patient Cooperation. Pressure applied around the neck or orbital area or in retracting the lids may increase pressure values.

Intraocular Inflammation. Anterior uveitis, either primary or secondary, causes decreased IOP, often below 5 mmHg. Lowered pressure is a sensitive but not exclusive indicator of the presence of uveitis.

Despite its disadvantages, the Schiøtz tonometer is most economical and suitable for use in small animal general practices. The more expensive applanation tonometers are more reliable and allow accurate differentiation of marginal increases in IOP.

Applanation Tonometry

The principle of applanation tonometry is that the force required to flatten a given area of a sphere is equal to the pressure within the sphere (Imbert-Fick law).

$$P = f/A$$

If the area is known (the size of the footplate) and the force is measured, the pressure can be calculated (Fig. 5–29). Numerous types of applanation tonometers have been used to measure IOP in domestic animals; these include Maklakoff, Draeger, Perkins, Goldmann, and Mackay-Marg types.

Of these, the Mackay-Marg (or guard-ring) type is the most useful in domestic animals (Figs. 5–30 and 5–31). Its advantages include:

1. It is accurate and easy to use.

2. It does not require the animal's head to be held vertically, although the probe must be held at right angles to the corneal surface.

3. Errors induced by different sizes and curvatures of corneas in different species are less important.

4. Because of the small instrument head, irregular or diseased corneal areas may be avoided and more accurate readings obtained from scarred corneas.

5. The probe tip is covered with a rubber cap, which is changed between uses and prevents transfer of infections.

6. Restraint required is minimal.

The major disadvantage of these instruments is cost, which limits their use to veterinary ophthalmologists or institutions. The instrument is much more accurate than the Schiøtz tonometer, and it is necessary for effective management of difficult glaucoma cases and adequate postoperative care after intraocular surgery.

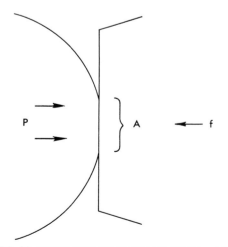

FIGURE 5–29. Applanation tonometry is based on definition of pressure—force per unit area. (Reproduced by permission from Moses, Robert A.: Intraocular pressure. In Moses, Robert A., and Hart, William M., Jr., editors: Adler's Physiology of the Eye, ed. 8, St. Louis, 1987, The C. V. Mosby Co.)

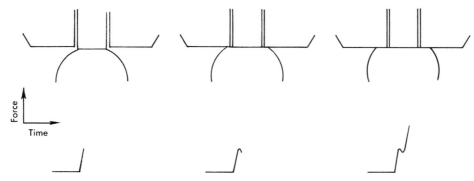

FIGURE 5–30. *Mackay-Marg tonometer. Left, Plunger supports both IOP and spring force of cornea. Center, Corneal bend is supported by footplate, and force on plunger decreases. Right, As tonometer is advanced, displaced aqueous raises IOP. Upper, Tonometer probe and cornea (grossly exaggerated). Lower, Record of tonometer plunger movement. (Reproduced by permission from Moses, Robert A.: Intraocular pressure. In Moses, Robert A., and Hart, William M., Jr., editors: Adler's Physiology of the Eye, ed. 8, St. Louis, 1987, The C. V. Mosby Co.)*

TONOGRAPHY

TONOGRAPHY is the study of aqueous outflow facility (see p 17). It is based on the observation that massage softens an eye because fluid is forced out through the drainage angle. This softening occurs to a lesser extent in a glaucomatous eye because aqueous is less able to pass out of the anterior chamber (i.e., outflow facility is decreased). In tonography the patient is restrained, usually in dorsal recumbency, under tranquilization, and a Schiøtz-type weight and plunger are placed on the cornea. The gradual reduction in IOP over a 4-minute period is measured graphically on a strip-chart recorder. The outflow facility coefficient (C) can be calculated (Chap 13).

GONIOSCOPY

In gonioscopy, the junction between the iris and the cornea—the drainage angle—is viewed directly. Gonioscopic examination is a routine part of the examination of patients suspected of having glaucoma or ocular hypertension, when tonometry is inconclusive. The technique is applicable to all domestic species but is most frequently used in dogs. In cooperative patients, topical anesthesia is usually sufficient; however, general anesthesia may be necessary in refractory animals (ketamine/diazepam is particularly useful).

In the normal eye, light rays that are reflected from the drainage angle enter the cornea from a posterior direction and undergo *total internal reflection* as in a prism (Fig. 5–32A–C). This occurs because of the difference in refractive index between the cornea and the surrounding air, and the high angle of incidence of the light rays from the drainage angle. (The angle of incidence is defined as the angle between the ray and the perpendicular to the reflecting surface of the cornea.)

By replacing the surrounding air with an optical medium (i.e., a goniolens) having an index of refraction

closely approximating that of the cornea, total internal reflection is avoided, and rays from the drainage angle can be viewed directly through the lens. Additional modifications may be made to the lens to provide magnification. Magnifying instruments may also be used (e.g., biomicroscope, gonioscope, head loupe, fundus camera). Many kinds of goniolenses are available, including the Koeppe, Cardona, Barkan, Zeiss, Allen-Thorpe, and Goldmann, in 17, 19, and 21 mm sizes. Two basic kinds are available—the direct lens (e.g., Koeppe; Fig. 5–33A), through which the angle is viewed directly, and the indirect lens (e.g., Goldmann; Fig. 5–33B), in which the image is viewed in a mirror. Low-pressure lenses[5] are very useful for veterinary use, as the lenses are held in place by low pressure, applied by a 2-ml syringe and column of saline solution.

Goniolenses are bonded to the cornea with a liquid medium (e.g., saline solution for low-vacuum lenses, methylcelluose solutions for non-vacuum lenses). The

---

5. Medical Laboratories, The Netherlands.

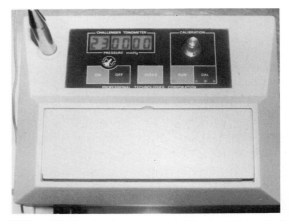

FIGURE 5–31. *The Challenger tonometer, a commercially available Mackay-Marg type.*

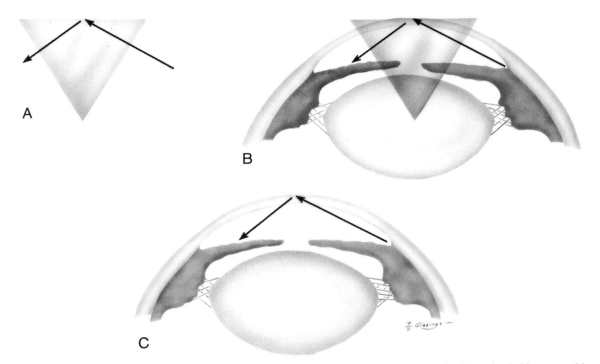

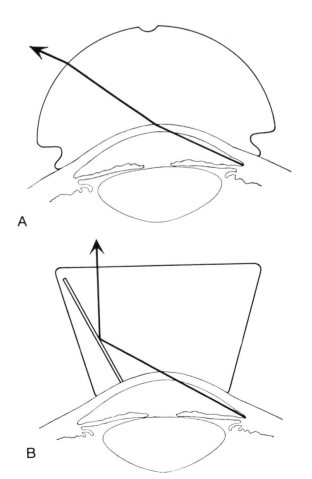

FIGURE 5–32. A, *Total internal reflection of a light ray in a prism.* B and C, *Total internal reflection of a light ray reaching the cornea from the drainage angle.*

FIGURE 5–33. A, *Diagram of light rays from the drainage angle, emerging through a Koeppe lens.* B, *Diagram of light rays emerging through a Goldmann lens.* (Reproduced by permission from Hoskins, H. Dunbar, Jr., and Kass, Michael A.: *Becker-Shaffer's Diagnosis and Therapy of the Glaucomas,* ed. 6, St. Louis, 1989, The C. V. Mosby Co.)

normal structures of the canine drainage angle are shown in Fig. 5–34.

Gonioscopy is used primarily to determine whether the angle is *open* or *narrow* (closed) or obstructed by mesodermal remnants, and to check for the presence of foreign bodies, tumors, and inflammatory exudates. The technique is used most frequently in dogs, but it is applicable to all species. In cats, the anterior chamber is deeper than in the dog, the angle of incidence is smaller, and total internal reflection does not limit the visible area of drainage angle as much.

BIOMICROSCOPY

The slit-lamp biomicroscope (Fig. 5–35) is an instrument for examining the eye with magnification (up to 40×) and illumination. Various combinations of

illumination and magnification are used to show different microscopic and optical features of the eye.

Because of the higher magnifications possible, many microscopic features (e.g., individual layers of the cornea) invisible to the naked eye may be examined and photographed. The slit-lamp biomicroscope allows pathological processes to be examined in much greater detail, allowing more accuracy in description, diagnosis, prognosis, and treatment. It is especially useful to examine the lids, lens, iris, cornea, conjunctiva, and third eyelid (i.e., the anterior segment). Estimates of width of the drainage angle and depth of the anterior chamber may be made; with optical modifications, the vitreous and retina may be examined. Several conditions (e.g., persistent pupillary membranes and cataracts), for which certificates of disease-free status are issued by veterinary ophthalmologists, require use of the slit-

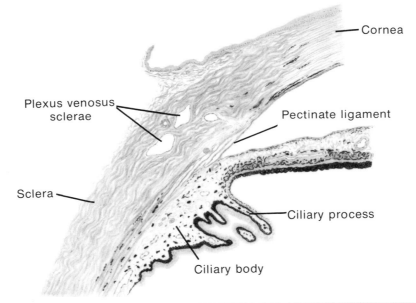

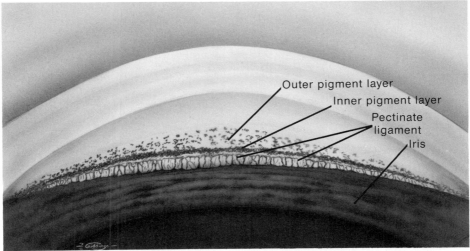

FIGURE 5–34. The normal canine drainage angle as viewed through a goniolens.

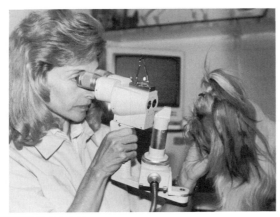

FIGURE 5–35. A Kowa portable slit-lamp biomicroscope in use. This model is also useful for large animal examinations.

lamp biomicroscope for complete evaluation. Because of the requirement for considerable training and skill in their use, slit-lamp biomicroscopes are usually found in specialty practices and teaching institutions.

RADIOGRAPHIC TECHNIQUES

Plain Films

Dorsoventral, lateral, anteroposterior, and oblique plain film radiographs of the orbit and surrounding region may reveal disease processes in and around the orbit and paranasal sinuses. Plain films are used before contrast techniques are commenced. Only contrast techniques that commonly yield clinically useful information are discussed.

Dacryocystorhinography

Dacryocystorhinography is the radiographic demonstration of the lacrimal canaliculi, lacrimal sac, and nasolacrimal duct by the injection of a radiographic contrast medium (Fig. 5–36). The technique is useful for demonstrating the sites of blockages that cannot be located by cannulation with a nylon thread passed either up or down the nasolacrimal duct. Contrast radiography often reveals the cause of obstructions (e.g., neoplastic inflammatory processes involving roots of the molar teeth, maxillary sinus, and nasal cavity). The technique is performed under general anesthesia, with the patient in lateral recumbency. A lacrimal cannula is inserted into the superior punctum, the inferior punctum is occluded by finger pressure, and 2 or 3 ml of diatrizoate meglumine and diatrizoate sodium (Hypaque or Renografin) is injected. Suitable lateral and dorsoventral exposures are made. Because of the small size of the lacrimal passages, care is taken to prevent excess contrast medium contaminating the facial hair and obscuring the passages. This can be limited by holding cotton over the punctum during injection and by inserting cotton into the external nares near the nasal meatus. The technique is equally applicable to large and small animals.

Orbital Venography[6]

Orbital venography is the most useful of the contrast techniques for examining the orbit, with the exception

---

6. See also Chap 18.

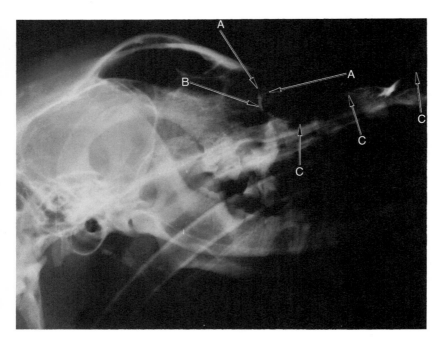

FIGURE 5–36. A lateral dacryocystorhinogram in a dog. A = lacrimal canaliculus; B, = lacrimal sac; C = nasolacrimal duct. (Courtesy of Dr. R. Wyburn.)

of computerized axial tomography (CAT scans). In this procedure, contrast medium is injected into the angularis oculi vein. From here, blood may return to the heart via the orbital venous system, to the cerebral and vertebral venous sinuses, or via the facial and external maxillary veins to the external jugular vein (Fig. 5–37). The latter route is minimized during radiography by occluding the external jugular veins with a tourniquet. The structures visible in a normal venogram are shown in Figure 5–38.

TECHNIQUE

Under general anesthesia, a tourniquet of thin rubber tubing is placed around the neck, just anterior to the

wings of the atlas. The area around the medial canthus of each eye is clipped anteriorly and ventrally for 3–4 cm and prepared with suitable surgical solutions (without iodine). The patient is placed with the head in lateral recumbency, neck extended, with the affected eye uppermost. An injection of 5–6 ml of a suitable IV contrast agent (Hypaque or Renografin) is placed, with a 20- or 22-gauge needle connected to a pediatric scalp vein infusion set, into the angularis oculi vein (Fig. 5–37). The film must be exposed as the injection is made, because the veins empty rapidly. The normal side may also be injected for comparison.

Lesions within the orbit cause displacement, compression, or collapse of one or more of the following veins:

1. superior ophthalmic vein

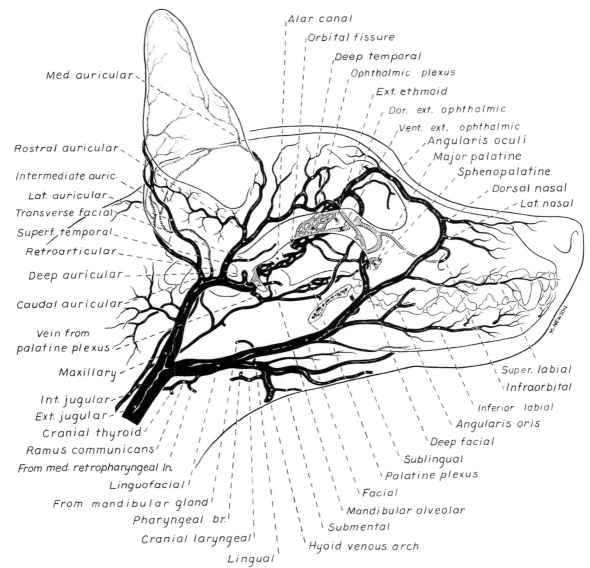

FIGURE 5–37. Superficial veins of the head. Lateral aspect. (From Evans HE, Christensen GC: Miller's Anatomy of the Dog, 2nd ed. WB Saunders Co, Philadelphia, 1979. © Cornell University 1964.)

A   LEFT LATERAL ORBITAL VENOGRAM

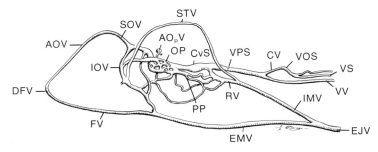

B   DORSAL ORBITAL VENOGRAM

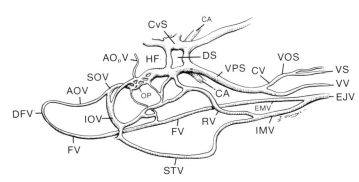

FIGURE 5–38. A, *Diagram of left lateral view of canine orbital venogram.* B, *Diagram of dorsoventral view of canine orbital venogram.* AOV = *angularis oculi vein;* AO$_p$V = *anastomosis of ophthalmic veins;* CA = *carotid artery;* CV = *condyloid vein;* CvS = *cavernous sinus;* DFV = *dorsal facial vein;* DS = *dorsum sellae;* EJV = *external jugular vein;* EMV = *external maxillary vein;* FV = *facial vein;* HF = *hypophyseal fossa;* IMV = *internal maxillary vein;* IOV = *inferior ophthalmic vein;* OP = *orbital plexus;* PP = *palatine plexus;* RV = *retroglenoid vein;* SOV = *superior ophthalmic vein;* STV = *superficial temporal vein;* VOS = *ventral occipital sinus;* VPS = *ventral petrosal sinus;* VS = *vertebral sinus;* VV = *vertebral vein. (Modified from Oliver JE: Cranial sinus venography in the dog. J Am Vet Rad Soc 10:70, 1969.)*

2. inferior ophthalmic vein
3. anastomotic branch between 1 and 2
4. orbital venous plexus

When the globe itself is enlarged, the vessels are rarely affected. Space-occupying lesions within the extraocular muscle cone cause disappearance or decrease in the characteristic "step" in the superior ophthalmic vein. Lesions in the lower part of the orbit displace the muscle cone and globe dorsally, causing displacement and constriction of the lumen of the superior ophthalmic vein rather than changes in the "step." Narrowing or constriction of the inferior ophthalmic vein or its anastomotic branch is associated with lesions in the ventral half of the orbit, outside the muscle cone.

Carotid Arteriography

Carotid arteriography is more difficult to perform than is orbital venography, and it gives less information of diagnostic importance. It is infrequently used in the diagnosis of orbital disease, as surgical exposure and selective catheterization of the internal carotid artery is necessary. Where orbital and intracranial lesions are suspected, the technique is more likely to yield useful information.

Contrast Orbitography

Air and radiopaque contrast agents may be injected into the orbit to outline lesions as radiolucent areas or filling defects. The most suitable technique in the dog

is injection of 2–3 ml of contrast agent (by Barth's method) into the orbit from beneath the zygomatic arch (Fig. 18–19).

CAT Scanning

CAT scans provide superior detail for localization of orbital lesions, but their availability is limited to teaching institutions and by cost. Iodinated contrast media do not improve localization of orbital tumors in dogs. Localization of brain lesions affecting vision may be significantly improved by this technique.

Localization of Foreign Bodies

It is often necessary to determine whether a foreign body is within the eye or in periocular tissues. Foreign bodies in periocular tissues may have penetrated orbital tissues or perforated the globe itself. Such objects may be localized by reference to a radiopaque marker placed in a known position. Simple markers consist of one or more concentric rings of stainless steel wire placed around the limbus. Radiographs are taken in different views and from different angles.

ELECTRORETINOGRAPHY[7]

Electroretinography is the study of electrical potentials produced when light falls onto the retina. Light

---

7. See also Chap 16.

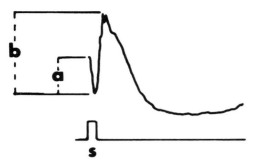

FIGURE 5–39. A, Normal single flash ERG from a dog. a = a-wave amplitude; b = b-wave amplitude; s = stimulus. (From Rubin LF: Atlas of Veterinary Ophthalmoscopy. Lea & Febiger, Philadelphia, 1974.)

of varying intensity, wavelength, and flash duration is directed onto the retina. Resulting potential differences are detected by electrodes implanted into a contact lens, amplified, and recorded on paper or on an oscilloscope screen for photography (Fig. 5–39). For accurate results the technique is performed under general anesthesia, and it is useful in all species. In dogs, xylazine and ketamine have little effect on the electroretinogram (ERG).

Electroretinography is a test of retinal but not visual function. It may be used to differentiate various retinal diseases, and it is frequently used before cataract extraction if the contralateral fundus is not visible.

ERGs are used for the following purposes.

1. Preoperative evaluation of retinal function before cataract extraction. This is necessary because of the frequent coexistence of retinal disorders with bilateral canine cataracts. If the patient is referred before the second lens becomes cataractous, fundoscopic examination of the remaining fundus eliminates retinal diseases and the ERG.

2. Diagnosis and differentiation of retinal disorders (e.g., specific rod, cone, or combined rod-cone diseases, sudden acquired retinal degeneration syndrome).

3. Early detection of progressive retinal degeneration before lesions are visible ophthalmoscopically. The ERG cannot be used to predict if an animal will develop such a disease; it can detect the disease at an earlier stage than can clinical examination. The age at which early detection is possible varies with the type of retinal degeneration and with the species and breed of the animal.

4. Investigation of unexplained visual loss (amaurosis) in which retinal lesions are not visible ophthalmoscopically, e.g., sudden acquired retinal degeneration syndrome.

ULTRASONOGRAPHY

In ultrasonography, high-frequency sound waves (500 MHz) above audible range are produced by passing an alternating electric current through a piezoelectric crystal. The waves are directed posteriorly through the eye from the cornea, and the echoes are detected, amplified, and displayed on an oscilloscope screen. In A-scan ultrasonography, the echoes are viewed as a series of peaks (Fig. 5–40A). Abnormalities are visible because reflecting surfaces within the eye are displaced from their normal position. In B-scan ultrasonography, a two-dimensional cross-section of the eye is obtained (Fig. 5–40B).

Ultrasonography is used to examine the contents of opaque eyes before surgery or other treatment. Direct corneal contact yields superior images of the posterior chamber. Indications include:

1. Detection of retinal detachments or other disease processes behind a cataractous lens or corneal opacity, if a history of trauma or other ocular findings suggest it. For instance, a cataract in a horse with small posterior synechiae or areas of pigment on the anterior lens capsule may be associated with recurrent equine uveitis with retinal detachments.

2. Detection of intraocular tumors or foreign bodies. Radiolucent materials are visible with ultrasonography.

3. Investigation of retrobulbar diseases.

Ultrasonography is used to examine the contents of the eye, when the media are opaque, or of the orbit.

FLUORESCEIN ANGIOGRAPHY

Fluorescein angiography may be used to investigate retinal and choroidal vascular patency, vessel wall permeability, and pigmentary abnormalities of the fundus. Vessels in areas of active inflammation and new vessels (neovascularization) show increased permeability to the dye.

When fluorescein is illuminated by light with a wavelength between 485 and 500 nm, it fluoresces with maximal emission between 520 and 530 nm. Fluorescein is injected intravenously, and the fundus is illuminated with the stimulating wavelength. The emitted light is photographed (Fig. 5–41). A series of approximately 30 photographs is taken in the first 30 seconds, followed by single photographs 20 and 30 minutes later. Circulation of the fluorescein is divided into

1. Choroidal phase—choroidal vasculature has filled.
2. Arteriolar phase—retina arterioles have filled.

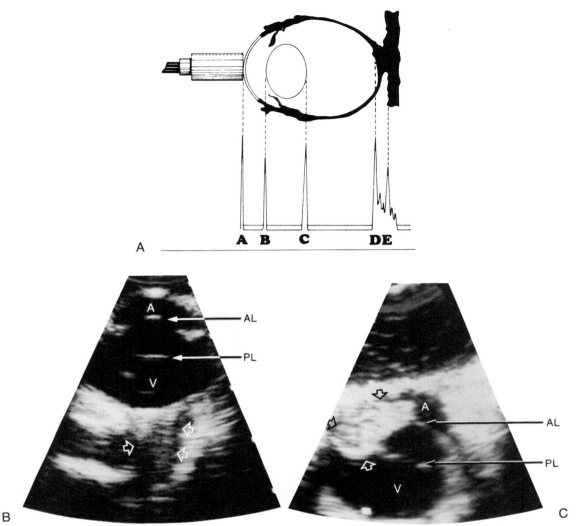

FIGURE 5–40. A, A-mode ultrasonogram of a normal canine eye, showing the transmitter pulse (A), anterior lens echo (B), posterior lens echo (C), posterior ocular wall echo (D), and retrobulbar echoes (E). (From Rubin LF, Koch SA: Ocular diagnostic ultrasonography. J Am Vet Med Assoc 153:1706, 1968.) B, Normal B-mode ultrasonogram of a canine globe and orbit in the horizontal plane. A real-time mechanical sector scanner (B-mode) with a 7.5-MHz transducer was used. A = anterior chamber; AL = anterior lens capsule; PL = posterior lens capsule; V = vitreous. Arrows delimit orbital contents. C, Ultrasonogram of a canine eye with a melanoma of the anterior uvea that has displaced the lens. A = anterior chamber; AL = anterior lens capsule; PL = posterior lens capsule; V = vitreous. Arrows delimit the anterior uveal mass. (B,C courtesy of Dr. J. Dziezyc.)

3. Arteriovenous phase—both arterioles and venules have filled.

4. Venous phase—arterioles have emptied and veins have begun to fill.

5. Late phase—certain tissues (e.g., optic nerve head) stain with fluorescein.

In the normal eye, fluorescein does not penetrate the endothelium of retinal or choroidal vessels but does pass the choriocapillaris. In disease states these relationships are altered. In interpretation of fluorescein angiograms, the first step is to determine whether the area under consideration represents *hyper-* or *hypofluorescence*. Fluorescence of the tapetum in domestic animals renders interpretation of fluorescein angiograms more difficult than in the human eye. The lower frequency of retinal vascular disease in domestic animals decreases the utility of the technique compared with the human eye.

For more detailed discussion of fluorescein angiography, numerous texts and atlases are available.

EVALUATION OF VISION

Although decussation of fibers from the nasal retina of each eye occurs in the optic chiasm, it is important not to confuse vision of objects in the right visual field

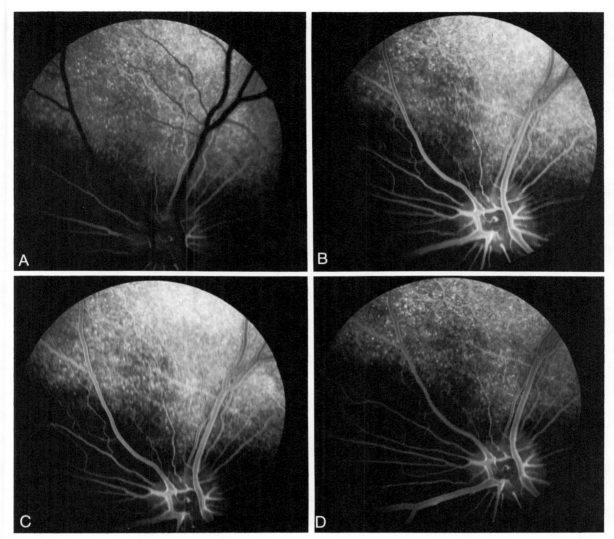

FIGURE 5–41. *Normal canine fluorescein angiogram. A, Choroidal phase. B, Arteriovenous phase. C, Venous phase. D, Late phase. (Courtesy of Dr. R. W. Bellhorn.)*

with vision by the right eye (and vice versa). Patients with a nonfunctional eye on one side may still retain vision in the visual field of that eye, because light from objects in that field falls onto the temporal retina of the remaining eye (Fig. 1–7). In horses, cattle, and sheep (where decussation is greater than in other domestic species), each eye is used predominantly for vision in its own visual field. A positive direct pupillary light reflex is not a reliable indicator of vision or normal retinal function.

A positive direct pupillary light reflex is not an indicator of vision. A negative direct pupillary light reflex is often associated with, but is not pathognomonic of, faulty vision.

Unfortunately, testing of vision in animals is subjective. No "percentage" of visual deficit should be quoted to an owner of an animal. Findings can be described as mild, moderate, severe, or total visual deficit. Each test must be interpreted by the clinician, considering the animal's personality, emotional state, and state of consciousness. During any of these tests, individual eyes may be tested by "patching" the remaining eye with a triangular black cloth eye patch, if the animal will tolerate it. Intolerance to a patch is more frequent in sighted animals.

Cotton Test

A small piece of cotton is dropped 20–30 cm in front and to one side of the patient. Most dogs and cats visually follow the object to the floor after one or two attempts. Some blind animals, especially cats, hear the cotton strike the floor and by reflex look in the direction of the sound. The test is performed in each visual field.

Obstacle Test

A variety of test obstacles (e.g., chairs, buckets) of different sizes and shapes are placed around a room or pen. With small animals, the owner stands on one side of the obstacles and calls the animal from the clinician, once only. Both the client and clinician remain still and quiet during the test. With horses, the patient is led through the maze on a long lead (3–4 m). Horses, cattle, and sheep that are unused to leading can be released in the pen or barn and their movements watched. If such a passive test is negative, the patient may be driven through the obstacles.

Obstacle tests are performed in lighted conditions (to test photopic vision) and in the dark (to test scotopic vision).

Scotopic obstacle tests are often sensitive indicators of rod dysfunction (e.g., rod-cone dysplasia in dogs, vitamin A deficiency in cattle).

Menace Reflex Test

In testing the menace reflex, the clinician makes a sudden threatening movement near the eye (with the other eye blindfolded) and observes the animal's response (e.g., blinking, head movements). Placid or highly trained animals show little response, and *care is necessary* in interpreting a lack of response, as the test is unreliable.

TABLE 5–4. Clinical Signs Associated with Visual Deficits

Dog
1. Bumping into unfamiliar objects
2. Hesitancy in unfamiliar surroundings and "smelling" along
3. Refusal to move
4. "Sudden" blindness on return to familiar surroundings after a short absence
5. Refusal to negotiate steps
6. Misjudging flight of a ball
7. Inability to find a downed bird
8. Inability to follow a lure (greyhounds)
9. Stopping during a race (greyhounds), especially under lights at night
10. Walking tentatively around walls
11. Staying very close to the owner
12. Refusal to go outside at night

Cat
1. Refusal to move
2. Hesitancy in unfamiliar surroundings and "smelling" along
3. Walking tentatively around walls

Horse
1. Bumping into walls, rails, and so on
2. High-stepping gait
3. Difficulty in negotiating steps
4. Difficulty in leading
5. Reluctance to pass through a gate

Cow, Sheep, Goat
1. Refusal to move
2. Separation from the herd
3. Carriage of the head close to the ground
4. Reluctance to pass through a gate

The eye is menaced from both nasal and temporal directions. Waving hands or objects in front of an animal is not a test of vision; air currents perceptible to the animal's sensory hairs frequently cause a positive reaction. To prevent air currents, the threatening motion can be performed behind a transparent sheet of plastic. Absence of the menace reflex is associated with diffuse degenerative lesions of the cerebellar cortex (deLahunta, 1983).

TABLE 5–5. Summary of Terms

Term	Definition
alopecia	absence of hair from an area in which it is normally found
anisocoria	pupils of different diameters
aphakia	absence of the lens
aphakic crescent	crescent of tapetal reflex seen between the pupillary margin of the iris and the edge of the lens in lens subluxation
aqueous flare	turbidity or opalescence of the aqueous caused by protein and cells
blepharospasm	complete or partial closure of the palpebral fissure owing to spasm of the orbicularis oculi muscle
cataract	partial or complete opacity of the lens or its capsule
chemosis	excessive edema of the conjunctiva
coloboma	congenital fissure of any part of the eye

TABLE 5–5. Summary of Terms *Continued*

Term	Definition
corectopia	an eccentric pupil
cornea plana	congenital flattening of the cornea
descemetocele	herniation or protrusion of Descemet's membrane through the anterior layers of the cornea
ectasia (scleral)	thinning of sclera—partial (localized) and total ectasia are distinguished
epiphora	abnormal overflow of tears down the face
exophthalmos	abnormal protrusion of the globe
glaucoma	clinical and pathological complex of ocular abnormalities caused by elevated intraocular pressure
glaucomatous cupping	abnormal depression in the optic disc associated with glaucoma
heterochromia iridis	difference in color between the two irides (plural form of iris) or between different parts of the same iris
hippus	abnormal exaggeration of the physiological rhythmic contraction and dilatation of the pupil that occurs independent of changes in illumination
hypopyon	accumulation of purulent material in the anterior chamber
iridodonesis	abnormal quivering or shaking of the iris in response to movement of the eye, occurring in lens subluxation when the iris loses support of the lens
iris bombé	total posterior synechia with anterior bowing of the iris, caused by accumulation of aqueous between the lens and the iris
keratic precipitates	focal precipitates of inflammatory cells on the corneal endothelium
keratoconus	conical protrusion of the cornea
keratoglobus	globular enlargement and protrusion of the anterior segment of the cornea in the absence of elevated intraocular pressure
lagophthalmos	inability to close the eyelids completely
lenticonus	conical protrusion of the anterior or posterior lens capsule
lentiglobus	globular enlargement and protrusion of the anterior or posterior lens capsule
leukocoria	a white pupil
luxation (lens)	displacement of the lens from the hyaloid fossa
microphakia	lens smaller than normal
microphthalmia	small size of the globe
miosis	contraction of the pupil
mydriasis	dilatation of the pupil
neovascularization	formation of new blood vessels
occluded pupil	obstruction of the pupil by a congenital or acquired membrane (pupillary membrane)
papilledema	edema of the optic papilla or disc
polycoria	more than one pupil
protopsis	same as exophthalmos
ptosis	drooping of the upper eyelid
pupillary block	blockage of the passage of aqueous between the pupillary border of the iris and the anterior lens capsule
secluded pupil	a complete, annular, posterior synechia that results from anterior uveitis and separates the anterior and posterior chambers of the anterior compartment
spherophakia	spherical deformation of the lens
staphyloma	stretching or protrusion of the fibrous coat of the eye (cornea or sclera) with the uveal tract (iris, ciliary body, or choroid) fused to the inner surface, and the whole lesion infiltrated with uveal pigment
subluxation (lens)	partial displacement of the lens from the hyaloid fossa, with part of the lens remaining in the fossa
synchysis	liquefaction of the vitreous
synechia	adhesion of the iris to the posterior surface of the cornea (anterior synechia) or lens (posterior synechia)
syneresis	shrinkage of the gel of the vitreous with release of fluid

Electrical potentials in response to a flash of light into the contralateral eye (the VISION EVOKED RESPONSE) may be recorded from the skin over the surface of the visual cortex. Although rarely used clinically, it can be used to evaluate central visual pathways. Clinical signs commonly associated with visual deficits are given in Table 5–4.

Retinoscopy

Retinoscopy allows evaluation of refractive errors, and whether they may be contributing to the visual state. It is often combined with an electroretinogram to determine retinal dysfunction.

SUMMARY OF TERMS

Many terms used in the description of clinical abnormalities were introduced in this chapter. Diseases and concepts covered in greater detail in later chapters are not included here. For review purposes, the definition in the right-hand column of Table 5–5 may be covered during self-testing.

OPTICS

A basic consideration of several optical principles is necessary to understand the eye's function as an optical instrument.

NATURE OF LIGHT

Light is electromagnetic radiation, which travels in straight lines. The eye is sensitive to a range of wavelengths, from 400 nm (violet) to 700 nm (red), although other wavelengths (infrared and ultraviolet) may enter the eye with undesirable effects in certain circumstances. The velocity at which light travels is variable, depending on the medium through which it is passing. The velocity of light in air is greater than that in glass and in most other transparent media.

When light strikes an object, any or all of several phenomena may occur, as shown in Figure 5–42. In reflection the ray returns to the original medium. The angle of incidence equals the angle of reflection (Fig. 5–43).

When light passes from a medium with a low refractive index (e.g., air) to one with a high refractive index (e.g., cornea), it is bent toward the normal to the surface (the line perpendicular to the surface, shown in Fig. 5–44). A surface that is convex in the direction of the incident light bends all rays toward the center line, bringing them to a focus.

When light passes between two media of the same refractive index, refraction occurs. The only tissues in the eye that refract light significantly are the cornea (air-cornea interface) and lens (aqueous-lens and lens-vitreous interfaces).

When light passes from a medium with a high refractive index to one with a low refractive index, it is refracted further away from the normal (Fig. 5–45). As the angle of incidence is increased under these conditions, a point is reached at which the refracted ray passes along the interface between the media (Fig. 5–45, second from right). If the angle of incidence is increased further, there can be no refraction and the ray is reflected back into the medium—the phenomenon of *total internal reflection*. This is why the drainage angle of the eye cannot be viewed directly (the rays attempt to pass from the cornea to air at a high angle of incidence and this phenomenon occurs) (see Fig. 5–32). This can be prevented by placing an object of higher refractive index—the goniolens—on the cornea; now, total internal reflection does not occur and light leaves the eye (Fig. 5–33).

PRISMS AND LENSES

When light passes through a prism, it deviates from its former direction as discussed previously. The extent

Text continued on page 123

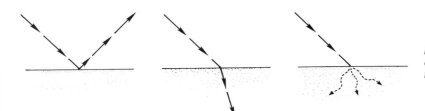

A Reflection **B** Refraction **C** Scattering

FIGURE 5–42. A, Ray is reflected. B, Ray enters second medium and is refracted. C, Ray is absorbed.

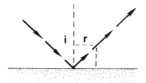

Reflection

FIGURE 5–43. In reflection, the angle of incidence (i, measured from dashed normal line) is equal to the angle of reflection (r, also measured from normal line).

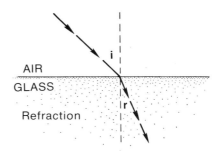

AIR

GLASS

Refraction

FIGURE 5–44. In refraction, the angle of incidence (i, measured from dashed normal line) is related to the angle of refraction (r, measured from normal line on other side of interface) by the refractive index.

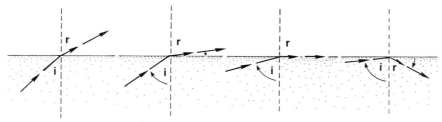

FIGURE 5–45. Refraction of ray passing from a medium with a high refractive index to one with a low refractive index. At a critical angle (which depends on the ratio between the refractive indexes), r becomes 90°. For all angles of incidence larger than the critical angle, total internal reflection occurs.

A

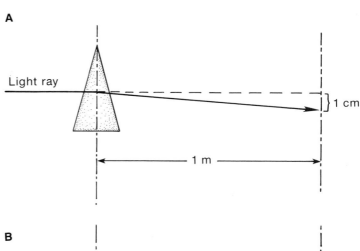

Light ray

1 cm

1 m

FIGURE 5–46. A, The effect of a prism of 1 D on a light ray. B, The effect of a prism of 5 D on a light ray. (From Severin GA: Veterinary Ophthalmology Notes, 2nd ed. Fort Collins, CO, 1976.)

B

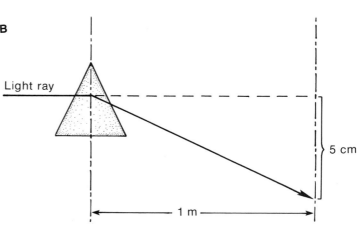

Light ray

5 cm

1 m

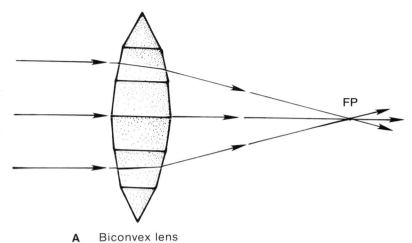

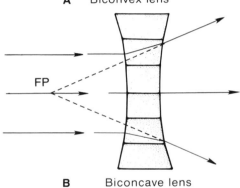

A   Biconvex lens

B   Biconcave lens

FIGURE 5–47. A, *Biconvex lens.* B, *Biconcave lens.* FP = *focal point.*

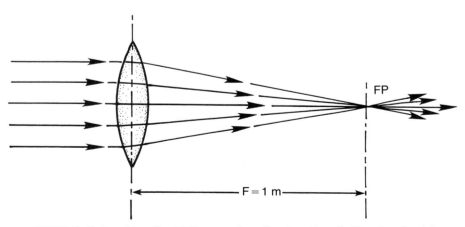

FIGURE 5–48. Focal length of 1-D convex lens: F = focal length; FP = focal point.

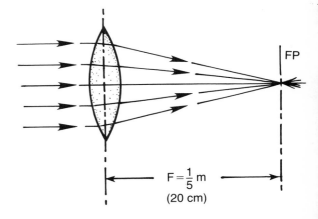

FIGURE 5–49. Focal length of 5-D convex lens.

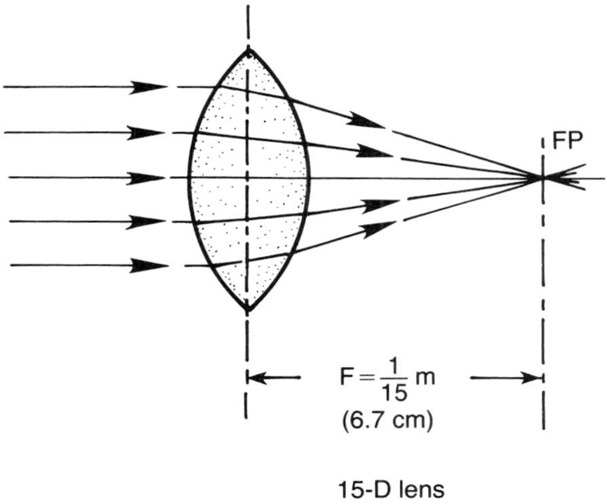

$F = \frac{1}{5}$ m
(20 cm)

5-D lens

FP

$F = \frac{1}{15}$ m
(6.7 cm)

15-D lens

FIGURE 5–50. Focal length of 15-D convex lens.

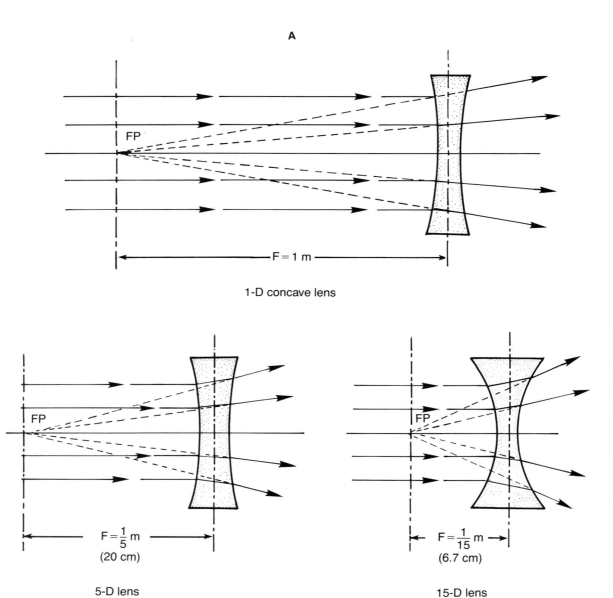

FIGURE 5–51. A, *Focal length of* − 1-D *concave lens.* B, *Focal length of* − 5-D *concave lens.* C, *Focal length of* − 15-D *concave lens.*

to which it deviates (the power of the prism) is measured in diopters: a prism of 1 D deviates a ray of light 1 cm at a distance of 1 m (Fig. 5–46).

A lens may be considered a series of prisms (Fig. 5–47). The focal point (FP) of a lens is the point at which parallel rays of light are brought together. Concave lenses cause divergence of the beams of light, producing a *virtual* focal point between the source of light and the lens. The power of lenses is also measured in diopters, defined now as the reciprocal of the focal length (F) (expressed in meters) (Figs. 5–48 to 5–51). That is,

$$D = \frac{1}{F} \text{ or } F = \frac{1}{D}$$

Convex (positive) lenses and concave (negative) lenses are contained in the direct ophthalmoscope head. Concave lenses are indicated by red numbers and convex lenses by black numbers on the dial. A simple test to determine whether a lens is positive or negative is to look through the lens at a stationary object and move the lens. If the object appears to move in the same direction as the lens, the lens is positive; if the object appears to move in the opposite direction, the lens is negative.

REFERENCES

Acland GM (1988): Diagnosis and differentiation of retinal disease in small animals by electroretinography. Semin Vet Med Surg 3:15.

Bedford PGC (1973): A practical method of gonioscopy and goniophotography in the dog and cat. J Sm Anim Pract 14:601.

Bellhorn RW (1973): Fluorescein fundus photography in veterinary ophthlmology. J Am Anim Hosp Assoc 9:227.

Bill A (1966): Formation and drainage of aqueous in cats. Exp Eye Res 5:185.

Blogg JR (1980): The Eye in Veterinary Practice. WB Saunders Co, Philadelphia.

Bryan GM (1965): Tonometry in the dog and cat. J Sm Anim Pract 6:117.

Carrington SD, et al (1987): Polarized light biomicroscopic observations on the precorneal tear film. 1. The normal tear film of the dog. J Sm Anim Pract 28:605.

Carrington SD, et al (1987): Polarized light biomicroscopic observations on the precorneal tear film. 3. The normal tear film of the cat. J Sm Anim Pract 28:821.

Cohen CM, Reinke DA (1970): Equine tonometry. J Am Vet Med Assoc 156:1884.

deLahunta A (1983): Veterinary Neuroanatomy and Clinical Neurology, 2nd ed. WB Saunders Co, Philadelphia.

Dixon RT (1974): The orbital venogram. Aust Vet Pract 4:159.

Dixon RT, Carter JD (1972): Canine orbital venography. J Am Vet Rad Soc 13:43.

Dziezyc J, Hager DA (1988): Ocular ultrasonography in veterinary medicine. Semin Vet Med Surg 3:1.

Dziezyc J, et al (1987): Two-dimensional real-time ocular sonography in the diagnosis of ocular lesions in dogs. J Am Anim Hosp Assoc 23:501.

Duke-Elder S, Leigh AG (1965): System of Ophthalmology, vol 7, Diseases of the Outer Eye, part 2. H Kimpton, London.

Gelatt KN, et al (1970): Radiographic contrast techniques for detecting orbital and nasolacrimal tumors in dogs. J Am Vet Med Assoc 156:741.

Gelatt KN, et al (1975): Evaluation of tear formation in the dog, using a modification of the Schirmer tear test. J Am Vet Med Assoc 166:368.

Gelatt KN, et al (1976): Fluorescein angiography of the normal and diseased ocular fundi of the laboratory dog. J Am Vet Med Assoc 169:980.

Hager DA, et al (1987): Two-dimensional real-time ocular ultrasonography in the dog—Technique and normal anatomy. Vet Rad 28:60.

Hawkins EC, Murphy CJ (1986): Inconsistencies in the absorptive capacities of Schirmer tear test strips. J Am Vet Med Assoc 188:511.

Heywood R (1971): Intraocular pressure in the beagle dog. J Sm Anim Pract 12:119.

Hoerlein B (1978): Canine Neurology, 3rd ed. WB Saunders Co, Philadelphia.

Kommonen B, Raitta C (1987): Electroretinography in Labrador retrievers given ketamine-xylazine anesthesia. Am J Vet Res 48:1325.

Lavach JD, et al (1977): Cytology of normal and inflamed conjunctivas in dogs and cats. J Am Vet Med Assoc 170:722.

LeCouteur RA, et al (1982): Computed tomography of orbital tumors in the dog. J Am Vet Med Assoc 180:910.

LeCouteur JD, et al (1983): X-ray computed tomography of brain tumors in cats. J Am Vet Med Assoc 183:301.

Lee R, Griffiths IR (1972): A comparison of cerebral arteriography and cavernous sinus venography in the dog. J Sm Anim Pract 13:225.

Lescure F (1963): L'angle camerulaine du chien. Etude goniophotographique. Proceedings XVII Worth Veterinary Congress, Hanover, Germany, vol 2:1001.

Magrane WG: Canine Ophthalmology, 2nd ed. Lea & Febiger, Philadelphia, 1971.

Manning R, et al (1977): The Schirmer test in equine: Normal values and the contribution of the glans nictitans. Proc Am Coll Vet Ophthalmol 8:101.

Martin CL (1969): Gonioscopy and anatomical correlations of the drainage angle of the dog. J Sm Anim Pract 10:171.

McClure JR, et al (1976): The effect of parenteral acepromazine and xylazine on intraocular pressure in the horse. Vet Med Small Anim Clin 71:1727.

Oliver JE (1969): Cranial sinus venography in the dog. J Am Vet Rad Soc 10:70.

Rubin LF (1967): Clinical electroretinography in animals. J Am Vet Med Assoc 151:1456.

Rubin LF (1974): Atlas of Veterinary Ophthalmoscopy. Lea & Febiger, Philadelphia.

Rubin LF, Koch SA (1968): Ocular diagnostic ultrasonography. J Am Vet Med Assoc 153:1706.

Rubin LF, et al (1965): Clinical estimation of lacrimal function in dogs. J Am Vet Med Assoc 147:946.

Severin GA (1976): Veterinary Ophthalmology Notes, 2nd ed. Fort Collins, CO.

Slatter DH (1973): Differential staining of canine cornea and conjunctiva with rose bengal and alcian blue. J Sm Anim Pract 14:291.

Startup FG (1969): Diseases of the Canine Eye. Baliere Tindall, London.

Vaughan D, Asbury T (1983): General Ophthalmology, 10th ed. Lange Medical Publications, Los Altos, CA.

Veith L, et al (1970): The Schirmer tear test in cats. Mod Vet Pract 51:48.

Woelfel CG, et al (1964): Intraocular pressure in vitamin A deficient Holstein male calves. J Diary Sci 47:655.

Yakely WL, Alexander JE (1973): Dacryocystorhinography in the dog. J Am Vet Med Assoc 159:1417.

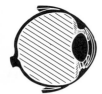

Principles of Ophthalmic Surgery

6

"No good physician quavers incantations
When the malady he's treating needs the knife."
—Sophocles *Ajax* 582

"I think all of us who have worked years in the profession understand that many skillful operators are not good surgeons."
—William J. Mayo (Surg Gynecol Obstet 67:535, 1938)

ANESTHESIA MONITORING PREOPERATIVE PREPARATION SURGICAL EQUIPMENT AND SUPPLIES	CARE AND STERILIZATION OF INSTRUMENTS PREVENTION OF SELF- MUTILATION	BASIC SURGICAL PROCEDURES COMMON OPHTHALMIC INSTRUMENTS

Attention to details, a correct diagnosis and choice of surgical procedure, the necessary instruments and equipment, and adequate training and experience in their use are necessary for acceptable results in ophthalmic surgery. Failure to complete seemingly minute pharmacological preoperative, procedural, or postoperative details may cause complications and poor or catastrophic results. As this discussion is primarily for nonophthalmologists, extensive details of intraocular surgery have been omitted, in favor of procedures applicable to general practice.

ANESTHESIA

In dogs and cats, general anesthesia is used for all but the most minor procedures. In cattle and horses, where assistance and facilities for prolonged general anesthesia are not always available, deep tranquilization and local anesthesia are suitable for minor procedures.

A useful anesthetic regimen in dogs and cats is

1. Minimal data base: Preoperative physical examination. All patients over 6 years of age receive a complete blood count, total body function chemistry profile, and thoracic radiographs.

2. Preoperative medication with atropine (0.05 mg/kg) and glycopyrrolate (10 μg/kg)[1] 30–40 minutes before induction, or intravenously at induction. The two are used together as glycopyrrolate may not always prevent bradycardia as effectively, but it is longer acting and superior in reducing salivary and bronchial secretions.

3. Induction with thiamylal sodium intravenously, and immediate intubation. In older or high-risk patients, induction with oxymorphone (0.1 mg/kg) to effect and diazepam (0.4 mg/kg) intravenously or isoflurane by mask is useful. Oxymorphone can be reversed postoperatively with naloxone (0.04 mg/kg) for rapid recovery. In cats, intravenous (IV) induction with equal volumes of ketamine and diazepam is more useful than is thiamylal or pentothal sodium and allows easier intubation.

4. Maintenance of anesthesia with methoxyflurane and oxygen, with nitrous oxide added if desired. In high-risk patients, isoflurane is useful but expensive.

---

1. Glycopyrrolate is most effective for preventing salivation and stabilizing heart rate, but it cannot be relied on alone for this purpose, hence the use of half the recommended dose of each agent.

124

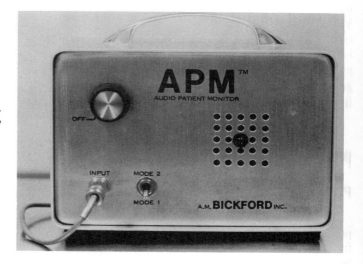

FIGURE 6–1. A battery-operated esophageal stethoscope, amplifier, and loudspeaker suitable for use with small and large animals.

Methoxyflurane[2] causes useful postoperative analgesia and tranquilization and reduces the risk of cardiac dysrhythmias or ventricular fibrillation that sometimes occur when intraocular epinephrine is used (*epinephrine syncope*). Methoxyflurane has the additional advantage of lowering intraocular pressure by 5–10 mmHg.

Preoperative administration of atropine, even in cats in which ketamine is subsequently used, does not reduce tear production to any clinically significant extent, and although useful, routine use of lubricating ointments as in humans is *not* mandatory in either dogs or cats. Lesions resulting from corneal drying in normal animals during anesthesia are rare.

In large animals, methoxyflurane is unsuitable because of the prolonged recovery time, so a combination of acepromazine, atropine, glyceryl guaiacolate, thiamylal sodium (or ketamine in horses), and halothane is used. In cattle, glyceryl guaiacolate is usually omitted. The following protocol is useful in horses:

1. preoperative physical examination

2. premedication with acepromazine (0.1 mg/kg) and atropine (0.02 mg/kg) 30–40 minutes prior to induction

3. induction of anesthesia with thiamylal sodium and glyceryl guaiacolate by slow IV infusion or IV ketamine.

4. maintenance of anesthesia with halothane and oxygen.

For techniques of local anesthesia suitable for use in large animals see p 93.

MONITORING

Because the head is covered with drapes during ophthalmic surgery, special care is required to monitor vital functions—heart rate and sounds, respiratory rate, and electrocardiogram (ECG)—during surgery. An amplified esophageal stethoscope[3] (Fig. 6–1), and ideally an oscilloscope[4] (Fig. 6–2), are used to check for

---

2. See Chap 3 for details of possible toxicity with flunixin meglumine.

3. APM (Audio Patient Monitor)—AM Bickford, Inc, E Aurora, NY.

4. Telectronics Pty Ltd, Sydney, Australia.

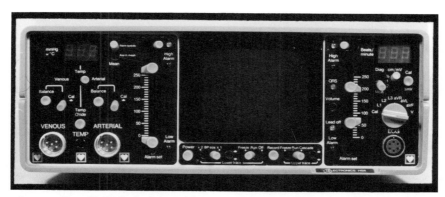

FIGURE 6–2. A cardiac monitor with ECG display and freeze capability, digital heart rate display, and adjustable alarms.

dysrhythmias induced by anesthetics, intraocular drugs, poor ventilation, or manipulation of the extraocular muscles or orbital contents (OCULOCARDIAC REFLEX). Young animals may be more susceptible to the oculocardiac reflex. The reflex is minimized by treatment before ophthalmic surgery with IV atropine or glycopyrollate and by keeping the patient adequately oxygenated, and the P_{CO_2} low. Statements that this reflex is not important in animals may be discounted.

PREOPERATIVE PREPARATION

Pharmacological Preparation

The eye often becomes rapidly inflamed after surgical procedures. Topical and systemic corticosteroids are frequently used for several days before ophthalmic surgery or cryosurgery in order to reduce miosis and protein release when the anterior chamber is opened or postoperative swelling, respectively. A preoperative IV bolus of corticosteroid has been shown experimentally to be synergistic with the effect of antiprostaglandins in reducing aqueous protein release in dogs, but the clinical advantages of such administration are unconvincing. Longer-term, topical preoperative corticosteroid therapy, plus flunixin (0.5 mg/kg) at anesthesic induction, yields satisfactory results. For details of antiprostaglandins see Chapter 3.

Complications seen with the use of corticosteroids are slow wound healing and decreased resistance to bacterial and fungal infections. To limit these effects, nonabsorbable suture (nylon or polypropylene) should be used in the globe where appropriate. Prophylactic antibiotics are bactericidal and are changed regularly during the pre- and postoperative periods.

ANTIBACTERIAL AGENTS

Even with aseptic surgical technique, pre- and postoperative antibiotic therapy is often used because

1. It is impossible to sterilize the conjunctival sac, lacrimal ducts, and tarsal glands. A considerable normal flora containing potential pathogens is present in all domestic animals (Tables 3–3, 3–5, and 3–7 to 3–9). Preoperative flushing of the conjunctival sac with sterile saline solution alone does *not* reduce the bacterial flora.

2. Local and systemic immunosuppression with corticosteroids is often necessary pre- and postoperatively in veterinary ocular surgery.

3. Domestic animals, especially normal dogs, frequently exhibit bacteremia with potential pathogens. The use of antibiotics is no excuse for lack of proper aseptic surgical technique.

Preoperative preparation with a broad-spectrum bactericidal agent(s), e.g., bacitracin, polymixin, and neomycin combinations, or dilute povidone-iodine solution, is advisable for elective procedures. Before intraocular procedures, ointments are avoided to prevent the entry of irritating oily material into the eye.

MYDRIASIS AND CYCLOPLEGIA

Pupillary dilatation and relaxation of the ciliary body are frequently desirable before intraocular procedures. Topical atropine, scopolamine, and phenylephrine are frequently used in different combinations. The use of topical medications by subconjunctival injection is not recommended.

Preparation for Surgery

A bland ointment or jelly (e.g., KY jelly, or Lacri-Lube) is placed in the conjunctival sac before hair removal. After preparation, the ointment and adherent hairs are removed. Alternatively, a scleral contact lens filled with methylcellulose or antibiotic solution may be used to protect the cornea. "Clipper burn" or traumatic dermatitis is carefully avoided, because it may cause postoperative irritation and scratching.

Cilia on the upper eyelid are trimmed and all hair removed by vacuum from the periorbital area. It is useful to flush the conjunctival sac with sterile saline solution, although this does not decrease bacterial contamination. Dilute povidone-iodine solution (1:25 to 1:50) placed in the conjunctival sac is a useful preoperative antibacterial agent, but it must be thoroughly flushed out before intraocular surgery. Great care may be necessary to prevent further damage when restraining an animal that has a penetrating ocular wound.

A variety of methods of skin preparation are used. Whatever agents are used, they must not be irritating to the eye. A successful and frequently used method is outlined here.

1. The area is cleaned with gauze sponges soaked in sterile saline solution until hair and gross contamination have been removed. Several drops of 1:25 povidone-iodine solution are instilled into the conjunctival sac.

2. Dilute povidone-iodine solution is used to disinfect the area. *Note:* Povidone-iodine solution (not scrub solution, which contains irritating detergents) is diluted with an equal volume of saline solution.

3. The surgical area is cleaned with 70% ethyl alcohol or 99% isopropyl alcohol, and the patient is moved to the operating room. The head is placed on a raised sandbag covered in plastic. If intraocular surgery is to be performed, alcohol may be omitted in order to limit irritation.

4. A final skin application of povidone-iodine is given, avoiding the conjunctival sac, and the eye is flushed with saline.

> The skin disinfectant *chlorhexidine* must not enter the conjunctival sac if it is used on the skin. It causes severe toxic keratitis.

DRAPING

The surgical field is draped with three field drapes and a drape with a circular fenestration (Fig. 6–3). A plastic adherent drape may be placed over the field first but is not necessary if preparation is adequate. All drapes should be double-thickness green cotton, cotton/ dacron, or water-impervious paper in order to lessen glare. The use of a rubber dental dam is unnecessary. Full aseptic precautions should be followed for the surgical procedure, including scrub suits, sterile gowns, gloves, masks, and head coverings. When dealing with penetrating injuries of the eye, starch powder is rinsed off the gloves with sterile saline solution in order to prevent the granules entering the eye and causing a foreign body reaction *(starch endophthalmitis)*. Cellulose sponges are preferable for absorbing blood as fibers from cotton-tipped applicators may enter the eye.

For minor ocular procedures (e.g., creation of third eyelid flaps), extensive aseptic precautions are unwarranted.

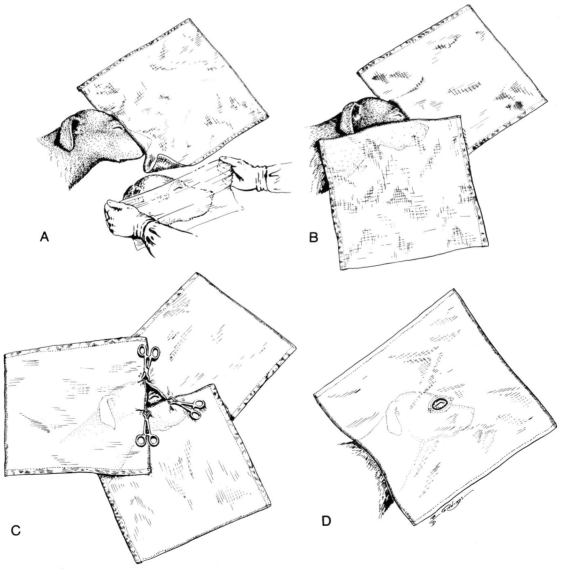

FIGURE 6–3. Draping for ocular surgery. A, The first field drape in position. B, The second field drape in position. C, The third field drape and Backhaus's towel clamps in position. D, The fenestrated eye drape in position.

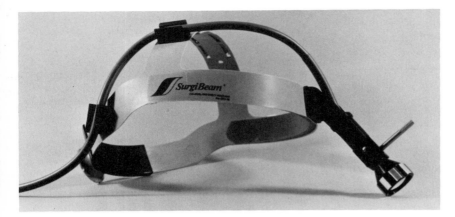

FIGURE 6–4. *Head-mounted fiberoptic spotlight.*

SURGICAL EQUIPMENT AND SUPPLIES

Illumination and Magnification

Ophthalmic surgery is performed with a focal light source in a semidarkened room in order to reduce reflections in the transparent media. For adnexal surgery a standard operating room light is adequate, but for fine work a head-mounted focusing light is useful (Fig. 6–4). Fiberoptic illumination does not cause heating and drying of delicate tissues.

For surgical procedures involving the cilia, lacrimal puncta, or globe, magnification is usually essential. For most purposes a simple head loupe of the kind used for ocular examination (Fig. 5–13) is used. A variety of loupes and loupe-light combinations are available. A combination of $1.5\times$ to $4\times$ and a working distance of 20–30 cm or more is suitable. For more intricate surgery (e.g., for distichiasis, corneal procedures), an operating microscope and appropriate microsurgical instruments (Fig. 6–5) are indispensable for optimal results.

Successful microsurgery requires considerable training and practice. Microsurgical instruments are smaller, more delicate, and more expensive, and they have matte surfaces to limit reflection.

Positioning

Ophthalmic surgery is performed from a sitting position, in a chair with armrests. The ideal is an ophthalmic operating stool with an armrest (Fig. 6–6), but a standard adjustable stool with sandbags placed on the table as armrests is adequate.

Hemostasis

Methods for hemostasis in general surgery are also useful in ophthalmic surgery; these include pressure with a cotton-tipped applicator, ligation, use of

1:80,000 epinephrine solution, and electrocautery. A good-quality electrosurgical unit (Fig. 6–7) is particularly useful if profuse hemorrhage is expected (e.g., in tumor excision, blepharoplastic procedures, or iridectomy). Units are available that blend both cutting and coagulating currents as desired, and more expensive units operate in a wet field. Hand-held battery-operated cautery units (Fig. 6–8) are ideal for minor but critical hemorrhage.

The use of an electrosurgical unit for epilation, even on the lowest power setting, may cause excessive tissue

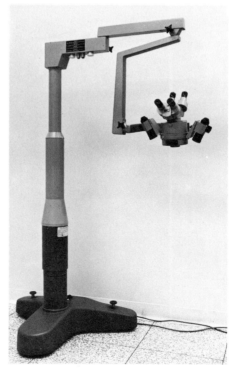

FIGURE 6–5. *An operating microscope with power-operated zoom, focus, tilt, and an assistant's headpiece.*

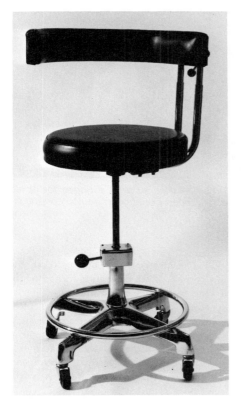

FIGURE 6–6. *Ophthalmic operating stool with armrest. (From Bistner SI, et al: Atlas of Veterinary Ophthalmic Surgery. WB Saunders Co, Philadelphia, 1977.)*

necrosis, cicatricial distortion and entropion, and iatrogenic chalazion (Fig. 6–9) and is contraindicated.

Cryotherapy

Cryotherapy is used for the selective destruction of neoplasms, treatment of glaucoma *(cyclocryotherapy)* and distichiasis *(cryoepilation)*, and occasionally grasping of

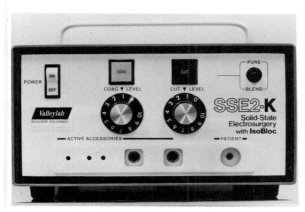

FIGURE 6–7. *An electrosurgery unit.*

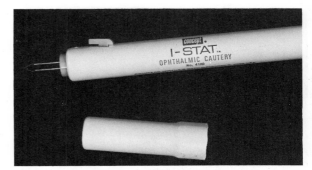

FIGURE 6–8. *A battery-operated, hand-held cautery. These units may be resterilized with ethylene oxide for repeated use.*

luxated lenses. Cyclocryotherapy and cryoepilation are major advances in ophthalmic surgery. General cryosurgical equipment may be used for periocular tumors, but for small lesions on the globe, ophthalmic cryosurgical units with a probe diameter of about 3 mm, cooled by nitrous oxide, are necessary (Fig. 6–10). For cyclocryotherapy, liquid nitrogen (Fig. 6–11) units give far superior results.

Miscellaneous Supplies

SPONGES

Care must be taken when using standard cotton surgical sponges to prevent lint from the sponge entering the eye (Fig. 6–12). For penetrating wounds, cellulose sponge wedges are recommended. For occasional use, autoclaved cotton-tipped applicators are useful for conjunctival hemorrhage but must not be placed inside the eye or near a penetrating wound.

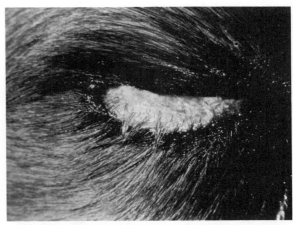

FIGURE 6–9. *Tissue necrosis in a dog, resulting from excessive use of an electrosurgical unit for epilation. (Courtesy of Dr. G. A. Severin.)*

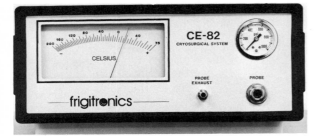

FIGURE 6–10. *Frigitronics N20 cryosurgical unit for direct ocular use. A temperature of −89°C is reached with this equipment. A large variety of probes are available, but the glaucoma and lens probes are most suited to veterinary use.*

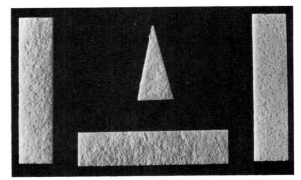

FIGURE 6–12. *Cellulose surgical sponges for ophthalmic use, especially when penetrating ocular wounds are present.*

IRRIGATING SOLUTIONS

Sterile physiological saline solution is suitable for external lavage. Balanced salt solution[5] is preferable for anterior chamber irrigation as it is less likely to cause endothelial damage. During ocular surgery the cornea is kept constantly moist. Sterile water should *never* be used near the eye because of toxic osmotic effects on cells and the danger of confusion with other solutions.

SUTURES

General principles of choice of suture material are

1. The suture should be as fine as is consistent with the surgeon's ability, training and equipment, and the patient being treated.

2. Suture materials that may touch the cornea must be soft and pliable.

3. Chromic gut is not used in the cornea. For buried sutures beneath the conjunctiva, chromic gut, polyglycolic or polyglactic acid or polydioxanone are suitable.

4. Absorbable materials are not used as the sole suture for a corneal or scleral wound, when nonirritant nonabsorbable materials are available. The use of braided synthetic absorbable material as the sole suture in an eye immunosuppressed for intraocular surgery is inadvisable unless the sutures are removed at the normal time. With braided sutures of these materials, acute infections with organisms not normally pathogenic may occur. The tendency for difficult infections with these materials has been recorded in other tissues.

5. If possible, use nonirritant fine materials in order to limit postoperative irritation.

Recommendations for suture materials are summarized in Table 6–1. Fine nylon sutures may be left in the cornea longer than silk, and these cause less inflammation. Polydioxanone (PDS) is an absorbable suture material, with a predictable rate of absorption. It causes little tissue reaction when buried in cornea and is

---

5. BSS—Alcon Laboratories, Fort Worth, TX.

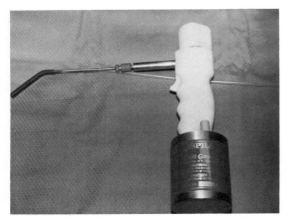

FIGURER 6–11. *A cryosurgical unit cooled by liquid nitrogen, with specific probes for cyclocryotherapy.*

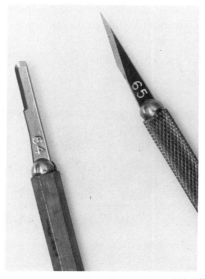

FIGURE 6–13. *Beaver handle with No. 64 and No. 65 blades.*

TABLE 6–1. Suture Material Selection

Tissue	Recommended Sutures	Size
Lids	Silk—soft and pliable	6/0, 4/0
	Nylon—nonirritating, but short sutures may be traumatic	6/0, 4/0, 3/0
Conjunctiva	Polydioxanone (PDS)	7/0, 6/0, 5/0
	Polyglactic acid (PGL)	
	Polyglycolic acid (PGA)	
	Chromic gut	6/0
Third eyelid	Silk	4/0
	Nylon	3/0, 4/0
Cornea	Nylon (preferred)	10/0, 9/0, 8/0, 7/0, 6/0 (10/0, 9/0—operating microscope)
	Silk	8/0, 7/0, 6/0
	PDS, PGA, PGL	9/0, 8/0, 7/0, 6/0

similar in this respect to monofilament nylon. For semipermanent tarsorrhaphy in treating infectious bovine keratoconjunctivitis in field situations, 0, 1, or 2 chromic gut may be used for convenience. The suture breaks in 2–3 weeks without the need for further handling. Tarsorrhaphy in horses requires a strong material because of the powerful orbicularis oculi muscle (medium Vetafil, 1/0 silk, or nylon is suitable).

NEEDLES

For corneal suturing, the micropoint spatula GS–9 needle (Ethicon) or cutting micropoint G–1, swaged to the suture, is recommended. For eyelids and third eyelid, a cutting PS–2 needle is recommended. Swaged-on needles cause less tissue trauma and are used routinely.

SCALPEL BLADES

Several methods may be used

1. Beaver handle with No. 64 or No. 65 blade (Fig. 6–13).

2. Standard No. 3 handle with No. 11 and No. 15 Bard-Parker blades (Fig. 6–14).

3. Swiss blade breaker and holder and sliver of razor blade (Fig. 6–15).

4. Special-purpose knives, e.g., von Graefe's cataract knife.

CARE AND STERILIZATION OF INSTRUMENTS

Ophthalmic instruments are extremely delicate and fragile and must be cared for accordingly. Instruments are individually cleaned and dried, preserving teeth,

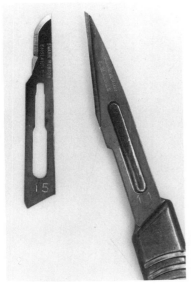

FIGURE 6–14. No. 3 handle with No. 11 and No. 15 blades.

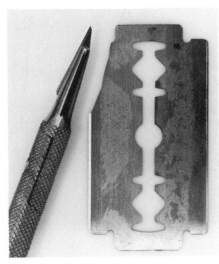

FIGURE 6–15. Swiss blade breaker and razor blade.

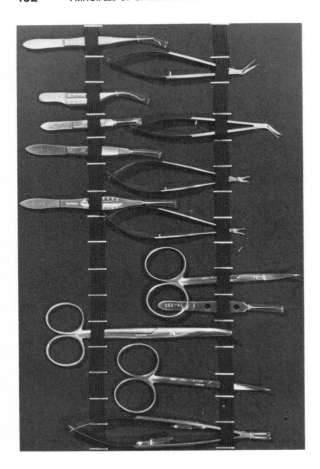

FIGURE 6–16. An instrument board for safe storage of instruments. (From Bistner SI, et al: Atlas of Ophthalmic Surgery. WB Saunders Co, Philadelphia, 1977.)

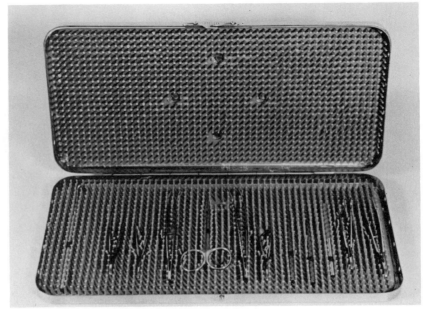

FIGURE 6–17. An instrument case with flexible rubber "fingers," suitable for autoclaving.

points, and cutting edges. Instruments are not placed together to be washed, as damage occurs. Tubular protective cuffs are placed over the ends of instruments during sterilizing. An ultrasonic instrument cleaner is useful to remove blood postoperatively.

Instruments may be protected in packs by racks, boards (Fig. 6–16), cloth wraps with individual compartments, or ideally, in an instrument case (Fig. 6–17).

Three methods of sterilization are commonly used:
autoclaving
ethylene oxide sterilization
dry heat sterilization

Ethylene oxide is the least damaging to instruments. Ethylene oxide is irritating and possibly carcinogenic, and instrument packs must be aired for 48 hours following sterilization before use. Staff must be protected from chronic low-level exposure, and monitoring of gas levels in the environment is advisable. The autoclave is commonly used, although over a long period corrosion and damage may occur to fine cutting edges, especially with poor-quality equipment or instruments. The dry heat sterilizer is useful for fine instruments but has the disadvantage of requiring 150°C for 1½ hours (160° damages fine edges).

PREVENTION OF SELF-MUTILATION

In dogs and cats especially, prevention of postoperative self-mutilation by a patient with a painful or pruritic lesion especially of the eyelids or adnexa may be essential. The most useful method is an Elizabethan collar (Fig. 6–18). Bandaging of the eye and dewclaws is less effective. Bandaging is infrequently necessary, because many painful lesions of the anterior segment of the eye are less irritating after a third eyelid flap or a

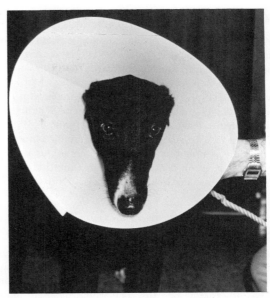

FIGURE 6–18. An Elizabethan collar to protect the eye from rubbing or scratching postoperatively. A plastic bucket, with a hole cut in the bottom, may be used in a similar manner but is not as effective.

conjunctival flap has been created. Tranquilization, e.g., diazepam or acetylpromazine, may be necessary in intractable dogs. In horses, cross-tying in a stall is useful to prevent rubbing.

BASIC SURGICAL PROCEDURES

The following procedures are used in the surgical treatment of many different ocular disorders. Their efficient and correct performance is necessary.

FIGURE 6–19. An adjustable Castroviejo speculum in position.

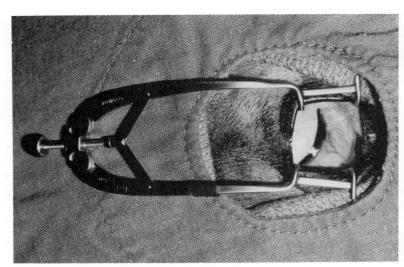

Exposure of the Globe

As in general surgery, good exposure is most important in ophthalmic surgery. The efforts required to expose animal eyes are due primarily to deviation of the eye in a ventromedial direction under anesthesia (reversed Bell's phenomenon), and the presence of the third eyelid. The retractors of Castroviejo, Vierheller, and Maumenee-Park are recommended (Figs. 6–19, 6–20, and 6–21). In some cases of restricted exposure, a canthotomy is necessary before retractors are used. For short procedures on conscious or tranquilized animals, or in horses, a hand-held retractor is useful (Fig. 6–22).

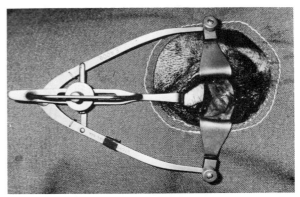

FIGURE 6–21. *A Maumenee-Park speculum in place. This speculum retracts in three directions.*

Canthotomy

A canthotomy is performed at the lateral canthus with straight Mayo's scissors (Fig. 6–23). The area may be infiltrated with epinephrine solution before incision in order to assist hemostasis. The orbital ligament must not be incised. The skin incision is 1–2 cm in length, and it can be facilitated by insertion of a speculum. On completion, the incision is closed accurately with two layers of simple interrupted sutures. The first layer of 4/0 chromic gut or equivalent is placed in the conjunctiva and subcutaneous tissues. The second layer is of 4/0 silk, with the first suture placed at the eyelid margin. Two-layered closure minimizes wound dehiscence. Accurate skin and lid margin apposition is essential to prevent disturbance to the lateral canthal ligament, causing an inversion of the lid margin.

Fixation of the Globe

In domestic animals, anesthesia causes an inferomedial rotation of the globe (reversed Bell's phenomenon), making exposure difficult. In cattle and dogs with long palpebral fissures or shallow orbits, the globe is readily placed in proptosis with a muscle hook or with curved Halsted's hemostats. Proptosis is suitable for simple surgical procedures, but fixation with sutures, small curved Oschner's forceps, or fixation forceps (see Fig. 6–29S) is preferable. Proptosis *must not be used* for intraocular procedures or if danger of perforation exists during the surgical procedure.

Fixation forceps or curved hemostats grasp the conjunctiva and Tenon's capsule in two or three places around the limbus, 1–2 mm from it. Fixation sutures, if used, are placed in the sclera superiorly and inferiorly 1–2 mm from the limbus (Fig. 6–24), using 6/0 silk and a fine cutting needle. The sutures are tagged with light hemostats or serrefines. Additional sutures may be placed laterally and medially. The superior rectus fixation suture used in humans is unsuitable in animals, because the muscle insertion is flatter and tendinous and makes a poor anchorage for the suture. Care must be taken to avoid scleral penetration with fixation sutures.

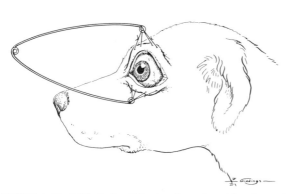

FIGURE 6–20. *A Vierheller lid retractor sutured in place. A single suture in each eyelid, extending the full length of the lid margin, may be used.*

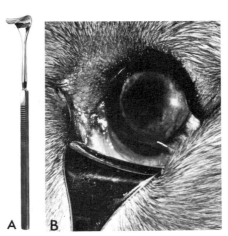

FIGURE 6–22. *A, A hand-held lid retractor. Several different sizes are available. B, Lid retractor in place.*

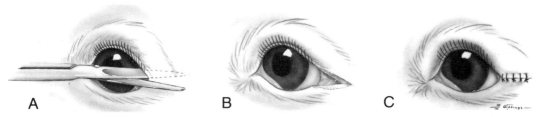

FIGURE 6–23. A, *Position of the scissors for canthotomy.* B, *The canthotomy performed.* C, *The incision accurately sutured, with the first suture placed at the lid margin.*

For more extensive fixation, a circular wire ring (Flieringa's ring) may be sutured around the limbus to prevent collapse of the globe during extensive intraocular procedures.

Third Eyelid Flap

The cornea is often covered during repair from inflammatory and pathological processes or after surgical or other trauma in order to facilitate healing, reduce pain, and prevent further injury. The technique is simple; when correctly performed it causes no discomfort to the animal; and it is a fundamental part of the clinician's armamentarium. Clients are warned in advance of the eye's postoperative appearance. A simple way to do this is to protrude the normal membrane with pressure on the globe through the upper lid.

In horses and cattle, a third eyelid flap is often combined with, or added to, a single temporary intermarginal tarsorrhaphy in order to add strength to the covering. In cattle, sutures of No. 0 to No. 1 chromic gut are used for this combined procedure. The sutures lose strength over 2–3 weeks and then break, preventing the need for suture removal and further handling of the animal.

In dogs and cats, the membrane may be sutured to the bulbar conjunctiva or the upper lid. The upper lid site has the advantage that the third eyelid moves as the globe moves, resulting in less relative motion between the corneal surface and the bulbar surface of the membrane. It has the disadvantage that sutures pull out of the conjunctiva sooner than they do from the upper lid.

If progression of healing must be checked in difficult

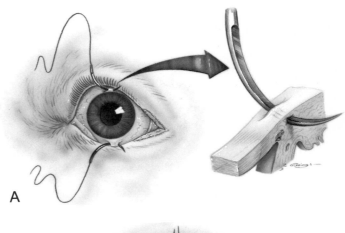

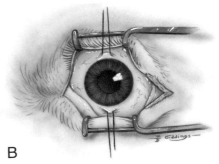

FIGURE 6–24. *Fixation of the globe.* A, *Placement of superior and inferior scleral fixation sutures. (Modified from Severin GA: Veterinary Ophthalmology Notes. Fort Collins, CO, 1976.)* B, *Fixation sutures "tagged" with serrefines or hemostats.*

A

B

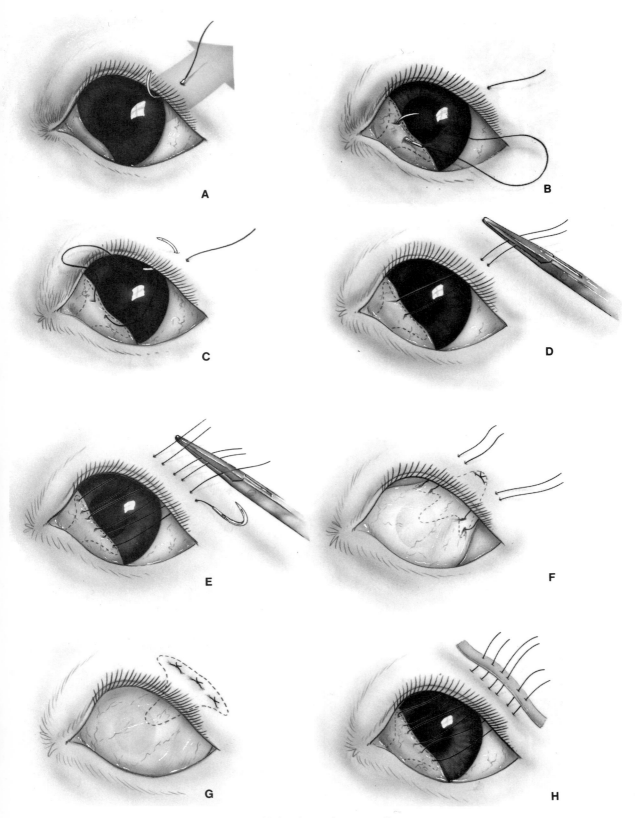

FIGURE 6–25 See legend on opposite page

cases, sterile monofilament nylon may be used, with long suture ends left through the upper lid so that the knot can be untied and the lesion checked. The knot is retied over a button and the flap replaced without the need for further anesthesia.

METHOD I—THIRD EYELID TO UPPER LID [6]
(Fig. 6–25)

Horizontal mattress sutures of 4/0 or 6/0 nylon or silk on a cutting needle are used (2/0 silk or nylon in horses and cattle). Sutures are placed in the normal direction of motion of the membrane, preventing undue tension on the sutures. The sutures are placed about 2 mm from the edge of the membrane, which is about 1 mm from the edge of the cartilage, generally where the line of pigmentation ceases in pigmented membranes. If there is excessive tension in the sutures, e.g., in brachycephalics, a piece of IV tubing split lengthwise or a small sterile button may be used (Fig. 6–25H, I) to distribute suture pressure. Unless the flap is to be removed and replaced, or in brachycephalic breeds in which excess tension is detected, buttons and tubing are unnecessary on the upper lid. If the sutures pull through the upper lid too soon they have been placed too tightly.

6. Modified from Severin GA: Veterinary Ophthalmology Notes, 2nd ed. Ft Collins, CO, 1976.

Some swelling may be present after the procedure, because of manipulation and needle penetration of the vascular upper lid, but this usually clears by 3–4 days. In small animals, flaps usually remain in place 3–4 weeks (most are removed after 10–14 days); in large animals, they remain for 1–2 weeks. If too much tension is present, perform a temporary intermarginal tarsorrhaphy as well.

A correctly placed third eyelid flap is one of the most useful surgical procedures available to the clinician.

Numerous conjunctival flaps for special circumstances are available.

METHOD II—THIRD EYELID TO SUPERIOR BULBAR CONJUNCTIVA [7]
(Fig. 6–26)

This method differs from method I:
1. The first suture is placed in the third eyelid rather than in the upper eyelid.
2. A soft suture material (silk) is always used,

7. Modified from Severin GA: Veterinary Ophthalmology Notes, 2nd ed. Ft Collins, CO, 1976.

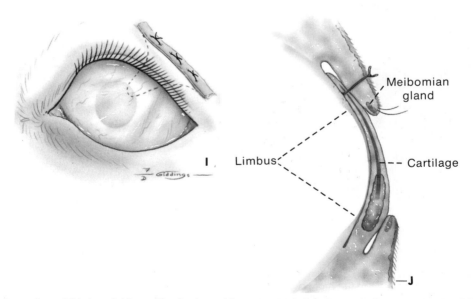

FIGURE 6–25. *Formation of third eyelid flap with attachment to upper lid. A, A cutting needle is directed through the upper lid, 2 mm from the margin. Tension in the sutures is in the direction of the normal movement of the third eyelid. B, The next bite is taken parallel to the eyelid margin, about 2 mm from the edge and 1 mm from the cartilage margin. The suture penetrates the cartilage (but does not go around the vertical part of the T). C, The horizontal mattress suture is completed by passing the needle point through the skin of the upper lid 2.5–3.0 mm from the first arm. D, The suture ends are tagged, and the remaining sutures are preplaced. E, The sutures are ready to be tied. F, The central suture is tied first. G, Sutures tied. H, The sutures are preplaced through a rubber band or a piece of IV tubing only if excess tension is present, as in brachycephalic breeds. I, The sutures are tied over the rubber band. J, The position of the flap in sagittal section. Note that the cornea is not in contact with the sutures. (Modified from Severin GA: Veterinary Ophthalmology Notes. Fort Collins, CO, 1976.)*

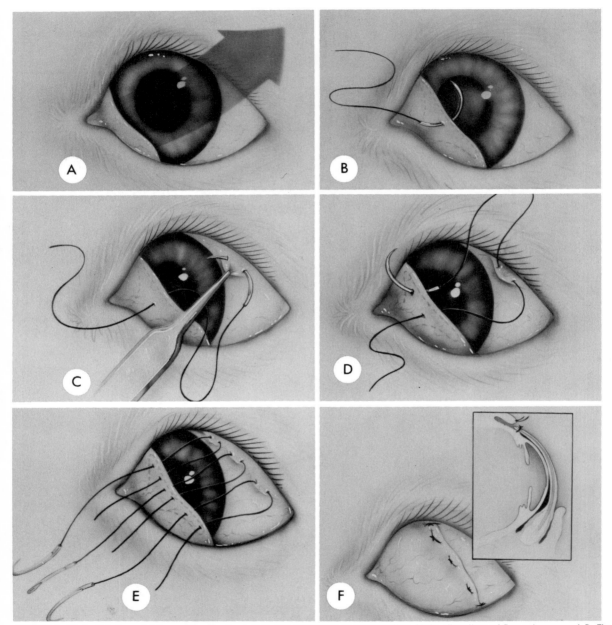

FIGURE 6–26. A, Third eyelid flap with attachment to superior bulbar conjunctive. Note direction of flap placement. B, The central suture is placed 2 mm from the margin. C, The conjunctiva is picked up 7 mm from the limbus, and a horizontal mattress suture is placed. D, The needle is passed back through the eyelid, 2 mm from the first arm of the suture. The remaining two sutures are placed. E, The sutures are tied in simple horizontal mattress suture with 5–10 mm ends. F, Inset, A sagittal section showing the flap in place. The cornea the sutures does not touch. (Modified from Severin GA: Veterinary Ophthalmology Notes. Fort Collins, CO, 1976.)

because the ends remain in the conjunctival sac for the duration of the flap.

3. Less motion occurs between the flap and the cornea, because the flap is free to move with the globe.

4. A tighter "bandage" and more support results, but the sutures pull out of the conjunctiva sooner than from the upper lid.

Table 6–2 shows the length of time flaps should remain in place.

In both methods of placing third eyelid flaps, the sutures may loosen after the 1st week, as swelling subsides. The sutures then rub on the cornea and produce erosions. If this occurs, remove the sutures and allow a few days for the cornea to heal.

COMMON ERRORS IN FORMING THIRD EYELID FLAPS

1. Rough handling and damage to the delicate edge of the membrane.

2. Failure to place sutures as described, resulting in disfiguring eversion of the membrane.

3. Incorrect placement of the sutures through the cartilage.

4. Use of too large a needle and suture material, causing inflammation, postoperative discomfort, and rubbing.

5. Failure to remove sutures if loosening and corneal erosion occur.

6. Failure to re-examine the eye when indicated (see the next list).

The following signs are indications for removal of the flap and for thorough clinical inspection:

1. Sudden onset of pain—rubbing, scratching.

2. Loss of appetite.

3. Sudden loss of fluid—serous, mucoid, or purulent discharge.

4. Change in the character of a discharge from mucoid or serous to purulent.

5. Evidence of pain—change in behavior or traumatic periocular dermatitis in the covered eye.

6. Persistent pyrexia and neutrophilia.

Tarsorrhaphy—Third Eyelid Flap in Cattle (Fig. 6–27)

In cattle infected with infectious bovine keratoconjunctivitis, protection of the cornea is an important part of treatment if corneal lesions are severe. Sutures

TABLE 6–2. Length of Time Third Eyelid Flaps Should Remain in Place

Condition	Dogs and Cats	Horses and Cattle
Normal eyes	7–14 days	3–10 days
Exophthalmos	7–10 days	3–7 days
Enophthalmos	10–14 days	5–10 days

of No. 1 chromic gut (No. 0 in calves) are placed to form both a tarsorrhaphy and a third eyelid flap. For both economic reasons and ease of treatment, the sutures are placed (without anesthesia) through the full thickness of the upper lid, including the outer surface of the third eyelid. A sharp cutting needle and a continuous suture pattern are used, but the sutures are cut and tied as simple interrupted sutures. The chromic gut breaks in 10–14 days, and suture removal is unnecessary.

Corneal coverage is an important part of treatment of severe ulcerative keratitis in cattle.

Inclusion of the third eyelid in the suture prevents sutures on the inner surfce of the eyelid from abrading the cornea.

Tarsorrhaphy

Tarsorrhaphy is surgical closure of the palpebral fissure. Temporary tarsorrhaphy is useful in protecting the cornea and supporting it during repair. It may be combined with a third eyelid flap (as described previously), or the two procedures may be performed independently at the same time for added security. Tarsorrhaphy may also be combined with a 360° conjunctival flap. An intermarginal suture technique (Fig. 6–28) must be used for tarsorrhaphy to corneal abrasion by sutures. In large animals 2/0 suture is used, and in small animals 4/0 is used. Either simple interrupted or horizontal mattress sutures may be employed.

COMMON OPHTHALMIC INSTRUMENTS (Fig. 6–29)

A basic set of instruments suitable for extraocular surgery and repair of corneal lacerations is listed here.

Instrument tray, 16″ × 12″, stainless steel
Saline solution bowl, 3″, stainless steel
Sponges, 3″
Sponges, cellulose
Lid speculum, Castroviejo's, Vierheller's, Maumenee-Park
Forceps, Castroviejo's
Tissue forceps, Adson-Brown
Corneal forceps, Colibri's
Scissors, strabismus
Scissors, Mayo's straight
Scissors, suture, Spencer's
Irrigating bulb, silicone
Fixation forceps, Elschnig-O'Brien
Scissors, corneal, McGuire's
Forceps, cilia
Hemostats, curved mosquito, Halsted's

Text continued on page 146

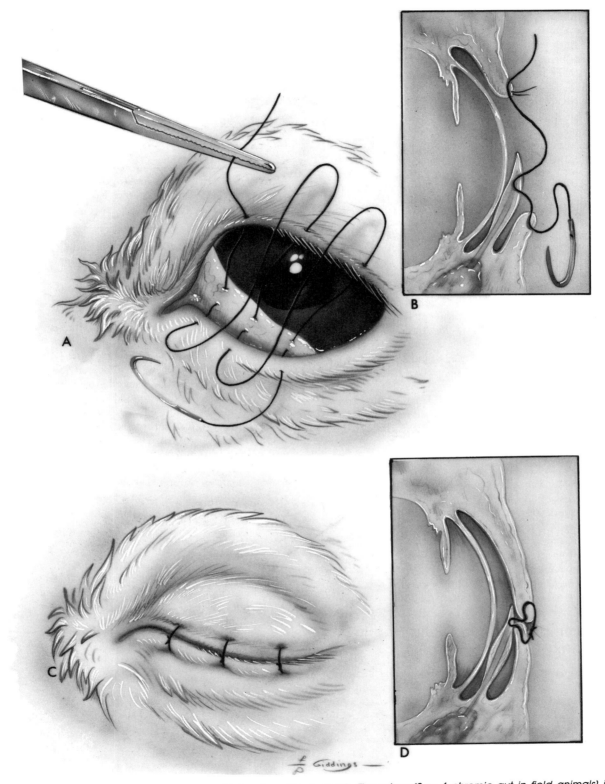

FIGURE 6–27. *Tarsorrhaphy and third eyelid flap in cattle. A and B, The suture (0 or 1 chromic gut in field animals) is inserted in a continuous manner from left to right. The suture emerges from the eyelid on the margin. A deep bite of the external surface of the third eyelid is taken. C and D, The continuous suture is cut, and three simple interrupted sutures are tied. (Modified from Severin GA: Veterinary Ophthalmology Notes. Fort Collins, CO, 1976.)*

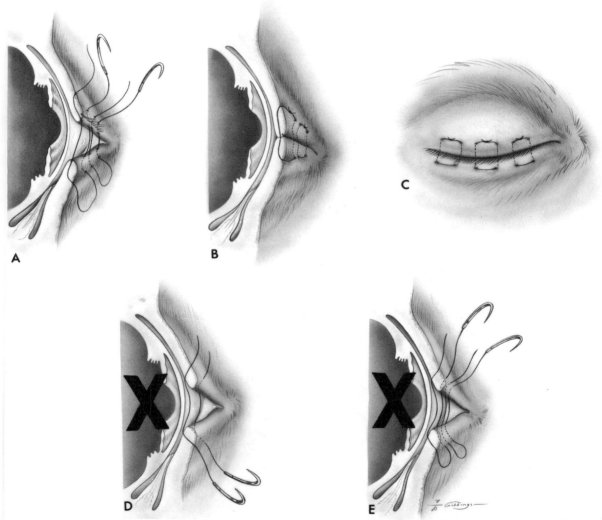

FIGURE 6–28. A, B, and C, Placement of interrupted intermarginal horizontal mattress sutures in temporary tarsorrhaphy. D and E, Incorrect suture placement, which results in corneal abrasions from the sutures. (Modified from Severin GA: Veterinary Ophthalmology Notes. Fort Collins, CO, 1976.)

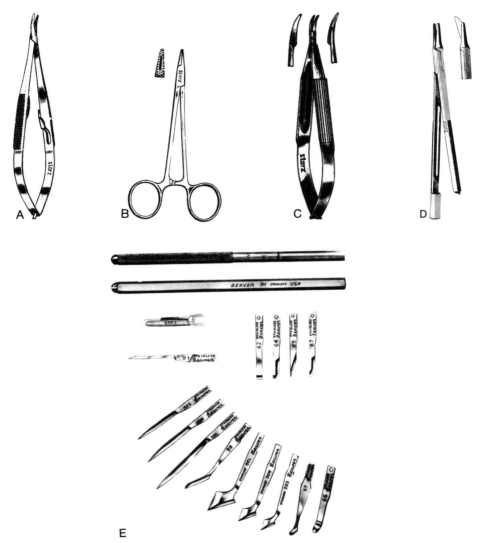

FIGURE 6–29. Common ophthalmic instruments. A, Castroviejo's curved needle holders. B, Derf's needle holders. C, Troutman's needle holders (microsurgery). D, Swiss blade breaker. E, Selection of Beaver's blades and handles.

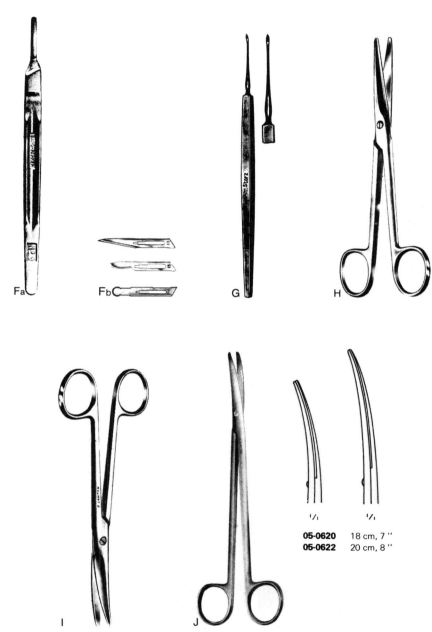

FIGURE 6–29 Continued F, Bard-Parker blades. G, Foreign body spud. H, Straight Mayo's scissors. I, Curved Mayo's scissors. J, Curved Metzenbaum's scissors.

Illustration continued on following page

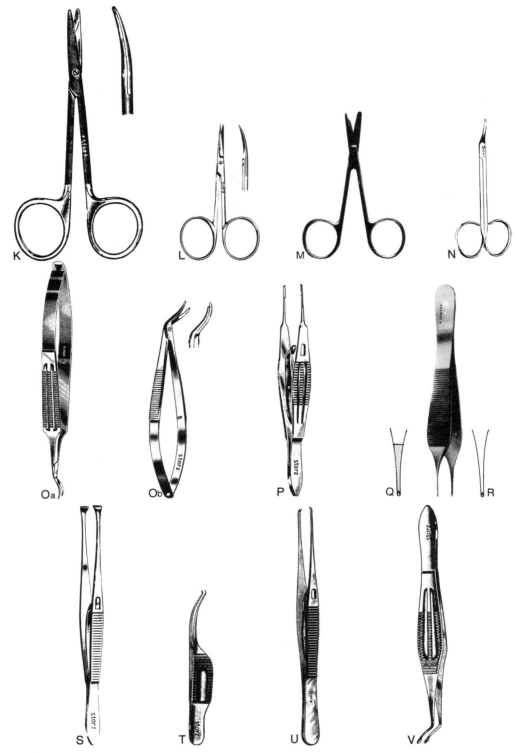

FIGURE 6–29 *Continued* K, *Strabismus scissors.* L, *Iris scissors.* M, *Spencer's suture scissors.* N, *McGuire's corneal scissors.* O, *Castroviejo's corneal scissors (left- and right-handed).* P, *Castroviejo's forceps with typing platforms.* Q, *Adson's tissue forceps (plain).* R, *Adson's tissue forceps (toothed).* S, *Von Graefe's fixation forceps.* T, *Colibri's forceps.* U, *Elschnig-O'Brien fixation forceps.* V, *Arruga's capsule forceps.*

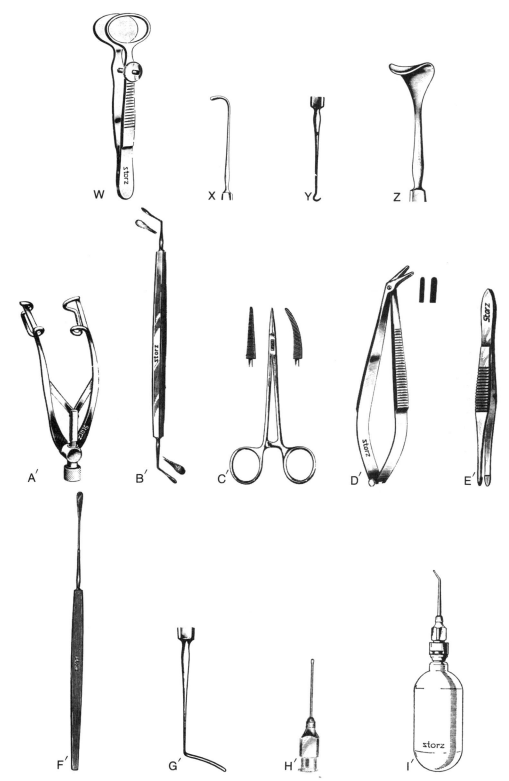

FIGURE 6–29 *Continued* W, *Chalazion forceps.* X, *Muscle hook.* Y, *Iris hook.* Z, *Lid retractor.* A', *Castroviejo's lid speculum.* B', *Martinez's corneal knife dissector.* C', *Halsted's curved hemostats.* D', *Scleral punch.* E', *Cilia forceps.* F', *Kimura spatula.* G', *Cyclodialysis spatula.* H', *Lacrimal cannula.* I', *Silicone irrigating bulb and anterior chamber needles.*

REFERENCES

Brightman AH, et al (1981): Effect of aspirin on aqueous protein values in the dog. J Am Vet Med Assoc 178:572.

Brightman AH, et al (1983): Decreased tear production associated with general anesthesia in the horse. J Am Vet Med Assoc 182:243.

Hamed LM, et al (1987): Hibiclens keratitis. Am J Ophthalmol 104:5.

Isenberg S, et al (1983): Chemical preparation of the eye in ophthalmic surgery. 1. Effect of conjunctival irrigation. Arch Ophthalmol 101:761.

Krohne SDG, Vestre WA (1987): Effects of flunixin meglumine and dexamethasone on aqueous protein values after intraocular surgery. Am J Vet Res 48:420.

Ludders JW, Heavner JE (1979): Effect of atropine on tear formation in anesthetized dogs. J Am Vet Med Assoc 175:585.

Magrane WG (1977): Canine Ophthalmology, 3rd ed. Lea & Febiger, Philadelphia.

Severin GA (1976): Veterinary Ophthalmology Notes, 2nd ed. Fort Collins, CO.

Short CE, Rebhun WC (1980): Complications caused by the oculocardiac reflex during anesthesia in a foal. J Am Vet Med Assoc 176:630.

Slatter DH (1985): Textbook of Small Animal Surgery, vol 2, chap 100. WB Saunders Co, Philadelphia.

Stallard HB (1973): Eye Surgery, 5th ed. John Wright, Bristol.

Varma S, et al (1981): Further studies with polyglycolic acid (Dexon) and other sutures in infected experimental wounds. Am J Vet Res 42:571.

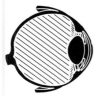

Eyelids

ANATOMY	ACQUIRED LID DISORDERS	SKIN DISEASES AFFECTING THE
FUNCTIONS OF THE EYELIDS	TUMORS OF THE EYELIDS	EYELIDS
PATHOLOGY		

ANATOMY

The skin on the outer surface of the eyelid is thinner and more mobile and pliable than elsewhere. Cilia (eyelashes) are present on the outer surface of the upper lid margin in dogs, horses, cattle, pigs, and sheep; a few cilia are present on the lower lids of horses, cattle, and sheep. The cat has no cilia. Modified sweat glands—the GLANDS OF MOLL—open onto the lid margin near the base of the cilia (Fig. 7–1). The GLANDS OF ZEIS (rudimentary sebaceous glands) open

into the follicles that produce the cilia. The tarsal (formerly meibomian) glands (Fig. 7–2) are much larger sebaceous glands that open posterior to the cilia. Their openings are visible grossly on the lid margin; a grayish-white secretion rich in phospholipids can be expressed with finger pressure. This secretion has two functions: it forms the SUPERFICIAL LIPID LAYER OF THE PRECORNEAL TEAR FILM, and it coats the eyelid margins to prevent overflow of tears. The superficial lipid layer has a high surface tension, adding stability to the film and lowering evaporation of the aqueous layer of the film.

The TARSAL GLANDS are embedded in the TARSAL

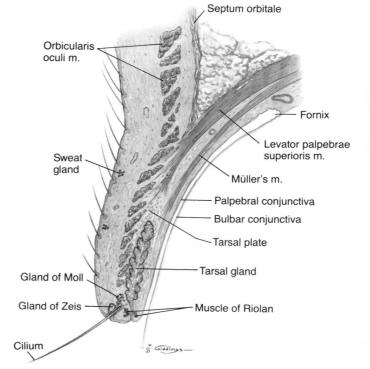

FIGURE 7–1. Anatomy of the normal eyelid.

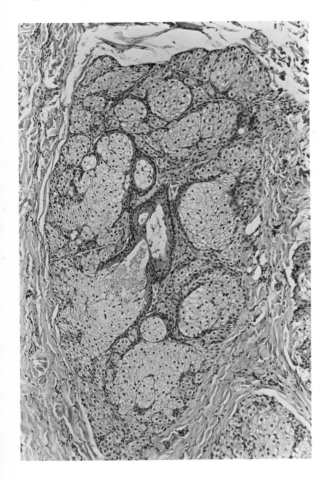

FIGURE 7–2. Photomicrograph of the tarsal (meibomian) glands, which open on the lid margin.

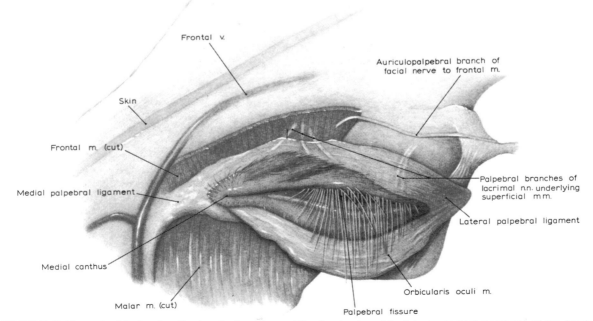

Frontal v.

Auriculopalpebral branch of
facial nerve to frontal m.

Skin

Frontal m. (cut)

Palpebral branches of
lacrimal n.n. underlying
superficial mm.

Medial palpebral ligament

Lateral palpebral ligament

Medial canthus

Orbicularis oculi m.

Malar m. (cut)

Palpebral fissure

FIGURE 7–3. View of orbit showing the terminal endings of the lacrimal and facial nerves and structures of the bovine eyelids. Note the position of the auriculopalpebral branch of the facial nerve for local anesthesia. (From Getty R: Sisson and Grossman's The Anatomy of the Domestic Animals, 5th ed, Vol 1. WB Saunders Co, Philadelphia, 1975.)

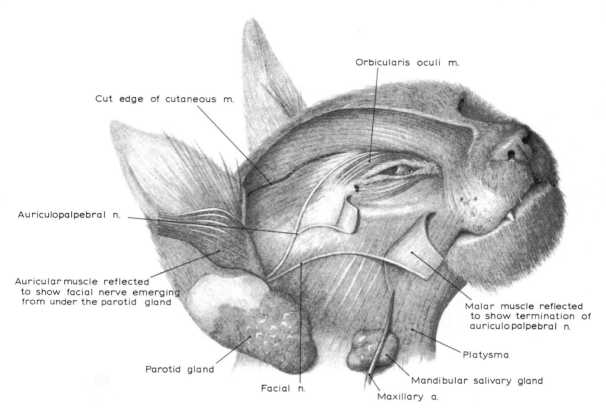

FIGURE 7–4. *Feline head with skin and part of frontal and malar muscles reflected. The diagram shows the course of the auriculopalpebral nerve and the position of the superficial glands. (From Getty R: Sisson and Grossman's The Anatomy of the Domestic Animals, 5th ed. WB Saunders Co, Philadelphia, 1975.)*

PLATE, a layer of fibrous tissue that gives some structural rigidity to the lid. The LACRIMAL PUNCTA lie on the inner surface of the eyelid 3–4 mm from the medial canthus, approximately opposite the last of the tarsal gland openings. The inner surface of the lid is lined with closely adherent palpebral conjunctiva. The OR-BICULARIS OCULI MUSCLE, which encircles and closes the PALPEBRAL FISSURE, lies anterior to the tarsal plate (Figs. 7–3 and 7–4). The orbicularis oculi is innervated by the PALPEBRAL NERVE, a branch of the facial (VII)

nerve. The general pattern and innervation of muscles surrounding the eyelids are similar in all species, although the names and relative development vary among species.

The orbicularis is anchored medially to the wall of the orbit by the MEDIAL PALPEBRAL LIGAMENT. The LACRIMAL SAC lies posterior and ventral to this ligament. A slip of the orbicularis, HORNER'S MUSCLE, passes behind the lacrimal sac to insert into the medial orbital wall. During contraction of the orbicularis oculi, fibers that insert into its lateral wall pull on it, creating a negative pressure within the sac, drawing tears into the sac (the so-called lacrimal pump). During relaxation of the orbicularis, pressure is placed on the sac, forcing tears down the nasolacrimal duct.

The orbicularis is anchored laterally by the RETRACTOR ANGULI OCULI LATERALIS. In cattle and sheep this structure is fibrous in nature and is known as the lateral palpebral ligament; in horses it is visible as a fibrous raphe within the orbicularis muscle. The medial and lateral attachments of the orbicularis oculi preserve the elliptical shape of the palpebral fissure and prevent it from becoming circular during contraction of the orbicularis. The upper lid is more mobile than the lower lid.

In addition to the orbicularis oculi with its medial and lateral attachments, provision is made to elevate the upper lid and depress the lower lid. The major elevators of the upper lid are the LEVATOR PALPEBRAE SUPERIORIS, which originates near the optic foramen, inserts into the tarsus (see Fig. 7–1), and is innervated by the OCULOMOTOR NERVE (III); and MÜLLER'S MUSCLE (sympathetically innervated), which lies posterior to the levator. The levator and SUPERIOR RECTUS muscles share common innervation, so that elevation of the eye by the superior rectus is coordinated with elevation of the upper lid (if not, the animal would see the inner surface of the upper lid on elevation of the globe). Minor elevators of the upper lid include the LEVATOR ANGULI OCULI MEDIALIS and FRONTALIS

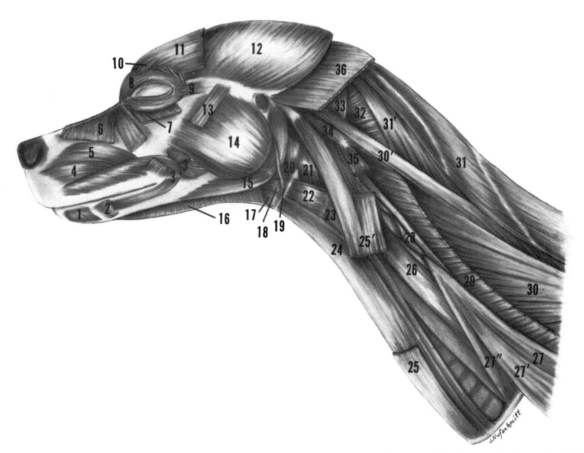

FIGURE 7–5. Deep muscles of the head and neck of the dog. Lateral view. (1 = Mentalis; 2 = orbicularis oris; 3, 3' = buccinator; 4 = caninus; 5 = levator labii maxillaris; 6 = levator nasolabialis; 7 = malaris; 8 = orbicularis oculi; 9 = retractor anguli oculi lateralis; 10 = levator anguli oculi medialis; 11 = frontalis; 12 = temporalis; 13 = zygomaticus; 14 = masseter; 15 = digastricus; 16 = mylohyoideus; 17 = geniohyoideus; 18 = hyoglossus; 19 = stylohyoideus; 20 = hyopharyngeus; 21 = thyropharyngeus; 22 = thyrohyoideus; 23 = sternothyroideus; 24 = sternohyoideus; 25, 25' = sternocephalicus; 26 = longus capitis; 27, 27' = scalenus dorsalis; 27" = scalenus medius; 28 = intertransversarii; 29 = serratus ventralis cervicus; 30, 30' = longissimus (cervicus capitis); 31, 31' = semispinalis capitis (biventer cervicis, complexus); 32 = obliquus capitis caudalis; 33 = obliquus capitis cranialis; 34 = rectus capitis lateralis; 35 = omotransversarius; 36 = splenius.) (From Getty R: Sisson and Grossman's The Anatomy of the Domestic Animals, 5th ed. WB Saunders Co, Philadelphia, 1975.)

MUSCLES, both innervated by the palpebral nerve (Fig. 7–5; see also Fig. 7–3).

The lower lid is depressed by the MALARIS MUSCLE, which is innervated by the DORSAL BUCCAL BRANCH OF THE FACIAL NERVE. Note that different branches of the facial nerve supply the orbicularis, which narrows the palpebral fissure, and the malaris, which widens it. Actions of the muscles of the eyelids are summarized in Figure 7–6.

Sensory Innervation of the Eyelids and Periocular Region

Sensory innervation for the dog, horse, and ox is shown in Figures 7–7 to 7–9 to allow location of blocking points and delineation of anesthesia or hyperesthesia in disease processes.

FUNCTIONS OF THE EYELIDS

Malfunction and poor conformation of the eyelids are very common causes of ocular disease in animals, especially because of destructive selection for detrimental but supposedly "desirable" features for the show ring (Table 7–1). Veterinarians must be aware of these manufactured features for the relief of pain, suffering, and potential blindness in their patients.

The lids protect the eye in the following ways:

1. Sensory and protective effects of the cilia on the upper eyelid.

2. Secretions of the tarsal glands and goblet cells

TABLE 7–1. Common Eyelid Disorders Due to Selective Breeding

Condition	Affected Breeds
Corneal exposure	Dog: Boston terrier, English bulldog, Lhasa apso, Pekingese, pug, Shih-Tzu Cat: Persian, Abyssinian
Trichiasis (including nasal fold trichiasis)	Dog: Chow chow, cocker spaniel, Lhasa apso, Maltese terrier, Pekingese, Shar Pei, Shih-Tzu Cat: Burmese, Persian
Ptosis and excess forehead skin	Dog: Bloodhound, chow chow, Shar Pei

Note: This table does *not* include hereditary conditions that may be eliminated or reduced in frequency by selective breeding.

within the conjunctiva contribute to the outer lipid and inner mucopolysaccharide layers of the precorneal tear film, respectively.

3. Physical protection against trauma, evaporation of tears, and distribution of the precorneal film by lid movements.

4. "Pumping" of tears down the nasolacrimal duct, preventing epiphora and promoting a precorneal film with uniform thickness and optical properties.

Interference with motor innervation of the lids may result in desiccation of the cornea, with severe secondary effects. If excess muscle tone is present in the orbicularis, resulting in blepharospasm and ENTROPION (rolling in of the lid), severe erosive lesions of the cornea may result from abrasion against the hairy external surface of the eyelid.

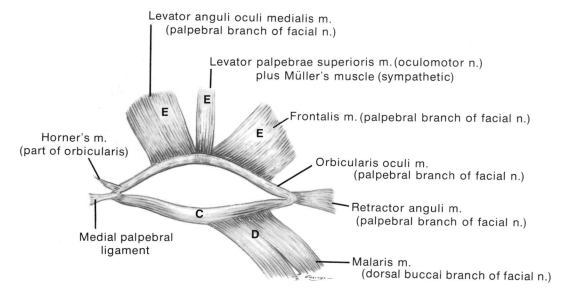

E—Elevate upper lid
D—Depress lower lid
C—Constrict palpebral fissure

FIGURE 7–6. Actions and innervations of the muscles of the eyelid.

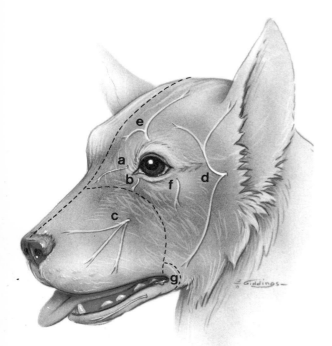

FIGURE 7–7. Sensory innervation of the canine periocular area: a = frontal nerve; b = infratrochlear nerve; c = infraorbital nerve; d = uriculotemporal nerve; e = lacrimal nerve; f = zygomatic nerve; g = mental nerve. (Redrawn from Westhues M, Fritsch R: Animal Anesthesia, Vol 1. Oliver & Boyd, London, 1964.)

In the newborn cat and dog, the lids open at 7–10 days of age. If they open too early (congenitally open eyelids), lesions occur similar to those caused by paralysis of the orbicularis in adult life. If the lids remain shut, infectious organisms may multiply in the accumulated secretions (OPHTHALMIA NEONATORUM).

PATHOLOGY

The eyelids show pathological reactions and diseases characteristic of skin, modified by numerous specialized structures within them. In addition, structural and pathological abnormalities of the lids frequently result in secondary ocular disease, especially of the conjunctiva and cornea. Metastases of primary lid neoplasms are frequently found in the parotid and maxillary lymph nodes in cattle.

Congenital Abnormalities

COLOBOMA

A coloboma (pl. colobomata) is a partial defect in a portion of an eyelid. It occurs in all species. It is most

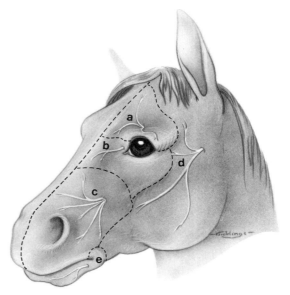

FIGURE 7–8. Sensory innervation of the equine periocular area: a = frontal nerve; b = infratrochlear nerve; c = infraorbital nerve; d = superficial temporal nerve; e = mental nerve. (Redrawn from Westhues M, Fritsch R: Animal Anesthesia, Vol 1, Local Anesthesia. Oliver & Boyd, London, 1964.)

common in cats, affecting the temporal portion of the upper lid, and in piebald and karakul sheep, affecting the middle area of the upper lid. In sheep and Burmese cats, colobomata are hereditary. Dermoids may be

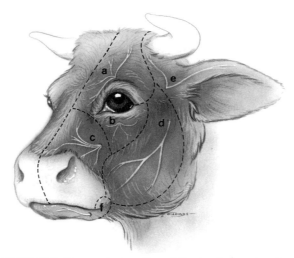

FIGURE 7–9. Sensory innervation of the bovine periocular area: a = frontal and infratrochlear nerves; b = zygomatic nerve; c = infraorbital nerve; d = superficial temporal nerve; e = cornual nerve; f = mental nerve. (Redrawn from Westhues M, Fritsch R: Animal Anesthesia, Vol 1, Local Anesthesia. Oliver & Boyd, London, 1964.)

seen in association with colobomata. Colobomata cause drying of the precorneal tear film with secondary corneal lesions, corneal irritation caused by hair around the edges of the defect rubbing on the cornea and conjunctiva, and if in the lower lid, epiphora because of escape of tears through the defect. The combined effects with time are corneal scarring, pigmentation, and pain.

Colobomata are repaired by a variety of blepharoplastic procedures, the choice depending on their size and position. Simple defects affecting less than one third of the lid margin are restored by removing the edges of the defect and closing as for a wedge excision of an eyelid lesion. Care is necessary in providing an eyelid margin. Larger defects require more extensive reconstructive procedures.

PROMINENT NASAL FOLDS

In Pekingese, pugs, English bulldogs, Boston terriers, and similar brachycephalic breeds, the nasal folds may be unusually protuberant. When this is combined with a shallow orbit and prominent globe, the hair on the skin folds irritates or even rubs the cornea; the result may include irritation, pigmentation, and epiphora, and in some cases, recurrent corneal ulceration. It may be effectively treated by removal of the folds or, if combined with partial drying, corneal exposure, and chronic keratitis, by reconstructive medial blepharoplasty. A careful inspection should be made for other causes of irritation (e.g., distichiasis, medial entropion). When inspecting young puppies of breeds at risk, look for conformational defects and advise the owner to observe the eyes carefully for signs of ocular disease as the animal matures.

Removal of Nasal Folds

Extra care is necessary with general anesthesia in brachycephalic breeds; the endotracheal tube is removed only after return of the laryngeal reflex. Both nasal folds are removed, either partially or totally (Figs. 7–10 and 7–11). In partial removal, only the medial portion of the fold is removed, where it touches the cornea, resulting in less alteration from the breed "norm" desired by some owners. The surgical site is routinely prepared, and the fold is removed with curved Mayo's scissors. Hemorrhage is usually minimal, and the wound is sutured with simple interrupted sutures of 4/0 silk placed 2.0 mm apart. In both methods the suture ends should be short enough to prevent corneal irritation. Sutures are removed 10 days later. Postoperatively an Elizabethan collar is used.

Entropion is often present in dogs with prominent nasal folds, at the medial end of both lids. If this is also present, medial blepharoplasty is the correction of choice, as it will often protect the cornea from the nasal folds as well, and their removal may not be necessary if too cosmetically objectionable to a particular owner.

Nasal Reconstructive Blepharoplasty

Indications. Medial entropion in brachycephalic breeds, chronic corneal drying due to exophthalmos, lagophthalmos, chronic corneal irritation after replacement of a prolapsed globe, chronic nasal pigmentary keratitis.

Nasal reconstructive blepharoplasty is a demanding technique and should not be performed by untrained or inexperienced persons. Difficulty may sometimes occur with wound dehiscence caused by tension and

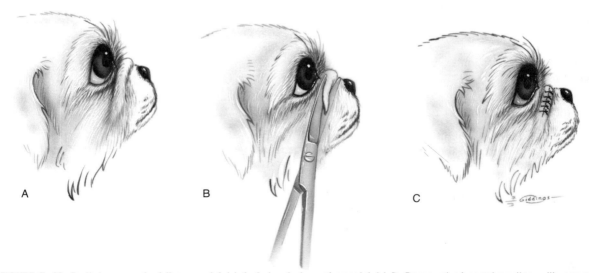

FIGURE 7–10. *Partial removal of the nasal fold. A, Lateral view of nasal fold. B, Removal of nasal portion with curved scissors. Note that the nasal portion of the fold is removed. C, The sutured wound with a small fold remaining that is more prominent laterally. The knots are placed on the anterior side of the incision in order to limit corneal contact. (Redrawn from Severin GA: Veterinary Ophthalmology Notes, 2nd ed. Ft Collins, CO, 1976.)*

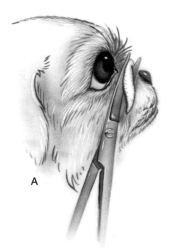 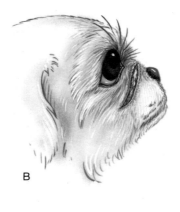 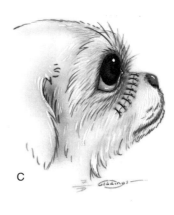

FIGURE 7–11. *Total removal of the nasal fold. A, Removal of the fold, starting laterally. B, The fold removed. C, The fold sutured. The knots are placed on the anterior side of the incision in order to reduce the chance of corneal contact. (Redrawn from Severin GA: Veterinary Ophthalmology Notes, 2nd ed. Ft Collins, CO, 1976.)*

constant movement of the operative site. The technique is illustrated in Figure 7–12. Important features of the method are avoidance of the lacrimal puncta, careful incision of the eyelid, reinforcement of the skin suture line by the underlying rotated conjunctival flap, postoperative support by tension sutures, and protection from the patient by a collar.

Disorders of the Cilia

There are three common disorders of cilia:

1. **DISTICHIASIS** (Fig. 7–13*B*): additional cilia emerging from the openings of the tarsal glands.

2. **ECTOPIC CILIA** (Fig. 7–13*C*): additional cilia arising in the tarsal glands and emerging through the palpebral conjunctiva.

3. **TRICHIASIS** (Fig. 7–13*D*): outer cilia and adjacent skin hairs pointing in an abnormal direction toward the cornea.

CLINICAL SIGNS OF CILIA DISORDERS

All the disorders have similar signs (Fig. 7–14).

1. Epiphora. Excess tearing and staining of facial hairs is usually present. The lacrimal puncta are flushed under local anesthesia to eliminate blockage as a cause. Epiphora is often present from an early age, and this helps differentiate cilia disorders from other conditions causing epiphora in later life.

2. Blepharospasm. Pain associated with constant irritation, causing blepharospasm and rubbing, is characteristic. In some dogs the pain and epiphora are intermittent.

3. Chronic conjunctival erythema. The surface vessels of the conjunctiva are engorged, and a reddish-pink capillary flush is present. It is unusual for disorders of cilia to be present without this sign. Conjunctival erythema caused by distichiasis must be distinguished from sensitive vessel syndrome. The superficial position of affected vessels may be demonstrated by constriction with topically applied epinephrine (Adrenalin) solution. Purulent conjunctivitis is unusual except in long-standing cases.

4. Corneal ulceration. Recent ulcers caused by cilia are usually shallow when stained with fluorescein, and they are frequently eccentrically placed on the cornea (corresponding to the position of the cilia). A thorough search for cilia is made, with magnification, under general anesthesia if necessary, in all cases of recurrent corneal ulceration. Ectopic cilia cause ulceration in dogs, cats, and horses.

5. Presence of cilia. The typical appearance of cilia in distichiasis is shown in Figure 7–15.

Adequate magnification is essential for detecting abnormal cilia.

A slit-lamp or operating microscope facilitates detection of abnormal cilia. Cilia may be white or pigmented, and considerable diligence may be necessary to find them. A few extra soft cilia and minor distichiasis are quite common in dogs, especially in poodles and cocker spaniels; without other confirming clinical signs they are not significant. Ectopic cilia sometimes do not emerge through the palpebral conjunctiva in dogs until middle age.

FREQUENCY

Disorders of cilia are most common in dogs. Trichiasis occurs in Pekingese in the temporal portion of

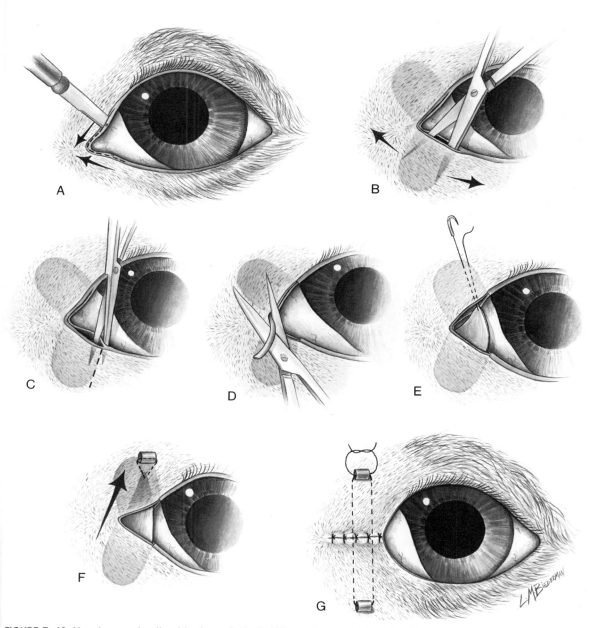

FIGURE 7–12. *Nasal reconstructive blepharoplasty. A, Lid margins are incised longitudinally from 2 to 3 mm temporal to the lacrimal punctum and anterior to the margins, to the nasal canthus. B, A pocket is made in each lid between the skin and the palpebral conjunctiva. C, An incision is made in the conjunctiva perpendicular to the lid margin at the temporal extremity of the inferior lid incision. D, The lid margins are excised adjacent to the lid incisions. E, A suture of 6/0 nylon is placed from the upper lid through the bulbar surface of the conjunctival flap. It exits the flap and passes back through the upper lid. F, The suture is tied over intravenous tubing. G, The lid margins are sutured with 6/0 nylon. A horizontal mattress tension suture is placed to support the skin sutures over plastic tubing both above and below. The same tubing is used above as was used for the earlier suture.*

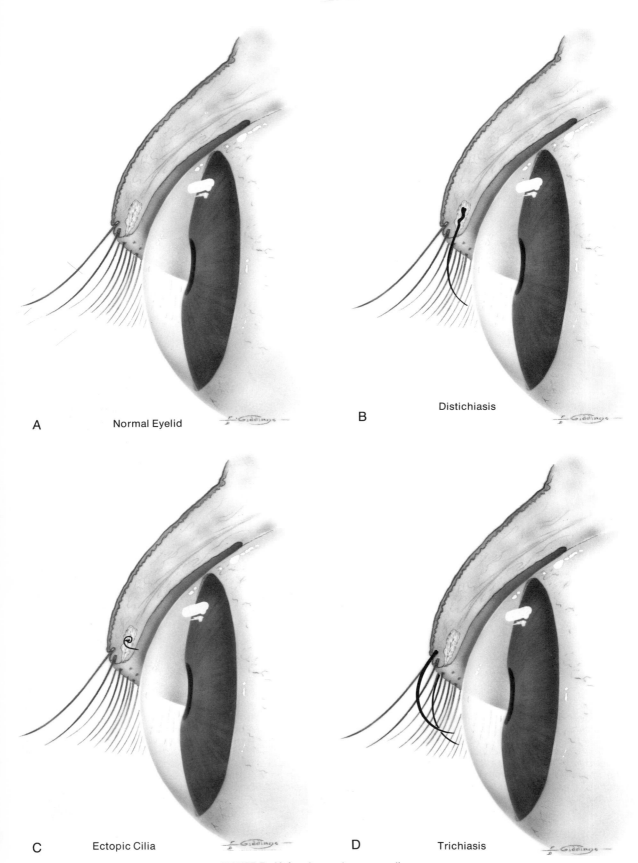

A   Normal Eyelid

B   Distichiasis

C   Ectopic Cilia

D   Trichiasis

FIGURE 7–13 See legend on opposite page

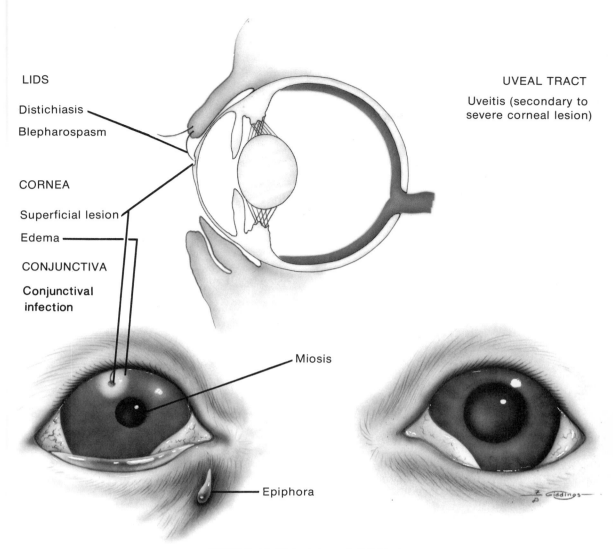

LIDS

Distichiasis

Blepharospasm

CORNEA

Superficial lesion

Edema

CONJUNCTIVA

Conjunctival
infection

UVEAL TRACT

Uveitis (secondary to
severe corneal lesion)

Miosis

Epiphora

FIGURE 7–14. Clinical signs of distichiasis.

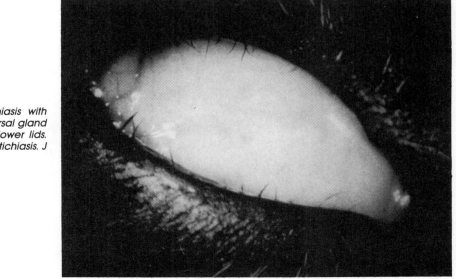

FIGURE 7–15. Severe distichiasis with
many cilia emerging from tarsal gland
orifices of both upper and lower lids.
(From Lawson DD: Canine distichiasis. J
Sm Anim Pract 14:469, 1973.)

FIGURE 7–13. A, A normal eyelid. Note the position of cilia in relation to the orifice of the tarsal gland. B, Distichiasis—extra
cilia emerge from the tarsal glands. C, Ectopic cilia—cilia arise from the tarsal glands but emerge through the palpebral
conjunctiva. D, Trichiasis—direction of the cilia and other external hairs is abnormal.

the upper lid and is frequent in the Shih-Tzu, Lhasa apso, and poodle. Cilia disorders affect both eyelids, although ectopic cilia are more frequent on the upper lid. Horses are sometimes affected, with acquired trichiasis being the most frequent disorder. The presence of cilia abnormalities is breed-related and familial.

PATHOGENESIS

Cilia rub the cornea, stimulating blepharospasm and increased tear production via the lacrimal reflex arc. Continual abrasion of the corneal epithelium during blinking results in loss of epithelium, and a superficial corneal ulcer may form. The corneal ulcer allows entry of fluid from the precorneal tear film into the corneal stroma, causing cloudy edema around the margins. The ulcer stimulates superficial corneal vascularization. Conjunctival irritation by the cilia causes erythema and chemosis in severe cases.

TREATMENT

Ectopic Cilia

Ectopic cilia are treated by resection of the affected cilium and tarsal gland under magnification. An elliptical Desmarres chalazion clamp with screw lock is placed around the cilium for hemostasis, and the lid is everted. The wedge is removed with a razor blade fragment (Fig. 7–16), leaving the lid margin intact if possible. Digital pressure for several minutes is sufficient to control hemorrhage. A topical broad-spectrum antibiotic preparation is applied 3 times daily for 5 days postoperatively. If correctly performed, this technique is highly effective and has few postoperative complications.

Focal tarsoconjunctival resection is the method of choice for removal of ectopic cilia.

Distichiasis (see Fig. 7–14)

Numerous methods have been advocated for the correction of canine distichiasis since its first description in 1967. Initially the "lid splitting" technique was used. However, because of postoperative cicatricial entropion, scarring of the lid margin, trichiasis, and epiphora, the technique was abandoned. Its successor—partial tarsal plate excision—has also been superseded by MICROCRYOEPILATION. Electroepilation of individual follicles can still be useful, but it is much less reliable and convenient than is cryoepilation.

Microcryoepilation (Fig. 7–17)

Microcryoepilation takes advantage of the selective susceptibility of hair follicles to extreme cold. A nitrous oxide cryoprobe is applied to the conjunctiva overlying the tarsal glands containing the offending cilia. The ice ball is observed under the operating microscope, as it advances over the line of the tarsal gland openings on the lid margin. A double freeze–thaw cycle is used. Initially the lid swells, and the tarsal gland undergoes cryonecrosis, which is visible histologically after 4 days. The lid is re-examined on the 14th day and any loose cilia are removed; by this time they are sitting in the gland unattached. The remaining tissues of the eyelid are unaffected. By 4 weeks, the tarsal gland has regenerated without the cilia.

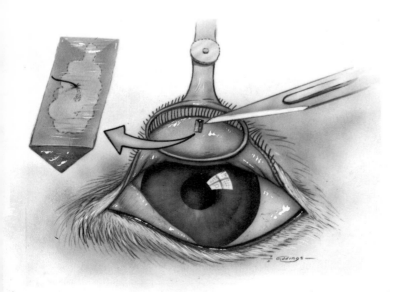

FIGURE 7–16. Ectopic cilium resection. The offending area of the lid is clamped with a Desmarres chalazion clamp for hemostasis, and the lid is everted. The wedge for resection is outlined.

2. Failure to appreciate the spherical nature of an ice ball, and the potential for inadequate freezing at depth when adjacent areas are frozen. Overlapping frozen areas avoids this.

3. Departure from the principles of controlled cryonecrosis—the ideal is a fast freeze–slow thaw with a double cycle.

4. Failure to accurately localize all aberrant cilia and immobilize the eyelid for therapy. Reference to published methods or appropriate training is recommended for inexperienced operators.

Simple epilation by forceps is a temporary measure, as the cilium regrows within 3–4 weeks. It can be useful to determine the clinical significance of a particular cilium. Occasionally cilia may appear at other follicles months or years later after any kind of treatment.

Electroepilation

The ideal electroepilator supplies direct current (1–5 ma) to the offending tarsal gland, destroying it by electrolysis. A fine needle (25 or 26 gauge) is used as the applying electrode, and it is passed down the follicle under magnification. Current is applied for 20–30 seconds. Easy removal of the cilium, which often adheres to the epilation needle, indicates follicle destruction. Low currents supplied by a small battery (see Fig. 6–8) prevent contraction of the orbicularis oculi and excess damage to surrounding structures and prevent postoperative scarring.

High-frequency alternating current supplied by electrosurgical units must *not* be used for epilation, as severe necrosis and scarring may result (see Fig. 6–9).

Trichiasis

Trichiasis is treated, depending on the location of the offending hairs, by

1. Regular trimming of the periocular hairs by the owner. This is often neglected by inexperienced owners, and it is important in breeds such as the poodle, Shih-Tzu, and Lhasa apso.

2. Cryoepilation of the offending hairs (see Fig. 7–17B). This method can be used anywhere around the lids, as it is especially useful at the medial canthus and where there are large numbers of hairs. The owner must be warned that the frozen area will be depigmented (Fig. 7–18). The pigment usually returns in 6–8 weeks even in darkly pigmented breeds. White hairs do not regain pigment.

3. Slight eversion of the eyelid margin. The "pinch" technique described for entropion repair is used, but

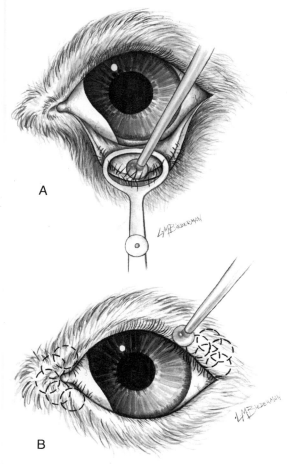

A

B

FIGURE 7–17. A, Microcryoepilation for distichiasis. The cilia are identified, and the tarsal gland from which they originate is isolated with a chalazion clamp; the lid is everted. The clamp is used to assist exposure and to slow thawing after freezing. The cryoprobe is applied over the tarsal gland from the conjunctival surface, and the ice ball is allowed to advance to the center of the eyelid margin, under microscopic control. A double freeze–thaw cycle is used. B, Cryoepilation for trichiasis. The probe is applied to the affected area, and overlapping areas of cryotherapy are used.

Postoperative swelling can be reduced by preoperative use of flunixin meglumine (0.5 mg/kg intravenous [IV]) and postoperative application of an antibiotic-steroid ointment. Some depigmentation of the lid margin may occur in dark animals, but most of this pigment returns by 6 weeks. The recurrence rate of cilia correctly epilated is negligible.

Failures with microcryoepilation may be attributed to

1. Use of a "counting" or timed technique to determine the size of the ice ball rather than actual, precise observation of the frozen area through the operating microscope.

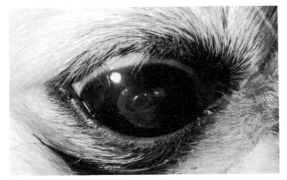

FIGURE 7–18. *Trichiasis. Darkly pigmented eyelids after cryotherapy, showing focal alopecia and loss of pigment. (Courtesy of Dr. G. A. Severin.)*

the piece of skin removed is much smaller; it is 2–3 mm from the eyelid margin and is restricted to the affected portion of the lid. In severe cases of cicatricial trichiasis (e.g., after injury), a resection of the entire lid thickness in the affected area may be necessary (see p 169).

Premature Opening of the Eyelids in Neonates

The eyelids in dogs and cats open at 7–10 days postpartum. Premature opening occurs infrequently in dogs and cats and results in corneal desiccation (the production of tears takes several weeks to reach adequate levels), keratitis, ulceration, and conjunctivitis. If left untreated, corneal perforation and endophthalmitis may occur.

Treatment consists of a temporary intermarginal tarsorrhaphy, which prevents evaporation of tears, aids in corneal healing, and prevents light damage to the developing retina. Bactericidal antibiotic ointment and artificial tears are administered frequently via a small gap left at the medial canthus. Sutures are removed after 7–10 days, but topical treatment may be necessary for an additional few days.

Entropion

Entropion, inward rolling or turning of the eyelid margin, is a common eyelid disorder. It may be congenital, spastic, or acquired. Congenital entropion occurs most frequently in dogs, horses, and sheep.

CLINICAL SIGNS (Fig. 7–19)

1. Epiphora.
2. Blepharospasm. The eyelid surface may be excoriated and white from constant contact with tears.
3. Rubbing at the affected area.
4. Corneal ulceration and vascularization in chronic cases.
5. Purulent conjunctivitis and discharge.
6. Photophobia.

7. Rolling in of the lid (Plate I*A*).

Note that in early cases, the signs may be intermittent and restricted to the area of the lid involved (usually the lower lateral lid).

DIFFERENTIAL DIAGNOSIS

The following conditions must be distinguished from entropion:

1. Other causes of epiphora: distichiasis, trichiasis, ectopic cilia, imperforate lacrimal puncta, dacryocystitis, corneal injuries, and coloboma in sheep.
2. Other causes of blepharospasm: distichiasis, ectopic cilia, corneal ulceration, and severe uveitis.
3. Enophthalmos and phthisis bulbi, causing an artificial appearance of entropion. Pain and epiphora are usually absent.

The diagnosis of entropion is usually not difficult, as inversion of the lid is evident. Congenital entropion usually affects both eyes, although occasionally only one eye is affected. The whole length of the lid may be affected in severe cases, but the affected area is usually restricted to one portion of the margin. The upper lid is less commonly affected than is the lower; in dogs, congenital entropion frequently affects the lateral part of the lower lid. This must be distinguished from **LATERAL ENTROPION**, which affects the lateral part of both the upper and lower lids, owing to a deficient retractor anguli oculi muscle (see the succeeding discussion).

In dogs, congenital entropion is common and is frequently hereditary in chow chows, English bulldogs, Irish setters, Labrador retrievers, Saint Bernards, and Shar Peis. Hereditary entropion is also common in golden retrievers, Great Danes, and Chesapeake Bay retrievers. Hereditary entropion often does not show up until later in life. In the chow chow, bullmastiff, and bloodhound the upper lid is often involved; correction may involve removal of redundant skin folds on the forehead.

In some breeds, especially Saint Bernards, the temporal lid may show entropion while the central part shows ectropion. Such lids can be repaired surgically, but experience and care are necessary in determining and performing the most appropriate techniques. Spastic entropion in dogs is caused by ocular pain and blepharospasm arising from corneal foreign bodies, ulceration, chronic conjunctivitis, blepharitis, and keratitis.

In horses, almost all entropion is congenital and occurs before 2 weeks of age. Acquired cicatricial entropion is not uncommon in adults after injury and is usually presented for cosmetic reasons.

Congenital entropion is common in lambs; it usually affects both eyes and most frequently involves the upper eyelid. Ovine entropion is hereditary, probably by a polygenic mode, and a large proportion of animals in a flock may be affected. Many cases resolve spontaneously without treatment. A thorough examination of the

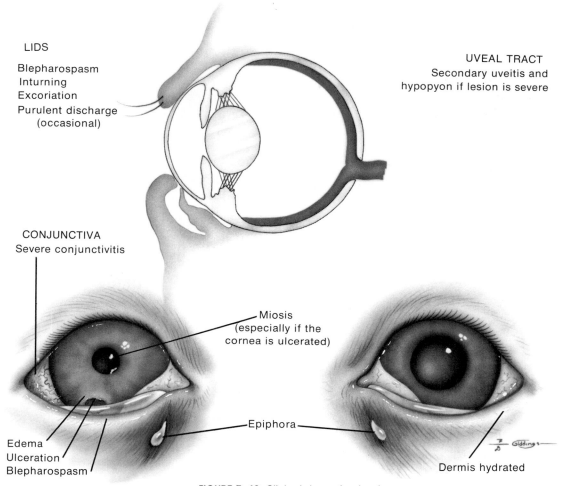

LIDS

Blepharospasm
Inturning
Excoriation
Purulent discharge
(occasional)

UVEAL TRACT
Secondary uveitis and
hypopyon if lesion is severe

CONJUNCTIVA
Severe conjunctivitis

Miosis
(especially if the
cornea is ulcerated)

Epiphora

Edema
Ulceration
Blepharospasm

Dermis hydrated

FIGURE 7–19. Clinical signs of entropion.

whole flock is required, as milder cases may go unnoticed.

Entropion is uncommon in cats, but it does occur in Persians. It is rare in cattle.

TREATMENT

The various methods of treating entropion are outlined here, although spastic entropion is discussed separately. The choice of technique depends on species, severity and position of the lid abnormality, and economic factors in lambs.

"Pinch" Technique (Fig. 7–20)[1]

This technique, when correctly performed, gives consistently good results in dogs and cats, in severe

acquired entropion in horses, and in valuable lambs. It is *not* necessary to remove orbicularis oculi muscle, as this increases hemorrhage, operating time, postoperative edema, and infection. Important factors in the success of this technique are

1. Use of fine suture material (6/0 silk or nylon in dogs and cats)
2. Minimal tissue trauma
3. Use of fine, swaged on, cutting suture needles
4. Lack of hemorrhage and trauma associated with hemostasis
5. Accurate control of skin resection

Before induction of anesthesia, the lid is everted manually and an estimate made of the amount of skin to be removed. Under anesthesia, a pair of curved Halsted's or Crile's forceps is placed on the area to be resected, 2–3 mm from the lid margin, and the amount of skin between the jaws is adjusted with toothed tissue forceps before crushing (Fig. 7–20A, B). The amount

---

1. This technique is sometimes incorrectly called the "Celsus-Hotz procedure," copied from human ophthalmology.

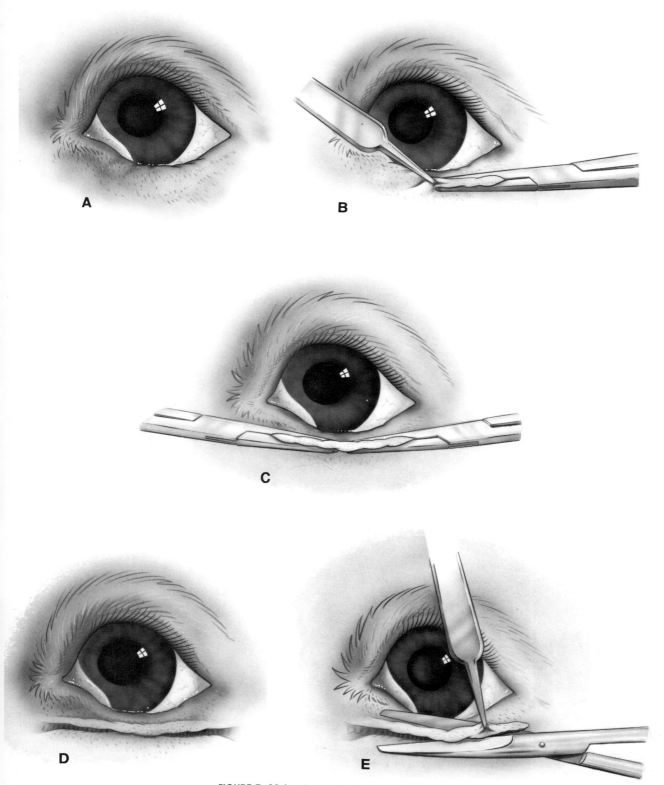

A

B

C

D

E

FIGURE 7–20 See legend on opposite page

of eversion is determined by the amount of skin removed and how close the incision is to the lid margin (the closer the incision the greater the effect). The hemostats are closed, the skin is crushed between the jaws, and the hemostats are removed (Fig. 7–20C, D). The strip of skin is grasped with forceps, held in the jaws of a pair of straight Mayo's scissors, and excised (Fig. 7–20E, F), beginning at the temporal canthus. The wound is carefully sutured with simple interrupted sutures of 6/0 silk (4/0 if the skin is thick) placed 1.5–2 mm apart (Fig. 7–20G). The sutures are removed after 10–14 days.

Correction of entropion in the Shar Pei should be performed by experienced persons only.

With uncontrollable and chronically affected patients with an established "itch-scratch" cycle, an Elizabethan collar is used.

The pinch technique is the operation of choice for correction of most entropion in dogs and cats and can be adapted to mild or severe cases. The resected areas correspond in location and extent to the affected portion of the lid.

Suture Technique (Fig. 7–21)

This method is used for correction of congenital entropion in foals if manual repositioning of the lid is unsuccessful, and in young Shar Pei puppies, up to 16–20 weeks of age, to avoid early reconstructive surgery in this breed. The lid edge is retracted with vertical mattress sutures that are left in place for 10–14 days (Fig. 7–21). A topical antibiotic ointment is used during this period. In Shar Peis, suturing may have to be repeated several times to prevent corneal lesions from occurring. Corrective surgery may be required later.

Injection Technique

This method is used for lambs, for economic reasons. In lambs, manual eversion of the lid alone is often successful if performed within 48 hours of birth. Various materials have been injected to evert the lower lid. An injection of sterile air (5–15 ml) along the affected area is often effective. (If air from sheep yards is used, injection of airborne spores of *Clostridium tetani* is present.) Other methods used for lambs include injection of procaine penicillin, stapling an elliptical piece of skin without suturing, and suturing as for the foal. As this condition is hereditary in lambs, affected animals are culled and breeding stock examined for evidence of entropion. Rams whose progeny are affected should be culled.

Trephine Technique (Fig. 7–22)

This method is a modification of the pinch technique. A local area of skin is removed with a dermal punch,

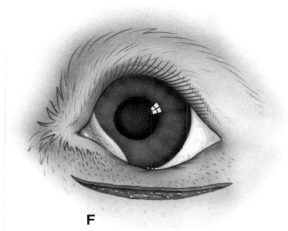 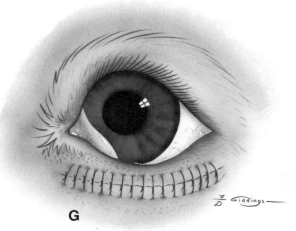

FIGURE 7–20. Pinch technique for entropion. A, Preoperative appearance of the entropion. B, The "rolled-in" area is everted, and the necessary amount of skin is placed between the forceps. C, The second pair of forceps is applied, and final adjustments are made before clamping. D, The forceps are removed. E, The strip of skin is excised, starting at the temporal canthus, including all of the clamped area. The strip is kept taut throughout the excision. F, The excised area with orbicularis oculi undisturbed. G, The incision sutured with simple interrupted sutures of 6/0 silk, 1.5–2.0 mm apart. A generous bite of tissue should be taken to prevent premature pulling out as the wound heals, but the sutures should not be tied tight, as postoperative edema may cause tearing of the surrounding tissue. (Redrawn from Severin GA: Veterinary Ophthalmology Notes, 2nd ed. Ft Collins, CO, 1976.)

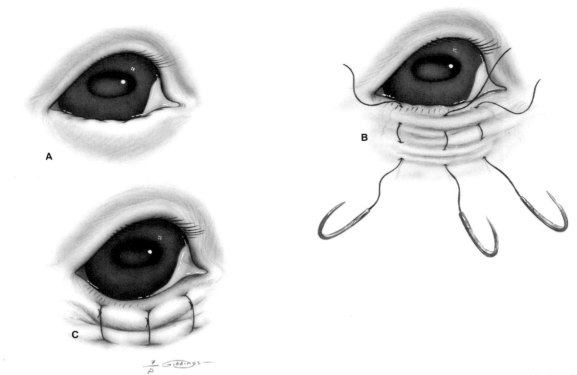

FIGURE 7–21. *Suture technique to correct entropion in foals and Shar Peis. A, Lower lid entropion in a foal. B, Insertion of the vertical mattress suture. The first bite is taken near the lid margin. Silk or nylon (2/0) is suitable. C, The sutures are tied, with the knots away from the eye. The sutures are removed after 10–14 days. In puppies, the sutures may remain for 14–21 days.*

resulting in a circular defect, which is sutured horizontally (Fig. 7–22). It is most useful for correction of entropion affecting a small area of the lid, in which a technique that everts the lid margin over its entire length may be undesirable (e.g., in Saint Bernards, in which the center of the lower lid is everted and the lateral part is inverted). The trephine method is convenient for localizing the correction. For lateral entropion affecting both upper and lower lids, the lateral canthal ligament (retractor anguli oculi muscle) is reconstructed.

OVERCORRECTION OF ENTROPION

If uncertainty exists about the extent of correction required, undercorrection with subsequent reoperation is preferable to overcorrection (cicatricial ectropion). For the first few days after surgery, when the tissues are swollen, the lid may appear overcorrected, but as swelling subsides (5–7 days) the correction can be evaluated. If a subsequent procedure is necessary for under- or overcorrection, and no corneal lesions are forming, wait 4–6 weeks before reoperating, until wound contraction is complete and the wound is stable.

Corneal lesions due to severe entropion usually resolve rapidly after surgical correction. The purulent secondary bacterial conjunctivitis often associated with entropion is treated with topical antibiotics.

If in doubt, entropion is undercorrected rather than overcorrected.

SPASTIC ENTROPION

Spastic entropion occurs with spasm of the ORBICULARIS OCULI MUSCLE following chronic painful ocular conditions that stimulate the palpebral or blink reflex. The condition occurs most frequently after painful corneal disorders (e.g., ulceration, trauma, uveitis) and skin and lid disorders (e.g., marginal blepharitis, lid tumors). Purulent blepharitis and conjunctivitis often follow, especially in long-haired dogs. Although treatment of the underlying condition sometimes relieves the spasm, surgical correction is often necessary. The pinch technique is frequently used, with local and systemic antibiotic cover given if secondary bacterial blepharitis or conjunctivitis is present. Because the condition is painful, a protective collar is used postoperatively.

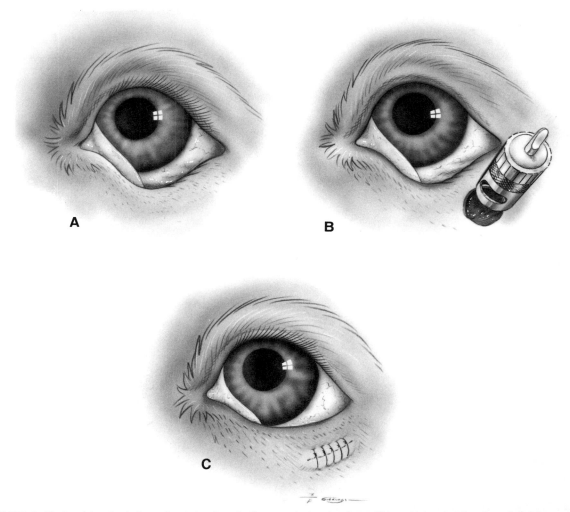

FIGURE 7–22. *Trephine technique for entropion. A, Uncorrected entropion with central ectropion in a Saint Bernard. B, Removal of a circle of skin opposite the everted lid with a 6 or 7 mm Keyes skin biopsy punch. C, The sutured incision. Increased skin tension helps correct the central ectropion. Note: For lateral entropion affecting both upper and lower lids, the lateral canthal ligament (or retractor anguli oculi muscle) is reconstructed.*

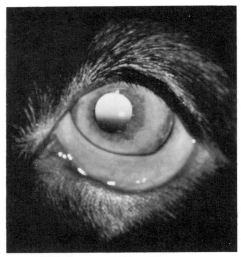

FIGURE 7–23. Hereditary ectropion.

Ectropion

Ectropion is eversion of the lower lid. It is distinguished from lagophthalmos in which the lids cannot meet but eversion is absent. The most common kinds are

1. CONGENITAL, HEREDITARY, or FAMILIAL ECTROPION. This type is usually breed-associated (e.g., Saint Bernard, bloodhound, cocker spaniel) and may be seen in dogs with loose facial skin (Fig. 7–23). Some ectropion is considered normal in particular breeds.

2. CICATRICIAL ECTROPION due to retraction of the lower eyelid by contraction of scar tissue from previous injuries or surgical procedures. It is most common in horses and dogs (Fig. 7–24) and may result in severe secondary ocular lesions.

3. INTERMITTENT ACQUIRED ECTROPION (physiological ectropion). This condition is poorly characterized

but not uncommon in larger hunting breeds (e.g., golden retriever, Irish setter, and Labrador retriever). Lid drooping occurs late in the day; the lids are normal in the morning. It is not associated with myasthenia of other muscles and should not be confused with typical myasthenia gravis. Surgical treatment is contraindicated, as entropion may follow. The disorder is cosmetic only and does not cause ocular lesions.

Surgical correction of intermittent acquired ectropion is contraindicated.

CLINICAL SIGNS

Clinical signs are shown in Figure 7–25.

TREATMENT

Ectropion is usually corrected surgically when it causes secondary conjunctival or corneal lesions (e.g., conjunctivitis, corneal vascularization or pigmentation, exfoliative blepharitis from epiphora) or for cosmetic improvement desired by the owner. Correction is required much less frequently than it is for entropion. Many animals tolerate slight ectropion with no ill effects. Cicatricial ectropion frequently results in unsightly cosmetic defects that justify correction even though secondary ocular lesions are not present.

A variety of techniques have been described for the correction of ectropion. Only commonly used methods suitable for the majority of cases are described here.

Trephination (Fig. 7–26)

Trephination is used for mild ectropion, especially when only a portion of the lid margin is affected. It

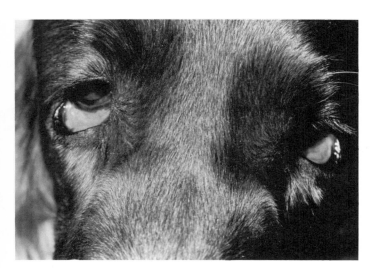

FIGURE 7–24. Cicatricial ectropion following extensive overcorrection of entropion.

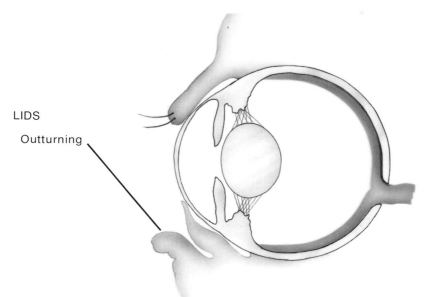

Corneal neovascularization and pigmentation in severe cases

LIDS

Outturning

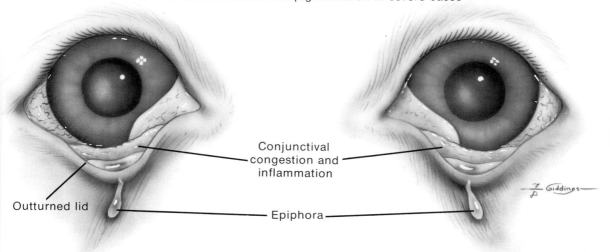

Conjunctival
congestion and
inflammation

Outturned lid

Epiphora

FIGURE 7–25. Clinical signs of ectropion.

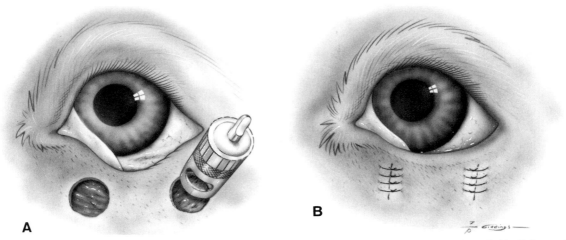

FIGURE 7–26. *Trephination for ectropion. A, Using a Keyes skin biopsy punch, several small circles of skin 5–7 mm in diameter are removed from the affected portion, 3–4 mm from the lid margin. B, The incision is sutured vertically with interrupted sutures of 4/0 or 6/0 silk or nylon. (Redrawn from Magrane WG: Canine Ophthalmology, 3rd ed. Lea & Febiger, Philadelphia, 1977.)*

may be combined with conjunctival resection if excess conjunctiva is present. Several small circles of skin are removed with a Keyes biopsy punch (5–7 mm), 3–4 mm from the lid margin (Fig. 7–26). The edges are sutured, and a vertical incision is left that tightens up the skin along the margin. The direction of suturing is at 90° to the direction for the similar method of correction for entropion. The incision is sutured with two or three sutures of 6/0 or 4/0 silk or nylon.

Modified Kuhnt-Szymanowski Procedure
(Fig. 7–27)

This method is suitable for most ectropion requiring surgical treatment, e.g., in undeformed eyelids, and is a triangular, full-thickness resection of the eyelid similar to that used for tumor removal. The resection is performed at the lateral area of the lower lid (Fig. 7–27).

Crile's forceps are placed into the conjunctival sac, vertically from the lateral canthus, and 1–2 mm of the tissue is lightly crushed as a marker. The lid margin is grasped with Adson-Brown forceps in the middle of the lid, and the excess lid is drawn laterally, tensing the lid margin and forming a fold adjacent to the crushed tissue. This allows accurate estimation of the amount of tissue to be removed. An incision is made at the lateral mark, the fold is drawn laterally, and a second incision is made through the lid margin to join the ventral end of the first incision. The fold, as a triangular piece of lid with its base on the margin, is removed and the skin sutured in two layers.

Conjunctival Resection (Fig. 7–28)

Excess conjunctiva may be removed alone or with other procedures for ectropion, to improve the cosmetic result. The procedure is similar to the pinch operation for entropion repair. Conjunctiva in the ventral fornix, anterior to the third eyelid, is grasped with fine forceps, elevated, and clamped with curved Halsted's or mosquito forceps for 30 seconds (Fig. 7–28). The clamps are removed, leaving an elevated ridge of tissue that is excised with tenotomy. Because conjunctiva heals rapidly, the incision is closed with a simple continuous suture of 6/0 absorbable suture, e.g., chromic gut.

Wharton-Jones Blepharoplasty (Fig. 7–29)

The Wharton-Jones or V-Y procedure is used for cicatricial ectropion, including ectropion resulting from wounds and tumor excision, and overcorrection of entropion. It is used when a small wedge excision is insufficient. It is better suited to correction of a broadly contracting scar than of a narrow band, when wedge excision is preferable. A triangular piece of skin with the base parallel and equal in length to the affected lid margin (Fig. 7–29) is outlined. The two lower sides of the triangle are incised, and the flap and its adjacent edges are fully undermined. Scar tissue beneath the flap is excised. The ventral incisions are sutured into a vertical line with simple interrupted sutures of 4/0 or 6/0 silk. The length of the vertical portion depends on how much elevation the lid margin requires to return it to its normal position. If the necessary correction is 4 mm, the vertical portion should be 6–7 mm long (the extra 2–3 mm allows for wound contraction). This

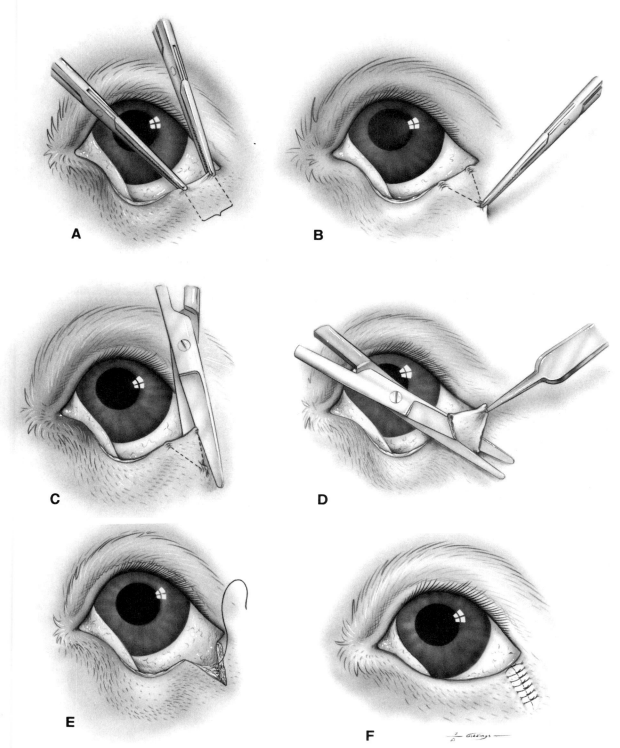

FIGURE 7–27. *Modified Kuhnt-Szymanowski procedure. A, The lid margin is marked laterally. B, An estimate of the amount of margin to be removed is made, and the lid is marked. The ventral end of the triangle is marked 10–14 mm below. C, The first incision is made with straight Mayo's scissors. D, The second incision is made. E, The triangular piece is removed. F, The conjunctiva is sutured with 6/0 absorbable suture and the skin with 6/0 silk or nylon.*

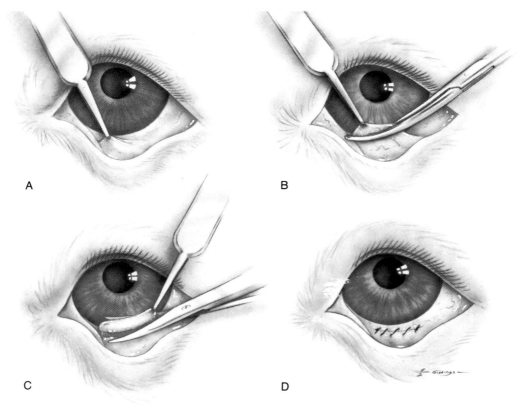

A

B

C

D

FIGURE 7–28. Conjunctival resection. A, Excess conjunctiva in the ventral fornix is elevated with fine forceps. B, The conjunctiva is grasped with curved mosquito forceps for 30 seconds. C, The fold is excised along the line of crushed tissue. The conjunctiva is held taut in the jaws of the scissors with fine forceps. D, The incision is closed with a simple continuous suture of 6/0 absorbable suture, e.g., chromic gut.

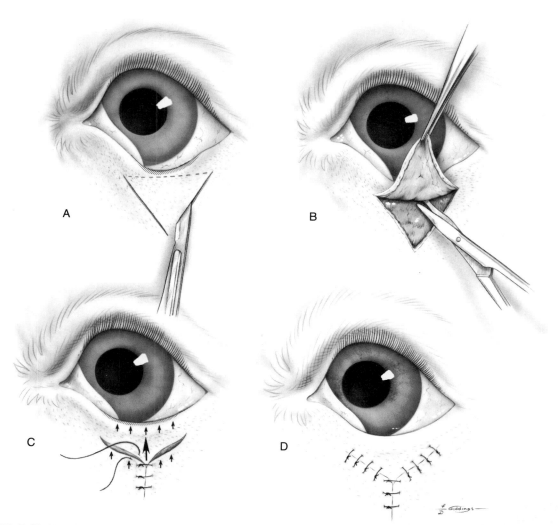

FIGURE 7–29. Wharton-Jones blepharoplasty. A, *Skin triangle outlined and incisions made.* B, *Skin flap elevated and dissected beneath.* C, *Vertical portion formed (defect + 3 mm).* D, *Completed Y incision sutured with 6/0 or 4/0 silk.*

vertical portion forces the triangle and lid margin superiorly. The horizontal arms are then closed.

Central Wedge Excision for Deformed Lids
(See Figs. 7–27 and 7–30)

When there is severe central ectropion due to either local cicatricial contraction or a deformity in the center of the lower lid, wedge excision at the lateral end is insufficient. Rather, a full-thickness wedge is removed from the center of the lid to include the fold of affected skin. As with all eyelid resections, the lid margin must be reconstructed accurately.

For broadly based cicatricial ectropion, a Wharton-Jones (V-Y) blepharoplasty is indicated. For a narrow cicatricial band or deformity, resection is preferable.

Combined Ectropion-Entropion
(Fig. 7–30)

Combined ectropion in the central lid and entropion at the lateral canthus occurs in the Saint Bernard, English bulldog, and cocker spaniel (Fig. 7–30). The condition may be caused by a deficiency in function of either the retractor anguli oculi muscle or the lateral palpebral ligament, and severe keratoconjunctivitis can result. The condition is corrected by either

1. Standard pinch technique for entropion and central lid excision or

2. Pinch technique for entropion, combined with construction of a lateral ligament from the orbicularis oculi muscle (Fig. 7–31). A lateral ligament supplement can be prepared with 4/0 nylon (Fig. 7–32).

In severe lateral entropion, method 2 (Fig. 7–32) is preferable.

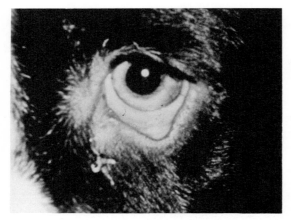

FIGURE 7–30. Combined ectropion-entropion in a Saint Bernard. (Courtesy of Dr. G. A. Severin.)

Euryblepharon

Euryblepharon is symmetrical enlargement of the palpebral fissure. There are two types: TRANSIENT JUVENILE and CONGENITAL.

TRANSIENT JUVENILE EURYBLEPHARON (EXOPHTHALMOS)

In this form, young dogs (particularly German shepherds) are affected with an apparent exophthalmos, usually noticed by the owner because of the obviously increased area of visible conjunctiva. The condition is usually bilateral, but occasionally only one eye is affected. The cause is unknown. In most cases no other ocular abnormalities are present, aside from a slight conjunctivitis due to exposure. In the absence of secondary lesions, treatment is unnecessary and resolution usually occurs in 2–3 months. Transient juvenile euryblepharon may be distinguished from other causes of acquired exophthalmos by

1. Occurrence in young dogs
2. Presence since birth and nonprogressive nature
3. Absence of secondary ocular lesions or pain
4. Spontaneous resolution
5. Lack of findings on orbital venography

Corticosteroids have been used to treat this condition, but a proven rationale is lacking.

CONGENITAL EURYBLEPHARON

The combination of a large palpebral fissure and shallow orbits with unusually apparent exophthalmos is seen in brachycephalic breeds (e.g., Boston terrier, Lhasa apso, pug, Pekingese, Shih-Tzu). Diagnosis is based on prominent globes, increased conjunctiva visible at the temporal limbus, and ease of creating partial proptosis by digital retraction of the lids. This defect and the increased evaporation of precorneal tear film and corneal exposure it causes, when combined with other abnormalities frequently seen in such breeds (e.g., prominent nasal folds and distichiasis), result in frequent recurrent corneal ulceration or chronic keratitis with pigmentation and vascularization.

Chronic ulcerative keratitis or keratitis with pigmentation and vascularization in brachycephalic breeds (chronic exposure keratitis syndrome) is caused by varying combinations of exophthalmos, euryblepharon, increased evaporation of the precorneal tear film, distichiasis, medial or nasal entropion, and prominent nasal folds.

Treatment

Congenital euryblepharon can be repaired surgically by shortening the palpebral fissure (Fig. 7–33; see also Fig. 7–12). This results in a narrower fissure with less

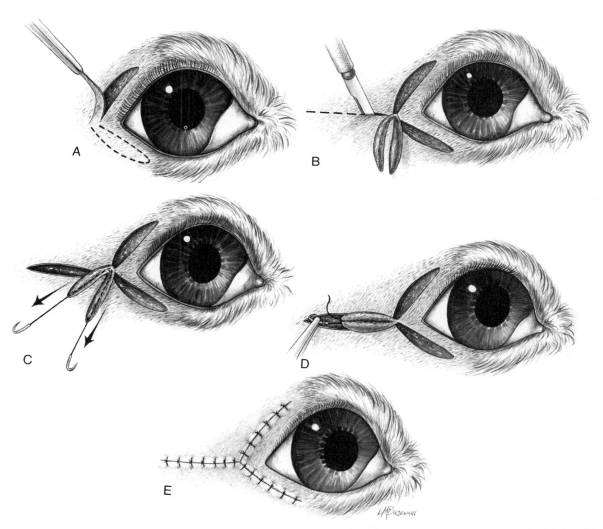

FIGURE 7–31. Lateral blepharoplasty for correction of combined entropion-ectropion. A, Folds of upper and lower lids are made to meet opposite the lateral canthus. B, Excision of folds. Skin incision is extended from the base of the skin incisions over the zygomatic arch. C, Strips of orbicularis muscle are dissected to terminate in a single base. One needle traverses the base and is turned and brought up through the opposite strip. The second needle is brought through the length of the other strip. D, The bundle is sutured to the periosteum of the zygomatic arch. E, Skin closure. (Redrawn from Magrane WG: Canine Ophthalmology, 3rd ed. Lea & Febiger, Philadelphia, 1977.)

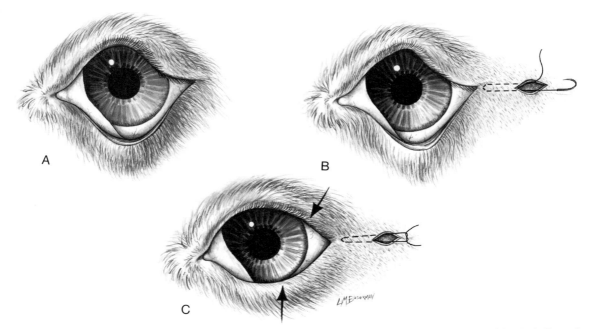

FIGURE 7–32. *Prosthetic lateral canthal ligament. The rolls of excess skin are removed as in Figure 7–31 A, B. A, Drooping of the lower lid. B, An access incision (1 cm) 2 cm lateral to the canthus is made. A 4/0 nylon suture is placed through the incision; it penetrates the canthal tissues and returns to the incision subcutaneously. C, The suture is tied, and the position of the canthus is adjusted by the tension in the suture. The knot is tied inverted, and the skin is closed with absorbable inverted subcuticular sutures.*

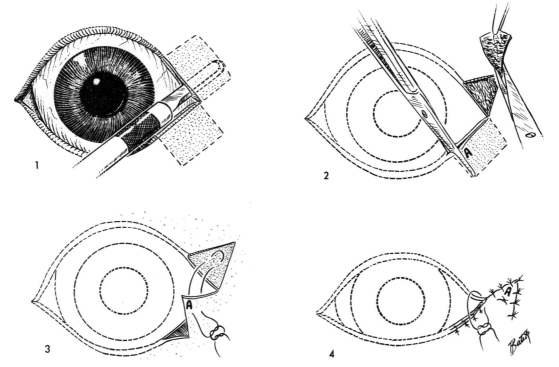

FIGURE 7–33. *1, The amount of palpebral fissure to be closed is estimated by pinching the lids closed at the lateral canthus. The upper and lower lids are split for the length of closure desired. The lid-splitting technique separates skin–orbicularis muscle from the underlying conjunctiva. 2, A cut (A) is made at the nasal end of the lid split in the lower lid, and the tarsal margin of this undermined lower lid flap is removed. A similar cut at the nasal end of the upper lid split is made, and the incision is extended outward and downward to end at the lateral canthus. This triangular piece of skin–orbicularis muscle is removed from the upper lid. 3, A double-armed 4/0 silk suture is used to place a mattress suture in the upper eyelid tarsoconjunctiva and through the lower lid skin-muscle flap. The lower lid is drawn up into the defect in the upper lid, and the mattress suture is tied. 4, Additional 6/0 silk sutures are used to secure the flap and re-create the lateral canthus. Care must be taken to close the lid-splitting defect in the lower lid. (From Bistner SI, et al: Atlas of Veterinary Ophthalmic Surgery. WB Saunders Co, Philadelphia, 1977.)*

corneal exposure and evaporation. The initial correction should be done nasally as the effect of closing the same amount of lid margin here is greater than it is at the lateral canthus. In severe cases, nasal and lateral correction may be required. Nasal reconstructive blepharoplasty is suitable in severely affected young dogs and in older dogs with progressive corneal lesions. It is also suitable for patients with postproptosis exophthalmos that does not resolve and causes lagophthalmos and secondary corneal lesions.

ACQUIRED LID DISORDERS

Injuries to the Eyelids

The eyelids have an excellent blood supply, and injuries heal rapidly when repaired correctly. Several facts are important:

1. Because of this rich blood supply, the lids are susceptible to severe edema and distortion after injury.

2. Bacterial flora in the conjunctival sac and surrounding area readily invade this damaged and edematous tissue.

3. Sutures in the eyelids must be soft and pliable, in order to prevent injury to the eye, or must be kept away from it.

4. During wound healing—especially if inflammation is present as a result of infection, tissue trauma, or large or tight sutures—severe pruritus often occurs, causing rubbing by the patient. Protective collars and bandaging may be necessary.

5. When an eyelid injury is examined, a thorough search is made for concurrent injuries to the cornea, sclera, and lacrimal passages in particular, and to the globe as a whole.

6. Although it is preferable to treat eyelid injuries as soon as possible, general treatment principles for an accident or emergency case should be followed and the patient's general condition stabilized before lid injuries are repaired.

TREATMENT

Immediate, intermediate, and delayed treatment for eyelid injuries are outlined in Table 7–2.

Simple Lid Laceration—Two-Layer Repair
(Figs. 7–34 and 7–35)

Most simple injuries can be converted to a V-shaped defect during débridement. Provided one third or less of the lid margin is missing, direct suturing may be used. If the defect is more extensive, an advancement flap (p 182) or other reconstructive procedure may be necessary. Details of the two-layer closure are shown in Figure 7–34. If trauma is severe, surrounding tissues have been damaged, or corneal coverage is desired, the healing surgical site may be "splinted" to the opposite lid margin (Fig. 7–35).

Injuries to Lacrimal Canaliculi

Lacerations and injuries may damage or sever the superior or inferior lacrimal canaliculi. If uncorrected,

TABLE 7–2. Immediate and Delayed Treatment of Eyelid Injuries

Immediate	Intermediate	Delayed
0–4 Hours After Injury	*Classified After Examination*	*After 12 Hours After Injury*
Repair as soon as possible, following regimen listed	Depends on severity, contamination, other life-threatening injuries, and so on	Repair within 24 hours, following regimen listed
1. Parenteral broad-spectrum antibiotics		1. Cleanse wound gently
2. General anesthetic		2. Treatment with suitable broad-spectrum antibacterial ointment or cream every 4 hours until infection controlled
3. Clean carefully with saline and povidone-iodine solution* (2:1)—*not* scrub, which contains detergent		3. Commence systemic antibiotics
4. Remove necrotic tissue but do not débride excessively		4. After infection is controlled treat as for a fresh wound
5. Suture by chosen method		5. Continue systemic antibiotics
6. Continue systemic antibiotics		6. Recheck during the healing period
7. Schedule a recheck examination during the healing period		7. Remove sutures in 14–21 days or earlier if healing completed
8. Remove sutures in 10–14 days		

Modified from Severin GA: Veterinary Ophthalmology Notes, 2nd ed. Fort Collins, CO, 1976.
*Betadine Solution—Purdue Frederick, Norwalk, CT.

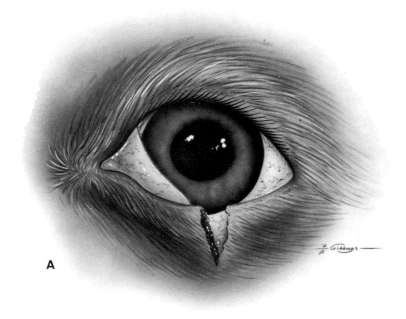

A

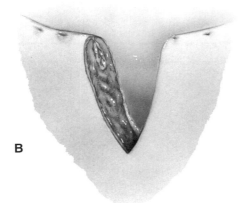

B

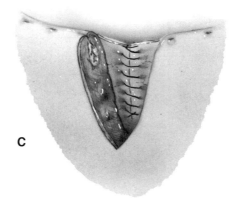

C

FIGURE 7–34. Simple two-layer repair. A, Initial injury before débridement. B, Wound after débridement and ready for suturing. C, The conjunctiva is sutured with 6/0 absorbable suture in a simple, continuous pattern. D, The marginal suture is placed first, in two separate bites. E, The second bite. F, The marginal suture is carefully tied to appose the margins. The knot lies along the margin. The wound is sutured with simple interrupted sutures of 6/0 silk, 2 mm apart. The first suture beneath the margin relieves tension on the marginal suture. G, The wound sutured. H, A figure-eight pattern may replace the first two sutures. I, The wound sutured using a figure-eight technique. (Redrawn from Severin GA: Veterinary Ophthalmclogy Notes, 3rd ed. Ft Collins, CO, 1976.)

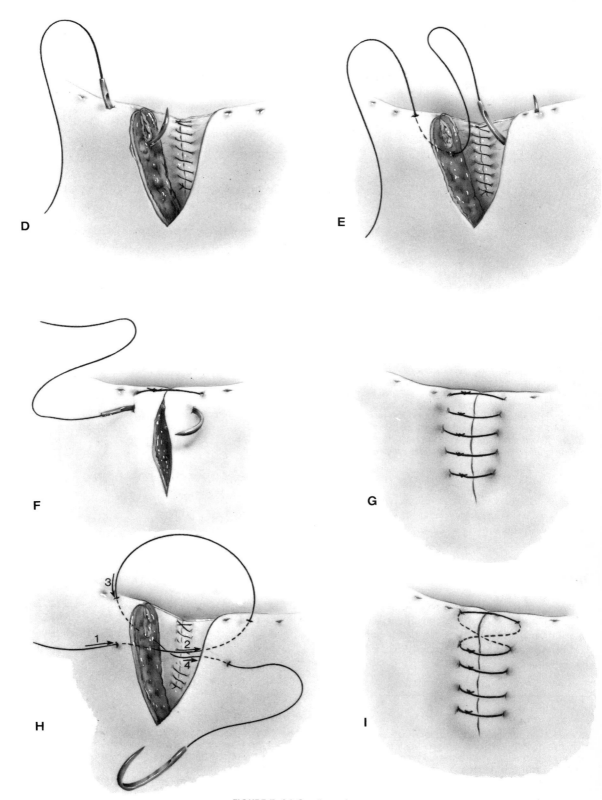

D

E

F

G

H

I

FIGURE 7–34 Continued

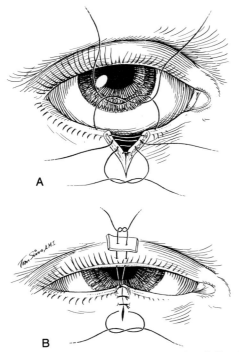

A

B

FIGURE 7–35. Simple two-layer closure with splinting. A, The conjunctiva is closed with either interrupted or continuous sutures of 6/0 absorbable suture, with buried knots. The splinting suture is placed along the lid margin and tied. B, The splinting suture is placed through the upper lid margin and tied over a piece of rubber or plastic or a small button. (From Paton D, Goldberg MF: Management of Ocular Injuries. WB Saunders Co, Philadelphia, 1976.)

drainage of tears causes epiphora. Although many animals with fusion of one punctum show no epiphora, especially if the inferior punctum and canaliculus remain patent, this is not constant or reliable.

TREATMENT

Every effort should be made to repair damage to either canaliculus as soon as possible after injury. The inferior canaliculus is most frequently injured in dog and cat fights. Immediate primary repair is performed by nasolacrimal catheterization (Fig. 7–36). If the

injury is presented too late, or if primary repair is unsuccessful, a new drainage canal to the nasal cavity can be created by conjunctivorhinostomy (see Chap 10).

Early and skilled repair of canalicular lacerations is necessary. Immediate referral to a veterinary ophthalmologist is frequently indicated.

Reconstruction of Simple Eyelid Defects

Defects in the eyelids after severe trauma and tumor resection frequently require the surgical placement of adjacent tissues for a functional and cosmetic result. As with lid injuries, plastic procedures may be performed immediately, or they may be delayed. With elective tumor excisions, reconstruction is performed immediately, although a second procedure is sometimes necessary later. After injury or cryosurgery, delayed treatment is preferred in order to allow 4–6 weeks for wound contraction. Many specialized techniques for lid repair have been described, but it is unnecessary to repeat them here. Methods of using the basic advancement flap for partial- and full-thickness defects are described. As extensive oculoplastic reconstructions are almost always elective in nature, specialist assistance is advisable.

ADVANCEMENT FLAP FOR PARTIAL-THICKNESS LESIONS (Fig. 7–37)

This method is appropriate for removal of marginal tumors and defects in which some conjunctiva remains. The following principles apply:

1. Only necessary layers are removed, consistent with total removal of the lesion.

2. In constructing the advancement flap, allowance is made for wound contraction, to prevent postoperative cicatricial ectropion.

3. Defects of one third or less of the lid margin can usually be repaired by simple suturing (see Figs. 7–34 and 7–35).

FIGURE 7–36. Nasolacrimal catheterization for canalicular laceration. A, Laceration of lid margin and canaliculus. B, A fine nylon (e.g., 2/0) thread is passed up the nasolacrimal duct from the nose. The superior punctum from which it normally emerges is occluded by finger pressure, and the thread is manipulated to emerge from the severed inferior canaliculus. C, A Worst probe is passed, and the suture is tied to it and pulled through the punctum (D). E, A polyethylene tube is passed over the nasal end of the suture and clamped with hemostats. The tube is carefully drawn up the nasolacrimal duct and through the severed canaliculus. F, The conjunctiva is closed with a simple continuous 6/0 absorbable suture. Two simple interrupted sutures are placed in the ends of the severed canaliculus. G, The defect is sutured as for a simple lid defect. The tube is sutured to the medial canthus and to the nose at its nasal end and remains in place for 2–3 weeks while the duct heals.

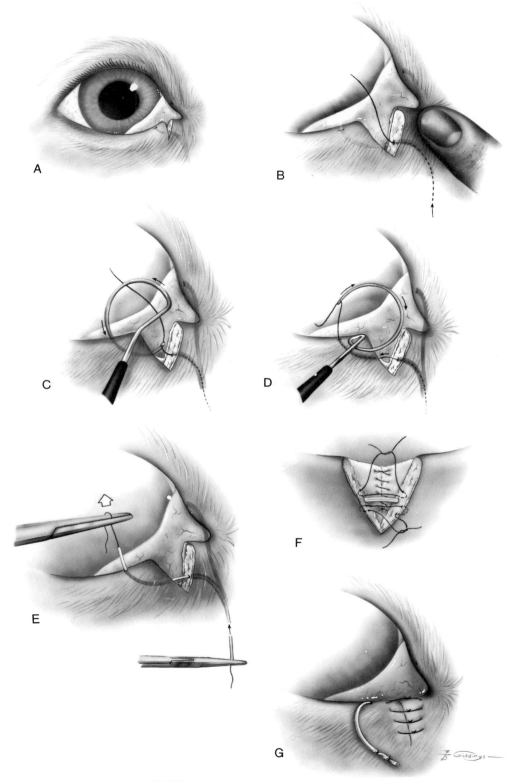

A

B

C

D

E

F

G

FIGURE 7–36 See legend on opposite page

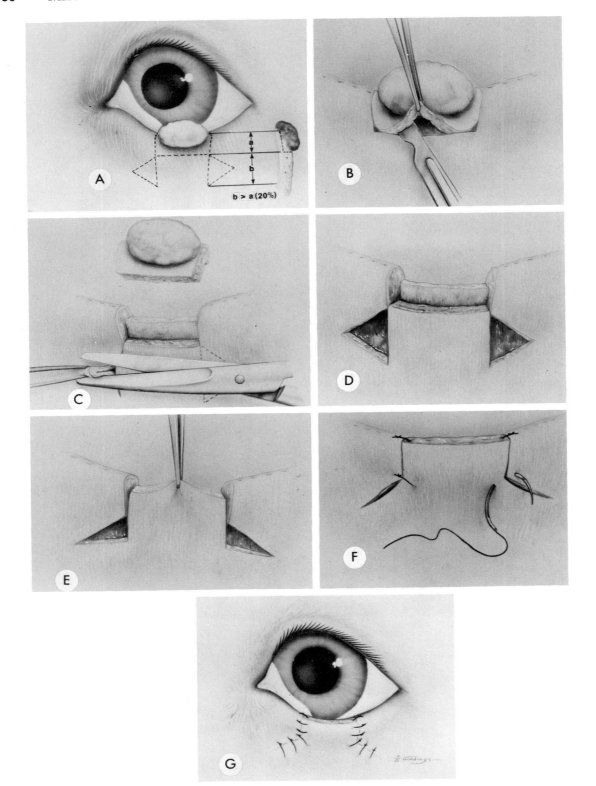

FIGURE 7–37 See legend on opposite page

ADVANCEMENT FLAP FOR FULL-THICKNESS LESIONS

If the defect or the lesion to be removed affects the full thickness of the lid margin, the conjunctiva may be replaced by transposition from the upper lid (Fig. 7–38). The tissue bridge to the upper lid is maintained intact for 10–14 days, until the repositioned conjunctiva establishes a blood supply. Transposition is necessary only for large defects, as the conjunctiva is mobile in the fornix and can be replaced over the inner surface of the lid and sutured, before the skin advancement flap is produced.

The intermarginal sutures are removed after 2–3 weeks, and the conjunctival flap is incised level with the edge of the lid margin.

Chalazion

A chalazion is an enlargement of a tarsal gland caused by blockage of the duct and inspissation of secretory products. It is a painless swelling that appears yellow white when viewed through the palpebral conjunctiva or skin (Fig. 7–39A). It is distinguished from a tarsal gland neoplasm by its hard nature, color, and failure to enlarge. If the gland ruptures, fatty sebaceous material escapes into the lid and causes a lipid granuloma that may be surrounded by fibrous tissue. Chalazion must also be distinguished from external hordeolum (stye) and internal hordeolum. Under topical or general anesthesia, the affected area is clamped with chalazion forceps, and a small incision is made into the mass through the palpebral conjunctiva. The contents are removed with a chalazion spoon (Fig. 7–39B).

External and Internal Hordeolum

External hordeolum is a purulent bacterial infection of a lash follicle and associated gland of Zeis. Internal hordeolum is a similar infection of a tarsal gland. Both are focal, painful, raised, reddened areas up to 10 mm in diameter on the lid margin. *Staphylococcus aureus* is most frequently responsible. Treatment consists of application of hot compresses until the infection "points," followed by surgical incision and drainage. (Manual expression is contraindicated, as the infection may be spread into surrounding tissues.) Appropriate systemic and local antibiotic therapy is begun. Localized lid abscesses are treated similarly.

Suppurative Tarsitis and Blepharitis

Infections of the lid margins occur frequently in dogs and are usually bacterial in origin. Although the onset is often associated with trauma to the lids, primary bacterial infections also occur, with *Staphylococcus aureus* being frequently responsible. Clinical signs include severe erythema and swelling of the lid margins, pruritus, pain (often severe), chemosis, and purulent conjunctivitis.

Hypersensitivity to bacterial antigens is implicated in the staphylococcal form based on clinical response to corticosteroids and on experimental reproduction of the disease in rabbits. Severe staphylococcal infections are often associated with either intermittent or previous keratoconjunctivitis sicca. Chronic *low-level* staphylococcal infection with release of toxins may cause keratitis of the superior half of the cornea with vascularization in dogs. Ribitol teichoic acid in the staphylococcal cell wall is believed to be responsible for the hypersensitivity. Chronic severe staphylococcal blepharitis requires patience and continued treatment for control.

TREATMENT

Uncomplicated Bacterial Blepharitis

1. Careful cleaning of lid margins and removal of purulent exudates with cotton soaked with warm saline solution or commercially available eye-cleaning kits.

2. Systemic doses of bactericidal antibiotics and topical application of antibiotic ointments, which may be carefully massaged into affected areas.

3. Prevention of self-mutilation with a protective collar.

Staphylococcal Blepharitis (Table 7–3)

1. Confirmation of staphylococcal involvement by careful collection of tarsal secretion into broth for culture and sensitivity testing.

FIGURE 7–37. Advancement flap for partial-thickness lesions. A, The tumor before excision. As the conjunctiva is not involved, it is not removed. Incisions are outlined by dotted lines. Vertical sides of the triangles are 20% longer than the vertical incisions adjacent to the tumor, to allow for wound contraction. B, A square or rectangular incision is made around the tumor. The tumor is dissected toward the lid margin. C, The tumor is removed and fixed. The triangle is elevated and excised. D, The triangles are removed and incisions completed. E, To reduce tension on the wound, undermine the surrounding tissues. The flap is advanced to the margin with no tension on it. F, Simple marginal sutures of 6/0 silk are placed. Sutures are placed at the corners of the incision to assist in accurate placement of subsequent sutures. G, Remaining sutures in place 2 mm apart. If the conjunctiva is mobile, it is sutured to the skin edge with a simple continuous suture. This helps prevent retraction of the advancement flap.

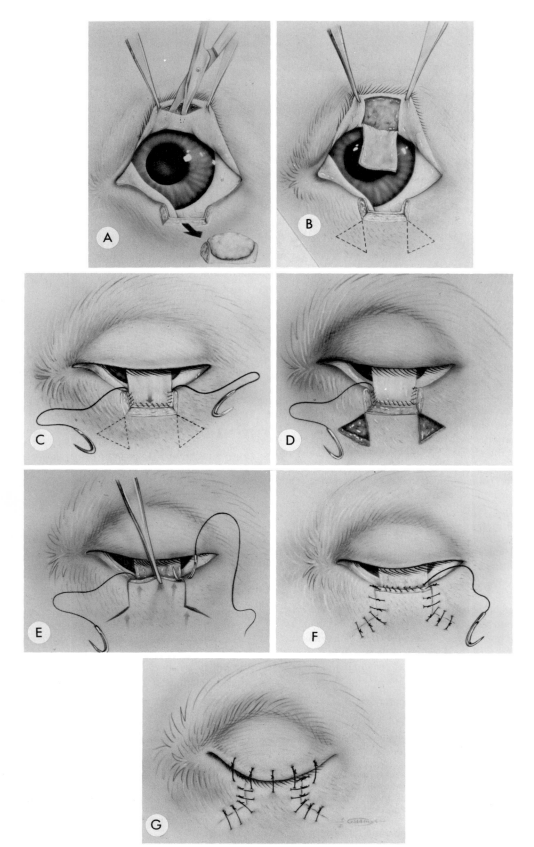

FIGURE 7–38 See legend on opposite page

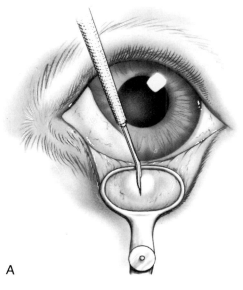

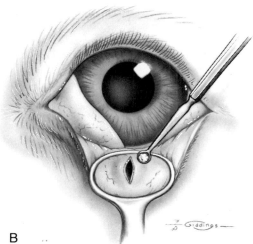

A

B

FIGURE 7–39. Treatment of chalazion. A, A chalazion clamp is applied, and the lesion is incised through the palpebral conjunctiva with a No. 11 blade. B, Removal of granulomatous material and secretion with a chalazion spoon.

2. Initial attempt to eliminate bacteria from the tarsal glands with appropriate topical and systemic antibiotics for 4 weeks.

3. In severe cases, corticosteroid therapy may be necessary with antibiotic therapy, if hypersensitivity is suspected.

4. Administration of appropriately prepared staphylococcal bacterin of animal origin.

Purulent blepharitis is also caused by fungi (e.g., *Microsporum canis, M. gypseum, Trichophyton mentagrophytes, Aspergillus niger*), which ususally cause a less severe inflammation that is resistant to antibacterial therapy.

TUMORS OF THE EYELIDS

Eyelid tumors are relatively common in all domestic species. The most common lid neoplasms are

Dog	tarsal adenoma, squamous papilloma, tarsal adenocarcinoma, and benign melanoma
Cat	squamous cell carcinoma (SCC)
Horse	SCC, equine fibrosarcoma
Ox	SCC

Squamous papillomas are common in older dogs, both on the lids and on the general body surface. They are generally less than 5–10 mm in diameter and are pedunculated. Surgical excision or localized cryotherapy is the treatment of choice. The sebaceous adenocarcinoma is similar in clinical behavior to the adenoma and rarely, if ever, metastasizes, even though it is histologically malignant. Benign and malignant melanomas of the canine eyelid occur in equal proportions and hence follow the general oncological clinical pattern of skin melanomas. All tumors of lids are regarded as malignant until proved otherwise by excisional biopsy.

Before considering details of tumor types in different species, the principles of tumor therapy are presented briefly.

Therapy

Better clinical responses in tumor treatment are often obtained using combination therapy, comprising

1. Surgical excision (including cryotherapy)

FIGURE 7–38. Advancement flap for full-thickness lesions. A, A full-thickness resection is performed. The edges of the excised block are examined histologically for evidence of neoplasia. The palpebral conjunctiva is undermined with strabismus scissors, toward the fornix. B, A conjunctival flap is formed slightly larger than the lower lid defect and is reflected toward the lower lid. C, The conjunctival flap is sutured into the defect with a double-armed suture of 6/0 absorbable suture. The suture is started in the center of the defect. D, Suturing of the conjunctival flap is completed, and triangles of skin for the advancement flap are excised. E, The skin flap is advanced, and marginal sutures of 6/0 silk are placed. F, Suturing of the advancement flap is completed, and the conjunctival flap is sutured to the edge of the advancement flap in a continuous pattern with the remainder of the double-armed suture. G, Several intermarginal sutures are placed between the lids to remove tension from the healing suture lines. (Modified from Severin GA: Veterinary Ophthalmology Notes, 2nd ed. Ft Collins, CO, 1976.)

TABLE 7–3. Therapy of Chronic Canine Staphylococcal Blepharitis

Severity	Diagnosis	Therapy
Early	Clinical signs, culture	1. Topical antibiotics 2. Systemic antibiotics (e.g., erythromycin until culture results received)
Moderate	Clinical signs, bacterial and fungal culture, conjunctival and skin scrapings	1. As for early type until culture results received (minimum therapy 14 days) 2. Topical and systemic dexamethasone (0.05 mg/kg once a day orally for 5 days then every 2nd day) for 4 weeks; withdraw systemic steroid only and observe for recurrence
Chronic or recurrent patients	As for moderate cases	1. As for moderate cases until response occurs, then discontinue systemic therapy 2. Continue topical antibiotic and corticosteroids 3. Bacterin injections at 1, 2, 3, 4 weeks until response occurs then decreasing frequency to every 2 weeks for 1–2 months, then every 3 weeks for 6 weeks, then monthly for 2 months, discontinue or continue depending on response

Courtesy of Dr. E. D. Chambers.

2. Radiation therapy
3. Chemotherapy
4. Immunotherapy

Surgical therapy is the major method of treatment of lid neoplasms.

Information from previous clinical studies often indicates that all four modes are not necessary in the treatment of every tumor type. Within any particular tumor type, variations in therapy may be chosen depending on malignancy, rate of growth, position, presence of metastases, local invasiveness, and response to previous and current therapy.

Rational tumor therapy requires an accurate histological diagnosis.

SURGICAL EXCISION

As much of the neoplasm as possible should be removed, including the regional lymph node if affected. Margins of the excised tissue are examined for evidence of neoplasia. If neoplastic cells are present in the edges of this tissue, excision has been incomplete. In neoplasms that invade extensively (e.g., SCC), complete surgical excision is not always possible.

The neoplastic cell mass is reduced ("debulking"), and additional methods are used to destroy remaining cells. Immunotherapy rarely cures a neoplasm, but it often gives dramatic results when the neoplastic cell mass has been suitably reduced first (equine sarcoids are an exception). For small tumors involving one third or less of the lid margin, a simple, full-thickness V excision is indicated (Fig. 7–40). As much of the lid margin as possible is retained.

In the treatment of tarsal adenoma/adenocarcinoma in dogs, correct surgical excision gives cosmetic results superior to those of cryotherapy. Cryotherapy may be used near the lacrimal canaliculi, and it does not damage them permanently.

RADIATION THERAPY

Because the eyelids are thick, gamma radiation is used most frequently and may be administered by radon or gold seeds (brachytherapy), removable cesium or cobalt implant, or x-ray therapy machine (teletherapy). Very small surface lesions may be treated with a strontium-90 ophthalmic applicator emitting beta radiation. Implants (brachytherapy) have the advantage of continuous treatment, and multiple manipulations are not required. A dose of 4000–5000 rads over 7–10 days is suitable for most neoplasms.

SCCs are the most sensitive to radiation of the commonly occurring lid neoplasms, although irradiation of other tumors not usually sensitive often results in clinical improvement. Presurgical irradiation of tumors may increase local recurrence of the tumor. Consequences of radiation therapy include skin erythema and loss or change in color of surrounding hair, keratopathy, keratoconjunctivitis sicca, uveitis, and cataract. Gavin and Gillette (1978) reported an overall cure rate for adnexal SCCs in horses of 74%, with excellent cosmetic results, with implantation of ^{60}Co or ^{137}Cs needles.

CHEMOTHERAPY

Chemotherapy agents (alkylating agents, antimetabolites, antibiotics, *Vinca* alkaloids, corticosteroids, enzymes) are not commonly used for the treatment of lid

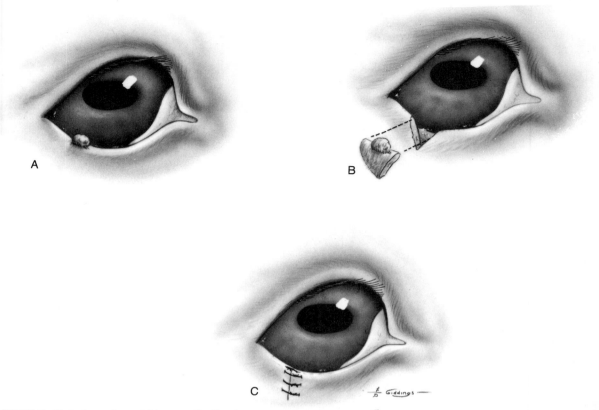

FIGURE 7–40. A, A small eyelid tumor affecting less than one third of the margin. B, The tumor and a surrounding area of normal tissue are removed by full-thickness V excision. C, The defect is closed with a marginal suture and simple interrupted sutures of 6/0 silk. The conjunctiva is closed with 6/0 absorbable suture with knots buried beneath the palpebral conjunctiva.

disorders, except in cases where the neoplasm has infiltrated extensively or is known to be especially sensitive (e.g., multiple histiocytoma, mastocytoma). Such agents are sometimes used to reduce the size of a tumor before surgical excision or radiation therapy.

Table 7–4 lists agents and dose rates related to body surface area or weight. Laboratory facilities for careful hematological monitoring must be available, as many

---

When using chemotherapy, clinicians must consider

1. The owner's wishes.
2. The patient's comfort and welfare.
3. The cost.
4. Very few animal tumor types have been shown by scientifically valid studies to respond to chemotherapy.
5. Many extravagant, unsupported, anecdotal claims are made for the effectiveness of chemotherapy in animal patients.

---

of these agents have severe side effects. For routine therapy, chemotherapy of lid tumors is rarely required. Appropriate safeguards against human exposure must be used when using these agents.

IMMUNOTHERAPY

Agents used to stimulate the immune system against neoplastic cells are of two types (Table 7–5):

1. Nonspecific immune stimulants. Thiabendazole, tetramisole, live and killed bacille Calmette-Guérin (BCG) extracts, live *Brucella abortus* vaccine (strain 19), and *Corynebacterium parvum* stimulate the entire immune system and are usually administered intramuscularly at various arbitrary dose rates and schedules.

2. Specific immune stimulants. BCG, *Corynebacterium parvum*, strain 19, and Freund's adjuvant have been injected into tumor masses to stimulate a cell-mediated response to tumor specific antigens.

A phenolized "vaccine" produced from SCCs in cattle has been used for treatment of the same lesion in the

TABLE 7–4. Cancer Chemotherapeutic Agents Used in Veterinary Practice

Agent	Unit	Cost (In US Dollars)	Route of Administration*	Dosage	Patient Toxicity	General Hazard	Effect on Skin	Manufacturer's Advice on Handling Precautions	Action on Contamination
Alkylating Agents									
Cyclophosphamide (Cytoxan) Bristol-Myers 25, 50 mg tablets 100, 200, 500 mg vials	25 mg tablet 50 mg tablet 100 mg vial	0.50 1.12 52.50	Oral mornings IV slow	2.2 mg/kg 3–4 days/ week 10 mg/kg, weekly	Bone marrow depression, cystitis, transitional carcinoma	Pro-drug, requires metabolism in liver before becoming cytotoxic, carcinogenic, and teratogenic	Irritation is rare	No special precaution	Wash thoroughly with water
Chlorambucil (Leukeran) Burroughs Wellcome 2 mg tablets	2 mg tablet	0.30	Oral	0.1–0.2 mg/kg, daily	Bone marrow depression	NA	NA	NA	NA
Melphalan (Alkeran) Burroughs Wellcome 2 mg tablets	2 mg tablet	0.63	Oral	0.1 mg/kg, daily for 10 days, then 0.05–0.1 mg/kg, daily	Bone marrow depression	Carcinogenic, mutagenic	Not a skin irritant	Gloves and dye shield	Solution of 3% sodium carbonate should be used if spilled
Busulfan (Myleran) Burroughs Wellcome 2 mg tablets	2 mg tablet	0.38	Oral	0.1 mg/kg, daily	Bone marrow depression, pulmonary fibrosis	NA	NA	NA	NA
Thiotepa Lederle 15 mg vials	15 mg vial	21.68	IV or intracavitary	Maximum systemic dosage, 9 mg/sq m; intracavitary, bladder: 5–10 mg diluted in 30 ml, allow contact 30 min, repeat weekly	Bone marrow depression	NA	NA	NA	NA
Cisplatin (Platinol) Bristol-Myers 10–50 mg vials	10 mg vial 50 mg vial	25.67 119.98	IV	30–50 mg/sq m every 3 weeks; pretreat with fluids 12 hours, 60 ml/kg, administer mannitol 0.5 gm/kg 30 min before drug therapy; slow drip 1–6 hours, follow with 12 hours fluid diuresis 60 ml/kg	Bone marrow depression, nephro-toxicity, local irritation	Carcinogenicity, mutagenicity, and teratogenicity suspected	Potentially allergenic	Gloves and mask necessary only if spilled	Wash thoroughly with water
Antimetabolites									
Methotrexate Lederle 2.5 mg tablets 25–50 mg vials	2.5 mg tablet 25 mg vial	0.56 6.65	Oral IV	2.5 mg/sq m, daily 0.3 to 0.8 mg/kg, weekly	Bone marrow depression	Teratogenic, carcinogenic, mutagenic	Irritant	Gloves	Wash with water, apply a bland cream for transient stinging; for systemic absorption of significant quantities, give calcium folinate (leucovorin); cover

TABLE 7–4. Cancer Chemotherapeutic Agents Used in Veterinary Practice *Continued*

Agent	Price Unit	Price Cost (In US Dollars)	Route of Administration*	Dosage	Patient Toxicity	General Hazard	Effect on Skin	Manufacturer's Advice on Handling Precautions	Action on Contamination
6-Mercaptopurine (6-MP, Purinethol) Burroughs Wellcome 50 mg tablets	50 mg	0.62	Oral	2 mg/kg, daily	Bone marrow depression	NA	NA	NA	NA
Azathioprine (Imuran) Burroughs Wellcome 25 and 50 mg tablets	50 mg	0.50	Oral	2.2 mg/kg, daily (dog)	Bone marrow depression	NA	NA	NA	Wash off quickly with water
5-Fluorouracil (5-FU) Roche 500 mg vials	500 mg vial	1.32	IV	5–10 mg/kg, weekly	Do not use in cats; bone marrow depression, central nervous system signs	Cytostatic	Minor local inflammation if skin is broken	No special precautions, but avoid contact with skin and mucous membranes	Flush affected parts with copious amounts of water
6-Thioguanine (6-TG) Burroughs Wellcome 40 mg tablets	40 mg	0.90	Oral	1 mg/kg, daily	Bone marrow depression	NA	NA	NA	NA
Cytosine arabinoside (Ara-C, Cytosar) Upjohn 100–500 mg vials	100 mg 500 mg	6.73 26.75	IV SC	100 mg/sq m, daily for 4 days; repeat cycle at 3-week intervals 30 mg/kg, weekly'	Bone marrow depression	Teratogenic; causes corneal speckling if applied to eyes for several days	Not absorbed through intact skin	No special precautions	Wash thoroughly with water
Antibiotics Bleomycin (Blenoxane) Bristol-Myers 15 unit vials	15 unit vial	121.94	IV, SC, IM	10 mg/sq m weekly, to maximum of 200 mg/sq m	Pulmonary fibrosis	Cytostatic	Locally toxic, allergenic	Gloves and mask	Rinse thoroughly with water, then wash with soap and water
Doxorubicin (Adriamycin) Adria Labs 10–50 mg vials	10 mg	28.34	IV	30 mg/sq m; repeat every 3 weeks to maximum cumulative dose of 200 mg/sq m	Bone marrow depression, cardiomyopathy	Antimitotic, cytotoxic	Irritant	Gloves	Wash with copious amounts of soap and water
Plant Alkaloids Vincristine (Oncovin) Lilly 1–5 mg vials	1 mg vial	29.54		0.5–0.8 mm sq m, weekly, or 0.02 mg/kg, weekly	Locally irritating, peripheral neuropathy	Suspected to be teratogenic	Irritant	Gloves	As for vinblastine

Table continued on following page

TABLE 7–4. Cancer Chemotherapeutic Agents Used in Veterinary Practice *Continued*

Agent	Price		Route of Administration*	Dosage	Patient Toxicity	General Hazard	Effect on Skin	Manufacturer's Advice on Handling Precautions	Action on Contamination
	Unit	Cost (In US Dollars)							
Vinblastine (Velban) Lilly 10 mg vial	10 mg	30.48	IV	3 mg sq m, weekly, or 0.1–0.4 mg/kg, weekly	Bone marrow depression, peripheral neuropathy	Suspected to be teratogenic	Irritant	Gloves	Wash thoroughly and immediately with large amounts of water, if accidental injection into SC* tissues, apply heparin cream to affected area
Miscellaneous Agents									
L-Asparaginase (Elspar) Merck, Sharp & Dohme 10,000 and 50,000 unit vials	10,000 unit vial	27.98	IV, IP, IM	400 units/kg, weekly	Anaphylaxis	Cytostatic	Not a skin irritant	No special precautions	Wash with water
Hydroxyurea (Hydrea) Squibb 500 mg tablets	500 mg	0.67	Oral	80 mg/kg every 3 days or 40 mg/kg, daily	Bone marrow depression	NA	NA	NA	NA

From Macy DW: Chemotherapeutic agents available for cancer treatment. *In* Kirk RW: Current Veterinary Therapy IX. Philadelphia: WB Saunders Co, 1986.

*SC = subcutaneous; IM = intramuscular; IP = intraperitoneal.

TABLE 7–5. Immunotherapeutic Agents

Agent	Route of Administration
BCG	IMS; intralesional
Thiabendasole	Oral
Tetramisole	IMS; oral
Brucella abortus (strain 19)	IM; intralesional
Corynebacterium parvum	IM; intralesional
Freund's adjuvant	Intralesional

eyelids. At present, all methods of immunotherapy are characterized by an empirical array of dose rates and schedules. Responses are often dramatic and well worth consideration for severe or nonresponsive neoplasms. Many chemotherapeutic agents are potent immunosuppressants, and ionizing radiation is lymphocytotoxic. When designing combination schedules, these methods should not overlap attempts at immunotherapy.

With the exception of equine sarcoid therapy, immunotherapy is rarely curative as the sole method of treatment.

CRYOTHERAPY

In cryotherapy, the lesion and a surrounding margin of normal tissue (together called the "ice ball") are frozen. This results in death of the cells, necrosis, and sloughing with healing by granulation. Temperature probes should be used in tissues on the margin of the area to be frozen where possible in order to ensure complete freezing. Without such probes, freezing is often inadequate, and tumors recur, requiring additional treatments.

The most effective method is a double freeze–thaw cycle, with the tissues frozen to −25°C and allowed to thaw to 20°C before application of the second freeze. After freezing, the tissues become swollen, edematous, and dark before necrosis and sloughing occur. Freezing

may be accomplished by application of a cold probe or by spraying liquid nitrogen onto the lesion after packing with surgical sponges impregnated with petroleum jelly. Freezing of tumors in laboratory animals causes increased antigenicity of the tumor cells and increased immunological response to the tumor.

HYPERTHERMIA

Hyperthermia uses the increased susceptibility of neoplastic cells to increased temperature, e.g., 42–46°C, which results in cell death. In veterinary ophthalmology, hyperthermia is sometimes used for the treatment of surface SCCs in cattle and horses. Tissue temperature is increased by application of localized, radiofrequency electrical energy with a commercially available probe.

SCC

SCC occurs in the eyelids of all species but is especially common in unpigmented areas of the lids in horses, cattle, and cats (Figs. 7–41 and 7–42). The tumor is associated with exposure to ultraviolet light and is more common in sunny or elevated areas and in animals with little pigmentation. In some elevated areas in Western states it is particularly common in horses. Although SCCs do metastasize to regional lymph nodes and eventually to the lungs, they are characterized initially by local invasiveness, and their degree of malignancy is generally low. In recent reports, rates of metastases of 10.2% and 15.4%, respectively, were recorded, an indication for early treatment in horses.

PATHOGENESIS

The pathogenesis of the lid lesion of SCC is shown in Figure 7–43. The invading neoplasms result in local inflammation with blepharitis and conjunctivitis.

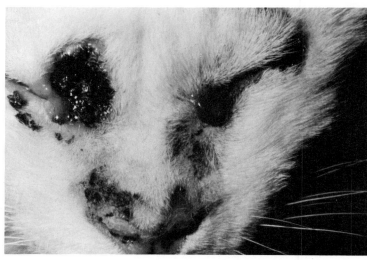

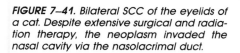
FIGURE 7–41. Bilateral SCC of the eyelids of a cat. Despite extensive surgical and radiation therapy, the neoplasm invaded the nasal cavity via the nasolacrimal duct.

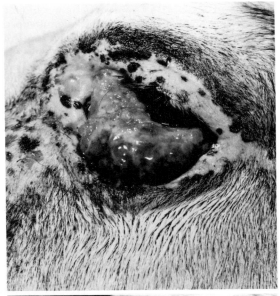

A

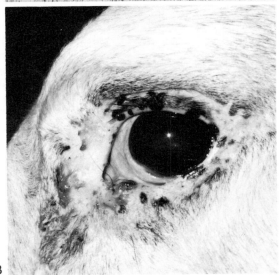

B

FIGURE 7–42. A, SCC in the lower eyelid of a 25-year-old mare. B, The same eye 4 weeks after cryotherapy. (From Hilbert BJ, et al: Cryotherapy of periocular squamous cell carcinoma in the horse. J Am Vet Med Assoc 170:1305, 1977.)

1. Acanthosis with focal ulceration
2. Papilloma

"Carcinoma in situ" (has not yet invaded the lamina propria of the epithelium) ⟶ Carcinoma

↓

Metastases ⟵ Local invasion and secondary infection

FIGURE 7–43. Pathogenesis of SCC in the eyelid.

CLINICAL SIGNS

1. Chronic ocular discharge, often purulent but responsive to antibiotics.
2. Periocular excoriation.
3. Chronic conjunctivitis.
4. Encrusted or hemorrhagic legions of the lids.

Diagnosis is confirmed by cytological scrapings and biopsy.

SCC must be distinguished from chronic conjunctivitis, for which it is frequently mistaken. Bilateral SCC also occurs frequently in certain geographical areas.

In horses the lids are less frequently affected than is the third eyelid. The limbus, conjunctiva, and sclera are frequently the primary sites. The mean age of affected horses is 9–10 years. In a survey of 49 equine cases, single lesions were found in the eyelids (14.3%), third eyelid (26.5%), and limbus (24.5%). Multiple lesions were found in one eye in 8.2%, and 16.3% of cases had bilateral lesions. In cattle, SCC occurs more commonly on the conjunctiva and third eyelid (75%) than on the lids (25%). In Herefords, pigmentation of the lids is associated with a lower incidence of neoplasms. Lid pigmentation is heritable. In addition, a further genetic susceptibility independent of lid pigmentation is present in cattle. (A more detailed discussion of ocular SCC in cattle is found in Chap 8.) Metastasis is greater from lesions on the lids and third eyelid than from the cornea or conjunctiva.

SCC is frequent in white cats, and it often occurs with multiple lesions of the lids, nares, and tips of the pinnae. It is the most common lid tumor in cats, horses, and cattle. SCC is uncommon in dogs, which represented only 2.5% of 202 cases noted in a survey of Krehbiel and Langham (1975).

TREATMENT

1. Small lesions (less than 1 cm in diameter)
   a. Surgical excision or cryotherapy.
   b. Follow-up radiation if the lesions recur.
2. Large or invasive lesions
   a. Surgical excision or cryotherapy.
   b. Follow-up radiation (brachytherapy if deep-seated) to a total dose of 50 Gy.
   c. Specific and nonspecific immunotherapy. In cattle the use of specific "vaccine" may be considered if available.

Equine SCC has a low metastasis and high local recurrence rate. The prognosis for cure depends more on the *commitment of the owner* to pursue treatment than on location or primary treatment (Schwink, 1988).

Fraunfelder and colleagues (1982a) recorded an 89% nonrecurrence rate in 20 tumors after local surgical excision and treatment of the surgical site with 25,000 rads of beta radiation extending 2 mm beyond the lesion edge in equine periocular SCC.

Tarsal Adenoma

The tarsal (sebaceous) adenoma is the most common eyelid tumor in dogs, occurring most frequently after middle age (Fig. 7–44 and Table 7–6). These tumors are uncommon in other species.

The tumors originate in the tarsal gland and—although many grow rapidly and appear histologically malignant—are clinically benign. The tumor mass may cause irritation and conjunctivitis, and it should be removed as soon as the diagnosis is made. For most tumors, a simple, two-layer, wedge excision is indicated. For small lesions, cryotherapy is effective. Correct surgical excision of larger lesions gives cosmetically superior results to those achieved with cryotherapy.

Tarsal adenomas of the canine eyelid must be completely excised. Simple incision along the eyelid margin is inadequate, as the tumor arises from the tarsal gland and will recur if not totally removed.

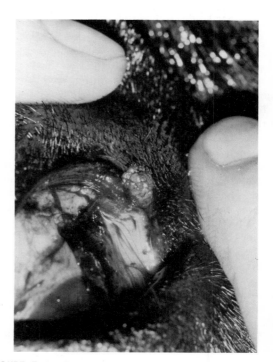

FIGURE 7–44. Tarsal adenoma arising within a canine eyelid.

TABLE 7–6. Frequency of Canine Eyelid Tumors

Classification	Total	Percentage
Sebaceous adenoma	58	28.7
Squamous papilloma	35	17.3
Sebaceous adenocarcinoma	31	15.3
Benign melanoma	26	12.9
Malignant melanoma	16	7.9
Histiocytoma	7	3.5
Mastocytoma	5	2.5
Basal cell carcinoma	5	2.5
Squamous cell carcinoma	5	2.5
Fibroma	4	2.1
Fibropapilloma	2	1.0
Lipoma	2	1.0
Adnexal carcinoma	1	0.5
Hemangiopericytoma	1	0.5
Malignant lymphoma	1	0.5
Neurofibroma	1	0.5
Neurofibrosarcoma	1	0.5
Atypical epithelioma	1	0.5
Undetermined	1	0.5
Total Benign	148	73.3
Total Malignant	54	26.7

From Krehbiel JD, Langham RF: Eyelid neoplasms of dogs. Am J Vet Res 36:115, 1975.

Equine Fibrosarcoma (Sarcoid)

Equine fibrosarcoma is the second most common tumor of the equine eyelid. Lesions may be present elsewhere on the face and body, but the tumor is often restricted to the eyelids (Fig. 7–45). Fibrosarcomas are nodular and lumpy beneath an intact skin and are usually well fixed to the overlying dermis and subcutaneous tissues. They must be distinguished from the lid lesions of habronemiasis in endemic areas. *Habronema* lesions are similar but usually ulcerate in their later stages, revealing a purulent center. They usually begin in the summer, when the flies that carry them are most numerous.

In a survey of 10 cases of fibrosarcoma, the mean age of the affected animals was 4.4 years, and there was no sex incidence. Because of the infiltrative nature, poor definition, and often advanced state of fibrosarcoma at clinical presentation, complete surgical excision is difficult, and recurrence is not infrequent. If surgical excision is used, a wide surrounding margin should be removed with reconstruction by a preplanned method.

Because of these difficulties, treatment by immunotherapy (BCG) is often useful as the first type of therapy, in the hands of experienced persons. If no response occurs, cryotherapy or radiation therapy can be used. If there is no recurrence 3 months after the final treatment, reconstructive surgical procedures can be commenced if required. Tumors that have been previously frozen do not respond as well to BCG cell wall fraction.

The following 12-month nonrecurrence rates have been reported:

^{222}Rn brachytherapy	92%
^{60}Co radiotherapy	58%
^{198}Au brachytherapy	83%
orthovoltage therapy	33%
BCG injection	100%

If radiation therapy is used, the rate of recurrence is higher if doses of less than 4000 rads are used.

Miscellaneous Tumors

VIRAL PAPILLOMATOSIS

Viral papillomas of the eyelids and conjunctiva occur in young dogs and cattle as part of oral or generalized papillomatosis. When continually moistened by tears, the tumors are grayish white and soft. The disease is

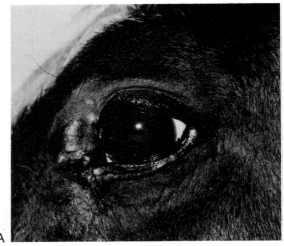

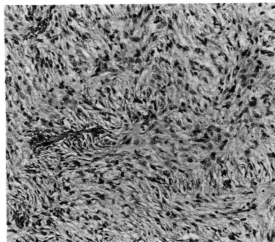

FIGURE 7–45. A, *Periocular lesions of equine fibrosarcoma (sarcoid). B, Histological appearance of fibrosarcoma. The lesion must be distinguished from schwannoma and fibroma.*

self-limiting, and excision is required only if the tumors are painful or causing secondary mechanical damage to the eye. The disease may be treated with systemic cyclophosphamide.

HISTIOCYTOMATOSIS

Masses of histiocytes occur rarely in canine eyelids. Two separate syndromes are recognized: multiple histiocytomatosis and proliferative keratoconjunctivitis syndrome.

Multiple Histiocytomatosis

Numerous pinkish, hairless masses grow around the eyelids and face and often ulcerate quickly (Fig. 7–46). The disease is treated by chemotherapy.

1. Oral dexamethasone (0.1–0.2 mg/kg), prednisolone (1–2 mg/kg) daily in divided doses, for 6–8 weeks or until obvious clinical effect. This treatment shortens the course of multiple histiocytomatosis, which is often self-limiting.

2. Cyclophosphamide orally (1–2 mg/kg every 2nd day) in the morning (see Chap 3 for details of administration), until regression begins (7–10 days). After the 5th day, total white cell count is monitored: if it is below 6000, the dosage is reduced by 50%; if it is below 400, dosage is stopped until the count reaches 6000, when 50% of the original dose is begun. The lid lesions usually heal without scarring.

Because of the combined immunosuppressant effects of cyclophosphamide and prednisolone, concurrent systemic antibiotic therapy may be warranted.

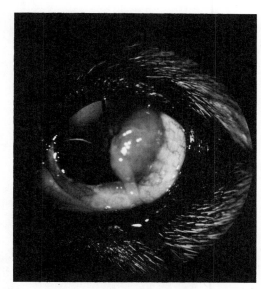

FIGURE 7–47. *Proliferative keratoconjunctivitis syndrome. A raised pink mass is present at the limbus. Lid lesions are less common in this disorder.*

Proliferative Keratoconjunctivitis Syndrome

This syndrome occurs more commonly in rough collies than in other dog breeds. It consists of

1. Raised pinkish masses at the limbus (Fig. 7–47).

2. Raised pinkish masses on the external surface of the third eyelid.

3. Corneal opacity as the limbal mass gradually spreads into the corneal stroma. The advancing lesion is frequently preceded by stromal accumulations of lipid.

4. Small pinkish lid masses. (Lid lesions are present in relatively few cases.)

This is not a self-limiting disease, as are most cases of multiple histiocytomatosis. Proliferative keratoconjunctivitis syndrome is discussed further in Chapter 8. Occasionally cases intermediate between the two syndromes of histiocytomatosis are encountered.

Less Common Neoplasms

Numerous tumors other than those mentioned occur in the eyelids of all domestic species but are not seen frequently enough to warrant specific consideration. All are treated in accordance with general surgical and oncological principles, using reconstructive and therapeutic methods presented previously.

SKIN DISEASES AFFECTING THE EYELIDS

Table 7–7 provides a comprehensive list of common skin disorders affecting the eyelids, clinical signs,

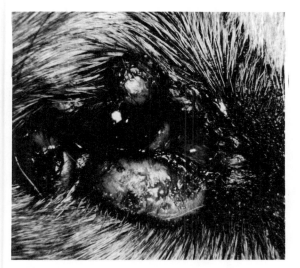

FIGURE 7–46. *Multiple histiocytomatosis in a young dog. Raised pink, hairless lesions are present in the eyelids and periocular dermis. (Courtesy of Dr. G. A. Severin.)*

Text continued on page 202

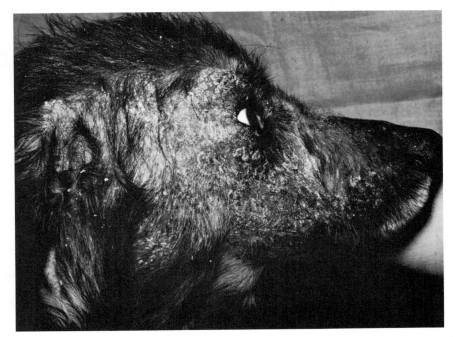

FIGURE 7–48. Canine seborrhea. (From Muller GH, et al: Small Animal Dermatology, 4th ed. WB Saunders Co, Philadelphia, 1989.)

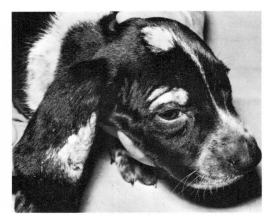

FIGURE 7–49. Ringworm in a dog (M. canis). (From Muller GH, et al: Small Animal Dermatology, 4th ed. WB Saunders Co, Philadelphia, 1989.)

FIGURE 7–50. Epidermolysis bullosa simplex in a 1½-year-old collie. Note the patchy alopecia, hypopigmentation, and crusts around lids and across the bridge of the nose in a "butterfly" pattern. (From Scott DW, Schultz RD: Epidermolysis bullosa simplex in the collie dog. J Am Vet Med Assoc 171:721, 1977.)

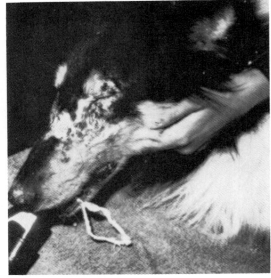

TABLE 7–7. Skin Diseases Affecting the Eyelids

Disorder	Clinical Signs	Diagnosis	Treatment	References
Parasitic				
Mites				
Sarcoptes scabiei (dog, horse, ox, sheep, pig)	Dermatitis with erythema, papules, alopecia, hemorrhagic crusts, and pruritus	Skin scrapings; KOH-sugar sedimentation; skin biopsy; pruritus	*Dog:* Acaricidal dips—lime-sulfur, malathion, ronnel, lindane, benzene hexachloride (BHC) (*Note:* Systemic corticosteroids limit self-inflicted trauma) *Horses and cattle:* 0.07% topical lindane	Muller et al, 1989 Blogg, 1975 Blood & Radostits, 1988 Dunne, 1970
Demodex spp (dog, ox, horse, sheep, goat, pig, cat)	*Dog:* Both localized and generalized forms occur around the eye of young dogs; areas of partial alopecia and mild erythema that show squamous debris may eventually become infected (Plat I*H*) *Cat:* Much milder and less common *Cattle and pigs:* Small hard nodules and pustules containing cheesy white material develop; in cattle the neck is affected first *Horses, dogs, sheep, and pigs:* The periocular area is an area of predilection	Skin scrapings; demonstration of the mite; hard nodules in bovine skin Distinguish from generalized pyoderma, dermatomycosis, acne, abrasions, allergic contact dermatitis, and localized seborrheic dermatitis in dogs, and from other parasitic dermatitides in farm animals	*Dog* 1. Localized—Rub acaricidal preparations daily into affected areas (e.g., benzyl benzoate, lindane, BHC, rotenone) 2. Generalized—See Muller & Kirk *Horse:* 3–5% sulfur ointment or acaricidal preparations daily *Ox:* Acaricidal dips and sprays are of doubtful use but may prevent spread In valuable animals, incise nodules and paint with tincture of iodine Recovery is usually spontaneous *Sheep and goats:* As for ox *Pig:* Lindane sprays and dips, selective culling	Muller et al, 1989 Blood & Radostits, 1988 Dunne, 1970
Notoedres cati (cat)	Partial alopecia, thickened, wrinkled skin with adherent gray crusts, and intense pruritus on head, face, and ears	Skin scrapings Differentiate from dermatomycosis and fight wounds	Clip hair from affected areas, bathe in warm, soapy water, then 2.5% lime-sulfur solution once every 10 days *Note:* Most acaricides are *toxic* to cats	Muller et al, 1989
Psoroptes equi *Psoroptes hippotis* *Psoroptes bovis* *Psoroptes ovis* *Psoroptes capri*	Pruritus, secondary dermatitis, anemia, weight loss, and alopecia in severe cases Eyelids are rarely affected alone For detailed descriptions of distribution of lesions, consult references	Identification of lice; clinical signs *P. hippotis* causes otitis externa	*Cattle, sheep, and goats:* Plunge dipping in 1.5% lime-sulfur, 0.06% lindane, 0.013% BHC, dieldrin, toxaphene (0.2—0.25%), or chlordane (0.25–0.4%) Quarantine affected animals *Horses:* 0.07% lindane, 0.1% BHC topically, and sprays as for cattle dips	Blood & Radostits, 1988 Dunne, 1970

Table continued on following page

TABLE 7–7. Skin Diseases Affecting the Eyelids *Continued*

Disorder	Clinical Signs	Diagnosis	Treatment	References
Lice *Linognathus setosus* (sucking dog louse) *Trichodectes canis* *Heterodoxus longitarsus* (biting dog louse) *Felicola subrostratus* (biting cat louse)	Excoriations, secondary dermatitis, and pruritus (especially around eyes, ears, and body openings) With sucking lice, anemia and debilitation	Identification of lice and nits Differentiate from seborrhea (Fig. 7–48) and canine or feline scabies	*Dog:* acaricidal baths (KFL, thionium, malathion, lindane); follow-up with 5% carbaryl powder (Sevin); repeat in 10 days Clip affected areas and bathe in warm soapy water before treatment *Cat:* KFL shampoo followed by dusting with 2% methoxychlor or 5% carbaryl powder (Sevin)	Muller et al, 1989 Soulsby, 1968
Linognathus ovillus (sucking face louse of sheep) *Linognathus vituli* (long-nosed sucking louse of cattle) *Haematopinus asini* (sucking louse of horses) *Haematopinus suis* (sucking louse of pigs) *Bovicola bovis* (biting louse of cattle) *Bovicola equi* (biting louse of horses)	Pruritus, secondary dermatitis, anemia, weight loss, and alopecia in severe cases Eyelids are rarely affected alone For detailed descriptions of distribution of lesions, consult references	Identification of lice; clinical signs	Dips of sodium arsenite, or sprays, dips, or dusts containing rotenone, pyrethrins, chlorinated hydrocarbons, or organophosphate insecticides Pour-on preparations of fenthion (Tiguvon) are also useful	Blood & Radostits, 1988 Dunne, 1970
Helminths *Habronema* spp (spread by *Musca* spp and *Stomoxys* spp) (horse)	Ulcerating nodules around eyelids and on nictitating membrane, especially in summer	Distribution of lesions, biopsy, identification of larvae in nodules Distinguish from squamous cell carcinoma and equine sarcoid	1. Local injection of fenthion (Tiguvon) into lesions 2. Systemic (IV) administration of Neguvon in saline solution, with atropine, for resistant cases 3. Surgical removal (rarely necessary)	
Ticks *Boophilus microplus* (cattle) *Haemophysalis* spp (cattle, sheep, goats) *Ixodes* spp (cattle, sheep, goats)	Small swollen areas with scabs Anemia, loss of weight Infections usually generalized	Lesions; removal of engorged tick for identification	Acaricides, chosen according to local resistance and previous usage	Blood & Radostits, 1988
Flies *Cuterebra* spp larvae (dog, cat)	Affect young pups and kittens in endemic areas Form large SC pocket that communicates with surface by fistula	Clinical signs	Surgical removal of larvae	
Lucilia cuprina, *Phormia*, *Protophormia*, and *Culliphora* spp larvae (sheep, cattle, dogs, cats, horses)	Primary fly strike uncommon around the eye Found in neglected wounds, neoplasms, wet wool Poll strike in rams may involve eyelids	Presence of larvae and removal for identification	Removal of larvae; clipping of wool or hair; débridement and surgical repair Topical BHC or lindane cream	Blood & Radostits, 1988

TABLE 7–7. Skin Diseases Affecting the Eyelids *Continued*

Disorder	Clinical Signs	Diagnosis	Treatment	References
Stomoxys calcitrans (stable flies) (horses, cattle)	Painful bites, with small scabs	Identification of fly	Removal of rotting organic matter; spraying of barns with insecticide, and use of fly repellents	
Musca domestica: M. vetustissima and autumnalis (horses, cattle)	Superficial dermatitis Conjunctivitis Epiphora	Presence of large numbers of flies	Removal of rotting organic matter, spraying of barns with insecticides, and use of fly repellents	Blood & Radostits, 1988
Lyperosia spp (buffalo and horn flies) (cattle, horses)	Found around eyes and on withers, shoulders, and flanks Cause dermatitis, loss of weight	Distribution—Australia, Southeast Asia, US, Africa	Sprays, dips, back-rubs, and pour-on preparations of insecticides and repellents	Blood & Radostits, 1988
Other Disorders				
Dermatomycosis (*Microsporum canis* and *gypseum; Trichophyton mentagrophytes* and *equinum*) (dog, cat, horse, cow)	Squamous lesions and alopecia around eyes, especially in pups (Fig. 7–49) In horses and cattle, numerous small scabs form	1. Demonstration of agent in scrapings 2. Culture 3. Wood's light examination 4. Skin biopsy and PAS stain Differential diagnosis: 1. Seborrhea 2. Demodicosis 3. Abrasions 4. Sporotrichosis (cattle)	*Topical:* Removal of scabs and treatment with local fungicides— tolnaftate ointment or paint (Tinactin); tincture of iodine; miconazole nitrate (Micotin, Conofite); haloprogin (Halotex); clotrimazole (Lotrimin); 10% thiabendazole paste *Oral:* griseofulvin (10 mg/ kg) (*Note:* teratogenic) *Dip or spray* in Captan (1:200 of 45%)	Muller et al, 1989
Streptotrichosis (*Dermatophilus congolensis*) (cattle, horses)	*Cattle:* Thick, horny, cream-brown crusts with granulation and purulent material underneath; found on head, neck, and body as multiple lesions *Horse:* Lesions spread to eyes from muzzle and may cause severe lacrimation and purulent discharge, sores are tender	Same as for dermatomycosis Lesions in cattle are usually multiple Differentiate in early stages from photosensitization, which occurs in unpigmented areas	*Cattle:* Administer parenteral sodium iodide or tetracycline (4 mg/kg for 3–5 days) or dip young calves in 1% CuSO$_4$ twice, 1 week apart *Horses:* Remove scabs and exudate, apply topical fungicides, and keep animal dry	Blood & Radostits, 1988
Primary seborrhea (dogs, horses)	Greasy, scaly patches around eyelids Usually also found elsewhere on the body No pruritus (Fig. 7–48)	Differential diagnosis: 1. Distinguish from secondary seborrhea 2. If pruritic in dogs, distinguish from atopic dermatitis or *Sarcoptes scabiei* 3. Scrapings and culture to eliminate demodicosis 4. Scaling and crusting distinguishes from the moist lid lesions of canine allergic inhalant dermatitis	1. Protect eyes with bland ointment (Lacri-Lube) 2. Wet the affected area thoroughly 3. Shampoo with coal tar or sulfur shampoo and rinse thoroughly 4. Rinse with bath oil emulsion 5. Repeat treatment as necessary	Muller et al, 1989 Anderson, 1974

Table continued on following page

TABLE 7–7. Skin Diseases Affecting the Eyelids *Continued*

Disorder	Clinical Signs	Diagnosis	Treatment	References
Pemphigus vulgaris (dog)	Erythema, then bulla formation and rupture around mucocutaneous junctions (Plate IF)—eyelids, anus, prepuce, ears, mouth Crusts and mats of hair form over bright red erosions Epiphora may be severe	1. Biopsy—characteristic suprabasilar cleft in epidermis 2. Distribution of lesions 3. Demonstration of autoantibodies to epidermal intercellular cement (fresh, frozen tissue) 4. Oral lesions are often the first sign 5. Lid lesions of allergic inhalant dermatitis often seasonal and associated with staining of paws, scratching, and lack of other severe mucocutaneous lesions	1. High doses of systemic corticosteroids 2. Systemic antibiotics if necessary 3. Oral cyclophosphamide 2 mg/kg, gradually reducing (WBC should not fall below 5000)	Muller et al, 1989 Hurvitz & Feldman, 1975 Stannard et al, 1975
Epidermolysis bullosa simplex (dog)	Alopecia, erythema, edema, ulcers, crusts, and pigmentary changes on face, lips, ears, and over body prominences; pruritus in Scotch collies or predisposed dogs of other breeds (Fig. 7–50) Hyper- or hypopigmentation often occurs in affected areas	Distribution of lesions; histopathology In nasal solar dermatitis, hypopigmentation is present, but pruritis is not marked; planum nasale is usually affected	Systemic corticosteroids, long term	Scott & Schultz, 1977
Pemphigus foliaceus (dog)	Scaling, eruptive dermatitis with bullae around mucocutaneous junctions, *but spreads to areas of normal skin* Mucosal involvement rare Face and eyelids affected	1. Histopathology (subcorneal cleft) 2. Lack of mucosal lesions 3. Demonstration of autoantibodies to epidermal intercellular cement (fresh, frozen tissue) 4. Presence of lesions far from mucocutaneous junctions distinguishes from *P. vulgaris*	Large doses of systemic corticosteroids	Halliwell & Goldschmidt, 1977
Dermatitis herpetiformis (dog)	Extreme pruritus, papules, vesicles, and pustules, with irregular, scaling erythematous eruptions sometimes following Present on feet, nose, head, ears, and trunk	1. Clinical signs 2. Biopsy and histopathology 3. Demonstration of deposits in skin by immunofluorescence 4. Response to dapsone treatment Distinguish from *Sarcoptes scabiei* and epidermolysis bullosa simplex (both of which show pruritus) and from pemphigus vulgaris and pemphigus foliaceus by distribution of lesions	1. Dapsone, 12.5 mg twice a day, CBC and serum enzymes (SGOT, SGPT, alkaline phosphatase) tested regularly to detect idiosyncratic reactions 2. Antibiotics as necessary	Halliwell et al., 1977

TABLE 7–7. Skin Diseases Affecting the Eyelids *Continued*

Disorder	Clinical Signs	Diagnosis	Treatment	References
Atopic dermatitis (allergic inhalant dermatitis) (dog)	More common in poodles, West Highland white terriers, Dalmatians, and wire-haired terriers Patient develops immediate type hypersensitivities between 1 and 3 years of age Signs include *scratching* (often seasonal in nature), erythema, conjunctivitis, moist ulcerative blepharitis, epiphora, and rust-colored staining of areas of white hair (Plate IG); allergic rhinitis and sneezing occur occasionally Conjunctivitis and blepharitis are often the major signs	1. Pruritus and seasonal incidence 2. Rust-colored areas of hair 3. Clinical signs 4. Allergy testing may be useful Distinguish from *Sarcoptes scabiei*, allergic contact dermatitis, seborrheic dermatitis, and other causes of conjunctivitis and epiphora; conjunctival scrapings are usually *negative* for eosinophils	1. Reduce exposure to pollens during pollen seasons 2. Minimize house dust 3. Topical corticosteroids in low doses (0.5% hydrocortisone) 4. Systemic corticosteroids 1 mg/kg of oral prednisolone three times a day for 2 days, twice a day for 2 days, then 0.5 mg/kg twice a day for 7 days Treat intermittently and repeat course as necessary	Muller et al, 1989 Anderson, 1974
Contact dermatitis (allergic) (all species)	Rarely confined to the periocular region unless secondary to topical drug treatment Neomycin preparations occasionally responsible—periocular dermatitis, blepharitis, and conjunctivitis may result from drug therapy with these agents	1. Clinical signs 2. Favorable response to withdrawal of drug 3. Patch testing— primary irritant contact dermatitis is rarely restricted to periocular area Distinguish from atopy, dermatomycosis, seborrheic dermatitis, solar dermatitis, insect bites	1. Withdrawal of drug or allergen 2. Antibiotics if necessary	Muller et al, 1989 Nesbitt & Schmitz, 1977
Hypopigmentation and nasal solar dermatitis (dog)	1. Collies most frequently affected, but all breeds susceptible 2. Occurs in unpigmented areas of eyelids, planum nasale, lips, and nares; congenital hypopigmentation may progress in some breeds before onset of dermatitis; hypopigmentation is exacerbated by the dermatitis 3. Alopecia and erythema develop with exudation, crusting, and ulceration in advanced lesions 4. Lesions progress, especially during summer 5. Neglected lesions may progress to squamous cell carcinoma	Distribution of lesions Differential diagnosis: 1. Nasal pyoderma (no hypopigmentation) 2. Contact dermatitis from feeding dishes (no ulceration of planum nasale; lips are simultaneously affected) 3. Neoplasms, dermatomycosis, trauma 4. Discoid lupus erythematosus in Shetland sheepdogs (extends further posteriorly) 5. Epidermolysis bullosa simplex (intense pruritus)	1. Limit exposure to sunlight 2. Tattooing of affected areas—mechanically or with ink mixed with hyaluronidase. Repeat tattooing may be necessary 3. Selective breeding *Note:* Affected areas heal with a thin, fragile, hairless, unpigmented epithelium	Muller et al, 1989

Table continued on following page

TABLE 7–7. Skin Diseases Affecting the Eyelids *Continued*

Disorder	Clinical Signs	Diagnosis	Treatment	References
Nasal fold pyoderma (dog)	Erythema and inflammation in the groove posterior to the nasal fold in Pekingese, pugs, English bulldogs, and Boston terriers Lacrimation caused by corneal irritation results in excoriation of skin in the groove	Presence and position of lesions Epiphora and corneal pigmentation are frequently concurrent	Surgical excision of the folds	Muller et al, 1989
Hypothyroidism (dog)	Seborrhea, secondary conjunctivitis, ptosis For general dermatological signs, consult references	1. Decreased uptake (less than 10%) of I^{131} 2. Depressed TSH response 3. Increased serum cholesterol 4. Thyroid biopsy 5. Serum thyroxine	1. Thyroid replacement therapy 2. Local antibiotics as necessary for conjunctivitis	Muller et al, 1989

TABLE 7–8. Differential Diagnosis of Feline Facial Dermatitis

Bacterial folliculitis–furunculosis
Fungal dermatitis
Demodicosis
Allergic dermatitis—food
Solar dermatitis—white area—squamous cell carcinoma
Seborrheic dermatitis
Pemphigus erythematosus
Pemphigus foliaceus
Pemphigus vulgaris
Systemic lupus erythematosus
Notoedric mange
Sarcoptic mange
Otodectic mange
Drug eruption
Eosinophilic plaque

From Manning TO, et al: Pemphigus diseases in the feline: Seven case reports and discussion. J Am Anim Hosp Assoc 18:441, 1982.

TABLE 7–9. Immune-Mediated Skin Diseases Affecting the Eyelids
TABLE BY DR. W. H. MILLER, JR.

Disease	Clinical Signs	Diagnostic Tests	Histological Features	Treatment*
Pemphigus vulgaris (dog, cat)	Vesicobullous, ulcerative disorder of oral cavity, mucocutaneous junctions, and skin	Skin biopsy immunofluorescence testing (DIT)	Suprabasilar clefting with acantholysis DIT: intercellular	Prednisolone: 1–3 mg/kg SID-BID Azathioprine (Imuran): Dog: 2 mg/kg PO every 24 hours Cat: 1.1 mg/kg PO every 48 hours Aurothioglucose (Solganal): 1 mg/kg IM once weekly after two test doses
Pemphigus vegetans (dog)	Vesicopustular, ulcerative disorder of oral cavity, mucocutaneous junctions, and skin	Skin biopsy DIT	Suprabasilar clefting ± intraepidermal eosinophilic microabscesses DIT: intercellular	Prednisolone: 1–3 mg/kg SID-BID Azathioprine (Imuran): 2 mg/kg PO SID
Pemphigus foliaceus (dog, cat, horse, goat)	Crusting, vesiculopustular eruption of skin, foot pads, and mucocutaneous junctions	Skin biopsy DIT	Intragranular or subcorneal clefting with acantholysis DIT: intercellular	Prednisolone: 1–3 mg/kg SID-BID Azathioprine (Imuran): Dog: 2 mg/kg PO every 24 hours Cat: 1.1 mg/kg PO every 24 hours Aurothioglucose (Solganal): 1 mg/kg IM once weekly after two test doses
Pemphigus erythematosus (dog, cat)	As in pemphigus foliaceus with lesions restricted to head and neck	Skin biopsy DIT Antinuclear antibody (ANA) test—50% positive	Intragranular or subcorneal clefting with acantholysis DIT: intercellular ± basement membrane	Prednisolone: 1–3 mg/kg SID-BID Azathioprine (Imuran): Dog: 2 mg/kg PO every 24 hours Cat: 1.1 mg/kg PO every 24 hours Aurothioglucose (Solganal): 1 mg/kg IM once weekly after two test doses
Bullous pemphigoid (dog, horse)	Vesicobullous, ulcerative disorder of oral cavity, mucocutaneous junctions, and skin	Skin biopsy DIT	Subepidermal clefting with no acantholysis DIT: basement membrane	Prednisolone: 1–3 mg/kg SID-BID Azathioprine (Imuran): Dog: 2 mg/kg PO every 24 hours Aurothioglucose (Solganal): 1 mg/kg IM once weekly after two test doses
Lupus erythematosus (dog, cat, horse)	Variable skin lesions alone (discoid lupus) or in combination with other organ involvement (systemic lupus) Seborrheic skin signs (alopecia, scaling, crusting) most common Face, foot pads, pressure points	Skin biopsy DIT ANA (negative in discoid lupus)	Interface dermatitis, which may be lichenoid, hydropic, or both DIT: basement membrane	*Systemic lupus:* Prednisolone: 1–3 mg/ kg BID *Discoid lupus:* Vitamin E: 200–400 IU BID Prednisolone: 2.2 mg/ kg SID Photoprotection
Vogt-Koyanagi-Harada–like syndrome (dog)	Uveitis with depigmentation of nose, lips, and eyelids	Skin biopsy DIT	Lichenoid interface dermatitis with numerous histiocytes DIT: negative	Prednisolone: 1–3 mg/kg SID-BID Azathioprine (Imuran): 2 mg/kg PO SID

Table continued on following page

TABLE 7–9. Immune-Mediated Skin Diseases Affecting the Eyelids *Continued*
TABLE BY DR. W. H. MILLER, JR.

Disease	Clinical Signs	Diagnostic Tests	Histological Features	Treatment*
Drug eruption (all species)	Lesions can mimic those of any skin disorders; skin lesions seen with topical or systemic drug administration	Spontaneous healing with drug withdrawal Skin biopsy	Variable	Withdraw drug, avoid cross-reactive drugs
Sterile pyogranuloma syndrome (dog)	Asymptomatic firm nodules or plaques of face, eyelids, or feet	Skin biopsy Negative bacterial and fungal cultures	Nodular to diffuse pyogranulomatous inflammation tracking appendages	Prednisolone: 2.2 mg/kg till resolved, then alternate-day therapy

*SID = once a day; BID = twice a day; PO = by mouth; IM = intramuscular.

diagnosis, and treatment and sources for further reference. Table 7–8 lists facial skin disorders that must be considered in differential diagnosis of feline blepharitis. Autoimmune disorders of the eyelids are discussed in Table 7–9.

Canine allergic inhalant dermatitis and conjunctivitis (atopy) are discussed in Chapter 8.

REFERENCES

Anderson W (1974): Canine Allergic Inhalant Dermatitis. W Anderson. Blue Island, IL.

Anderson WN (1974): A treatment regimen for seborrhea of dogs. J Am Vet Med Assoc 164:1111.

Banks WC, England RB (1973): Radioactive gold in the treatment of ocular squamous cell carcinoma in cattle. J Am Vet Med Assoc 163:745.

Bedford PGC (1971): Eyelashes and adventitious cilia as causes of corneal irritation. J Sm Anim Pract 12:11.

Bedford PGC (1973): Distichiasis and its treatment by the method of partial tarsal plate excision. J Sm Anim Pract 14:1.

Blogg JR (1975): The Eye in Veterinary Practice. VS Supplies, Melbourne, Australia.

Blood DC, Radostits OM (1988): Veterinary Medicine: A Textbook of Diseases of Cattle, Sheep, Pigs, Goats, and Horses. WB Saunders, Philadelphia.

Campbell LH, McCree AV (1977): Conjunctival resection for the surgical management of canine distichiasis. J Am Vet Med Assoc 171:275.

Chambers ED, Severin GA (1984): Staphylococcal bacterin for treatment of chronic staphylococcal blepharitis in the dog. J Am Vet Med Assoc 185:422.

Chambers ED, Slatter DH (1984): Cryotherapy (N₂D) of canine distichiasis and trichiasis: An experimental and clinical report. J Sm Anim Pract 25:647.

Crowley JP, McGloughlin P (1963): Hereditary entropion in lambs. Vet Rec 75:1104.

Dunne H (ed) (1970): Diseases of Swine, 4th ed. Iowa State University Press, Ames.

Farris HE, Fraunfelder FT (1976): Cryosurgical treatment of ocular squamous cell carcinoma of cattle. J Am Vet Med Assoc 168:213.

Fox SA (1970): Ophthalmic Plastic Surgery, 4th ed. Grune & Stratton, New York.

Fraunfelder HC, et al (1982a): ⁹⁰Sr for treatment of periocular squamous cell carcinoma in the horse. J Am Vet Med Assoc 180:307.

Fraunfelder HC, et al (1982b): ²²²Rn for treatment of periocular

fibrous connective tissue sarcomas in the horse. J Am Vet Med Assoc 180:310.

Gavin PR, Gillette EL (1978): Interstitial radiation therapy of equine squamous cell carcinoma. J Am Vet Rad Soc 19:138.

Gelatt KN, et al (1974): Conjunctival squamous cell carcinoma in the horse. J Am Vet Med Assoc 165:617.

Halliwell REW, Goldschmidt MH (1977): Pemphigus foliaceus in the canine: A case report and discussion. J Am Anim Hosp Assoc 13:431.

Halliwell REW, et al (1977): Dapsone for the treatment of pruritic dermatitis (dermatitis herpetiformis and subcorneal pustular dermatosis) in dogs. J Am Vet Med Assoc 170:697.

Helper LC, Magrane WG (1970): Ectopic cilia of the canine eyelid. J Sm Anim Pract 11:185.

Hilbert BJ, et al (1977): Cryotherapy of periocular squamous cell carcinoma in the horse. J Am Vet Med Assoc 170:1305.

Hurvitz AI, Feldman E (1975): A disease in dogs resembling human pemphigus vulgaris: Case reports. J Am Vet Med Assoc 166:585.

Johnson BW, et al (1988): Non-surgical correction of entropion in Shar Pei puppies. Vet Med 83:482.

Krehbiel JD, Langham RF (1975): Eyelid neoplasms of dogs. Am J Vet Res 36:115.

Lane JG (1977): The treatment of equine sarcoids by cryosurgery. Equine Vet J 9:127.

Latimer C, Dunstan RW (1987): Eosinophilic plaque involving eyelids of a cat. J Am Anim Hosp Assoc 23:649.

Lavach JD, Severin GA (1977): Neoplasia of the equine eye, adnexa and orbit—A review of 68 cases. J Am Vet Med Assoc 170:202.

Lawson DD (1973): Canine distichiasis. J Sm Anim Pract 14:469.

Littlejohn AI (1969): A defect in the upper eyelid in a flock of piebald sheep. Vet Rec 85:189.

Liu D, et al (1984): Cryosurgical treatment of the eyelids and lacrimal drainage ducts of the rhesus monkey. Course of injury and repair. Arch Ophthalmol 102:934.

Manning TO, et al (1982): Pemphigus diseases in the feline: Seven case reports and discussion. J Am Anim Hosp Assoc 18:433.

Miller WW (1988): Aberrant cilia as an aetiology for recurrent corneal ulcers: A case report. Equine Vet J 20:145.

Mondino BJ, et al (1987): A rabbit model of staphylococcal blepharitis. Am J Ophthalmol 105:409.

Moses RA (1970): Adler's Physiology of the Eye, 5th ed. CV Mosby Co, St Louis.

Muller GH, et al (1989): Small Animal Dermatology, 4th ed. WB Saunders Co, Philadelphia.

Murphy JM, et al (1979): Immunotherapy in equine sarcoid. J Am Vet Med Assoc 170:202.

Nesbitt GH, Schmitz JA (1977): Contact dermatitis in the dog: A review of 35 cases. J Am Anim Hosp Assoc 13:155.

Owen RA, Jagger DW (1987): Clinical observations on the use of

BCG cell wall fraction for treatment of periocular and other equine sarcoids. Vet Rec 120:548.

Prince JH, et al (1960): Anatomy of Histology of the Eye and Orbit in Domestic Animals. Charles C Thomas, Springfield, IL.

Roberts SM, et al (1986): Prevalence and treatment of palpebral neoplasms in the dog—200 cases (1975–1983). J Am Vet Med Assoc 189:1355.

Schwink K (1988): Factors influencing morbidity and outcome of equine ocular squamous cell carcinoma. Equine Vet J 19:198.

Scott DW, Schultz RD (1977): Epidermolysis bullosa simplex in the collie dog. J Am Vet Med Assoc 171:721.

Severin GA (1976): Veterinary Ophthalmology Notes, 2nd ed. Fort Collins, CO.

Soulsby EJL (1968): Helminths, Arthropods and Protozoa of Domesticated Animals. Williams & Wilkins, Baltimore.

Stannard AA, et al (1975): A mucocutaneous disease in the dog, resembling pemphigus vulgaris in man. J Am Vet Med Assoc 166:575.

Strafuss AC: Squamous cell carcinoma in horses. J Am Vet Med Assoc 168:61.

Van Kampen KR, et al (1973): The immunologic therapy of squamous cell carcinoma. Am J Obstet Gynecol 166:569.

Wyman M (1971): Lateral canthoplasty. J Am Anim Hosp Assoc 7:196.

Wyn-Jones G (1978): Treatment of periocular tumours of horses using radioactive gold 198 grains. Equine Vet J 11:3.

8

Conjunctiva

ANATOMY AND PHYSIOLOGY	CONGENITAL ABNORMALITIES	ACQUIRED CONJUNCTIVAL
PATHOLOGICAL REACTIONS	CONJUNCTIVITIS	DISORDERS
CLINICAL SIGNS OF		
CONJUNCTIVAL DISEASE		

Diseases of the conjunctiva are the most common of all eye disorders.

ANATOMY AND PHYSIOLOGY

The CONJUNCTIVA is a mobile mucous membrane covering the inner surfaces of the lids, inner and outer surfaces of the third eyelid, and the anterior portion of the globe adjacent to the limbus (Fig. 8–1). The space lined by the conjunctiva is called the CONJUNCTIVAL SAC. The PALPEBRAL CONJUNCTIVA is tightly bound to the inner surface of the lids. In the dorsal FORNIX the conjunctiva is supported by an anterior extension of the muscle sheath of the levator palpebrae superioris and dorsal rectus muscles. This band moves the loose conjunctiva of the fornix with the globe and prevents it from falling down over the cornea. The bulbar conjunctiva is loosely attached to the episclera over the globe and anchored more firmly near the limbus.

The conjunctiva consists of three layers (Fig. 8–2):
1. precorneal tear film
2. epithelium
3. substantia propria
   a. glandular layer
   b. fibrous layer

The PRECORNEAL TEAR FILM is an essential protective layer whose disappearance results in severe changes in the conjunctiva. It is secreted by the lacrimal gland, gland of the third eyelid, and tarsal glands and goblet cells of the conjunctiva, and it is continuous with the film covering the cornea. Mucoid secretion from the goblet cells of the conjunctiva gathers in the superior and anterior inferior fornices as the MUCOUS THREAD. The mucous thread migrates medially, gathering dust particles and cells for eventual disposal down the

nasolacrimal duct or onto the surface of the skin at the medial canthus. In animals with a deep inferior fornix (e.g., Irish setter, Doberman), the normal mucous thread may be particularly prominent, accumulating as a grayish gelatinous mass at the medial canthus.

CONJUNCTIVAL EPITHELIUM is nonkeratinized and columnar, and it contains numerous mucus-producing goblet cells (see Fig. 8–2). The glandular layer of the SUBSTANTIA PROPRIA contains numerous lymphocytes that, when stimulated by antigens, form active follicles. These follicles are present throughout the conjunctiva, but they are particularly numerous on the bulbar surface of the third eyelid. The fibrous layer lies beneath the glandular layer and is adjacent to the unstriated fibers of Müller's muscle. The arterial supply of the conjunctiva is prolific and comes from

1. peripheral arcades of the lids
2. marginal arcades of the lids
3. anterior ciliary arteries

The superficial conjunctival vessels overlie the deeper, straighter anterior ciliary vessels near the limbus, although the two systems communicate. When engorged, the conjunctival vessels give a fiery red appearance, whereas the ciliary vessels are an intense rosy pink (*ciliary flush*). The superficial conjunctival vessels terminate in loops or arcades at the limbus. It is from these loops that "endothelial budding" occurs in response to corneal disease, resulting in *superficial corneal vascularization*. *Deep corneal vascularization* originates from the deeper ciliary vessels. Two layers of lymphatic drainage are present—one adjacent to the superficial conjunctival vessels and one in the deeper fibrous layer. The conjunctiva is the most exposed mucous membrane in the body. To respond rapidly to noxious stimuli, it has well-developed defense mechanisms, because of which it has been compared with an everted lymph node (Fig. 8–3). It is frequently necessary to distinguish between injection of ciliary and conjunctival vessels in

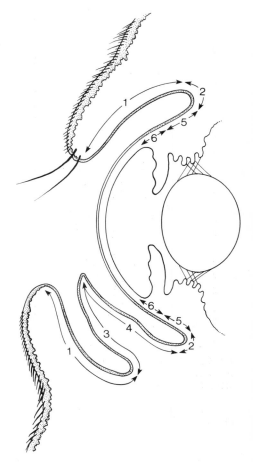

FIGURE 8–1. *Areas of the conjunctiva: 1 = palpebral; 2 = fornix; 3 = anterior third eyelid; 4 = posterior third eyelid; 5 = bulbar; 6 = limbal.*

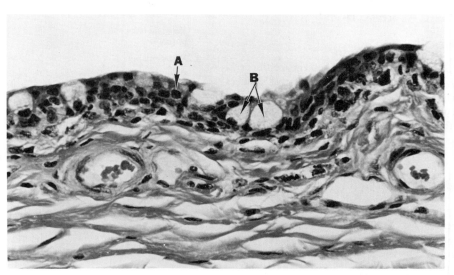

FIGURE 8–2. *Normal conjunctiva. A = columnar epithelial cells; B = goblet cells. Substantia propria lies beneath the epithelium and contains numerous spaces and blood vessels of significance in the formation of chemosis.*

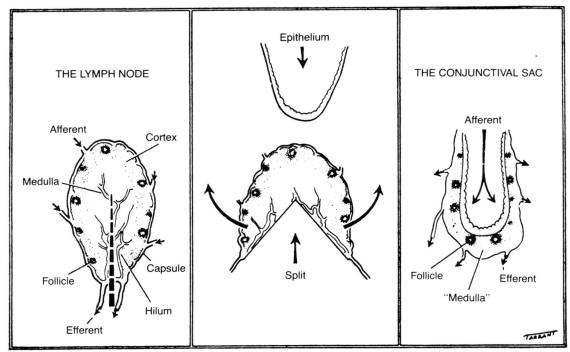

FIGURE 8–3. *The relationship between the lymph node and the conjunctival sac. (Reproduced by permission from Duke-Elder, Sir Stewart, editor: System of Ophthalmology. Vol VIII. Diseases of the Outer Eye. Part 1. St Louis, 1965, The CV Mosby Co. [BR Jones].)*

the differential diagnosis of conjunctivitis and uveitis (Table 8–1).

Ciliary injection and conjunctival injection frequently coexist.

PATHOLOGICAL REACTIONS

Wound Healing

Simple, uncomplicated wounds of the conjunctiva heal rapidly. Within a few hours, conjunctiva attaches to the episclera, and healing by epithelial sliding and mitosis occurs. The phases of inflammation follow rapidly, with clinical healing of simple lacerations in 24–48 hours. Denuded areas of bare sclera are also re-epithelialized rapidly.

Conjunctivitis

Acute conjunctivitis is characterized by
1. hyperemia
2. cellular exudates
3. edema (chemosis)

Identification of cells in the exudate is often useful in differentiating the possible cause of conjunctivitis (Table 8–2).

Inflammatory membranes may form as conjunctivitis becomes chronic (e.g., mycoplasma conjunctivitis in

TABLE 8–1. Differentiation of Ciliary and Conjunctival Injection

Conjunctival Vessels	Ciliary Vessels
1. Bright red in color	1. Pinkish red in color or darker red
2. Conjunctiva affected	2. Cornea, iris, ciliary body, and sclera affected
3. Vessels in fornix conjunctiva affected	3. Vessels at and near limbus affected
4. Vessels dilated and tortuous	4. Vessels small and straight
5. Vessels mobile	5. Vessels stationary
6. Pupil usually normal	6. Pupil dilated or constricted
7. Mucoid, mucopurulent, or purulent discharge with adhesion of lid margins	7. Epiphora often present
8. Lack of corneal involvement	8. Cornea dull—edema or deposits
9. Lens and vitreous transparent	9. Lens and vitreous often opaque
10. Intraocular pressure normal	10. Intraocular pressure often increased or decreased
11. Cleared by topical epinephrine (1:100,000)	11. Topical epinephrine still leaves a "muddy" appearance or has no effect
12. Separate vessels distinguishable	12. Separate vessels indistinguishable without magnification

TABLE 8–2. Differentiation of Conjunctivitis by Cell Type in Exudate

Cell Type	Type of Conjunctivitis
Neutrophils	Bacterial or acute
Lymphocytes and mononuclears	Viral, chlamydial, or chronic
Goblet cells	Chronic
Basophils and eosinophils	Allergic (these cell types are rarely seen in allergic conjunctivitis in animals)
Keratinized epithelial cells	Chronic conjunctivitis of any cause; deficiency of precorneal tear film

cats). True membranes consist of cellular debris and fibrin, are firmly attached to the underlying epithelium, and when removed, leave a raw, bleeding surface. Pseudomembranes consist of similar material that is not adherent and is easily removed.

As conjunctivitis becomes chronic, goblet cells increase in number, the epithelium proliferates and is thrown into folds (papillary hypertrophy), and it becomes velvety in appearance. Neutrophils and lymphocytes infiltrate the substantia propria and epithelium. Metaplasia of the conjunctiva may occur with chronic vitamin A deficiency, especially in chickens. Active lymphoid follicles are frequently formed (Fig. 8–4) and are visible in clinical patients.

Lymphoid follicles indicate chronic antigenic stimulation. They are not a specific disease.

CLINICAL SIGNS OF CONJUNCTIVAL DISEASE

The accurate observation and interpretation of conjunctival signs are important in the *differential diagnosis of the "red eye"* (Fig. 8–5). Too frequently, conjunctivitis is diagnosed and treated when the underlying disorder continues, destroying vision or the eye.

1. *Ocular discharges.* Mucopurulent discharges are the most common sign of conjunctival disease and are associated with infectious processes or keratoconjunctivitis sicca. Epiphora alone is rarely a sign of primary conjunctival pathology unless accompanied by other signs, e.g., increased production of mucus, follicle formation, erythema, blepharospasm. Eyelid margins may stick together overnight with severe discharges. Change in color of the mucous thread from transparent or gray to yellow is due to accumulations of inflammatory cells and cellular debris within it.

2. *Chemosis* (edema of the conjunctiva). Chemosis may be caused by any stimulus and results in acute inflammation. It is especially common in acute allergic conjunctivitis, toxic injuries, and trauma.

3. *Hyperemia.* Active hyperemia imparts a bright red appearance to the conjunctiva. Conjunctival and ciliary engorgement must be distinguished. Passive hyperemia is associated with altered venous drainage from the area; examples are the increased central venous pressure in ventricular septal defect and obstruction of drainage by cervical neoplasms via internal and external jugular veins. Passive hyperemia may also arise from inflammation of a nearby tissue (e.g., the ciliary body), although the conjunctiva itself is not involved. Transitory vasodilatation of conjunctival vessels occurs fre-

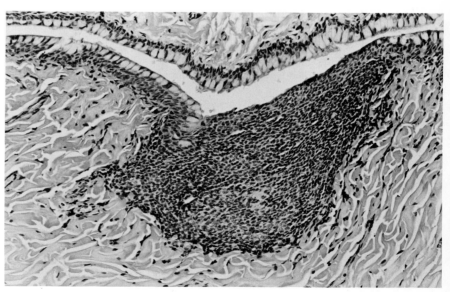

FIGURE 8–4. Conjunctival lymphoid follicle in chronic conjunctivitis.

Ocular discharge

Chemosis

Hyperemia

Pallor

Hemorrhage

Emphysema

Follicle formation

Pruritus

Abnormal swellings

FIGURE 8–5. Clinical signs of conjunctival pathology.

quently in excited dogs (SENSITIVE VESSEL SYNDROME) and should not be confused with inflammatory hyperemia. Topical ophthalmic anesthetics may also cause conjunctival vasodilatation.

Conjunctival inflammation is rarely present in the absence of erythema and hyperemia.

---

4. *Pallor.* Pallor is commonly associated with anemia (Plate I*H*). Hematological investigation and fecal examination are warranted.

5. *Hemorrhage.* Subconjunctival extravasations and ecchymoses are frequent. Ecchymoses are present in many severe, acute, systemic inflammations and septicemias, in blood dyscrasias (e.g., platelet and clotting disorders), and after trauma. Large subconjunctival hemorrhages are usually traumatic in origin. The hemorrhage is resorbed over 7–10 days and changes successively from bright red to dark red, yellow, and white.

6. *Emphysema.* Small gas bubbles beneath the conjunctiva occasionally occur after head trauma involving the paranasal sinuses. Air escapes into the orbit when the bony walls of the cavity are breached and migrates to the conjunctiva via the fascial planes of the periorbita. Provided no further air is added, absorption is uneventful and takes 7–14 days.

7. *Follicle formation.* Lymphoid follicles frequently occur after antigenic stimulation in chronic inflammatory disorders. Slight epiphora and follicle formation are often the only signs of mild allergic conjunctivitis (e.g., in allergic inhalant dermatitis [AID] syndrome, or atopy). Follicles are normally present on the bulbar surface of the third eyelid, but following stimulation they may appear in other parts of the conjunctiva.

8. *Pruritus.* Conjunctivitis is frequently associated with pruritus, although the history provided by the owner plus secondary lesions (e.g., periocular alopecia and erythema, stained or matted hair on the medial aspect of the metacarpus) may be the only indication. Deep ocular pain, as in glaucoma or uveitis, is more likely to cause the patient to rub its face on the carpet or lawn or to cause changes in behavior or appetite. Superficial pruritus usually causes rubbing motions with the paws and, if very severe, blepharospasm.

9. *Abnormal swellings.* Swellings and infiltrates are examined for color, rate of growth, position, and attachment to conjunctiva, sclera, or adjacent structures.

CONGENITAL ABNORMALITIES

Dermoid

Dermoids (dermolipomas) are congenital tumor-like masses of normal tissue arising in the conjunctiva, often at the lateral limbus and frequently overlying the limbus (Fig. 8–6). The mass infrequently involves the third eyelid or eyelid and may rarely coexist with an eyelid coloboma. Dermoids contain many of the elements of normal skin—epidermis, dermis, fat, sebaceous glands, and hair follicles—and frequently there is hair growing from the surface. This hair causes conjunctival and corneal irritation, which results in epiphora and keratitis. Dermoids usually grow slowly, if at all. In Hereford cattle, dermoids are inherited, with recessive and polygenic genetic characteristics being reported.

Treatment for dermoids is careful surgical excision by conjunctivectomy and dissection down to bare sclera. If the lesion extends onto the cornea, the prognosis for removal without residual scar formation is guarded and depends on the depth of the lesion. Some deep corneal dermoids cannot be removed without leaving a scar, although superficial keratectomy is successful in many cases. Some small dermoids cause no clinical signs.

CONJUNCTIVITIS

Conjunctivitis is inflammation of the conjunctiva. It is characterized by erythema and hyperemia, chemosis, discharge, infiltration with leukocytes, and follicle formation. In the past, conjunctivitis has been classified in many ways, based on duration, nature of discharge, appearance, and etiology. Whenever possible, an etiological diagnosis should be attempted as a basis for rational therapy.

Classification

The three categories in Table 8–3 are used to describe the type of conjunctivitis present. Of the three methods of classification, etiology is the most important. Classification by duration or by appearance is useful in

TABLE 8–3. Three Methods of Classification of Conjunctivitis

Etiology	Duration	Appearance
Bacterial	Acute	Mucoid ("catarrhal")
Fungal	Subacute	Purulent
Viral	Chronic	Mucopurulent
Parasitic		Hemorrhagic
Allergic		Follicular
Toxic or chemical		Membranous
Foreign body		Pseudomembranous
Precorneal tear film deficiency		

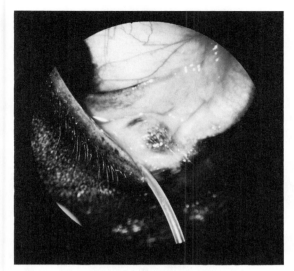

FIGURE 8–6. A conjunctival dermoid with protruding hairs.

and bacteria (Gram-stained). The types of cells commonly encountered are shown in Figure 8–7, and the cell types found in the different types of conjunctivitis are listed in Table 8–4. Exfoliative cytology is approximately 90% accurate in the diagnosis of bovine squamous cell carcinoma (SCC). In examination of scrapings, intracytoplasmic melanin granules should not be confused with other inclusions (e.g., *Chlamydia* in cats and sheep). Scrapings may be used to determine the malignancy of cells associated with conjunctival masses, e.g., SCC in cattle.

Conjunctival Biopsy

A small sample of conjunctiva can be obtained under topical anesthesia (1 drop every 30 seconds for 3 minutes) by elevating the bulbar conjunctiva with Adson's tissue forceps and removing it with strabismus scissors. Pre- and postbiopsy application of 10% phenylephrine helps control hemorrhage. The sample is pinned flat to cardboard and fixed for histological processing. Equine conjunctival samples may be examined sliced, incubated in saline solution at 37°C, and the supernatant examined for *Onchocerca* microfilariae.

describing the stage of conjunctivitis present, but it adds little to understanding the etiology.

DIAGNOSTIC METHODS

Bacterial Culturing

Cultures are usually performed only after initial antibiotic therapy has been unsuccessful. Culture swabs should be moist (saline solution), and the sample plated onto blood agar or into nutrient and thioglycollate broth as soon as possible. For a list of the most frequent organisms and antibiotics, see Chapter 3.

Conjunctival Scrapings

For method of collection, see Chapter 5. Scrapings are examined for cellular alterations (Giemsa-stained)

Differential Diagnosis

PRIMARY VERSUS SECONDARY CONJUNCTIVITIS

Diagnosis of conjunctivitis based on the clinical signs of erythema, discharge, chemosis, and follicle formation is simple. Beyond this, it must be determined if the conjunctivitis is primary or secondary.

Because of the close anatomical relationship between conjunctiva and cornea, conjunctival and corneal disorders often coexist, or diseases may spread from conjunctiva to cornea. It is important for diagnosis and therapy to determine the degree of corneal involvement,

TABLE 8–4. Cellular Response Associated with Specific Conjunctivitides*

Disease	Cellular Response
Acute bacterial conjunctivitis	Predominantly neutrophils, few mononuclear cells, many bacteria, degenerating epithelial cells
Chronic bacterial conjunctivitis	Predominantly neutrophils, many mononuclear cells, degenerate or keratinized epithelial cells, goblet cells, bacteria may or may not be seen, mucus, fibrin
Feline herpesviral conjunctivitis	Pseudomembrane formation, giant cells, fibrin, erythrocyte, neutrophils and mononuclear cell numbers depend on stage of infection
Feline mycoplasmal conjunctivitis	Predominantly neutrophils, fewer mononuclear cells, basophilic coccoid or pleomorphic organisms on cell membrane
Feline chlamydial conjunctivitis	Predominantly neutrophils, mononuclear cells in subacute cases are increased in numbers, plasma cells, giant cells, basophilic cytoplasmic inclusions early in the disease
Keratoconjunctivitis sicca	Epithelial cells keratinized, goblet cells, mucus, neutrophilic response marked if there is much infection, bacteria
Canine distemper	Varies with stage of disease: early—giant cells, and mononuclear cells; later—neutrophils, goblet cells, and mucus; infrequent intracellular inclusions
Allergic conjunctivitis	Eosinophils, neutrophils may be marked, basophils possible

From Lavach JD, et al: Cytology of normal and inflamed conjunctivas in dogs and cats. J Am Vet Med Assoc 170:772, 1977.

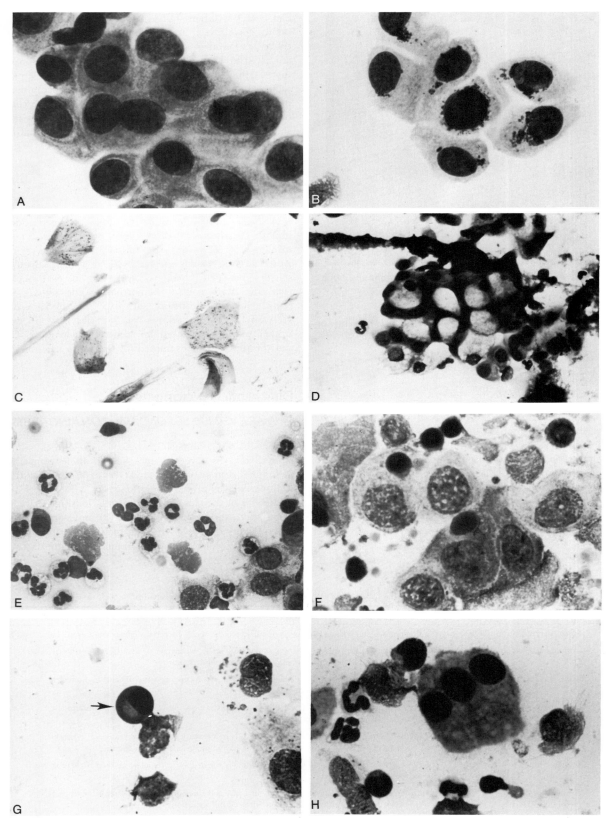

FIGURE 8–7 See legend on opposite page

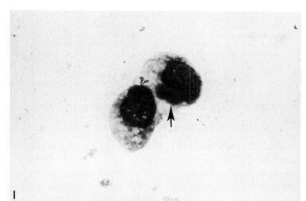
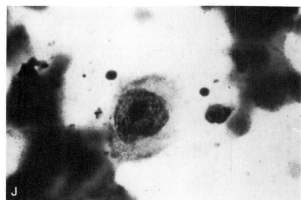

FIGURE 8–7. Cell types found in different types of conjunctivitis. A, Epithelial conjunctival cells from a normal dog. The cells are found in sheets and are round to oval, with a large nucleus. B, Conjunctival epithelial cells containing melanin granules. Melanin occurs in varying amounts and may be identified as dark green to black granules after Giemsa's staining. C, Keratinized epithelial cells. These cells are abnormal in large numbers. D, Conjunctival goblet cells. Goblet cells contain a large amount of mucus, which displaces the nucleus to the periphery. E, Scraping from a dog with acute bacterial conjunctivitis. Large numbers of neutrophils and degenerating epithelial cells are present. F, Scraping from a kitten with herpesvirus infection. Mononuclear cells predominate, but viral inclusions are not visible. G, Plasma cell. This finding is abnormal but not associated with any specific disease. H, Multinucleated cell in a scraping from a dog with distemper. Neutrophils, mononuclear cells, and degenerating epithelial cells are also present. I, Chlamydial inclusion in the cytoplasm of an epithelial cell from a cat with acute conjunctivitis. J, Neoplastic epithelial cell from a cat with squamous cell carcinoma of the lid margin. The cell is unusually large and vacuolated. (From Lavach JD, et al: Cytology of normal and inflamed conjunctivas in dogs and cats. J Am Vet Med Assoc 170:722, 1977.)

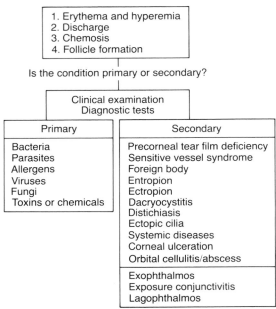

FIGURE 8–8. *Steps in the diagnosis of conjunctivitis.*

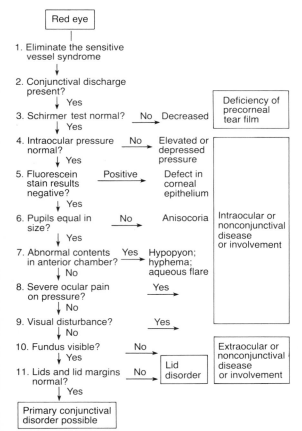

FIGURE 8–9. *Differentiation of conjunctivitis from other eye diseases. (See also "Differential Diagnosis of the Red Eye," Chap 21.)*

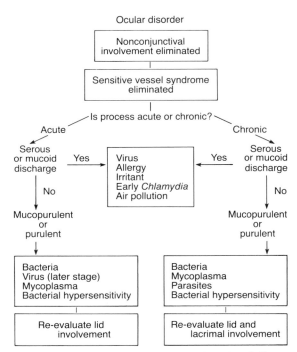

FIGURE 8–10. *Differential diagnosis of conjunctivitis.*

because if severe corneal pathology is ignored, blindness may ensue. Figure 8–8 shows the different types of primary and secondary conjunctivitides, and Figures 8–9 and 8–10 provide a guide for the differentiation of conjunctivitis from other ocular disorders. Once the correct cause has been determined (Table 8–5), reference to details of specific disorders in different species is necessary. (Characteristics of the major types of conjunctivitis in feline, equine, and bovine diseases are shown in Tables 8–6 to 8–9.)

SENSITIVE VESSEL SYNDROME

SENSITIVE VESSEL SYNDROME is a condition in which the conjunctival vessels appear engorged, usually tem-

TABLE 8–5. Irritative Factors Causing Conjunctivitis

Exogenous	Endogenous
Foreign bodies	Deficiency of precorneal
Dust	tear film
Sand	Entropion
Smoke	Distichiasis
Smog	Trichiasis
Industrial pollution	Ectopic cilia
Low humidity	Ectropion
Allergens	Prominent nasal folds
Wind	Lagophthalmos
Water (hunting dogs)	Prominent globes
Plant toxins (e.g., ergot)	Ocular exposure

Modified from Martin CL: Conjunctivitis—Differential diagnosis and treatment. Vet Clin North Am 3:367, 1973.

porarily, in the absence of disease. It occurs in dogs, especially of the smaller breeds, and occasionally cats, and it is frequently seen associated with the excitement of travel to a veterinarian or during examination. A similar phenomenon occurs after resolution of previous uveitis, when minor subsequent stimulation may result in erythema out of proportion to the insult. This can be seen after cataract surgery, in the absence of uveitis, and it must be distinguished from significant recurrent uveitis. Affected vessels usually remain engorged for a short time only and do not persist.

Treatment of Conjunctivitis

After determination of the etiology and treatment of nonconjunctival factors (e.g., correction of lid defects, removal of foreign bodies, replacement of deficient tear film, protection from exogenous factors), the following therapeutic agents are employed:

1. *Antibiotics.* Drops and ointments are the most frequently used methods of administration. For rationale of antibiotic choice, see Chapter 3.

2. *Corticosteroids.* These are used in noninfectious disorders after correction of nonconjunctival factors, when an immune or allergic cause is suspected. However, corticosteroids are not a routine part of conjunctivitis therapy, in the absence of a specific diagnosis.

3. *Cleansing agents.* Frequent cleaning by flushing, e.g., twice a day, of the conjunctiva and eyelid margins is a useful part of therapy of many conjunctival disorders. Many commercial solutions are available, but those not containing boric acid are preferable for public health reasons. Flushing may be followed by application of a bland protective ointment.

4. *Mast cell stabilizers.* Sodium cromoglycollate is used topically to treat canine allergic inhalant conjunctivitis and other nonspecific causes of ocular atopy.

5. *Nonsteroidal anti-inflammatory agents.* Topical flurbiprofen (Ocufen) has been advocated for ocular inflammatory disease, but specific indications in animals are currently poorly defined.

6. *Astringents.* Zinc sulfate drops have been used in mild conjunctivitis, often combined with mild vasoconstrictors. Although widely available, objective evidence of effectiveness is not convincing.

7. *Vasoactive agents.* Sympathetic agents in low concentration (e.g., 0.125% phenylephrine) may be used to reduce erythema and chemosis in acute conjunctivitis or allergy. If there has been no improvement within 5–7 days, the etiology should be questioned.

Bacterial Conjunctivitis

Primary bacterial conjunctivitis is more frequent in dogs, cattle, and sheep, although *Moraxella* spp have been isolated from horses with conjunctivitis in both North America and Australia. (Infectious Bovine and Ovine Keratoconjunctivitis are discussed in Chap 11.) In dogs, *Staphylococcus aureus*, *S. epidermidis*, and strep-

tococci are most frequently isolated (Tables 3–3 and 3–4), although these organisms are frequently found in normal eyes. Other factors besides the type and number of organisms and their virulence are obviously involved—e.g., lid conformation, immune status, and irritant factors. Frequently conjunctivitis is one of a spectrum of conditions that may be present, including otitis externa, hypothyroidism, generalized seborrhea, and pyoderma. Often control of these disorders is more appropriate than are attempts at complete cure, which may be unrealistic. Acute bacterial conjunctivitis is usually unilateral and responds well to treatment in 3–4 days, provided predisposing factors are removed.

Chronic bacterial conjunctivitis is often secondary. Examination of the lids, lid margins, and nasolacrimal system, measurement of tear production and intraocular pressure, and fluorescein staining are routine. Chronic forms are often bilateral and frequently associated with lid abnormalities or with infections in the ear and skin (e.g., in the Saint Bernard, bulldog, cocker spaniel, and chow chow). Successful treatment depends on improvement of the patient's general condition and associated infections.

TREATMENT

1. Topical broad-spectrum antibiotics (see Chap 3 for choice of antibiotic and steps to be taken in chronic cases).

2. Removal of crusts and exudates by soaking with saline-moistened cotton or commercial eye-cleaning kits.

3. Systemic antibiotic therapy in severe or chronic cases.

4. Expression of tarsal glands in chronic cases.

5. Prevention of self-mutilation with an Elizabethan collar.

6. Use of artificial tear solutions if tear production has been decreased by chronic conjunctivitis, and as a general supportive measure.

7. Combination antibiotic-steroid therapy is sometimes useful in very chronic conjunctivitis but should not be used routinely.

"Follicular Conjunctivitis"

In the author's opinion this condition does not exist as a separate entity. Lymphoid follicles enlarge as a result of antigenic stimulation, the source of which should be eliminated if possible, and the enlargement inhibited with appropriate medications. Although copper sulfate crystals, surgery, or sterile gauze has been advocated for removal of lymphoid follicles from the inner surface of the third eyelid in chronic conjunctivitis, this is rarely necessary or indicated. This method assumes the follicles are the cause rather than the result of the conjunctivitis. Careful removal of these follicles in very severe cases does not appear to be harmful and may be advantageous when combined with standard methods of therapy.

Seasonal Equine Conjunctivitis

In horses, a chronic conjunctivitis and blepharitis occurs in summer, associated with constant irritation from flies (*Musca domestica*). Mucopurulent discharge, epiphora, and moist eyelid margins are the usual signs. Treatment consists of local antibiotic preparations, application of corticosteroids to conjunctiva and eyelid margins in severe cases, and use of insecticides (e.g., gamma benzene hexachloride ointment), fly repellants, and fly veils. In very severe cases, insect-proof stabling is sometimes necessary. In some areas this "summer conjunctivitis" is due to release of *Habronema* larvae by feeding flies.

Mycotic Conjunctivitis

Mycotic conjunctivitis is uncommon in all species and tends to be chronic. Exudates are less profuse and drier in nature and form crusts around the eyelid margins. The most common organisms involved are *Candida* spp, *Aspergillus* spp, and yeasts. The history is usually one of chronic conjunctivitis with little or no response to previous antibiotic or antibiotic-steroid therapy. Diagnosis is by culture and cytology. Mycotic keratitis in horses usually lacks conjunctival involvement.

TREATMENT

A variety of antifungal agents have been used, depending on the sensitivity of the organism.
1. Pimaracin (Natacyn) drops frequently
2. Amphotericin B—125 µg subconjunctivally every 2nd day for 2–3 weeks, or 0.015% drops 3–6 times daily
3. Nystatin ointment or nystatin in artificial tears (200,000 units/15 ml)

Viral Conjunctivitis

Conjunctivitis is caused by a variety of viruses in all species. The following factors should be kept in mind:
1. Although the conjunctiva is frequently an important portal of entry of systemic viral diseases, it is not always the site of severe pathology or predominant clinical signs.
2. Conjunctivitis is present in both mild and severe forms in numerous systemic diseases (e.g., infectious bovine rhinotracheitis, canine distemper).
3. Very severe viral conjunctivitis is frequently responsible for the most obvious clinical signs, although other systems may be involved (e.g., herpetic conjunctivitis in cats).

4. Not all viruses isolated from the conjunctiva are pathogenic, nor is their significance completely understood. For example, adenoviruses have been found in cattle afflicted with infectious bovine keratoconjunctivitis (IBK).

CANINE VIRAL CONJUNCTIVITIS

Canine Distemper

Conjunctivitis is frequently present in the early stages of distemper, appearing as severe erythema and serous discharge combined with tonsillitis, pharyngitis, pyrexia, anorexia, and lymphopenia, especially in young pups. Cytoplasmic inclusion bodies in epithelial cells are difficult to find in conjunctival scrapings, but viral antigen may be detected by immunological methods. In advanced stages of distemper, there is characteristically a chronic bilateral conjunctivitis, the cornea is dull, Schirmer tear test readings are lowered, and bilateral mucopurulent rhinitis is present. Secondary bacteria (e.g., *S. aureus*) are usually present. The disease must be distinguished from a similar set of oculonasal signs that frequently occur in atypical infectious tracheobronchitis ("kennel cough") in dogs, in which coughing and signs of tracheitis are absent. Lack of severe systemic disease, early resolution or response to therapy, and history of association with dogs showing signs of respiratory disease are useful differentiating features.

Treatment
1. Local and systemic antibiotics
2. Tear replacement solutions and removal of crusts
3. Therapy for systemic disease (refer to standard texts)

Adenovirus

Adenovirus I (infectious canine hepatitis) and adenovirus II (infectious tracheobronchitis) can cause conjunctivitis in dogs, although the former is rare. Marked bilateral hyperemia and serous or seromucous exudate are present. Age, vaccination history, recent contacts and environment, and systemic signs differentiate both of these diseases from canine distemper, except in severe complicated tracheobronchitis. In addition to treatment of the systemic disease, topical antibiotic therapy is indicated to prevent and control bacterial infection. Topical use of antiviral agents is ineffective. Ocular lesions of infectious canine hepatitis are discussed in Chapter 11.

FELINE VIRAL CONJUNCTIVITIS

Viruses, *Chlamydia* spp, and *Mycoplasma* spp cause an array of conjunctivitides in cats. Although frequently manifested in association with severe upper respiratory

TABLE 8–6. Differential Diagnosis of Feline Conjunctivitis and Respiratory Disease Complex

	Rhinotracheitis (FVR)	Caliciviral Disease (FCV)	Reovirus Infection (FRI)	Pneumonitis (FPN)	Mycoplasma and Other Infections
Agent	Feline herpesvirus I	Feline caliciviruses (picornaviruses) numerous strains	Reovirus	*Chlamydia psittaci* (*Miyagawanella felis*; *Bedsonia felis*)	*Mycoplasma* spp, *Staph. pyogenes*, *Strep. pyogenes*, *P. multocida*, *B. bronchiseptica*, and others
Signs:					
Severity	Regularly more severe	Mild to moderate; subclinical infections common	Mild	Mild	Subclinical infections common
Ocular	Lacrimation, conjunctivitis, chemosis, occasionally keratitis	Lacrimation, sometimes conjunctivitis	Lacrimation	Conjunctivitis can be follicular	Conjunctivitis
Nasal	Serous or mucopurulent discharge, sneezing	Serous discharge, occasional sneezing; ulceration of external nares	Nasal discharge rare	Nasal discharge rare	None or purulent
Oral	Occasional small vesicles and ulcers in buccal epithelium	Frequent ulceration on anterior dorsal margin of tongue *and* hard palate, gingivitis	None	None	None
Other	Coughing, abortion, skin ulcers, central nervous system signs	Paw erosions	None	None	None
Course	2–4 weeks	7–10 days	1–26 days	Often chronic or recurrent	May be chronic
Incubation (natural infection)	2–10 days	1–9 days	4–19 days	6–15 days	Usually secondary
Immunity	Initially low and transient; can be boosted and become persistent	Some strains produce broad cross-protection clinically but allow reduced viral multiplication	Unknown	Weak, transient	Weak, transient
Diagnosis	Demonstration of intranuclear inclusions in early conjunctival smears; tissue culture isolation; FA test*	Tissue culture isolation, FA test*	Tissue culture isolation, SN test,† HA test‡	Conjunctival smears Giemsa-stained to show elementary bodies; CF test§	Culture
Inclusions	Intranuclear inclusions in respiratory epithelial cells, conjunctiva, and so on	None	Paranuclear cytoplasmic	Intracytoplasmic elementary bodies in conjunctival epithelial cells	None
Carrier state	Latent phase with periodic excretion after stress	Continuous shedding until self-clearance	Probable	Yes	Yes
Morbidity	High	High	50%	Variable	Variable
Mortality	High in kittens, aged, or immunodepressed	Variable; may be moderate in young kittens	Very low	Very low	Very low
Maternal antibody	<9 weeks	<11 weeks	Unknown	Unknown	Unknown
Prophylaxis	Live modified vaccine	Live modified vaccine	None	Live modified vaccine	None
Treatment	Symptomatic, supportive with antibiotics	Symptomatic, supportive with antibiotics	Symptomatic	Tetracyclines locally and systemically	Antibiotics

From Kirk RW: Current Veterinary Therapy VI, p 1284. WB Saunders Co, Philadelphia. Modified from Panel Report, Colloquium on Feline Diseases. J Am Vet Med Assoc 158:838–839, 1971.
*FA test = fluorescent antibody test.
†SN test = serum-neutralizing test.
‡HA test = hemagglutinating antibody test.
§CF test = complement-fixing test.

tract infections, conjunctivitis may also occur alone. Major features of the types of conjunctivitis and systemic syndromes caused by various microorganisms (feline herpesvirus 1, feline calicivirus, reovirus, *Chlamydia psittaci, Mycoplasma* spp, and others) are shown in Table 8–6.

Significant Features

Overall clinical signs of the complex are sneezing, fluctuating fever, ocular and nasal discharges, anorexia, depression, and salivation. The signs are more severe in kittens. Other important features are

1. With the exceptions of *Chlamydia* and *Mycoplasma*, the responsible organisms are highly infectious.

2. Ulcerative glossitis and gingivitis are usually associated with *feline calicivirus. Feline herpesvirus 1* causes occasional small vesicles and ulcers on the buccal epithelium.

3. Severe herpesvirus infections in young kittens frequently result in permanent corneal scarring. Conjunctival cicatrization may involve or destroy the lacrimal puncta, causing persistent epiphora. Creation of a conjunctivorhinostomy is the only definitive treatment.

4. Chlamydial conjunctivitis is usually unilateral, progresses to the other eye, and is not associated with severe rhinitis or glossitis.

5. Recovered cats may be carriers of feline herpesvirus and feline calicivirus for several months, making control difficult. Fully recovered asymptomatic queens may infect newborn kittens.

6. Conjunctivitis and rhinitis usually begin concurrently, with lacrimation followed by mucoid exudate after 1 or 2 days, becoming purulent and copious thereafter. The lids often stick together in feline herpesvirus infection, with frequent ulceration of lid margins.

7. The initial chemosis in feline herpesvirus and calicivirus may be so severe as to suggest a traumatic or toxic etiology.

8. Ulcerative keratitis with corneal perforation occurs frequently in feline herpesvirus infection (Table 8–7). Recurrences of dendritic keratitis associated with sinusitis and rhinitis are not uncommon in mature cats, especially Siamese and Abyssinians.

All cats and kittens with upper respiratory tract infection should receive a thorough eye examination to ensure that ulcerative keratitis or corneal perforation is not present.

Treatment

1. Antimicrobial therapy, depending on the responsible organism and secondary bacteria. Use of systemic

TABLE 8–7. Ocular Syndromes Due to Feline Herpesvirus

Age	Signs and Course
2–4 weeks	Severe ocular lesions, rhinitis, tracheitis, bronchopneumonia, and hepatic necrosis; severe ulcerative keratitis often present
4–6 months	Acute conjunctivitis and upper respiratory tract infection; course: 10–14 days
>6 months	Ulcerative dendritic keratitis and upper respiratory tract infection

From Bistner SI, et al: Ocular manifestations of feline herpesvirus infection. J Am Vet Med Assoc 159:1223, 1971.

and local tetracyclines or chloramphenicol is helpful in chlamydial conjunctivitis. Idoxuridine is recommended in feline herpesvirus 1 infection, although controlled studies of its efficacy are lacking.

2. Supportive therapy, including:

   a. Frequent cleaning of eyelid margins followed by application of a suitable antibiotic ointment.

   b. Forced feeding and fluid therapy by nasogastric tube.

   c. Administration of B-complex vitamins.

Severe feline herpesvirus 1 infections may persist for 2–4 weeks, requiring constant treatment.

Equine Viral Conjunctivitis

Viral conjunctivitis in horses, as in cats, is frequently associated with upper respiratory tract infections. The most common diseases are equine viral rhinopneumonitis, parainfluenza, and influenza. Details are shown in Table 8–8.

Bovine Viral Conjunctivitis

Infectious bovine rhinotracheitis (IBR) and malignant catarrhal fever (MCF) are the only common major viral diseases resulting in conjunctivitis. Numerous exotic diseases (e.g., Rift Valley fever, foot-and-mouth disease) cause conjunctivitis in ruminants, in addition to the more important systemic signs. Reference should be made to standard veterinary texts for details. Table 8–9 lists the clinical features of IBR and MCF in comparison with those of infectious bovine keratoconjunctivitis (IBK).

Chlamydial Conjunctivitis

Chlamydia psittaci causes significant conjunctivitis in cats and sheep. Chlamydial polyarthritis and conjunctivitis have been described in a foal, but the condition is not widespread. In cats, the conjunctivitis is initially unilateral, but usually spreads to the other eye within 7 days. Rhinitis may also be present. Initially, the

TABLE 8–8. Comparative Features of Oculorespiratory Syndromes in Horses: Clinical Summary

Feature	Equine Viral Rhinopneumonitis (EVR)	Parainfluenza	Influenza	Strangles	Equine Viral Arteritis (EVA)
Conjunctivitis	+ Slight	+ Slight	—	Rare, mild only	+ + Purulent, petechia, edema
Etiology	EVR virus	Parainfluenza 3	Influenza A/Equi 1	*Streptococcus equi* (virus may be associated with it)	EVA virus
General	Mild disease; emphasis on respiratory tract in young; abortion in adult	Mild to moderate disease	Mild disease; emphasis on coughing	Severe disease; emphasis on suppuration	Severe disease; emphasis on subcutaneous edema
Incubation period	2–10 days	3–8 days	2–3 days	4–8 days	1–6 days
Fever	39.5–40.5°C	38.5–40.0°C	38.5–41.0°C	39.5–40.5°C	39.5–41.0°C
Nasal discharge	Serous; may become purulent	Seropurulent, moderate to marked	Slight, serous only	Serous, then copiously purulent	Serous; may become purulent
Cranial lymphadenitis	+ Slight	+ Slight (may be marked in PGM influenza 3)	+ Slight	+ Abscessation with secondary fever	+ Slight
Cough	+ Slight	+ Slight	+ + Hacking, dry	+ + + Moist, severe	+ + Moderate
Respiratory distress	—	May be marked in foals	Severe in complicated cases and in young foals	Severe if lymph node obstruction or pneumonia present	+ + + In severe cases
Limb edema	Rare	—	Present in complicated cases	Occurs in atypical cases with lymph node obstruction	+ In stallions, edema of prepuce and scrotum also
Appetite	Good	Poor (pharyngitis)	Fair to good	Poor	Poor
Diarrhea	—	—	—	—	+ + In severe cases jaundice also
Abortion	Up to 90% at 8–10 months; some as early as 5 months Often no respiratory signs	—	—	—	+ + Up to 50%
Miscellaneous	Inapparent infection common	Rhinovirus may infect human attendants	Heavy mortality in newborn foals Influenza A/Equi 2 transmissible to humans	Involvement in many organs in some atypical cases	Severe depression
Course	2–5 days Cough up to 3 weeks	7 days Rhinitis and bronchitis may persist	7 days Cough and rhinitis may persist to 3 weeks	10–21 days	3–8 days Some deaths
Clinical pathology	Virus in nasal discharge Serum antibodies at 12 days and after Leukopenia	Virus in nasal discharge (pharynx preferred) Serological tests ?	Virus in nasal discharge Serological tests ?	*Streptococcus equi* in nasal swabs — Leukocytosis	Virus in blood at fever peak — Leukopenia
Treatment	Secondary bacteria only	Secondary bacteria only	Secondary bacteria only, especially in foals	Penicillin, tetracyclines	Secondary bacteria only
Control	Vaccine available, but of doubtful value	No vaccine	Successful killed vaccine	Vaccine	Tissue culture vaccine under examination

Modified from Blood DC, et al: Veterinary Medicine, 7th ed. Balliere Tindall, London, 1989.
+ = mild; + + = moderate; + + + = severe.

TABLE 8–9. Bovine Diseases with Ocular Manifestations

Feature	Infectious Bovine Rhinotracheitis (IBR)	Malignant Catarrhal Fever (MCF)	Infectious Bovine Kerotoconjunctivitis (IBK)
Conjunctival signs	Acute erythema and serous discharge (variable—may be sole sign of disease in some outbreaks) Distinguished from IBK by lack of corneal lesions or minute size of peripheral lesions	Mucopurulent conjunctivitis and eyelid edema, blepharospasm, conjunctival injection	Marked inflammation and erythema with mucopurulent discharge in later stages Lacrimation, photophobia, blepharospasm
Corneal signs	—	Peripheral corneal opacity (edema) moving centrally and becoming diffuse	Severe central ulceration and opacity
Anterior chamber signs	—	Hypopyon, panophthalmitis	Hypopyon
Etiology	IBR (herpes) virus	Herpesvirus	*Moraxella bovis* (?)
General	Decreased milk yield Occurs mostly after 6 months of age Encephalitic form in young animals	Extreme depression, anorexia, agalactia Nervous signs: nystagmus in late stages In peracute disease, fever, dyspnea, and acute gastroenteritis, with death occurring in 1–3 days	Rupture of cornea and endophthalmitis occur in a minority Anorexia and agalactia occur in acute stages More common in summer months
Incubation period	3–7 days (up to 21 days)	3–8 weeks	Variable
Mortality	Beef cattle, 6–12% Dairy cattle, 3% (Higher in encephalitic form)	60–100%	None
Morbidity	Beef cattle, 20–30% Dairy cattle, 8% (Higher in encephalitic form)	Usually isolated animals, but occasionally up to 50%	Variable, depending on previous exposure Calves affected more frequently
Respiratory signs	Nasal discharge and hyperemia, shallow fast respiration, cough, respiratory distress on exercise	Profuse mucopurulent nasal discharge, dyspnea	None
Gastrointestinal signs	Salivation; no mucosal lesions	Necrosis of nasal and buccal mucosa, lips and gums, and muzzle; salivation	None
Course	Rapid recovery	Prolonged course or early death	Spontaneous recovery in many cases by 5–6 weeks Residual lesions may be severe
Fever	Positive 42°C	Positive 41–41.5°C; may persist for weeks	None
Clinical pathology	Serum neutralization test Bacterial swabs of nasal exudate useful in chronic cases	Moderate leukocytosis Whole-blood nasal swabs and lymph node tissue are collected for transmission experiments	Numerous leukocytes and gram-positive cocci seen on smear *Moraxella, Neisseria* may be isolated
Abortion	Positive after illness or vaccination	—	—
Epidemiology	Occurs in large groups of cattle	Both sporadic and explosive outbreaks	Outbreaks may be explosive or restricted to a few animals
Control	Immunity after attack lasts 3 months Isolation of sick animals Vaccination	Separation of affected animals and of cattle from sheep	Separation of affected animals
Treatment	Broad-spectrum antibiotics	—	Tarsorrhaphy, subconjunctival antibiotics
Diagnosis	Signs restricted to upper respiratory tract and eye	Nasal, oral, and ocular lesions with fever, lymph node enlargement, and terminal encephalitis	Clinical signs and culture

conjunctiva is grayish pink, and lacrimation is increased. Within 2 days, mucous exudate forms, becoming purulent soon after. Conjunctival edema decreases, the membrane thickens, follicles form on the anterior medial surface of the third eyelid, and conjunctival hyperplasia becomes chronic. If untreated, the disease may last for months.

Kittens with neonatal conjunctivitis may be infected by a carrier queen. Immunity to infection is short-lived, and some animals may remain carriers. Chlamydial conjunctivitis is diagnosed by its clinical signs, a history of exposure to groups of cats, and the demonstration of characteristic intracytoplasmic elementary bodies in scrapings of epithelial cells. The disease responds well to topical treatment with chloramphenicol or tetracycline, especially in the early stages.

A similar chlamydial conjunctivitis occurs in sheep, with polyarthritis and associated lameness. This condition is distinguishable from infectious ovine keratoconjunctivitis (IOK) by the presence of lameness and lack of corneal lesions. Diagnosis and treatment are similar to the feline form, although systemic antibiotics may be indicated in valuable animals.

Chlamydial conjunctivitis also occurs in pet birds and in the Australian koala, in which a high proportion of the population may be affected by chronic keratoconjunctivitis and infertility. Different strains of *Chlamydia psittaci* are responsible for infection of the conjunctiva and genitalia. Stress is believed to play a major role in the pathogenesis in koalas. Many koalas harbor the organism but lack clinical signs. Diagnosis is by culture rather than by the ELISA (enzyme-linked immunosorbent assay) test, which lacks sensitivity.

Mycoplasmal Conjunctivitis

Mycoplasmas cause conjunctivitis in cats, and suggestions have been made that they are implicated in IOK and IBK and in many other types of infectious conjunctivitides in other animals. The feline condition is well described by Cello (1971).

The condition may be differentiated clinically from chlamydial and viral conjunctivitis. Initially a unilateral serous or mucoid discharge is present, which extends to the other eye within a week. The conjunctiva is frequently pale, and a pseudomembrane may form on the external surface of the third eyelid. Untreated, the disease has a self-limiting course of about 4 weeks.

In conjunctival scrapings, coccoid or coccobacillary organisms—which may be differentiated from pigment granules—may be seen in clusters on or near the surface of epithelial cells. Neutrophils are the most common cell type present. Mycoplasmal conjunctivitis is thus differentiated from viral and chlamydial conjunctivitis by the pale conjunctiva, presence of a pseudomembrane, and neutrophils on smears. Treatment is by topical application of chloramphenicol or erythromycin.

Parasitic Conjunctivitis

Parasites that may cause conjunctivitis in various species are shown in Table 8–10.

Allergic Conjunctivitis

Because of the exposed position of the conjunctival sac and the content of lymphoid tissue, allergic conjunctivitis frequently occurs after the entry of antigens into the sac. The response is elicited by many different kinds of antigens and can occur in all species. The clinical signs include:

1. erythema and hyperemia
2. serous discharge
3. chemosis
4. concurrent inflammation of the nasal cavity, ears, pharynx, and gums

Eosinophils are usually not present in smears, although lymphocytes and plasma cells may be seen.

TABLE 8–10. Parasitic Conjunctivitis

Parasite	Species Affected	Treatment and Prevention
Thelazia spp	Dog, cattle, horse, pig, sheep, deer, cat, human	1. Removal under local anesthesia 2. Topical echothiophate (Phospholine Iodide)
Onchocerca cervicalis	Horse	1. Systemic diethylcarbamazine citrate (2–4 mg/kg) 2. Systemic ivermectin
Habronema megastoma	Horse	1. Fly repellants, traps, poisons, and screened stalls; sanitary disposal of manure 2. Local injection of fenthion 3. Systemic injection of ivermectin or Neguvon 4. Daily application of glycerine to the conjunctiva
Oestrus ovis	Sheep	1. Mechanical removal 2. Systemic organophosphates (e.g., Neguvon) 3. Local injection of fenthion
Oxyspirura mansoni	Poultry, especially turkeys	1. Removal of parasites 2. Removal of cockroaches (intermediate host)

Secondary bacterial conjunctivitis may occur after inflammation has been initiated by an antigen. It has been suggested that toxins produced by bacteria (e.g., *S. aureus*) present in the conjunctival sac or tarsal glands may initiate allergic conjunctivitis. Food allergy also results in allergic conjunctivitis in calves.

Treatment

1. Local corticosteroid therapy with the dose as low as will control the condition. In mild cases dilute, low-potency steroids may be used intermittently (e.g., 0.5% hydrocortisone drops twice daily).
2. Systemic corticosteroids in severe cases.
3. Local antibiotic preparations if secondary bacterial conjunctivitis is present. (*Note*: Neomycin itself occasionally causes allergic conjunctivitis, although this is insufficient to prevent routine use.)

CANINE ALLERGIC INHALANT DERMATITIS (ATOPY)[1]

Etiology

Inhalation of plant pollens, molds, house dust, and other antigens, especially during periods of peak pollen production, is thought to cause canine allergic inhalant dermatitis (CAID). The condition frequently shows seasonal fluctuation and is exacerbated by any condition that tends to increase skin irritability. IgE immunoglobulins are formed in response to the antigen and are believed to fix to skin and conjunctival tissues. Subsequent exposure to antigen, and consequent antigen-antibody interaction, results in inflammation and clinical signs.

Clinical Signs

1. Serous ocular discharge.
2. Conjunctival erythema.
3. Intense pruritus, causing secondary dermatitis, on the face, axilla, and feet.
4. Paw-licking and staining of hair on paws.
5. Blepharitis.
6. Occasional sneezing and rhinitis.
7. A triad of dry skin, seborrheic dermatitis, and infectious dermatitis is often present in severe cases of CAID. Hematological examination frequently reveals eosinophilia. Intradermal testing may help to outline the responsible antigen.

Treatment

1. Removal or limitation of antigenic exposure.
2. Local corticosteroid applications in as low a dose and for as short a period as will control the inflammation.

---

1. See also Chap 19.

3. Systemic oral corticosteroids (e.g., prednisolone) in short courses when allergic reactions occur. The dose should be as low as possible. Long-acting parenteral preparations should be avoided.
4. If the disease is prolonged, topical corticosteroids, moist compresses of aluminum acetate (Burow's solution), prevention of self-trauma, and soothing baths.

Topical and systemic antihistamines are of very limited use in the treatment of allergic conjunctivitis.

ACQUIRED CONJUNCTIVAL DISORDERS

Conjunctival Emphysema

Emphysema (air beneath the conjunctiva) is recognized by subconjunctival swellings and crepitus (Fig. 8–11). It is caused by the entry of air onto the periorbita from surrounding paranasal sinuses, usually after traumatic damage to the sinus walls. The presence of subconjunctival air is an indication for thorough radiographic study of the sinuses and a complete ocular examination. Depending on the severity of the initial trauma, subconjunctival hemorrhages and intraocular damage may also be present. In the absence of more severe lesions, the air is usually resorbed in 7–14 days. A systemic antibiotic should be administered to prevent orbital infection with normal flora from the damaged sinus.

Drug Plaques

Certain repository medications (e.g., methylprednisolone) leave unsightly, creamy-white subconjunctival plaques months after injection in some animals. The material in these plaques may also incite local conjunctivitis adjacent to the material. In such cases, surgical excision under a short-acting general anesthetic is indicated.

Conjunctival Lacerations

Severe lacerations of the conjunctiva may be seen after trauma and fights. The conjunctiva heals very rapidly, and small lacerations usually require short-term topical antibiotic therapy only. More severe lacerations are flushed with saline solution to remove foreign material, sutured with 6/0 Vicryl, and treated with topical antibiotics.

Proliferative Keratoconjunctivitis Syndrome in Collies

Synonym: "fibrous histiocytoma"

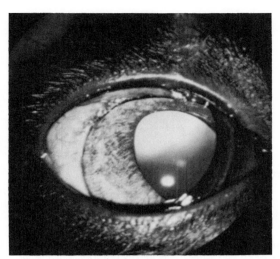

FIGURE 8–11. Subconjunctival emphysema. (From Bryan GM: Subconjunctival emphysema in a cat. Vet Med Small Anim Clin 72:1087, 1977.)

Clinical Signs

1. Raised (up to 5 mm), yellow-red, subconjunctival masses at the temporal limbus (see Fig. 7–47). The nasal and ventral limbi and the third eyelid are occasionally affected.

2. Thickening, infiltration, and occasionally depigmentation of the margin and anterior surface of the third eyelid. The lesion may protrude anteriorly up to 4 mm.

3. Mild conjunctivitis.

4. Corneal opacity as the lesion advances into the corneal stroma. Crystalline opacities (presumably of cholesterol and triglycerides) and corneal edema may precede the lesion in the stroma.

The syndrome occurs predominantly in collies. The etiology is unknown, but the condition is more common in poorly pigmented animals exposed to intense sunlight. The lesions are bilateral but not symmetrical. The lesions consist of masses of histiocytes and fibrocytes.

Differential Diagnosis

The syndrome must be distinguished from the following disorders: ocular nodular fasciitis, systemic and palpebral histiocytomatosis, neoplasia, exuberant granulation tissue, Überreiter's syndrome (different breed predisposition), and secondary lipid keratopathy.

Course of the Disease

Without treatment, the condition is progressive and often leads to blindness. Long-term treatment is usually necessary for control, although some cases show regression after 12 months' treatment. Some cases do not respond despite therapy and progress to eventual blindness. The presence of a large, fast-growing limbal mass at initial presentation is cause for guarded prognosis.

Treatment

1. Limitation of exposure to sunlight.

2. Subconjunctival (nonrepository) and topical corticosteroid therapy as frequently as necessary to control the condition (cure is unlikely). In the initial stages, systemic treatment is useful.

3. Surgical removal of large protuberant masses.

4. Beta radiation over the limbal lesion (4000 rads repeated as necessary).

5. Cryotherapy has been suggested as an effective method for resistant cases, but it is not uniformly successful.

6. Azathioprine can be used orally, especially when lid masses are also present or when other treatments fail.

Because of the chronic course of and difficulty in controlling this disease, treatment by a veterinary ophthalmologist is advised.

Conjunctival Neoplasms

Of the conjunctival neoplasms, SCC is the most common. Others commonly recorded include hemangioma and hemangiosarcoma, papilloma, and mastocytoma in dogs. (SCC of the lids and conjunctiva is discussed in Chap 7.) Solar radiation has been suggested as a cause of SCC, telangiectasia, hemangioma, and invasive hemangiosarcoma of the nonpigmented limbal conjunctiva in dogs housed in the open at high elevation (1500 m) in Colorado. Similar lesions occur in dogs at elevation in the Reno-Tahoe area.

BOVINE SCC

SCC of the eye and adnexa is one of the most frequent and important ocular conditions affecting cattle.

Breed Incidence

SCC affects Herefords most frequently, but it also occurs in shorthorns and Friesians. It is uncommon in breeds with pigmented conjunctiva and lids but may occur in any breed. The incidence in Hereford herds may reach 10%. Most animals are affected at between 7 and 9 years of age; SCC is rare in those younger than 4 years.

Etiology

The exact etiology is unknown. The incidence of SCC is much higher in areas of high sunlight or altitude, where exposure to ultraviolet radiation is greater. The relationship among ultraviolet radiation, hypopigmentation, and increased incidence suggests that ultraviolet radiation is the cause in a susceptible animal. About 75% of cases occur in animals lacking pigment in the eyelids, third eyelid, or conjunctiva. Lid pigmentation is highly heritable and is present at birth, whereas conjunctival pigmentation has a lower heritability and is not fully developed until 5 years of age. Selection for lid pigmentation has been used as a control measure. Although IBR virus and other viral particles have been demonstrated in SCC lesions, an etiological relationship has not been established.

Clinical Signs and Pathogenesis

For the globe and third eyelid, the plaque is the initial precursor lesion (Fig. 8–12). The plaques are grayish-white areas of thickened epithelium, occurring most frequently at the nasal and temporal limbus. Papillomas are the next stage and have a similar distribution, but the surface is roughened and the mass is frequently pedunculated or freely moveable. The base often merges with an underlying plaque. On the lids, the precursor lesion is the keratoma, a dirty-brown, horn-like structure up to 3 cm long, which occurs near the hairline at the mucocutaneous junctions and is more common in older animals. Carcinoma in situ may arise from any of these lesions; this term is used for the stage before the neoplastic cells have penetrated the lamina propria of the epithelium to become an SCC.

The surface of carcinomas may be roughened or papillary (Fig. 8–13), hemorrhagic, or ulcerated. Both the precursors to SCC and the disease itself are usually unilateral (10% are bilateral). Ocular lesions outnumber lid lesions by a ratio of 3:1, whereas lesions of the third eyelid account for less than 5% of the total lesions. Precursor lesions are not uncommon at less than 4 years of age, whereas SCC is more common at 7–9 years, and

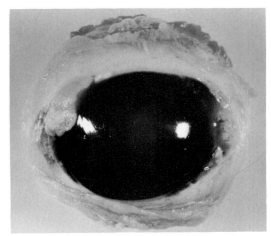

FIGURE 8–13. SCCs at the nasal and temporal limbus in a Hereford eye. Note the papillary or granular surface.

it is rare at less than 5 years. This is expected for a progressive precursor lesion.

Fifty per cent of precursor lesions present at the end of one summer may disappear by the next summer.

After invasion of surrounding periocular and orbital tissues, metastasis occurs to the parotid lymph node, followed by spread to the atlantal or retropharyngeal nodes, anterior cervical chain or tracheal lymph ducts, jugular vein, and finally wide hematogenous infiltration. The rate of progression of SCC is variable, with lesions ranging from slow-growing to highly malignant and rapidly fatal, depending on the individual case. Both cell-mediated and humoral immunity to tumor antigens have been demonstrated. Common antigens between tumors are probable.

Differential Diagnosis

SCC must be distinguished from the following conditions:

1. IBK (appearance of corneal lesions, age, sudden onset, and epidemic nature)
2. Penetrating injuries (appearance)
3. Dermoid (congenital and nonprogressive)
4. Lymphosarcoma (exophthalmos, hematology, clinical signs, and elevated serum lactate dehydrogenase [LDH])

Biopsy or cytological scraping of suspicious lesions is usually diagnostic (Fig. 8–14) with up to 90% accuracy having been reported. The latter method, using Papanicolaou's stain, is useful for early results and can usually be performed by a human pathology laboratory.

Globe, Third Eyelid

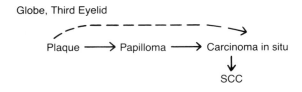

FIGURE 8–12. Clinical signs and pathogenesis of SCC at various ocular sites.

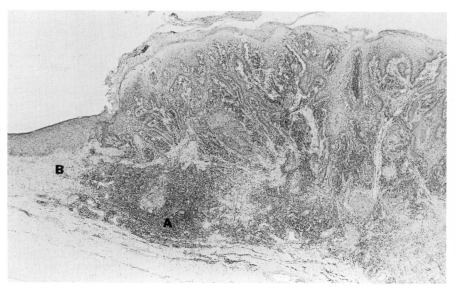

FIGURE 8–14. Section of the SCC shown in Figure 8–13. Numerous lymphocytes (A) are present in the base of the lesions. Sheets of squamous cells (B) are infiltrating the corneal and scleral stroma.

Control

1. Selective breeding for lid and corneoscleral pigmentation, which are genetically related and heritable.
2. Use of breeding animals whose progeny have not developed SCC.
3. Selection of animals based on lid pigment at birth.

Treatment

Treatment for individuals depends on the value of the animal and the stage of the disease. Immunotherapy and cryotherapy have extended the therapeutic choices available. The efficacy of immunotherapy was foreshadowed by a knowledge of the high spontaneous-regression rate of precursor lesions and the extensive infiltration of lesions with lymphocytes seen so frequently on histological examination. Studies have demonstrated the possibility of a shared antigen between the plaque and the malignant lesions. Table 8–11 provides a list of treatment options for the four stages of SCC.

Economic and radiological health complications limit the use of radiotherapy in many developed countries. Nevertheless, the susceptibility of tumors to and the good cure rates achieved with radiotherapy—often as the sole treatment—mandate its use when economic, experience, and safety requirements can be met. Regarding cryotherapy, in a large study using a double freeze–thaw cycle to $-25°C$, an overall cure rate of

TABLE 8–11. Treatment of Squamous Cell Carcinoma

Stage	Type of Lesion	Treatment Options
Stage I	Precursor lesions	1. Local cryotherapy or hyperthermia 2. Surgical removal ($\pm$ tissue destruction by electrosurgery) 3. Follow 1 and 2 by local radiation therapy (25,000 rads) over the site
Stage II	SCC of lids, third eyelid, cornea, or conjunctiva, without globe or orbital invasion	1. Local cryotherapy or hyperthermia (<5 cm in size) 2. Immunotherapy (saline-phenol tumor extract if available) 3. Radiotherapy; ^{90}Sr for conjunctiva and cornea; cesium, gold, or radon seeds, or cobalt implants for third eyelids and lids 4. Repeat treatments if lesions recur
Stage III	Globe or orbital invasion	1. Enucleation and orbital exenteration 2. Immunotherapy 3. Radiotherapy (radon, cesium, cobalt implants)
Stage IV	As for stage III, plus lymph node involvement	As for stage III

97% was achieved, and even quite large lesions responded well. Immunotherapy (saline-phenol tissue extract) caused regression in 84% with complete disappearance in 13.5% of cases in which immunotherapy was the only treatment method used. Treatment with bacille Calmette-Guérin (BCG) cell wall vaccine injected into the tumor caused regression in 71% of affected animals.

Cryotherapy has the advantages of simplicity and rapidity, economy, analgesia, minimal preoperative and postoperative treatment, repeatability, and minimal side effects. It promises to become the treatment of choice, with even higher cure rates available when it is used together with immunotherapy, radiotherapy, and surgery. A detailed study of various combination therapies in properly staged tumors is necessary in order to determine the most economic and effective combination. Misdorp and associates (1985) found block resection to be superior to intralesional BCG in cattle.[2]

CANINE CONJUNCTIVAL PAPILLOMATOSIS

Papillomas usually occur on the eyelids or mucocutaneous junctions. For those arising from the conjunctiva, the most important differential diagnosis is SCC. The relationship to oral and cutaneous papillomatoses is not established. The oral and cutaneous forms are caused by different papillomaviruses. Surgical removal or cryotherapy is the treatment of choice, especially if the lesion is causing pain by rubbing, or it is cosmetically objectionable. Recurrence has been observed, presumably due to seeding of surrounding tissues with virus or tumor cells, and after attempted removal by electrosurgery. Spontaneous regression of ocular papillomas has not been recorded.

EQUINE CONJUNCTIVAL ANGIOSARCOMA

Conjunctival angiosarcomas occur in aged horses, grow slowly, and metastasize despite excision and radiation therapy. They are diagnosed definitively by factor VIII:RAg.

REFERENCES

Anderson DE (1963): Genetic aspects of cancer with special reference to cancer of the eye in the bovine. Ann NY Acad Sci 108:948.

Anderson W (1975): Canine Allergic Inhalant Dermatitis. Ralston Purina Co, St Louis.

Atluru D, et al (1982): Tumor associated antigens of bovine cancer eye. Vet Immunol Immunopathol 3:279.

Banks WC, England RB (1973): Radioactive gold in the treatment of ocular squamous cell carcinoma of cattle. J Am Vet Med Assoc 163:745.

Barkyoumb SD, Leipold HW (1984): Nature and cause of bilateral ocular dermoids in Hereford cattle. Vet Pathol 21:316.

---

2. *Author's note:* This study was performed by cancer researchers, without regard to the practical effect of BCG on tuberculin testing in cattle.

Bistner SI, et al (1971): Ocular manifestations of feline herpesvirus infection. J Am Vet Med Assoc 159:1223.

Blogg JR, Slatter DH (1977): Proliferative keratoconjunctivitis in the collie. Proc Am Coll Vet Ophthalmol 8:89.

Blood DC, et al (1989): Veterinary Medicine, 7th ed. Balliere Tindall, London.

Bonney CH, et al (1980): Papillomatosis of conjunctiva and adnexa in dogs. J Am Vet Med Assoc 176:48.

Bryan GM (1977): Subconjunctival emphysema in a cat. Vet Med Small Anim Clin 72:1087.

Carter JD (1973): Medial conjunctivoplasty for aberrant dermis of the Lhasa apso. J Am Anim Hosp Assoc 8:242.

Cello RM (1971): Clues to differential diagnosis of feline respiratory infections. J Am Vet Med Assoc 158:968.

Cockram FA, Jackson ARB (1974): Isolation of a chlamydia from cases of keratoconjunctivitis in koalas. Aust Vet J 50:82.

Cockram FA, Jackson ARB (1981): Keratoconjunctivitis of the koala, *Phascolarctos cinereus*, caused by *Chlamydia psittaci*. J Wildl Dis 17:497.

Duke-Elder S (1965): System of Ophthalmology, vol 8, part I, Diseases of the Outer Eye. H Kimpton, London.

Duke-Elder S (1970): Parson's Diseases of the Eye, 15th ed. Churchill Livingstone, Edinburgh.

Duke-Elder S, Wybar KC (1961): System of Ophthalmology, vol 2, The Anatomy of the Visual System. H Kimpton, London.

Farris HE, Fraunfelder FT (1976): Cryosurgical treatment of ocular squamous cell carcinoma of cattle. J Am Vet Med Assoc 168:213.

Fledderus A, et al (1988): Conjunctivitis, red nose, and skin hypersensitivity as signs of food allergy in veal calves. Vet Rec 122:633.

French GT (1959): A clinical and genetic study of eye cancer in Hereford cattle. Aust Vet J 35:474.

Girjes AA (1988): Two distinct forms of *Chlamydia psittaci* associated with disease and infertility in *Phascolarctus cinereus* (koala). Infect Immun 56:1897.

Grier RL, et al (1980): Treatment of bovine and equine ocular squamous cell carcinoma by radiofrequency hyperthermia. J Am Vet Med Assoc 177:55.

Hacker DV, et al (1986): Ocular angiosarcoma in four horses. J Am Vet Med Assoc 189:200.

Hargis AM, et al (1978): Tumor and tumor-like lesions of perilimbal conjunctiva in laboratory dogs. J Am Vet Med Assoc 173:1185.

Hoffman D, et al (1978): An evaluation of exfoliative cytology in the diagnosis of bovine ocular squamous cell carcinoma. J Comp Pathol 88:497.

Huntington PJ, et al (1987): Isolation of a *Moraxella* spp. from horses with conjunctivitis. Aust Vet J 64:118.

Jennings PA, et al (1979): Bovine ocular squamous cell carcinoma: Lymphocyte response to phytohaemagglutinin and tumor antigen. Br J Cancer 40:608.

Johnson BW, et al (1988): Conjunctival mast cell tumors in two dogs. J Am Anim Hosp Assoc 24:439.

Kainer RA, et al (1980): Hyperthermia for treatment of ocular squamous cell tumors in cattle. J Am Vet Med Assoc 176:356.

Kleinschuster SJ, et al (1977): Regression of bovine ocular carcinoma by treatment with a mycobacterial vaccine. J Natl Cancer Inst 58:1807.

Klostlin RG, Jonek JE (1986): Cancer eye in German spotted cattle. Occurrence, treatment methods and results. Tieraztl Prax 14:477.

Kuchroo VK, Spradbrow PB (1985): Tumour-associated antigens in bovine ocular squamous cell carcinoma: Studies with sera from tumour-bearing animals. Vet Immunol Immunopathol 9:23.

Kuchroo VK, et al (1983): Serum blocking factors in bovine ocular squamous cell carcinoma demonstrated by inhibition of erythrocyte rosette augmentation. Cancer Res 43:1325.

Last RJ (1968): Wolff's Anatomy of the Eye and Orbit, 6th ed. WB Saunders Co, Philadelphia.

Lavach JD, et al (1977): Cytology of normal and inflamed conjunctivas in dogs and cats. J Am Vet Med Assoc 170:722.

Martin CL (1973): Conjunctivitis—Differential diagnosis and treatment. Vet Clin North Am 3:367.

Misdorp W, et al (1985): Clinico-pathological aspects of immuno-therapy by intralesional injection of BCG cell walls or live BCG in bovine ocular squamous cell carcinoma. Cancer Immunol Immunother 20:223.

Monlux AW, et al (1957): The diagnosis of squamous cell carcinoma of the eye in cattle. Am J Vet Res 18:5.

Nesbitt GH (1978): Canine allergic inhalant dermatitis: A review of 230 cases. J Am Vet Med Assoc 172:55.

Ott RL (1972): A practitioner's complete guide to upper respiratory infections in cats. Feline Pract 2:10.

Prince JH, et al (1960): Anatomy and Histology of the Eye and Orbit in Domestic Animals. Charles C Thomas, Springfield, IL.

Russel WO, et al (1956): Studies on bovine ocular squamous cell carcinoma. I. Pathological anatomy and historical review. Cancer 9:1–52.

Saunders LZ (1971): Pathology of the Eye of Domestic Animals. Parey, Berlin.

Spradbrow PB, et al (1977): Immunotherapy of bovine ocular squamous cell carcinomas. Vet Rec 100:376.

Swango LJ, et al (1970): A comparison of the pathogenesis and antigenicity of infectious canine hepatitis virus and the A26–61 virus strain (Toronto). J Am Vet Med Assoc 156:1687.

Trevor-Roper P (1974): The Eye and Its Disorders, 2nd ed. Blackwell, Oxford.

Vogt DW, Anderson DE (1964): Studies on bovine ocular squamous cell carcinoma. Heritability of susceptibility. J Hered 55:133.

Waldham DG, et al (1982): Use of endotoxin and mycobacterial fractions in treating malignant epithelioma of the bovine eye. US Anim Hlth Assoc Proc 81:64.

Weigler BJ, et al (1988): Aspects of epidemiology of *Chlamydia psittaci* infection in a population of koalas *(Phascolarctos cinereus)* in southeastern Queensland. J Wildl Dis 24:282.

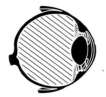

9

Third Eyelid

ANATOMY AND PHYSIOLOGY	PROTRUSION OF THE GLAND	TRAUMA TO THE THIRD EYELID
EXAMINATION	OF THE THIRD EYELID	FOLLICULAR CONJUNCTIVITIS
UNPIGMENTED THIRD EYELID	NEOPLASMS AFFECTING THE	MISCELLANEOUS DISORDERS
EVERSION OF THE THIRD EYELID	THIRD EYELID	

ANATOMY AND PHYSIOLOGY

The third eyelid is a mobile protective structure lying between the cornea and the lower eyelid, in the nasal portion of the inferior conjunctival sac (Fig. 9–1).

In domestic animals the third eyelid reaches its greatest development in horses and ruminants, in which it can sweep across the eye. The musculature controlling the third eyelid is vestigial in domestic species, the membrane moving passively across the eye when the globe is retracted by M. RETRACTOR BULBI (abducens nerve). Movement is in a superotemporal direction, toward the orbital ligament. The position of the third eyelid is also partially determined by sympathetic tone in the orbital smooth muscles. Interruption to this sympathetic supply, as in Horner's syndrome, results in prominence of the third eyelid and enophthalmos (posterior placement of the globe within the orbit).

The third eyelid consists of the following parts:
1. T-shaped cartilaginous skeleton
2. Gland of the third eyelid

3. Conjunctival covering on bulbar and palpebral surfaces
4. Superficial lymphoid follicles on the bulbar surface

The horizontal part of the T lies parallel to and 1.5 mm from the edge of the membrane, at right angles to the direction of motion, and is embedded in the gland of the third eyelid at its base (Fig. 9–2). The entire cartilage gives rigidity to the third eyelid. The gland of the third eyelid is seromucoid and produces about 50% of the normal precorneal tear film. The base of the gland and the cartilage are secured by a poorly defined fascial retinaculum to the region of the ventral oblique and rectus muscles and the periorbita surrounding them. The cartilage is covered on both bulbar and palpebral surfaces by adherent conjunctiva. Lymphoid follicles, pinkish red in color, are normally present beneath the bulbar conjunctiva (Fig. 9–3). In the pig and certain laboratory animals a deeper portion of the gland of the third eyelid is found within the orbit (HARDER'S GLAND). Harder's gland is absent in other domestic species.

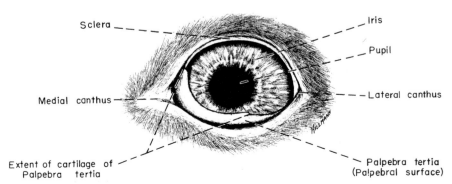

FIGURE 9–1. Diagram of the eye showing the third eyelid. (From Evans HE, Christensen GC: Miller's Anatomy of the Dog, 2nd ed. WB Saunders Co, Philadelphia, 1979. © Cornell University 1964.)

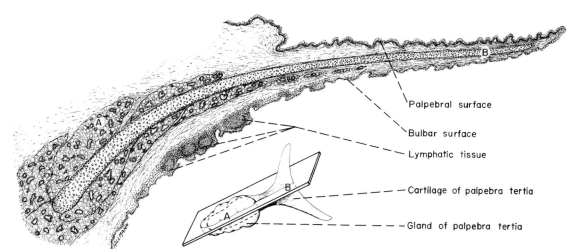

FIGURE 9–2. Histological section of the third eyelid. (From Evans HE, and Christensen GC: Miller's Anatomy of the Dog, 2nd ed. WB Saunders Co, Philadelphia, 1979. © Cornell University 1964.)

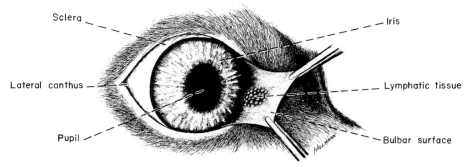

FIGURE 9–3. Diagram of everted third eyelid showing normal lymphoid follicles. (From Evans HE, Christensen GC: Miller's Anatomy of the Dog, 2nd ed. WB Saunders Co, Philadelphia, 1979. © Cornell University 1964.)

The third eyelid has three important functions:
1. Production of fluid for the precorneal tear film
2. Distribution of the precorneal tear film
3. Protection of the cornea, especially in grazing animals when the head is down, and in all animals when the corneal and palpebral reflexes are activated and the globe is retracted by m. retractor bulbi

Removal of the third eyelid causes:
1. Increased corneal exposure, drying of the cornea, corneal trauma, and chronic keratitis
2. A chronic conjunctivitis that is often purulent and frequently resistant to treatment
3. Decreased tear production, which contributes to problems 1 and 2.

EXAMINATION

The palpebral surface of the third eyelid is easily examined by applying digital pressure on the globe, through the upper lid. The bulbar surface is examined under topical anesthesia with von Graefe's or similar fixation forceps. The palpebral surface and margin are usually pigmented in dogs. Absence of this pigment reveals normal well-vascularized conjunctiva, which is frequently mistaken by owners for protrusion or inflammation. It is not pathological and does not require surgical correction. The third eyelid protrudes or appears prominent in the following disorders:
1. Horner's syndrome (unilateral protrusion) (see Chap 17)
2. Third eyelid protrusion syndrome (haws syndrome) (see Chap 17)
3. Space-occupying orbital lesions that push the membrane across the eye passively, by increasing pressure within the orbit
4. During tranquilization, e.g., with acetylpromazine
5. Shrinkage or retraction of the globe, as in enophthalmos, dehydration, and phthisis bulbi

---

The third eyelid is a useful and important structure. The only indications for its removal are *severe, irreparable trauma* and *histologically confirmed malignant neoplasia.*

The third eyelid is frequently infiltrated or thickened during other disorders of conjunctiva and cornea. In chronic immune-mediated keratoconjunctivitis syndrome of Überreiter it is often either infiltrated with lymphocytes and plasma cells or thickened and depigmented along the margin. During various kinds of conjunctival and corneal inflammation, reddish lymphoid follicles on the bulbar surface of the membrane are usually hypertrophic. This normal response to antigenic stimulation is distinguished from abnormal follicles (usually white in color) on the palpebral surface of the membrane in follicular conjunctivitis (Chap 8).

UNPIGMENTED THIRD EYELID

Breeders frequently present normal animals with unpigmented third eyelid margins for evaluation and removal. Such eyelids are normal, and surgical intervention is not indicated. When such eyes become inflamed for other reasons, the unpigmented membrane may appear more visible, as the conjunctival vasculature is not obscured by pigment.

EVERSION OF THE THIRD EYELID

Eversion of the third eyelid refers to rolling out of the margin of the membrane owing to abnormal curvature of the vertical portion of the cartilaginous T (Fig. 9–4). The condition may be unilateral or bilateral, and although it is most commonly seen in young dogs, it occasionally develops in middle-aged dogs. Eversion may develop because of a greater rate of growth of cartilage on the inner surface of the T. It is more common in Weimaraners, Saint Bernards, Newfoundlands, and Irish setters. A hereditary basis has been suggested in German short-haired pointers and other breeds. Injuries and improper suturing of the third eyelid may also result in eversion.

Eversion of the third eyelid is corrected surgically because of its undesirable cosmetic appearance and resultant secondary conjunctivitis and keratitis in some animals.

Treatment

The deformed cartilage only is removed, via a surgical approach from the bulbar surface, preferably under operating microscopic control. The affected cartilage is usually found near the junction of the two arms of the T (Fig. 9–5). A topical antibiotic solution may be used for 3–5 days after surgery.

PROTRUSION OF THE GLAND OF THE THIRD EYELID

Synonyms: prolapse, adenitis, hyperplasia, adenoma of the nictitans gland, "cherry eye" (colloquial)

The gland of the third eyelid protrudes from behind the third eyelid as a reddish mass (Fig. 9–6). This is thought to result from a defect in the retinaculum that binds the nictitans to the periorbita, allowing the gland

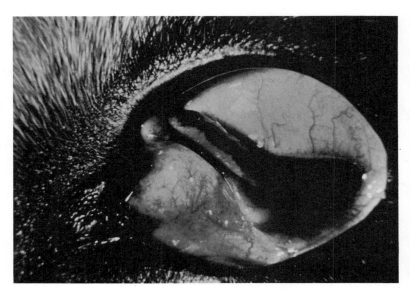

FIGURE 9–4. Eversion of the cartilage of the third eyelid.

to evert while remaining attached to the nictitans cartilage. Abrasion and drying of the exposed gland result in secondary inflammation and swelling. Hyperplasia, neoplasia, and primary inflammation are not the cause of this condition.

Because of inflammation, resulting irritation, and cosmetic appearance, the gland is replaced. If the gland is severely infected, preoperative treatment with topical antibiotics is advisable for 2–4 days. Nonspecific therapy with antibiotic-steroid combinations will not result in resolution of protrusion. Occasionally, in the early stages, a prolapsed gland returns to its normal position by manipulation or without assistance. Prolapsed glands of the third eyelid should not be removed, as a significant contributor to precorneal tear film production is also removed, and keratoconjunctivitis sicca is frequently seen in such animals, often years later. Uncontrolled anecdotal reports by proponents of removal must be ignored in favor of patient welfare. Partial removal of the gland is justifiable in treating the tear-staining syndrome, under specific circumstances (see Chap 10).

Treatment

Prolapsed gland of the third eyelid is treated by surgical replacement. The original method of suturing to the globe inferiorly (Blogg, 1979) has been superseded by the superior method of Kaswan and Martin (1985) in which the gland is sutured to the periosteum of the inferior orbital margin (Fig. 9–7). (The former technique had a higher rate of recurrence owing to difficulty in suturing to the tough sclera, and a risk of globe penetration.) The technique should be performed only by persons skilled in the method.

Prolapsed glands of the third eyelid are treated by replacement, *not* by excision. For best results, only experienced surgeons should attempt the technique.

NEOPLASMS AFFECTING THE THIRD EYELID

Squamous cell carcinoma is the most frequent neoplasm affecting the third eyelid in all species (Fig. 9–8). Unpigmented membranes are more susceptible. Numerous other neoplasms affecting the third eyelid (e.g., mastocytoma, lymphosarcoma, fibrosarcoma) have been described, but these are rare.

Treatment

1. Surgical removal of the affected area and a small margin of surrounding tissue is the method of choice. Consistent with complete removal of the neoplasm, as little tissue as possible is removed, in an attempt to retain as much functional membrane as possible (Fig. 9–9). Surgical excision is preferable to cryotherapy, as it can be more accurately controlled.

2. Radiation. Squamous cell carcinoma, mastocytoma, and lymphomatous infiltration are all susceptible to radiotherapy. A dose of 40–50 Gy is applied with a strontium-90 applicator to the surgical site and the surrounding area. The underlying globe is protected with a lead shield, to absorb radiation that passes through the membrane.

Text continued on page 234

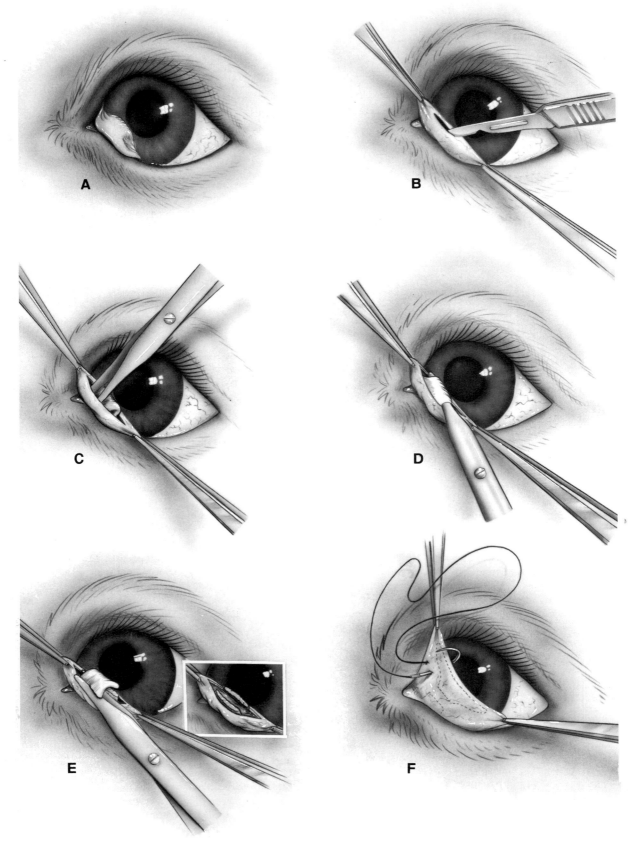

FIGURE 9–5 *See legend on opposite page*

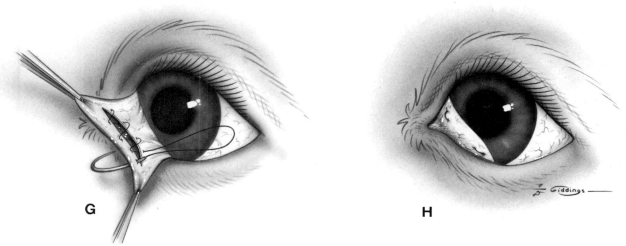

FIGURE 9–5. Treatment of eversion of the third eyelid. A, Eversion of the third eyelid. B, The cartilage is immobilized with fixation forceps, and a superficial incision is made through the bulbar conjunctiva covering the deformed cartilage. C, The bulbar and palpebral conjunctiva are carefully dissected from the deformed cartilage with strabismus scissors (rounded tips). D and E, The scissors are placed under the cartilage, and the deformed piece is removed. Care is taken to avoid puncturing the palpebral conjunctiva. F, The deformed cartilage has been removed. The incision is sutured with 6/0 absorbable suture, with the knot tied on the outside to prevent corneal abrasion. G, A simple continuous pattern is used. H, The suture is passed through to the palpebral surface and the knot tied.

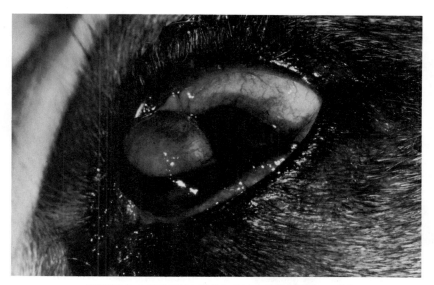

FIGURE 9–6. Protrusion of the gland of the third eyelid.

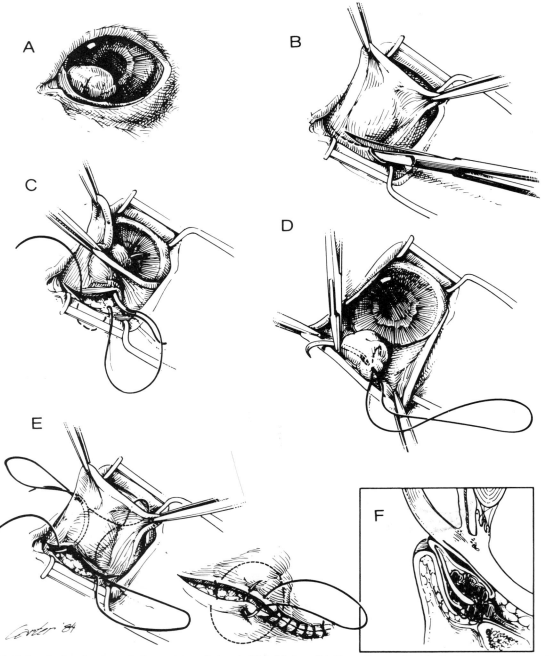

FIGURE 9–7. Surgical replacement of a prolapsed gland of the third eyelid. (From Kaswan RL, Martin CL: Surgical correction of third eyelid prolapse in dogs. J Am Vet Med Assoc 186:83, 1985.)

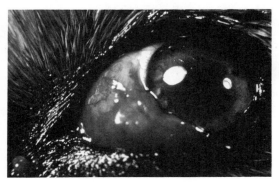

FIGURE 9–8. Squamous cell carcinoma of the third eyelid in an 8-year-old saluki. The lesion did not recur after surgical removal, as in Figure 9–9, and treatment with beta radiation. (Patient referred by Dr. Richard Glassburg.)

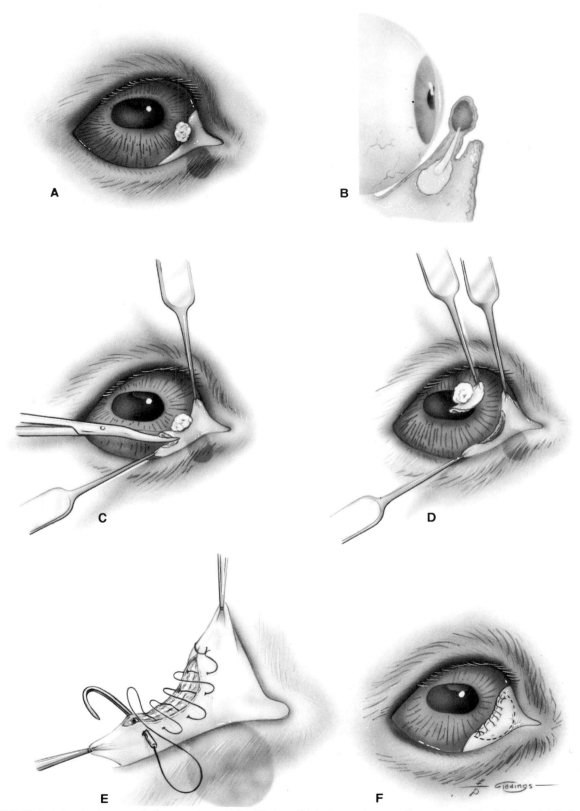

FIGURE 9–9. Surgical removal of a neoplasm of the third eyelid. A, A neoplasm on the margin of the third eyelid. B, Cross-section of (A) showing relative positions of the neoplasm and the gland of the third eyelid. C and D, The membrane is grasped with fixation forceps, and the mass plus a 2 mm margin is removed with strabismus scissors. E, The bulbar and palpebral portions of the conjunctiva are sutured over the edge of the cartilage with 6/0 absorbable suture. F, The edge after suturing is completed. The area for radiotherapy is outlined. (Modified from Severin GA: Veterinary Ophthalmology Notes, 2nd ed. Ft Collins, CO, 1976.)

3. Hyperthermia may be used for surface lesions not involving the cartilage of the third eyelid.

TRAUMA TO THE THIRD EYELID

Traumatic injuries to the third eyelid occur as a result of fights, foreign body penetration, and surgical intervention. Conjunctival tears only do not require suturing. If the membrane is perforated, the bulbar and palpebral conjunctiva are sutured, with the knots remaining on the bulbar surface (Fig. 9–10). In severe injuries when some of the membrane must be removed, the surrounding bulbar and palpebral conjunctiva overlying the third eyelid are mobilized and sutured to the edge of the third eyelid (Fig. 9–11). Although some retraction takes place during healing, a functional third eyelid can often be retained.

Whenever the third eyelid is damaged, surgically or otherwise, an attempt is made to retain or reconstruct a functional membrane and margin. The oral mucous membrane grafting technique of Kuhns (1977) is useful for replacing previously excised third eyelids. In the author's experience, a graft survival rate of about 60% may be expected.

FOLLICULAR CONJUNCTIVITIS[1]

Conjunctivitis with follicles on either the palpebral or bulbar surface of the third eyelid has been discussed as a conjunctival disorder.

MISCELLANEOUS DISORDERS

Habronemiasis

Nodules of habronemiasis occur occasionally on the palpebral surface of the third eyelid of horses, especially near the medial canthus. Lesions are more common on the lids.

---

1. See Chap 8.

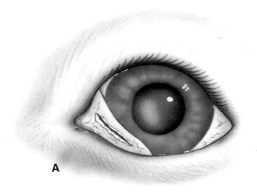
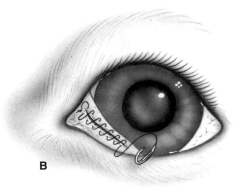
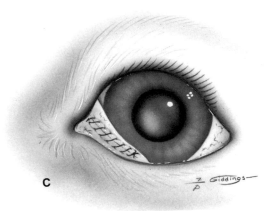

FIGURE 9–10. Suturing a tear in the third eyelid.

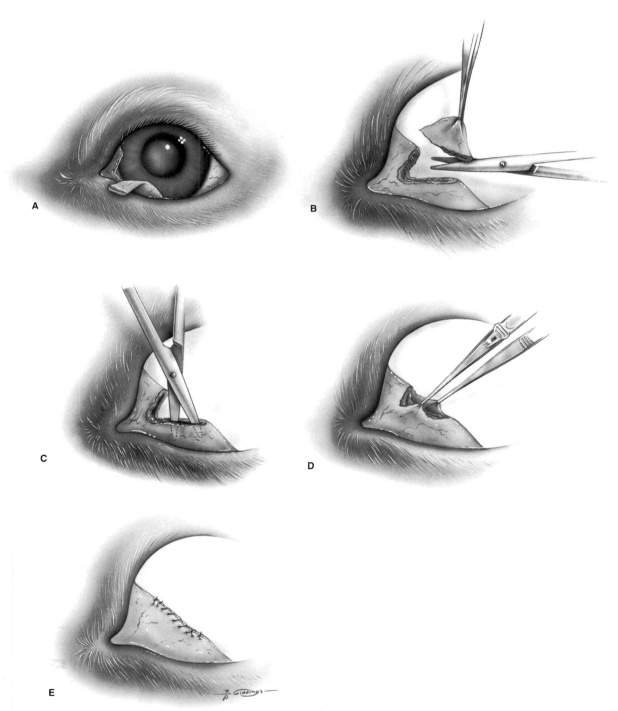

FIGURE 9–11. Repair of a severely torn third eyelid. A, Torn third eyelid. B, The traumatized piece is removed. C, The bulbar and palpebral conjunctiva are mobilized with strabismus scissors. D, The mobilized conjunctiva is drawn up. E, The mobilized conjunctiva is sutured with continuous 6/0 absorbable suture, with the knots tied on the external surface.

Eosinophilic Nodules in Horses

Circumscribed, red nodules consisting of an almost pure population of eosinophils with scattered macrophages occur on the third eyelid of horses in tropical and subtropical areas. Parasites have not been demonstrated on histological section. The lesions do not recur after excision, and the etiology is unknown.

Conjunctival Third Eyelid Thickening

Thickening of the conjunctiva of the third eyelid may be seen in the proliferative keratoconjunctivitis syndrome in collies, and chronic immune-mediated keratoconjunctivitis of Überreiter, and as a result of solar irritation in nonpigmented membranes in horses and dogs.

Protrusion of the Third Eyelid

Protrusion of the third eyelid may be seen in Horner's syndrome (see Chap 17), and in feline third eyelid protrusion syndrome (Chap 17).

The techniques for forming third eyelid flaps are discussed in Chapter 6.

REFERENCES

Blogg JR (1979): Surgical replacement of a prolapsed gland of the third eyelid ("cherry eye")—A new technique. Aust Vet Pract 9:75.

Buykmichi N (1975): Fibrosarcoma of the third eyelid in a cat. J Am Vet Med Assoc 167:934.

Crafts GA, Pulley LT (1975): Generalized cutaneous mast cell tumor in a cat. Feline Pract 5:57.

Evans HE, Christensen GC (1979): Miller's Anatomy of the Dog, 2nd ed. WB Saunders Co, Philadelphia.

Kaswan RL, Martin CL (1985): Surgical correction of third eyelid prolapse in dogs. J Am Vet Med Assoc 186:83.

Kuhns EL (1977): Oral mucosal grafts for membrana nictitans replacement. Mod Vet Pract 58:768.

Martin CL (1970): Everted membrane nictitans in German short-haired pointers. J Am Vet Med Assoc 157:1229.

Severin GA (1976): Veterinary Ophthalmology Notes. 2nd ed. Fort Collins, CO.

Lacrimal System

10

ANATOMY AND PHYSIOLOGY
DISTURBANCES OF LACRIMAL
FUNCTION
NEOPLASIA

ANATOMY AND PHYSIOLOGY

The lacrimal system consists of
1. Lacrimal gland and gland of the third eyelid
2. Accessory lacrimal glands
3. Precorneal tear film (PTF)
4. Mucous threads
5. Lacrimal puncta and canaliculi (Fig. 10–1)
6. Nasolacrimal duct (Fig. 10–2)
7. Nasal puncta

LACRIMAL GLAND AND GLAND OF THE THIRD EYELID

The gland of the third eyelid lies on the inner surface of the third eyelid (see Chap 9). The lacrimal gland is flattened and tubuloalveolar and lies over the supero-temporal part of the globe (Fig. 10–3). In the dog it lies beneath the ORBITAL LIGAMENT and supraorbital process of the frontal bone and is related to the medial surface of the zygomatic bone (Fig. 10–4). The position is similar in species with a fully enclosed bony orbit.

Lacrimal secretions enter the superior conjunctival fornix via numerous microscopic ducts. The PRECORNEAL TEAR FILM (PTF) moves across the cornea by the effects of blinking and movement of the third eyelid, with removal via the LACRIMAL PUNCTA.

ACCESSORY LACRIMAL GLANDS (Fig. 10–5)

The accessory lacrimal glands, which are near the lid margins and contribute to the PTF, are
1. Tarsal glands
2. Glands of Moll (modified sweat glands)
3. Glands of Zeis (modified sebaceous glands associated with the cilia)

PTF

The PTF covers the cornea and conjunctiva (Fig. 10–6). It consists of three layers, differing in composition, and is about 7 μ thick. The MIDDLE or AQUEOUS LAYER, consisting predominantly of water derived from the lacrimal gland and gland of the third eyelid, serves
1. To flush foreign material from the conjunctival sac
2. To lubricate the passage of lids and third eyelid over the cornea
3. To provide a medium for the transference of atmospheric oxygen, inflammatory cells (attracted by chemotactic influences during inflammation), and antibodies (IgA) to the cornea
4. To give a smooth surface to the cornea for optimal optical efficiency

The OUTER SUPERFICIAL LAYER is composed of oily materials and phospholipids from the tarsal glands and the glands of Zeis along the lid margin. It has two functions:
1. To limit evaporation of the aqueous layer
2. To bind the PTF to the cornea at the lid margins and prevent overflow by its high surface tension

Drugs containing preservatives with detergent properties and commercial shampoos remove this layer and cause severe corneal drying and focal ulceration in brachycephalic breeds.

The INNER MUCOID LAYER consists of mucoproteins derived from the conjunctival goblet cells. Because of the hydrophilic, lipophobic nature of the aqueous layer, a medium is necessary to bind the PTF to the corneal surface, which, in contrast, is lipophilic and hydrophobic. The mucoprotein molecules are thought to be bipolar, with one end lipophilic (associated with the corneal epithelium) and one end hydrophilic (associated with the aqueous layer). The mucoid layer binds the aqueous layer to the cornea.

MUCOUS THREADS

The mucous threads lie in the superior and inferior conjunctival fornices and are accumulations of mucus from the goblet cells. The threads migrate nasally in a

237

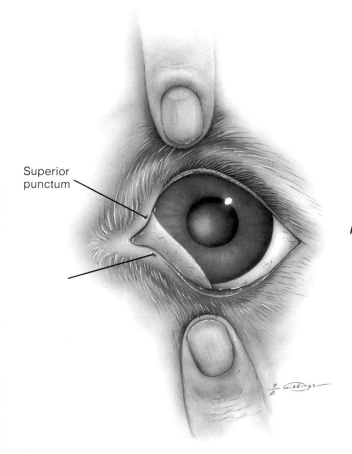

Superior
punctum

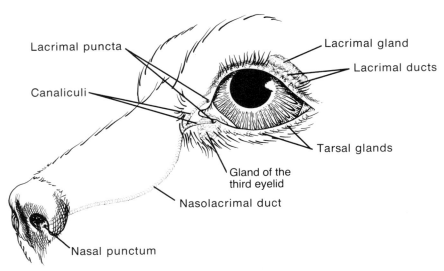

FIGURE 10–1. The superior and inferior lacrimal puncta.

Lacrimal puncta

Canaliculi

Lacrimal gland

Lacrimal ducts

Tarsal glands

Gland of the
third eyelid

Nasolacrimal duct

Nasal punctum

FIGURE 10–2. Components of the nasolacrimal system.

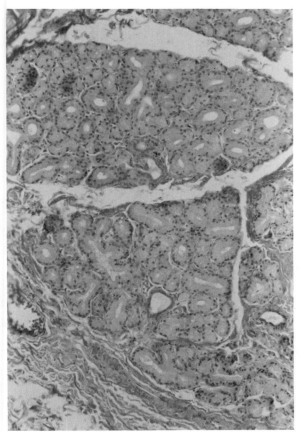

FIGURE 10–3. Tubuloalveolar structure of the canine lacrimal gland.

predictable fashion, collecting debris from the conjunctival sac. Vacuoles within the threads contain debris and exhibit enzymatic activity. Dehydrated remnants of these threads are frequently found on the skin at the nasal canthus in the morning ("sleep" or "sleepy seeds"). These accumulations are normally grayish and translucent and may be quite large in animals with deep conjunctival fornices (e.g., Irish setters, Doberman pinschers). Without signs of conjunctival inflammation or epiphora, larger accumulations are normal if they are grayish or translucent. Increased quantities are often a sensitive indicator of early inflammation, e.g., recurrence of allergic conjunctivitis or keratoconjunctivitis sicca (KCS). If objectionable to owners, normal accumulations may be removed daily with cotton. Change in color of the mucous thread to green or yellow is a reliable indicator of the presence of inflammatory cells and mandates a careful clinical examination.

Accumulations of normal mucus are frequently mistaken by owners for signs of ocular disease. Yellowish or green mucus,

however, is a sign of inflammatory cells in the mucus.

LACRIMAL PUNCTA, CANALICULI, NASOLACRIMAL DUCT, AND NASAL PUNCTA

The INFERIOR and SUPERIOR PUNCTA lie on the inner conjunctival surface of the eyelids, near the nasal limit of the tarsal glands (see Fig. 10–2).

The LACRIMAL CANALICULI (SUPERIOR and INFERIOR) lead to a variable dilatation in the common nasolacrimal duct—the LACRIMAL SAC. The lacrimal sac varies in size; in some animals it is only a slight dilatation in the duct. The sac lies within a depression in the lacrimal bone called the LACRIMAL FOSSA (Fig. 10–7).

From the lacrimal sac, the NASOLACRIMAL DUCT passes via a canal on the medial surface of the maxilla to open in the nasal cavity (Fig. 10–8). In dogs the opening is ventrolateral near the attached margin of the alar fold; in horses it is ventral on the mucocutaneous junction; and in cattle it is more lateral. In cattle and horses the nasal opening is readily visible and can be cannulated, but in the dog it can be seen only after exposure with a speculum or other suitable instrument. In the dog the nasolacrimal duct frequently has an opening into the nasal cavity between the lacrimal sac and the nasal opening, although the remainder of the duct is intact.

Approximately 25% of the PTF is lost by evaporation. The remainder passes into the puncta and via the canaliculi, sac, and duct to the nasal cavity. A large proportion of the PTF accumulates in the inferior fornix as the LACRIMAL LAKE. Most of this fluid enters the inferior punctum by capillary attraction and by movements of the lids. During contraction of the orbicularis oculi, the wall of the sac is tensed, creating a lower pressure within the lumen and causing tears to enter. This mechanism is called the LACRIMAL PUMP.

Innervation

Innervation of the lacrimal gland and control of secretion are complex, and the exact details are undetermined in domestic animals. Fibers from the ophthalmic division of the trigeminal nerve, facial nerve, and pterygopalatine ganglion, and sympathetic fibers from the carotid plexus have been traced to the lacrimal gland.

DISTURBANCES OF LACRIMAL FUNCTION

There are two categories of lacrimal dysfunction.
1. Failure to produce a normal PTF (or one of its

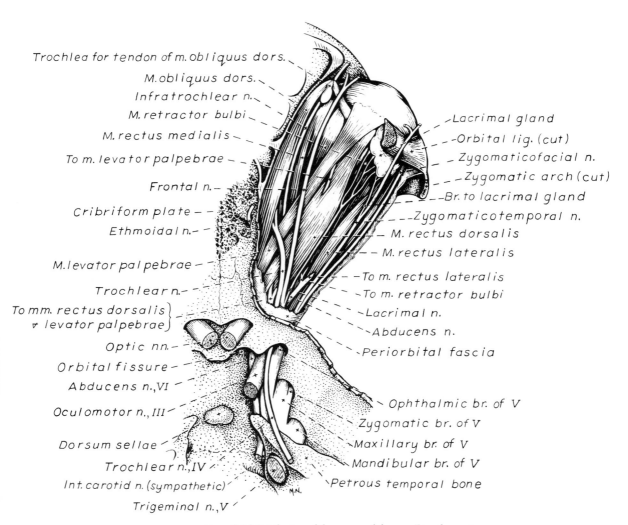

Trochlea for tendon of m. obliquus dors.
M. obliquus dors.
Infratrochlear n.
M. retractor bulbi
M. rectus medialis
To m. levator palpebrae
Frontal n.
Cribriform plate
Ethmoidal n.
M. levator palpebrae
Trochlear n.
To mm. rectus dorsalis ꝶ levator palpebrae
Optic nn.
Orbital fissure
Abducens n., VI
Oculomotor n., III
Dorsum sellae
Trochlear n., IV
Int. carotid n. (sympathetic)
Trigeminal n., V

Lacrimal gland
Orbital lig. (cut)
Zygomaticofacial n.
Zygomatic arch (cut)
Br. to lacrimal gland
Zygomaticotemporal n.
M. rectus dorsalis
M. rectus lateralis
To m. rectus lateralis
To m. retractor bulbi
Lacrimal n.
Abducens n.
Periorbital fascia
Ophthalmic br. of V
Zygomatic br. of V
Maxillary br. of V
Mandibular br. of V
Petrous temporal bone

Superficial distribution of the nerves of the eye. Dorsal aspect.

FIGURE 10–4. Superficial distribution of the nerves of the canine eye. Dorsal aspect. Note the position of the lacrimal gland beneath the orbital ligament. (From Evans HE, Christensen GC: Miller's Anatomy of the Dog, 2nd ed. WB Saunders Co, Philadelphia, 1979. © Cornell University 1964.)

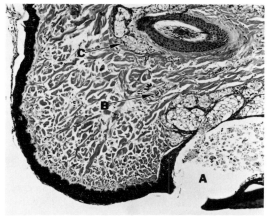

FIGURE 10–5. *The accessory lacrimal glands of the lid margin: (A) tarsal gland duct; (B) glands of Moll; (C) glands of Zeis.*

components), usually resulting in secondary conjunctivitis and keratitis.

2. Inability of the drainage system to remove the tears produced. This may be caused either by *obstruction* of the drainage system or by *overproduction* of tears. The clinical signs depend on the relative amounts of tears produced and drained away.

Examination

The techniques for examination of lacrimal disorders have been discussed in Chapter 5. The reader is referred to the following specific tests:

Schirmer tear test
Fluorescein passage test
Nasolacrimal cannulation and flushing
Dacryocystorhinography
Rose bengal stain

The fluorescein passage test is reliable only when positive. Because of communications between the nasolacrimal duct and the nasal cavity, false-negative results occur, although the duct is patent.

Disorders Characterized by Epiphora

Obstruction of the nasolacrimal duct is distinguished from reflex lacrimation and overproduction due to chronic irritation of the cornea or conjunctiva.

CONGENITAL ATRESIA, ECTOPIA, AND IMPERFORATE PUNCTA

In dogs imperforate puncta are not uncommon. The condition is congenital and is characterized by epiphora (diagnosed by inability to cannulate or probe the puncta with a lacrimal cannula or fine nylon thread). Detailed examination under general anesthesia with the operating microscope is advisable. In most cases obstruction consists of a layer of conjunctiva over the lumen, but occasionally obstructions are present in other parts of the nasolacrimal duct. The overlying conjunctiva may be removed by elevating it with liquid under pressure (Fig. 10–9) or by retrograde probing with fine nylon (2/0) from the nasal opening (Fig. 10–10).

In foals, the nasal meatus may be covered with mucosa, or additional or abnormally positioned openings may be present. The lumen of the duct is distended with saline solution via the lacrimal puncta or with a plastic cannula, and the mucosa is dissected off until the lumen is entered. The meatus is cannulated with plastic tubing, which is sutured in place for 7–10 days. Daily application of a topical antibiotic-corticosteroid preparation is advisable for 3–4 days after removal of the tube. A variety of diverse congenital anomalies of the nasolacrimal duct occur in all species, but all are rare.

In young cats, the most common cause of apparent congenital lacrimal obstruction is cicatrization due to *Herpesvirus felis* infection during severe viral rhinotracheitis.

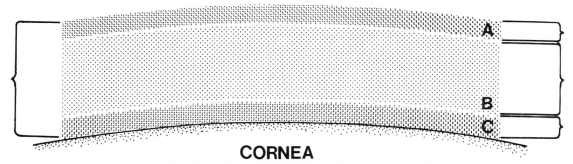

CORNEA
FIGURE 10–6. *Precorneal tear film. A, Superficial lipid layer. B, Aqueous layer. C, Inner mucoid layer.*

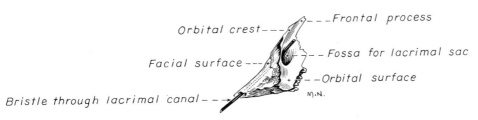

FIGURE 10–7. Left canine lacrimal bone. Lateral aspect, showing lacrimal fossa. (From Evans HE, Christensen GC: Miller's Anatomy of the Dog, 2nd ed. WB Saunders Co, Philadelphia, 1979. © Cornell University 1964.)

DACRYOCYSTITIS

Dacryocystitis is inflammation within the lacrimal sac and nasolacrimal duct. It occurs most frequently in dogs and cats and less frequently in horses. Although foreign bodies (e.g., grass awns and concretions of mucopurulent material) can often be expressed, the primary cause is usually unknown. The infected focus within the proximal portion of the duct may reinfect the conjunctival sac, resulting in chronic unilateral conjunctivitis of unexplained etiology.

Chronic dacryocystitis may cause recurrent unilateral conjunctivitis with no other apparent clinical signs.

Clinical Signs

1. Thick mucopurulent exudate at the medial canthus. The exudate may have layers of purulent and clear material or gas bubbles within it.
2. Mild conjunctivitis.
3. Epiphora.
4. Expression of mucopurulent material from a punctum as a result of flushing of the punctum or manipulation of the nasal canthus. This area is often painful to the touch or, in other cases, totally painless.
5. Painful, erythematous dermatitis at the medial canthus in some cases.
6. Abscessation of the sac in severe cases. In chronic cases, this abscessation may cause a large cavity to form.
7. History of recurrent unilateral conjunctivitis with temporary responses to topical antibiotics and attempted flushing.

Diagnosis

Diagnosis is based on clinical signs, especially expression of purulent material from the puncta. The exact site of the obstruction may be determined by either cannulation or dacryocystorhinography.

Treatment

Passage of a Nasolacrimal Catheter

Because of the tendency for dacryocystitis to recur, definitive surgical catheterization (Fig. 10–11) is indicated. Although daily flushing and topical medication are effective in some cases, they are less reliable and there is a greater chance of recurrence. The tube is left in place for 2–3 weeks. The inserted tubes rarely cause patient discomfort unless they become loose. For the first few days the uncannulated punctum is flushed daily with an antibiotic solution, and a topical anti-

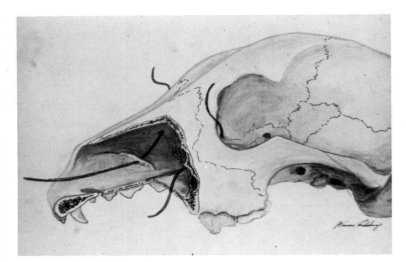

FIGURE 10–8. Cutaway drawing of canine skull, showing the lacrimal fossa, lacrimal foramen, and relative position of the nasolacrimal duct. (From Severin GA: Veterinary Ophthalmology Notes, 2nd ed. Ft Collins, CO, 1976.)

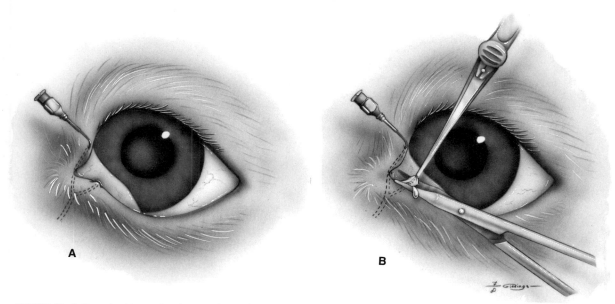

A

B

FIGURE 10–9. Repair of imperforate punctum using pressurized fluid. A, The opposing punctum is cannulated, and pressure is applied via a saline solution–filled syringe to elevate the obstructing conjunctiva over the other punctum. The use of methylene blue solution aids location of the bleb. Some loss of saline solution occurs down the nasolacrimal duct. B, The tissue is grasped with fine forceps and incised with strabismus scissors. Antibiotic-corticosteroid preparations are applied in order to prevent scarring and obstruction for 7–10 days. Daily dilatation and flushing may be necessary for a few days in order to prevent closure.

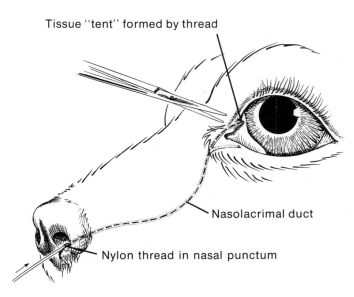

Tissue "tent" formed by thread

Nasolacrimal duct

Nylon thread in nasal punctum

FIGURE 10–10. Retrograde probing of imperforate punctum. The nasal meatus of the nasolacrimal duct is probed, using nylon (2/0). The probe is passed up in order to elevate the obstructing conjunctiva, which is excised. This procedure is most useful for the superior punctum, as it is more difficult to pass a probe into the inferior punctum from the nasal end.

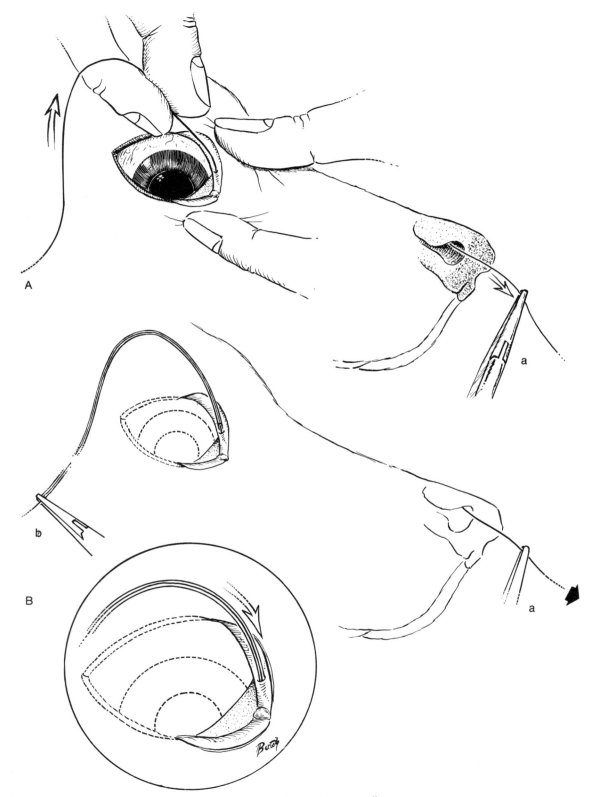

A

B

FIGURE 10–11 See legend on opposite page

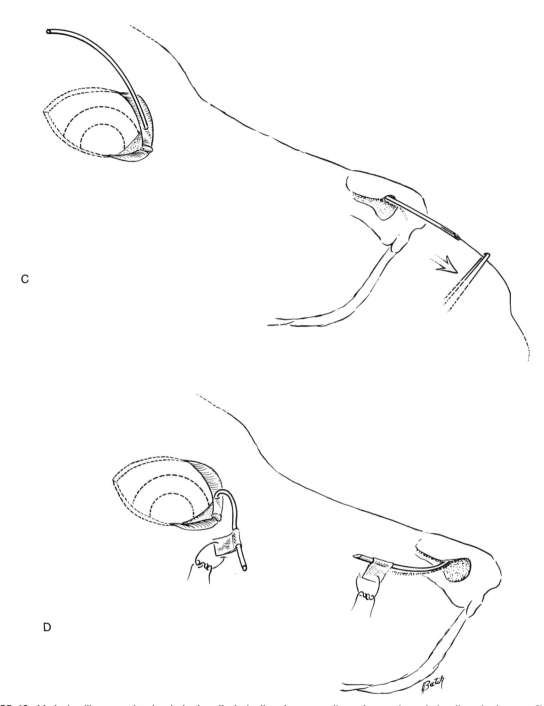

C

D

FIGURE 10–11. *Indwelling nasolacrimal duct catheterization for correction of recurring obstruction. A, A monofilament nylon thread (2/0 with a smooth melted end) is passed via the superior punctum to emerge from the nose. If an obstruction is present in the sac, the duct is threaded from the nasal end and the thread is manipulated to emerge from the superior punctum. B, Fine polyethylene (PE90) or polyvinyl tubing with a beveled end is passed over the thread. Halsted's forceps are clamped behind the tubing, which is pulled from the nasal end by forceps on the thread. In horses larger tubing is used. C, Care is taken as the tubing enters the punctum. Note: The inferior punctum may also be used if threading via this punctum is used. The tubing is pulled down the nasolacrimal duct, past any obstructions. D, The tube is sutured in place for 2–3 weeks. Although rarely necessary, protective collars will prevent mutilation by the patient. (From Bistner SI, et al: Atlas of Veterinary Ophthalmic Surgery. WB Saunders Co, Philadelphia, 1977.)*

biotic is used. If abscessation of the sac or severe dermatitis is present, systemic and skin antibiotics are added.

Dacryocystotomy

For patients in which a catheter cannot be passed owing to the obstruction, the lacrimal sac may be exposed ab externo, through an incision parallel to the lower lid, followed by removal of the outer surface of the lacrimal bone with a Hall surgairtome over the sac, flushing of the sac, and placement of the catheter. In some chronically affected animals, a cavity may develop in the region of the sac. If the catheter is left in place, and antibiotic therapy is continued, the space usually fills with fibrous tissue and a patent duct remains. This may take several months.

CICATRICIAL NASOLACRIMAL DUCT OBSTRUCTION

In cats, especially kittens, after severe upper respiratory tract viral infections, scarring and blockage of the nasolacrimal ducts and puncta are not uncommon. If the puncta and ducts cannot be cannulated, conjunctivorhinostomy or drainage procedures to the oral cavity (conjunctivobuccostomy) are the only remedy, except for removal of a portion of the gland of the third eyelid, which risks inducing keratoconjunctivitis sicca (KCS). Conjunctivorhinostomy and conjunctivobuccostomy are usually performed by a veterinary ophthalmologist, in animals without evidence of active conjunctivitis or chronic respiratory disease.

If recurrent respiratory disease is present, serological tests for feline leukemia virus and a careful examination for evidence of herpetic keratitis are performed. Recurrent upper respiratory tract infection and keratitis with occasional sinusitis are common in Siamese and Abyssinian cats.

Treatment

Conjunctivorhinostomy

In conjunctivorhinostomy a communication is made from the medial conjunctival sac to the nasal cavity, and it is kept open with a stent of plastic tubing until healed (Fig. 10–12). The method is most suitable for dogs lacking lacrimal drainage, but it can be used in cats. In cats the opening tends to become obstructed with scar tissue, and the stent is left in longer (8–12 weeks) before initial removal. During the postoperative period the patient is maintained on topical antibiotics, and the stent is cleaned frequently. During this postoperative period, the eye is checked weekly if possible, to ensure the stent is not causing ocular irritation, e.g., by pressing on the cornea through the third eyelid.

Conjunctivobuccostomy

Conjunctivobuccostomy is an alternative method of providing lacrimal drainage (Fig. 10–13).

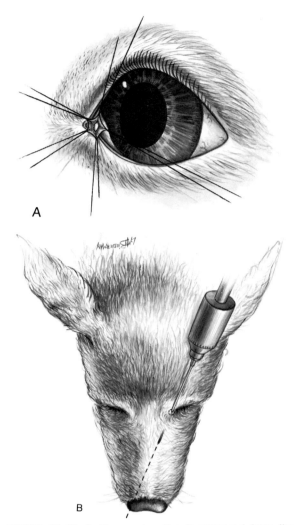

FIGURE 10–12. A, The conjunctiva is removed from the inferior nasal area overlying the lacrimal bone. B, A communication is made from the conjunctival sac to the nasal cavity with a Steinmann orthopedic pin. The pin is directed toward the contralateral external nares but is advanced only until it enters the nasal cavity.

TEAR-STAINING SYNDROME IN DOGS

The miniature and toy poodles and the Maltese terrier are most commonly affected (Fig. 10–14). The hair and skin around the medial canthus are stained brown from constant epiphora. The staining is believed to be due to lactoferrin-like pigments in the overflowing tears. Epiphora may result from folds of conjunctiva that prevent entry of tears into the puncta (Bistner et al, 1977). The condition is usually present from birth. Although generally it is a cosmetic defect, it may progress, causing local dermatitis. Although conjunctivitis and tonsillitis are occasionally present with the tear staining, this is not the rule. Some patients also have allergic conjunctivitis.

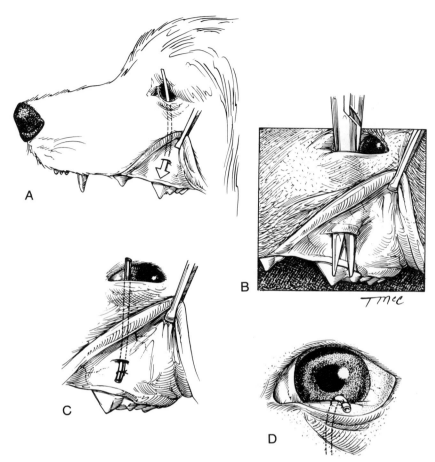

FIGURE 10–13. Conjunctivobuccostomy. A, Direction of the final drainage canal. B, A canal is made from the inferior conjunctival fornix to the oral cavity with straight hemostats. C, A tube is passed and sutured to the oral mucosa. D, The upper end of the tube is sutured to the skin in the region of the nasal canthus so as not to rub on the cornea. The tube is left in place for a minimum of 2 months. (From Lavach JD: Lacrimal system. In Slatter DH [ed]: Textbook of Small Animal Surgery. WB Saunders Co, Philadelphia, 1985.)

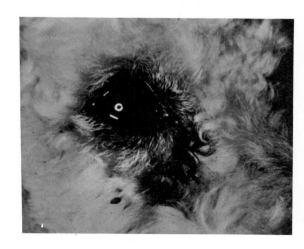

FIGURE 10–14. Chronic tear-staining syndrome in a miniature poodle.

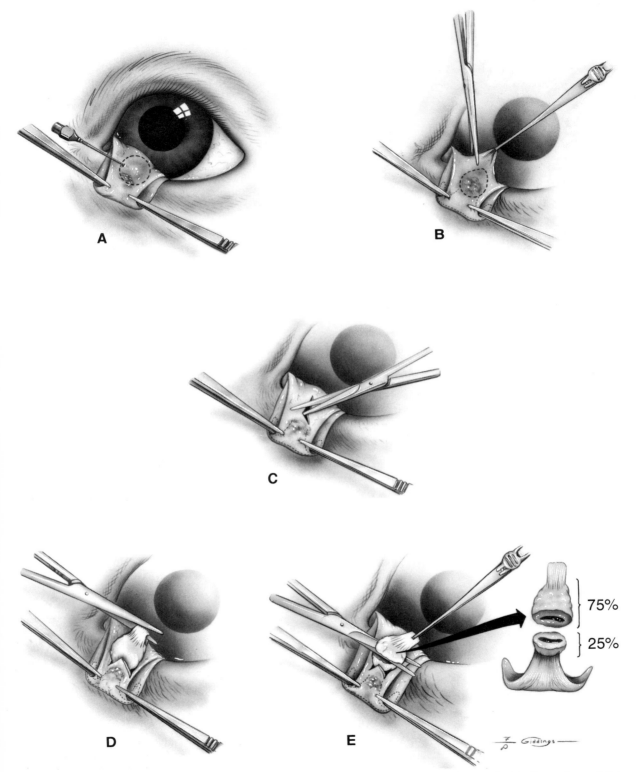

FIGURE 10–15. *Partial removal of the gland of the third eyelid.* A, *Fixation forceps are applied to the edges of the cartilaginous T portion of the third eyelid.* B, *The gland is exposed by traction, and 0.25 ml of 1:10,000 epinephrine solution is injected subconjunctivally for hemostasis (avoid with halothane anesthesia).* C, *With strabismus scissors, the conjunctiva is incised at the base of the gland.* D, *The gland is exposed by blunt subconjunctival dissection.* E, *Sixty to 75% of the gland is removed. (Redrawn from Severin GA: Veterinary Ophthalmology Notes, 2nd ed. Ft Collins, CO, 1976.)*

Treatment

1. Partial removal of the gland of the third eyelid results in permanent improvement (Fig. 10–15). As this procedure permanently removes a portion of the tear production mechanism, it is performed only if Schirmer readings exceed 14 mm/min, to avoid causing KCS. This procedure is not used indiscriminately as a substitute for full ophthalmic investigation of epiphora.

2. Oral tetracycline, 5 mg/kg once daily, provides definite short-term improvement. Staining normally reappears 2–3 weeks after cessation of therapy. The mode of action of tetracyclines in preventing tear staining is unknown, but there is no toxic effect on the lacrimal gland or gland of the third eyelid, and Schirmer values are unaltered.

OTHER CAUSES OF EPIPHORA

Other causes of epiphora include:
1. Prominent nasal folds
2. Entropion
3. Cilia disorders
4. Allergic inhalant dermatitis and conjunctivitis

Epiphora also occurs frequently in brachycephalic Persian cats. Treatment is the same as for canine tear-staining syndrome.

Deficiency of PTF

Deficiency of the aqueous phase is most frequent, but lipid or mucoid layers may also be reduced. A deficiency of the mucoid layer occurs in dogs, resulting in dry corneas with irregular surfaces but with normal or slightly subnormal Schirmer values above 10 mm/min. Defects in the PTF are visible biomicroscopically. This condition is treated with synthetic mucin-like drugs (polyvinylpyrrolidone).[1]

Deficiency of the aqueous phase of the PTF is a common disorder in dogs that occurs occasionally in cats and horses and leads to xerosis (abnormal dryness) and KCS. Failure of secretion is distinguished from deficiencies of the aqueous phase associated with Addison's disease (hypoadrenocorticism), congenital open eyelids (increased evaporation), failure of the eyelids to close (increased evaporation) as in facial paralysis and exophthalmos, and neurotrophic keratitis (decreased secretion due to interruption of the trigeminal reflex arc).

KCS

Etiology

1. Drug-induced. Phenazopyridine and sulfadiazine have caused KCS in dogs. Phenazopyridine, a urinary

analgesic, causes KCS after 7–10 days in most dogs, but not in cats. Long-term administration (3–4 months) of sulfadiazine is necessary before KCS occurs, and then only in a proportion of dosed animals. Older animals are more susceptible to permanent lacrimal gland damage by sulfadiazine. Other sulphonamides, e.g., sulfasalazine (used for chronic colitis in dogs), also cause KCS in dogs, but not all drugs of the group do so. 5-amino salicylic acid (5-ASA), a derivative of sulfasalazine, is the active constituent in the treatment of colitis and also causes KCS in dogs. It is also available as an independent drug. Neither sulfasalazine nor 5-ASA is approved for use in dogs.

2. Surgically-induced. KCS results clinically from removal of prolapsed glands of the third eyelid and experimentally from removal of both glands of the third eyelid and lacrimal glands.

3. Idiopathic. The majority of cases are in this category, both in dogs and in the infrequent affected cat. Electron microscopic studies on the lacrimal gland and gland of the third eyelid of a 9-year-old cocker spaniel with untreated KCS of 3 years' duration and a concurrent fatal tonsillar squamous cell carcinoma revealed reduced numbers of cytoplasmic secretory granules of the glandular cells in both glands, without autoimmune involvement, indicating that senile atrophy of the glands is one cause of this group.

4. Autoimmune. The etiology in up to 30% of idiopathic cases may be associated with autoimmune destruction of the lacrimal gland and gland of the third eyelid, as such glands show infiltration with lymphocytes, and serological evidence is suggestive. As in humans, animals with KCS may also be affected with a variety of autoimmune-related disorders, including xerostomia (salivary gland involvement), hypothyroidism, diabetes mellitus, polymyositis and polyarthritis, chronic generalized and interdigital pyoderma, glomerulonephritis, and ulcerative colitis. It is probable that some of this observed adenitis is caused by the KCS with ascending infection via the excretory ducts to the conjunctival sac.

5. Orbital and supraorbital trauma affecting the glands directly or via their nerve supply.

6. Canine distemper. Canine distemper virus affects the lacrimal gland and gland of the third eyelid and may result in temporary or permanent dysfunction.

7. Locoweed poisoning in cattle, sheep, and horses.

8. Other causes. Numerous unproven causes have been proposed. Vitamin A deficiency does *not* cause clinical KCS in dogs as it does in humans.

KCS is a *common and important ocular disease* in dogs. It should be suspected whenever chronic conjunctivitis or keratitis is present.

---

1. Adsorbotear—Alcon, Ft Worth, TX.

Pathogenesis (Fig. 10–16)

Xerosis (dryness) causes a mucopurulent conjunctivitis with diffuse infiltration of subconjunctival tissues by neutrophils and lymphocytes. Initially, superficial followed by deep keratitis occurs with vascularization and mixed inflammatory cell infiltration of the corneal stroma. Ulceration and descemetocele formation are not uncommon. In chronic cases, pigmentation and keratinization of the cornea may occur (see Fig. 10–17). Staphylococcal infection of the conjunctiva, tarsal glands, and eyelids, sometimes with hypersensitivity, is frequent. Vascularization of the cornea usually occurs throughout 360°, an important differentiating feature from vascularization due to staphylococcal hypersensitivity, in which the superior half of the cornea is affected.

Breed Predisposition

KCS occurs more frequently in the Shih-Tzu, Lhasa apso, Pekingese, poodle, English bulldog, West Highland white terrier, cocker spaniel, and miniature schnauzer.

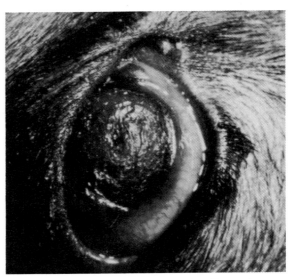

FIGURE 10–17. *Keratinization of the conjunctiva and cornea in a long-standing case of KCS in an aged terrier cross. (From Severin GA: Keratoconjunctivitis sicca. Vet Clin North Am 3:407, 1973.)*

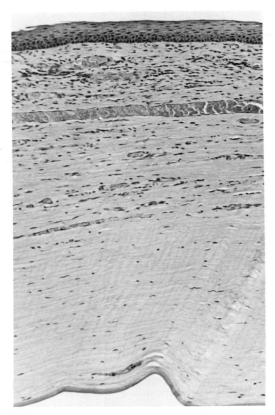

FIGURE 10–16. *Corneal section from an 8-year-old collie cross with chronic KCS. Note the superficial and deep vascularization and inflammatory infiltrate.*

Clinical Signs (Figs. 10–17 and 10–18)

The signs of KCS depend on whether the condition is bilateral or unilateral, acute or chronic, temporary or permanent.

1. Blepharospasm. Blepharospasm, accompanied by enophthalmos, is often the first sign, and it results from the pain and discomfort caused by deficiency of PTF.

2. Mucoid and mucopurulent discharge. When the aqueous phase of the PTF is absent, mucus accumulates and is not washed down the lacrimal system. The mucus differs from that in conjunctivitis; it is thick and stringy and adheres to the conjunctiva and cornea in ropy strands. As the KCS becomes chronic, a mucopurulent conjunctivitis occurs, with dried exudate present around the eyelid margins.

3. Corneal ulceration (Fig. 10–19). In severe or acute cases, epithelium is lost, especially in the center of the cornea. Mucopurulent material may adhere to the ulcer. Ulceration is revealed by fluorescein staining. In chronic cases, corneal perforation and endophthalmitis may occur.

4. Corneal vascularization and pigmentation. In chronic cases, superficial and deep corneal vascularization and pigmentation occur.

5. Dry, lusterless cornea and conjunctival erythema. The dry appearance of the cornea due to lack of PTF is characteristic.

6. Dry ipsilateral nostril. The nares and nostril are usually dry on the affected side.

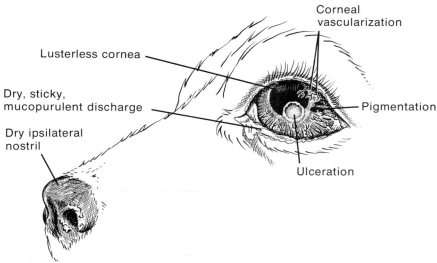

FIGURE 10–18. Clinical signs of KCS.

7. Chronic staphylococcal infection. Chronic infection, sometimes with hypersensitivity, often occurs, although not all such cases are due to KCS. KCS is included in the differential diagnosis of such cases until proved otherwise.

Intermittent KCS occurs occasionally, and frequent observations with Schirmer testing are necessary for diagnosis. In the author's experience, unilateral cases in dogs are more often intermittent. Many patients show fluctuations of Schirmer values above and below the normal lower limit of 10 mm/min. Clinical signs are more frequent at hot, dry times of the year when the values are near low-normal, and tear evaporation is greatest.

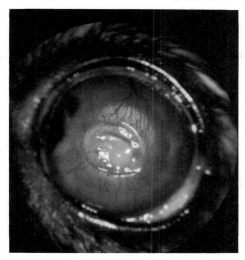

FIGURE 10–19. Corneal ulceration in KCS. This patient had been treated with a mixture of antibiotics and corticosteroids while the ulceration was present.

Diagnosis

The diagnosis of KCS is suggested by clinical signs and confirmed by the Schirmer tear test, and rose bengal staining if necessary. Normal, suspicious, and abnormal values are listed in Table 5–2. Rose bengal stains conjunctival cells and mucus a bright rose red when devitalized by xerosis. All patients with the disease should have a complete hematological and serum chemistry profile performed in order to evaluate systemic effects of concurrent autoimmune-related diseases such as diabetes mellitus, hypothyroidism, hypoadrenocorticism, polyarthritis and polymyositis, rheumatoid arthritis, and immune-mediated skin disorders.

Natural Course of the Disease

KCS caused by drugs, systemic diseases, and orbital and supraorbital trauma usually resolves spontaneously in 45–60 days. Some patients, however, do not recover. The majority of idiopathic cases do not improve without treatment, and often progress with painful and blinding results.

Failure by owners to treat adequately and consistently is a frequent cause of poor therapeutic results in KCS. The cost, convenience, aims, and alternatives for therapy must be discussed with the owner at the start of and throughout therapy.

Treatment

Both medical and surgical methods may be used. With consistent medication, most patients can be

TABLE 10–1. Constituents of Compound KCS Medication

Constituent	Amount
Gentamicin, parenteral solution	50 mg (usually 1 ml)
Acetylcysteine, 20% solution	6 ml
Pilocarpine, 2% solution	6 ml
Adsorbotear	6 ml

Modified from Severin GA: Veterinary Ophthalmology Notes, 2nd ed. Ft Collins, CO, 1976.

managed medically, but owners are often not able to administer medication as frequently as needed. The method of long-term treatment depends on the expected course of the disease and the owner's wishes. Medical treatment is initially used in all patients.

Medical Therapy

The aims of medical therapy are as follows:
1. Replacement of the PTF
   Agents: synthetic mucins,[2] artificial tears[2]
2. Stimulation of normal secretion
   Agent: pilocarpine
3. Control of secondary infection
   Agents: gentamicin, chloramphenicol succinate
4. Removal of excess mucus
   Agent: acetylcysteine[3]
5. Inhibition of collagenase in ulcerative corneal lesions
   Agent: acetylcysteine[3]
6. Presumed inhibition of immune mechanisms
   Agent: topical cyclosporine[4] (actual method of action unknown)

Agents 1–5 are conveniently mixed in one solution, which is stored in a stock bottle in the refrigerator by the client to prevent contamination (acetylcysteine is stable at room temperature for the normal storage periods involved). A 15-ml dropper bottle is maintained at room temperature and refilled periodically. Pilocarpine solutions containing polyvinyl alcohol as a base should *not* be used. As therapy progresses, individual constituents may be varied to suit the patient, but the formula given here should be used initially.

2. Adsorbotear—Alcon Laboratories, Ft Worth, TX.
3. Mucomyst—Mead Johnson Laboratories, Evansville, IN.
4. Sandimmune—Sandoz Pharmaceuticals, E Hanover, NJ. *Note:* Cyclosporine is not officially approved for ocular or veterinary use.

Failure of therapy with compound KCS medication is usually due to substitution of constituents by the compounder (Table 10–1) or to infrequent usage by the owner.

In individual animals, acetylcysteine may cause irritation; this is relieved by decreasing the concentration in the overall mixture. When choosing an artificial tear, preparations containing methylcellulose derivatives are preferable to those with polyvinyl alcohol, which is often irritating to canine patients. A broad-spectrum antibiotic, stable in aqueous solution, is included in the mixture. In the past, oral pilocarpine was used to stimulate tear production, but topical medication is more effective and lacks the systemic side effects of oral pilocarpine.

For the first 2 days, medication is administered hourly during the day, followed by every 2 hours for the next 2 days, then every 4 hours (Table 10–2). Cyclosporine may be added to the regimen once daily in the evening. The eye is washed each morning with a commercial eye wash, and lubricating ointment is placed in the eye at night. The patient is examined at 1 month, and the frequency of therapy may be decreased if Schirmer values are higher. Some patients require only 1–2 drops daily.

If severe ulceration is present, topical therapy is used for 2–3 days; if the ulcer does not improve, a third eyelid flap is applied and topical therapy continued for 10–14 days, by which time ulceration is usually resolved. Some patients require immediate surgical therapy if corneal rupture is imminent, and such high-risk patients are best referred to an ophthalmologist.

Once the patient is stabilized, intermittent topical dexamethasone may be used, e.g., twice daily for 1 week each month, to decrease accumulated scarring. The need for continuous steroid usage indicates failure of therapy. Patients should *not* be placed on continuous antibiotic-steroid mixtures.

After 30 days, Schirmer readings are reassessed and frequency of KCS medication altered if necessary. If the readings have not reached 10 mm/min, the original frequency is continued until 90 days. Eye lubricant and wash are continued as long as therapy is required. The exact place of cyclosporine in canine KCS therapy remains to be evaluated.

TABLE 10–2. Treatment Regimen for KCS

Day	Compound KCS Medication	Cyclosporine Drops	Sterile Eye Lubricant	Sterile Eye Wash
1 and 2	Hourly	SID* at night	SID* at night	BID†
3 and 4	Every 2 hours	SID* at night	SID* at night	BID†
4–30	QID‡	SID* at night	SID* at night	SID*–BID†

*SID = once a day.
†BID = twice a day.
‡QID = four times a day.

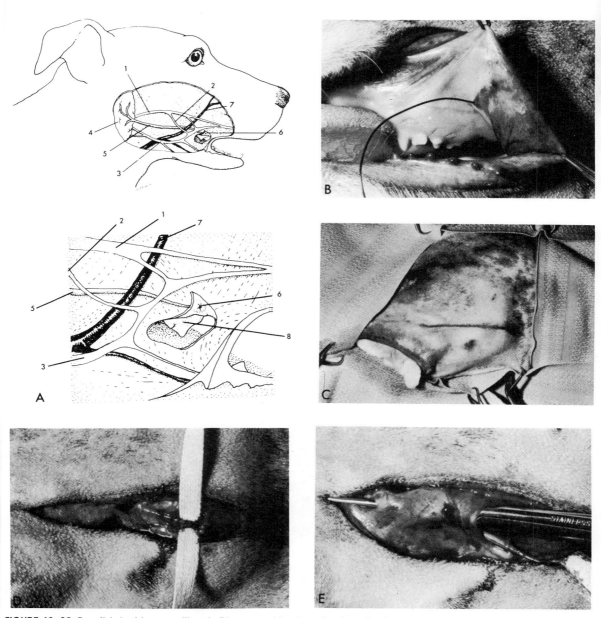

FIGURE 10–20. Parotid duct transposition. A, Diagram of the face (top) and enlargement of area where duct enters mouth (bottom). Dorsal buccal nerve (1); anastomosis of dorsal buccal and ventral buccal nerves (2); ventral buccal nerve (3); parotid salivary gland (4); parotid duct (5); papilla of parotid duct (6); facial vein (7); upper carnassial tooth (8). B, Monofilament nylon suture marker in place in the parotid duct. C, Cotton soaked with 1:750 aqueous benzalkonium chloride placed over the parotid duct papilla. The course of the duct is marked on the skin. D, Umbilical tape passed beneath parotid duct so that the duct can be manipulated without damaging it with forceps. E, Completed dissection beneath the facial vein and branches of buccal nerve with blunt scissors.

Illustration continued on following page

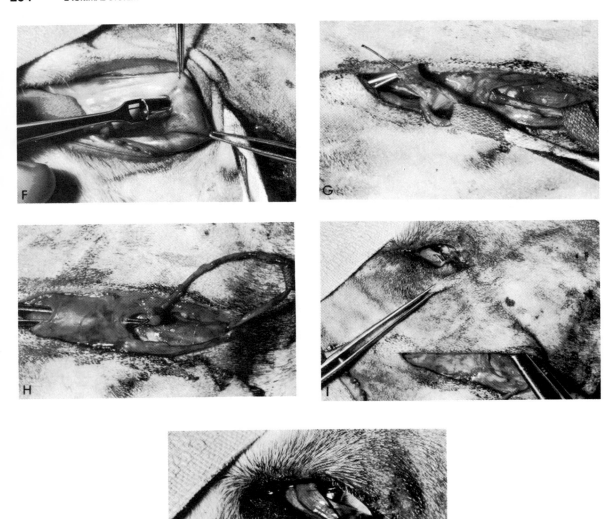

FIGURE 10–20 *Continued* F, *Position of biopsy punch to cut mucous membrane plug containing parotid papilla and duct. G, Pulling parotid duct and papilla into facial wound. H, Parotid duct dissected free to the angle of the mandible. I, Tunneling to the lower lateral fornix with blunt delicate scissors. J, Oral mucous membrane plug with parotid duct papilla positioned for suturing to the conjunctiva. (From Severin GA: Keratoconjunctivitis sicca. Vet Clin North Am 3:407, 1973.)*

A minimum of 3 months of medical therapy is desirable before considering surgical therapy, as some dogs regain tear production during this time. If surgical treatment is performed too early, epiphora may result when tear production returns, requiring surgical reversal. By the end of 3 months, the owner has often decided in favor of either medical or surgical treatment. For long-term medical treatment, acetylcysteine and antibiotics may be deleted or reduced from the regimen. For patients that fail to respond by increased tear production, or that develop sensitivity to pilocarpine, or for whose owners topical treatment is inconvenient, surgical therapy is a viable alternative.

Surgical Therapy

Parotid Duct Transposition

The parotid duct conducts saliva from the parotid gland to an oral papilla near the carnassial tooth. In this procedure the duct and papilla are mobilized and transferred to the conjunctival sac to provide substitute lubrication. The technique is technically demanding and requires precision and practice to be performed correctly.

Because of potential complications (occurring in 9–37% of cases, as reported by various authors) parotid duct transposition should be undertaken only by a competent surgeon experienced in the technique, and only after medical treatment has been evaluated for 3 months.

Before surgical intervention, function of the parotid gland and patency of the duct are confirmed by placing several drops of 1% atropine onto the oral mucosa and observing the papilla for secretion. (*Note:* 1 per cent atropine—a parasympatholytic agent—is bitter and acts as a sialagogue in these circumstances.) Under general anesthesia, the oral cavity is cleaned and packed with gauze soaked in povidone-iodine solution. The lateral surface of the face is prepared for surgery, and the parotid papilla is cannulated with 2/0 nylon (colored) with a smooth blunt end (Fig. 10–20A). This cannula facilitates later identification and manipulation of the duct. Because of a right-angle bend in the duct as it enters the papilla, perseverance may be necessary in order to effect cannulation. Grasping the papilla and moving it rostrally reduces the bend and makes passage of the nylon easier. Because of the incidence of complications, the "blind" subcutaneous approach should be avoided.

POSTOPERATIVE TREATMENT. Until a regular supply of parotid secretion is established, artificial tears (preferably those containing a synthetic mucin) and topical antibiotics are used 3–4 times daily. Small, regular amounts of food (e.g., a dry dog biscuit every hour or so at the owner's convenience) are used to aid in establishing a continuous supply of secretion until skin sutures are removed at 10 days.

OPERATIVE AND POSTOPERATIVE COMPLICATIONS. Postoperative subcutaneous edema is common for the first few days and can be limited by careful suturing of the oral mucosal incision to prevent saliva from entering the wound.

The most severe complication is severing the duct from the papilla. This results in scar formation and constriction around the junction with the conjunctiva. If the end of the duct is opened by incising along both sides for 2–2.5 mm, a wider opening with less chance of constriction can be obtained. Careless or traumatic handling of the duct with instruments results in cicatricial constriction and obstruction. Microsurgical resection and anastomosis of obstructions is possible but cannot be relied on to repair the results of poor surgical technique.

Accumulations of whitish crystalline material may occur on both the lid margins and the cornea. These accumulations cannot be prevented and are not painful, but they occasionally result in severe blepharoconjunctivitis and blepharospasm. They can be reduced by frequent applications of ethylenediaminetetra-acetic

acid (EDTA) drops. Irritation may be relieved with artificial tears when it is especially severe, but ligation of the parotid duct is rarely necessary. If glandular function returns after transposition, epiphora can result. This may be prevented in the majority of patients by adequate medical evaluation before surgery is attempted. If it should occur, ligation of the duct or retransposition to the mouth is curative.

NEOPLASIA

Neoplasms of the lacrimal gland are rare in dogs and are manifested as space-occupying lesions, which can be removed by suitable orbital approaches (see Chap 18). Lacrimal adenocarcinoma has a good prognosis if removed early while it is still localized. Conjunctival neoplasms may invade the nasolacrimal duct and spread to the nasal cavity (Fig. 7–41); likewise, neoplasms in the nasal cavity may invade the nasolacrimal duct. Space-occupying nasal lesions may obstruct the nasolacrimal duct, causing epiphora. Cryotherapy may be used near the lacrimal puncta and canaliculi, without causing permanent obstruction.

REFERENCES

Aguirre GD, et al (1971): Keratoconjunctivitis sicca in dogs. J Am Vet Med Assoc 158:1566.
Baker GJ, Formston C (1968): An evaluation of transplantation of the parotid duct in the treatment of keratoconjunctivitis sicca in the dog. J Sm Anim Pract 9:261.
Barnett KC (1986): Keratoconjunctivitis sicca and the treatment of canine colitis. Vet Rec 119:363.
Barnett KC, Joseph EC (1987): Keratoconjunctivitis sicca in the dog following 5-aminosalicylic acid administration. Hum Toxicol 6:377.
Beaumont PR (1976): Excessive lacrimation in the dog. Vet Rec 97:180.
Bistner SI, et al (1977): Atlas of Veterinary Ophthalmic Surgery. WB Saunders Co, Philadelphia.
Bryan GM, Slatter DH (1973): Keratoconjunctivitis sicca induced by phenazopyridine in dogs. Arch Ophthalmol 90:310.
Carrington SD, et al (1987): Polarized light biomicroscopic observations on the precorneal tear film. 2. Keratoconjunctivitis sicca in the dog. J Sm Anim Pract 28:671.
Carwadine PC, Templeton R (1976): Excessive lacrimation in the dog. Vet Rec 97:245.
Covitz D, et al (1977): Conjunctivorhinostomy: A surgical method for the control of epiphora in the dog and cat. J Am Vet Med Assoc 171:251.
Evans HE, Christensen GC (1979): Miller's Anatomy of the Dog, 2nd ed. WB Saunders Co, Philadelphia.
Glen JB, Lawson DD (1971): A modified technique of parotid duct transposition for the treatment of keratoconjunctivitis sicca in the dog. Vet Rec 88:210.
Harker DB (1970): A modified Schirmer tear test technique. Vet Rec 86:196.
Harvey CE, Koch SA (1971): Surgical complications of parotid duct transposition in the dog. J Am Anim Hosp Assoc 7:122.
Heider L, et al (1975): Nasolacrimal duct anomaly in calves. J Am Vet Med Assoc 167:145.

Helper LC (1970): The effect of lacrimal gland removal on the conjunctiva and cornea of the dog. J Am Vet Med Assoc 157:72.

Helper LC, et al (1972): Surgical induction of keratoconjunctivitis sicca in the dog. J Am Vet Med Assoc 165:172.

Joyce JR, Bratton GR (1973): Keratoconjunctivitis sicca secondary to fracture of the mandible. Vet Med Sm Anim Clin 68:619.

Kaswan RL, et al (1984): Keratoconjunctivitis sicca: Histopathologic study of nictitating membrane and lacrimal glands from 28 dogs. Am J Vet Res 45:112.

Kaswan RL, et al (1985): Keratoconjunctivitis sicca: Immunological evaluation of 62 cases. Am J Vet Res 46:376.

Laing EJ, et al (1988): Dacryocystotomy: A treatment for chronic dacryocystitis in the dog. J Am Anim Hosp Assoc 24:223.

Latimer CA, Wyman M (1984): Atresia of the nasolacrimal duct in three horses. J Am Vet Med Assoc 184:989.

Latimer CA, et al (1984): Radiographic and gross anatomy of the nasolacrimal duct of the horse. Am J Vet Res 45:451.

Lavach JD (1985): The lacrimal system. In Slatter DH (ed): Textbook of Small Animal Surgery. WB Saunders Co, Philadelphia.

Lavach JD, et al (1984): Dacryocystitis in dogs: A review of 22 cases. J Am Anim Hosp Assoc 20:463.

Lavignette AM (1966): Keratoconjunctivitis sicca in a dog treated by transposition of the parotid salivary duct. J Am Vet Med Assoc 148:778.

Lundvall RL, Carter JD (1971): Atresia of the nasolacrimal meatus in the horse. J Am Vet Med Assoc 159:289.

Peruccio C (1982): Incidence of hypothyroidism in dogs affected by keratoconjunctivitis sicca. Proc Am Coll Vet Ophthalmol 14:37.

Rickards DA (1973): Nasolacrimal abscess in the cat. Feline Pract 3:32.

Rubin LF, Aguirre GD (1967): Clinical use of pilocarpine for keratoconjunctivitis sicca in dogs and cats. J Am Vet Med Assoc 151:313.

Rubin LF, et al (1965): Clinical estimation of lacrimal gland function in the dog. J Am Vet Med Assoc 147:946.

Sansom J, et al (1985): Keratoconjunctivitis sicca in the dog associated with the administration of salicylazosulphapyridine (sulphasalazine). Vet Rec 116:391.

Schmidt G, et al (1970): Parotid duct transposition: A follow-up study of sixty eyes. J Am Anim Hosp Assoc 6:235.

Severin GA (1972): Nasolacrimal duct catheterization in the dog. J Am Anim Hosp Assoc 8:13.

Severin GA (1973): Keratoconjunctivitis sicca. Vet Clin North Am 3:407.

Slatter DH (1973): Keratoconjunctivitis sicca in the dog produced by oral phenazopyridine hydrochloride. J Sm Anim Pract 14:749.

Slatter DH, Blogg JR (1978): Keratoconjunctivitis sicca associated with sulfonamide administration in dogs. Aust Vet J 54:444.

Slatter DH, Davis WJ (1974): Toxicity of phenazopyridine: Electron microscopical studies on canine lacrimal and nictitans glands. Arch Ophthalmol 91:484.

Testoni FJ, et al (1977): Anatomy and cannulation of the parotid duct in the dog. J Am Vet Med Assoc 170:831.

Thun R, et al (1975): Effect of tetracycline on tear production in the dog. J Am Anim Hosp Assoc 11:802.

Todenhofer H (1969): Toxische Nebenwirkungen von Sulfadiazin (Debenal, Sulfatidin) be Anwendung als Geriatrikum fur Hunde. Deutsch Tieraerztl Wschr 76:14.

Van Kampen KR, James LF (1971): Ophthalmic lesions in locoweed poisoning of cattle, sheep and horses. Am J Vet Res 32:1293.

Veith LA, et al (1970): The Schirmer tear test in cats. Mod Vet Pract 51:48.

11

Cornea and Sclera

ANATOMY	NEOPLASIA	ACQUIRED SCLERAL DISEASES
PHYSIOLOGY	ACQUIRED CORNEAL DISEASES	SURGICAL PROCEDURES
PATHOLOGICAL RESPONSES	DEGENERATIVE AND	
CONGENITAL DISEASES	DYSTROPHIC KERATOPATHIES	

ANATOMY

The outer coat of the eye consists of the opaque SCLERA and the anterior, transparent CORNEA. The zone of transition between the cornea and the sclera-conjunctiva is called the LIMBUS. In domestic species the horizontal diameter of the cornea is greater than the vertical diameter. The corneal thickness varies among species but is usually less than 1.0 mm. Canine and bovine corneas are thickest at the center, the equine cornea is thickest at the limbus, and the feline cornea is variable. When performing keratectomy from the limbus in species with the greatest thickness in the center, care is taken to avoid removing excessive tissue.

The cornea has five layers (Fig. 11–1):
1. Precorneal tear film
2. Epithelium and its basement membrane
3. Stroma
4. Descemet's membrane (basement membrane of the endothelium)
5. Endothelium

The CORNEAL EPITHELIUM is simple, squamous, and nonkeratinized, of variable thickness, with the basic pattern of basement membrane, basal epithelial cells, wing cells, and squamous surface cells (Fig. 11–2).

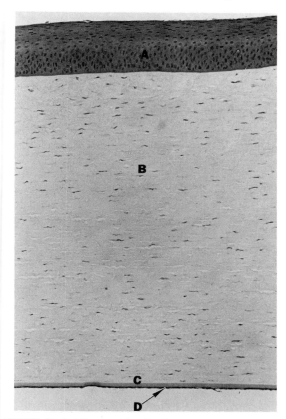

FIGURE 11–1. Microscopic structure of the cornea: A = epithelium; B = stroma; C = Descemet's membrane; D = endothelium.

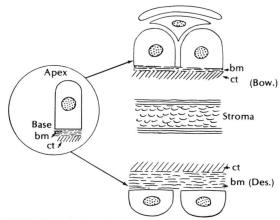

FIGURE 11–2. Basic structure of the cornea. Note that in domestic animals a Bowman membrane is absent. bm = basement membrane; ct = connective tissue; Bow. = Bowman's membrane; Des. = Descemet's membrane. (From Fine BS, Yanoff M: Ocular Histology. Harper & Row, New York, 1972.)

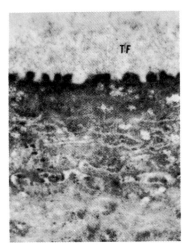

FIGURE 11–3. Electron micrograph of the corneal surface. Precorneal tear film (above) is attached to surface microvilli, which can be observed below. (From Fine BS, Yanoff M: Ocular Histology. Harper & Row, New York, 1972.)

Basal cells contain a nucleus, mitochondria, and Golgi's complex, and they are attached to the basement membrane by HEMIDESMOSOMES. As basal cells divide, daughter cells are forced toward the surface, become flattened as WING CELLS, and gradually lose their organelles. The surface cells possess small villous projections that anchor the deep mucoid layer of the precorneal tear film (Figs. 11–3, 11–4, and 11–5).

The STROMA is composed of fibrocytes, keratocytes, collagen, and ground substance, and it makes up 90% of the corneal substance. The parallel collagen fibrils form interlacing sheets, or lamellae, with occasional interspersed lymphocytes, macrophages, and neutrophils. The regular spacing of stromal collagen fibrils maintains corneal transparency and distinguishes stroma from the collagen in scar tissue and sclera (Figs. 11–6 and 11–7). The replacement time of stromal collagen varies with species, but it may extend to years. Keratocytes are capable of synthesizing collagen, glycosaminoglycans, and mucoprotein of the ground substance.

DESCEMET'S MEMBRANE is the basement membrane of the endothelium and is laid down throughout life, increasing in thickness with age. Descemet's membrane lies posterior to the stroma and anterior to the endothelium (Fig. 11–8), and it is composed of extremely fine collagenous filaments (Fig. 11–9). It is elastic, and if ruptured, the ends curl back into the anterior chamber (see Fig. 11–15). Eventually endothelial cells secrete a new membrane to fill small defects produced by such penetrating wounds. Descemet's membrane does not stain with fluorescein, and it appears as a dark, transparent, outwardly bulging structure in the center of a deep corneal ulcer or wound that is about to rupture.

The ENDOTHELIUM is one cell thick and lies posterior to Descemet's membrane, lining the anterior chamber.

Because of high metabolic activity, endothelial cells contain numerous mitochondria (see Fig. 11–8). The endothelium has a limited capability to replicate depending on age and species and when endothelium is lost the defect is replaced by migration of existing adjacent cells. The endothelium of the young dog has considerable regenerative capacity, with a monolayer forming 6 weeks after 90% destruction. With advancing age, the number of endothelial cells decreases. The endothelium is of particular relevance as trauma during surgery, even though not perceptible, and inflammation, e.g., uveitis, reduce the number of endothelial cells. The normal canine endothelial cell density in young dogs is approximately 2800/sq mm.

Loss of corneal endothelium, beyond the ability of surrounding cells to compensate, usually causes permanent corneal edema and opacity.

PHYSIOLOGY

Cornea

The cornea is the most powerful optical refracting surface in the eye and is transparent. Both transparency and curvature are maintained by anatomical and cellular features.

Corneal transparency is based on
1. Lack of blood vessels and cells
2. Lack of pigment
3. Control of water content
4. A smooth optical surface (provided by the precorneal tear film)
5. A regular, highly organized arrangement of collagen fibrils, which eliminates scattered light by destructive interference.

Metabolism of glucose provides most of the energy requirements of corneal tissues. About two thirds is metabolized via the Embden-Meyerhof pathway and the Krebs cycle, and the remaining third via the hexose monophosphate shunt (Fig. 11–10). Because the cornea is avascular, oxygen is available from four sources (Fig. 11–11):
1. Aqueous
2. Precorneal tear film and the atmosphere
3. Limbal capillary plexus
4. Palpebral conjunctival capillaries

The endothelium receives most of its oxygen from aqueous, but atmospheric oxygen is the major source for the remainder of the cornea. By a variety of

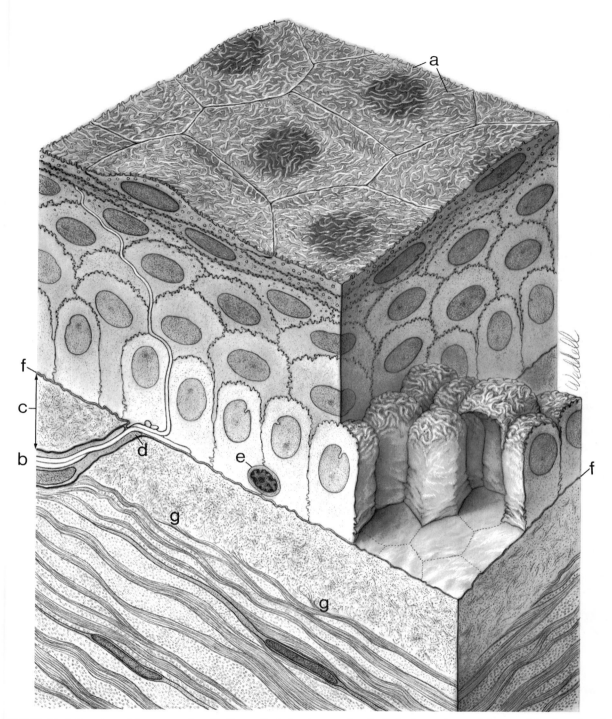

FIGURE 11–4. Drawing of the corneal epithelium with its five layers of cells. Note the polygonal shape of the basal and surface cells and their relative size. The wing cell processes fill the spaces formed by the dome-shaped apical surface of the basal cells. The turnover time for these cells is about 7 days, and during this time the columnar basal cell is gradually transformed into a wing cell, then into a thin flat surface cell. The intercellular space separating the outermost surface cells is closed by a zonula occludens that prevents the precorneal tear film from entering the corneal stroma. The cell surface has an extensive net of microplicae (a) and microvilli, which help retain the precorneal tear film.

A corneal nerve (b) passes through the irregular layer (c); it loses its Schwann sheath near the basement membrane (d) of the basal epithelium. The nerve then passes between the epithelial cells toward the superficial layers as a naked nerve. A lymphocyte (e) is seen between two basal epithelial cells. The basement membrane is seen at (f). (From Hogan MJ, et al: Histology of the Human Eye. WB Saunders Co, Philadelphia, 1971.)

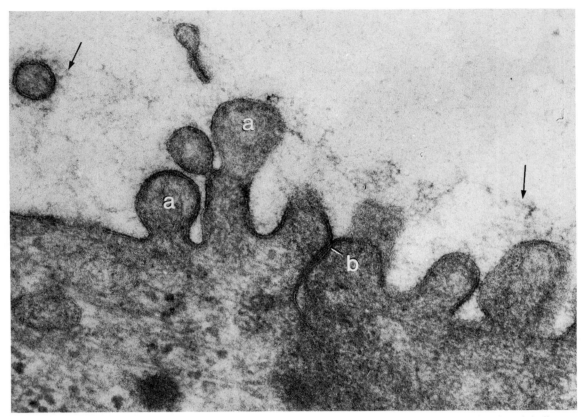

FIGURE 11–5. Corneal epithelium, surface cell. Microplicae and microvilli (a) protrude from the cell surface into the space occupied by the precorneal tear film. Fine filamentous strands are observed (arrow) within this space. A zonula occludens (b) is constantly found in this position. It probably extends for 360° around the intercellular space. (× 105,000.) (From Hogan MJ, et al: Histology of the Human Eye. WB Saunders Co, Philadelphia, 1971.)

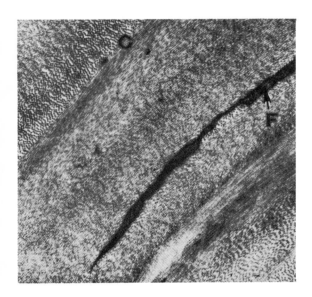

FIGURE 11–6. Interlacing lamellae crossing at right angles in a canine cornea. The lamellae consist of regularly spaced collagen fibrils (C) separated by ground substance. A process of a keratocyte (F) is present between lamellae. (From Shively JN, Epling GP: Fine structure of the canine eye: Cornea. Am J Vet Res 31:713, 1970.)

FIGURE 11–7. The corneal stroma. A, Fibroblast. This diagram shows six fibroblasts lying between the stromal lamellae. The cells are thin and flat, with long processes that contact fibroblast processes of other cells lying in the same plane. There is almost always a 200 Å wide intercellular space separating the cells. Unlike fibroblasts elsewhere, these cells occasionally join each other at a macula occludens. B, Lamellae. The cornea is composed of a very orderly, dense, fibrous connective tissue. Its collagen, which is a very stable protein having a half-life estimated at 100 days, forms many lamellae. The collagen fibrils within a lamella are parallel to each other and run the full length of the cornea. Successive lamellae run across the cornea at an angle to each other. Three fibroblasts are seen between the lamellae. C, The theoretical orientation of the corneal collagen fibrils. Each of the fibrils is separated from its fellows by an equal distance. Maurice has explained the transparency of the cornea on the basis of this very exact equidistant separation. As a result of this arrangement the stromal lamellae form a three-dimensional array of diffraction gratings. Scattered rays of light passing through such a system interact with each other in an organized way, resulting in the elimination of scattered light by destructive interference. The mucoproteins, glycoproteins, and other components of the ground substance are responsible for maintaining the proper position of the fibrils. D, Orientation of the collagen fibrils in an opaque cornea with the orderly positions of the fibrils disturbed. Because of this disarrangement, scattered light is not eliminated by destructive interference, and the cornea is hazy. Edema in the ground substance also produces clouding of the cornea by altering the interfibrillar distance. (From Hogan MJ, et al: Histology of the Human Eye. WB Saunders Co, Philadelphia, 1971.)

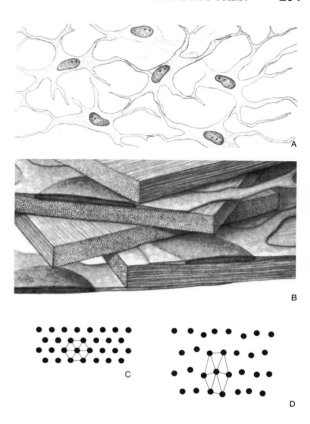

processes, water tends to enter the cornea. Energy-dependent control of the entry of water or maintenance of a state of deturgescence is important to transparency. The endothelial cells are the major site of this "fluid pump," which moves water from the stroma to the aqueous against the intraocular pressure, which forces water into the cornea. The epithelium is also important in control of water content of the stroma. Interference with the oxygen supply to the epithelium (e.g., by an impermeable contact lens) causes anaerobic glycolysis, build-up of lactic acid and water, and corneal edema. The removal of water by the epithelium and endothelium is balanced by the tendency of collagen and mucopolysaccharides in the stroma to attract water. Both the endothelium and epithelium contain large amounts of Na^+- and K^+-activated ATPase associated with the sodium pump. If the corneal epithelium is removed, water enters the stroma from the precorneal tear film and gross swelling occurs, until a new layer of epithelium has covered the area and fluid balance is restored. Fluid may be temporarily removed from the cornea by bathing it with a hypertonic solution, such as 5% NaCl solution or ointment.

Alterations to the *amount of water* in the cornea (corneal edema, which causes swelling and separation of the collagen fibril lattice); *arrangement of the collagen fibrils* (irregular arrangement in scar tissue); *lack of blood vessels*; and *optical surface* (removal of epithelium or

precorneal film) all affect corneal transparency. The effect of altered spacing between collagen fibrils can be demonstrated readily by pressing on the globe. This increases intraocular pressure, distorts the lattice, and causes corneal opacity. When pressure is released, transparency returns. This mechanism differs from opacity in corneal edema due to elevated intraocular pressure (glaucoma), in which endothelial damage and elevated pressure cause increased stromal water.

Factors that alter the collagen lattice, optical surface, or type of collagen—e.g., corneal edema, loss of epithelium or precorneal tear film, elevated intraocular pressure, damage to endothelium, formation of scar tissue—also reduce corneal transparency.

Sclera

The SCLERA is the largest portion of the fibrous coat of the eye. The sclera has three layers (Fig. 11–12): the EPISCLERA, THE SCLERA PROPER, and the LAMINA FUSCA. The episclera is composed of a dense, highly vascular layer that binds TENON'S CAPSULE (fascia bulbi) to the sclera. Collagenous fibers within the episclera

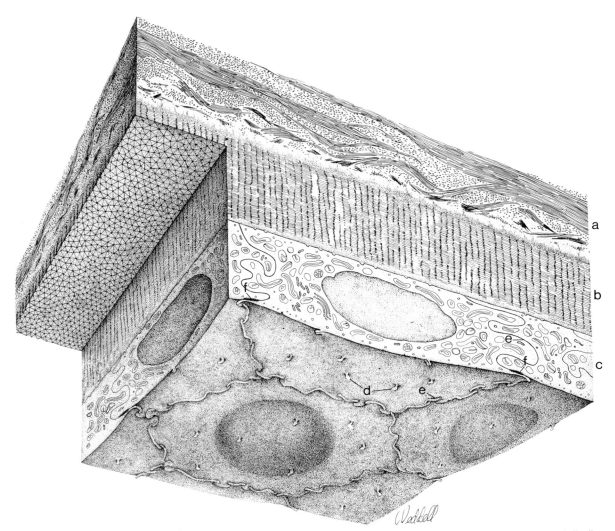

FIGURE 11–8. The deep cornea, showing the deepest corneal lamellae (a), Descemet's membrane (b), and endothelium (c). The deeper stromal lamellae split, and some branches curve posteriorly to merge with Descemet's membrane. Descemet's membrane is seen in meridional and tangential planes. The endothelial cells are polygonal in shape, measuring approximately 3.5 μm in thickness and 7 to 10 μm in length. Microvilli (d) protrude into the anterior chamber from the posterior cell, and the marginal folds (e) at intercellular junctions project into the anterior chamber. The intercellular space near the anterior chamber is closed by a zonula occludens (f). The cytoplasm contains many intercellular rod-shaped mitochondria. (From Hogan MJ, et al: Histology of the Human Eye. WB Saunders Co, Philadelphia, 1971.)

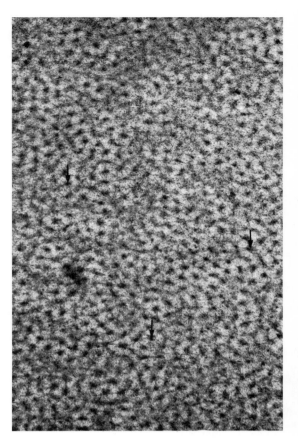

FIGURE 11-9. Descemet's membrane, tangential section. Descemet's membrane is composed of extremely fine collagenous filaments that have a uniform distribution. (From Hogan MJ, et al: Histology of the Human Eye. WB Saunders Co, Philadelphia, 1971.)

blend into the superficial scleral stroma. Anteriorly, the episclera thickens and blends with Tenon's capsule and subconjunctival connective tissue near the limbus. The sclera is composed of collagen fibers and fibroblasts. The collagen fibers differ in size and shape and run in different directions in different parts of the globe. The scleral collagen fibrils differ from those in the cornea

by their considerable variation in diameter and by the absence of fixed spacing between them. The lamina fusca is the zone of transition between the sclera and the outer layers of the UVEA (the vascular coat). The

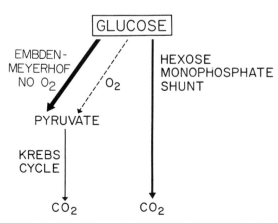

FIGURE 11-10. Pathways of glucose metabolism in the cornea. (From Scheie HG, Albert DM: Textbook of Ophthalmology, 9th ed. WB Saunders Co, Philadelphia, 1977.)

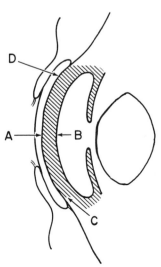

FIGURE 11-11. Sources of oxygen available to cornea: A = precorneal film; B = aqueous humor; C = limbal capillaries; D = palpebral conjunctival capillaries. (From Scheie HG, Albert DM: Textbook of Ophthalmology, 9th ed. WB Saunders Co, Philadelphia, 1977.)

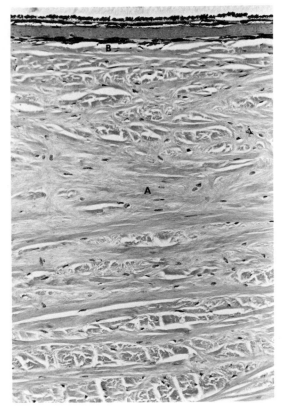

FIGURE 11–12. Layers of the canine sclera: A = scleral stroma; B = lamina fusca.

lamina fusca contains scleral collagen bundles that separate and intermingle with widely separated bundles in the choroid and ciliary body. Between the bundles, melanocytes and pigmented macrophages are present. The zone of transition between the sclera and the cornea is the LIMBUS. The optic nerve enters the eye through the sclera via a sieve-like perforation—the LAMINA CRIBROSA—at the posterior pole. (Fig. 11–13). The SHORT POSTERIOR CILIARY ARTERIES and NERVES pierce the sclera around the nerve and enter the choroid. The LONG POSTERIOR CILIARY ARTERIES and NERVES pierce the sclera near the nerve and pass horizontally around the eye to the CILIARY BODY. ANTERIOR CILIARY ARTERIES and VORTEX VEINS enter and leave the sclera anteriorly in the area overlying the ciliary body.

The sclera is opaque. The following features account for this difference between sclera and cornea:

1. Variation in size and orientation of collagen fibrils
2. Lower mucopolysaccharide content
3. Variation in water content
4. Lack of regular arrangement and spacing of collagen fibrils

PATHOLOGICAL RESPONSES[1]

Several priorities of the cornea affect its response to pathological processes. Because of its *avascularity* and *compact construction,* pathological reactions tend to be sluggish, chronic, and intractable. Variable factors such as fluid balance and state of deturgescence, together with the regular arrangement of collagen fibrils, are responsible for the precarious state of transparency. Changes that would be mild in other tissues—e.g., edema, slight scar formation, or change in tissue tension—may greatly alter transparency and are more significant in the cornea.

Corneal disorders are of three categories:

1. Exogenous
2. Extension from other ocular tissues
3. Endogenous

Exogenous insults, e.g., trauma from eyelid disorders, must first pass or damage the corneal epithelium, which—despite its special properties and precarious position—is an effective barrier to bacteria, because of its unique sensitivity and impervious superficial cells.

1. Modified from Duke-Elder S, Leigh AG: System of Ophthalmology, vol 7, part 2, Disease of the Outer Eye. H Kimpton, London.

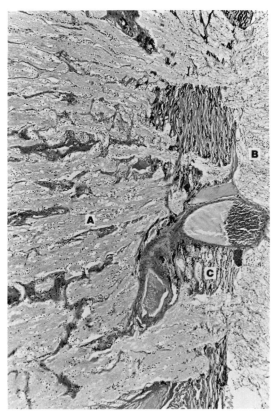

FIGURE 11–13. Canine lamina cribosa: A = optic nerve; B = optic disc; C = lamina cribrosa.

With the exception of *Moraxella bovis,* bacteria rarely cause primary keratitis in animals. Once the epithelium has been breached, microorganisms readily establish themselves and spread within the avascular stroma. The efficiency of the epithelial barrier is indicated by the frequency of pathogenic bacteria in the normal conjunctival sac of domestic animals (Chap 3) and by the lack of consequences.

The extension of disease processes from other ocular tissues is a common course of corneal disorders. Examples are the entry of infectious canine hepatitis virus into the cornea from the aqueous, the effects of uveitis (including corneal edema), and the infiltration of corneal stroma by inflammatory cells and blood vessels in canine immune-mediated keratoconjunctivitis syndrome (Überreiter's).

Endogenous disorders, e.g., corneal dystrophies, affect the cornea less frequently than do exogenous disorders and processes by extension, but they are still frequent.

Normal Corneal Healing

EPITHELIUM

The corneal epithelium has great regenerative capacity. Within a short time after an injury, cells surrounding the margin of a lesion slide in to cover the affected area (Fig. 11–14). An entire cornea can be covered in 4–7 days or less. Once the cells have covered the defect,

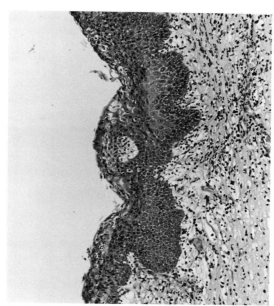

FIGURE 11–15. *Epithelial facet and associated subepithelial inflammatory cell infiltration after a superficial injury in a canine cornea.*

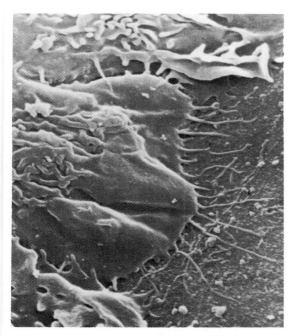

FIGURE 11–14. *Filopodia extending from an epithelial cell over bare basement membrane at the edge of an epithelial defect. (From Pfister RR: The healing of corneal epithelial abrasions in the rabbit: A scanning electron microscope study. Invest Ophthalmol 14:648, 1975.)*

mitosis occurs and the multilayered epithelial surface is reconstituted. During sliding, melanocytes from the limbus may be carried into formerly transparent areas. Small deficiencies in underlying stroma may be filled with epithelial cells, forming an *epithelial facet* (Fig. 11–15).

STROMA

Superficial stromal defects are filled by epithelial facets. In deeper defects, the epithelium soon covers the surface but infiltration and regeneration occur in the stroma beneath. Because regeneration is incomplete, overall corneal thickness is usually reduced.

Uncomplicated stromal wounds undergo avascular healing, but in infected or destructive lesions, vascularized healing occurs, as in other sites in the body.

Avascular Healing

Avascular healing of corneal stroma occurs in the following way:

1. Neutrophils infiltrate and surround the lesions under chemotactic influences. These cells reach the lesion through the tear film and the stroma from limbal conjunctival vessels.

2. Keratocytes in the immediate area die. In surrounding areas, keratocytes transform to fibrocytes and migrate to the damaged area, where they synthesize collagen and mucopolysaccharides of the ground substance. An epithelial covering aids these processes, and if it is absent, healing is slower.

3. About 48 hours after injury, macrophages invade the lesion, remove cellular debris, and transform into keratocytes at a later stage. The collagen fibrils laid down throughout the regenerating stroma are irregular and decrease corneal transparency. Within the ensuing weeks, the density of the scar decreases but does not disappear. Scar resolution is greater in the bovine and feline corneas than it is in other species. A standardized 7 mm corneal defect to a depth of one third of the corneal stroma in the equine cornea heals in a median time of 11 days, provided topical antibiotics are used. Clinical observations suggest that healing times in dogs and cats are less.

Vascular Healing

In vascularized healing of destructive lesions, cellular infiltration is more extensive, and the area is invaded by blood vessels originating from the limbal plexus (see Fig. 11–19). Granulation tissue is laid down and forms a more dense scar than that formed in avascular healing. Eventually the blood vessels collapse but do not disappear; they remain as "ghost vessels" and are visible biomicroscopically with a slit-lamp biomicroscope. Irregularities in the surface are filled by the epithelial reaction mentioned previously. Corneal nerves damaged by the lesion gradually regenerate, and sensation returns slowly to the affected area.

ENDOTHELIUM

Because of its elasticity, Descemet's membrane retracts when damaged and curls toward the anterior

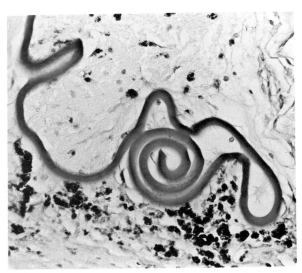

FIGURE 11–16. Retraction of Descemet's membrane in a canine cornea after rupture by a perforating injury due to a cat's claw. Note melanocytes in the area of the scar from an anterior synechia (periodic acid–Schiff stain).

chamber (Fig. 11–16), exposing a small area of stroma. Neighboring endothelial cells slide in to cover the area, and a new Descemet membrane is laid down. In extensive lesions, endothelium may not cover the area, and an area of swollen and edematous stroma persists. The endothelium itself is a very delicate tissue; if it is widely damaged, permanent opacity often results. Endothelial regenerative capability varies with species. Many substances and influences, including advancing age, drugs, phacoemulsification, lens removal, and trauma with surgical instruments cause loss of endothelial cells. If possible, reconstruction of the anterior chamber with balanced salt solution results in less loss of cells than with air.

Protection of the endothelium is the major reason for using sodium hyaluronate (viscosurgery) in the anterior chamber during intraocular surgery. It is used in human ophthalmic surgery to limit endothelial damage during insertion of intraocular lenses. Cost limits its use in veterinary ophthalmic surgery, in which methylcellulose is used more frequently.

EFFECTS OF CORTICOSTEROIDS ON CORNEAL HEALING

Corticosteroids inhibit epithelial regeneration, infiltration with inflammatory cells, fibroblastic activity, and endothelial regeneration. The strength of the resulting healed wound is lessened, collagenases are potentiated up to 15 times, and the risk of infection is greatly enhanced (Fig. 11–17). Although topical corticosteroids do not appreciably decrease wound strength of surgically induced corneal wounds, their use is not recommended without specific indications.

Corneal Reactions to Disease

Although there are numerous specific keratopathies, the majority of clinically important lesions exhibit one of the following major reactions:
1. Edema
2. Vascularization
3. Scar formation
4. Pigmentation
5. Cellular infiltration
6. Accumulation of an abnormal substance within the cornea

EDEMA

Edema results when excess fluid accumulates within the stroma and forces the collagen lamellae apart, accumulates when the regulating functions of the epithelium and endothelium are disturbed, either by removal or by functional alteration. On examination the cornea appears hazy blue, either in localized areas, as around an injury, or throughout, as in endothelial

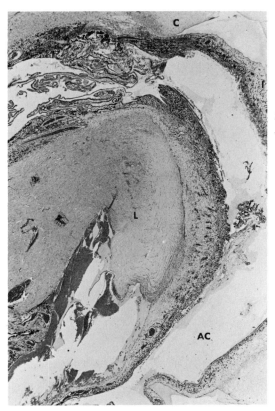

FIGURE 11–17. Ruptured descemetocele, endophthalmitis, and disorganization due to infection by Pseudomonas spp after treatment of a minor corneal wound with subconjunctival corticosteroids in a dog. (See also Plate II E). C = cornea; I = iris; L = lens; AC = anterior chamber.

dysfunction (e.g., glaucoma). Corneal edema is usually reversible if fluid balance is re-established and the underlying cause is removed. Chronic corneal edema may result in vascularization or, less commonly, bullous keratopathy. In bullous keratopathy, fluid-containing vesicles form in the epithelium, and recurring ulceration may develop. Corneal edema can be caused by oral phenothiazine administration in cattle, after exposure to sunlight (see also Chap 3).

Corneal edema can be cleared temporarily for examination with hypertonic solutions (e.g., 5% NaCl solution or ointment, 40% glucose, glycerine).

VASCULARIZATION

The normal cornea contains no blood vessels. Vessels invade the corneal stroma in response to various pathological processes and in vascularized stromal healing. Corneal vascularization may be either superficial (Plate IIIA; Fig. 11–18) or deep (Plate IIIB). Superficial vessels occur in the anterior third of the stroma and are continuous with the conjunctival circulation at the limbus. They branch more than deep vessels do, although in central corneal lesions the part of the vessel near the limbus may be straight. Superficial vessels are bright red rather than the darker red of deep vessels. Deep vessels are usually short and straight, and they branch less and are dark red. They are continuous with the ciliary circulation and disappear at the limbus. The depth of the invading vessels is some indication of the depth of the initiating corneal lesion. The sequence of vascularization is shown in Figure 11–19.

In complicated stromal lesions, especially when the stimulus in the cornea persists, vessels may not collapse, but further vascularization and granulation tissue formation occurs. In general, vascularization is beneficial (e.g., in stromal repair after prolapse of the globe in the dog), but vessels result in decreased transparency, ingrowth of pigment, and in some cases, transport of antibodies and inflammatory cells that reduce corneal transparency. For these reasons, control of vascularization during the repair process is often attempted after an epithelial cover is achieved, with corticosteroids and beta radiation. Beta radiation can be used in the absence of corneal epithelium.

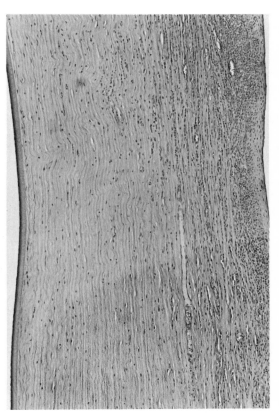

FIGURE 11–18. Superficial corneal vascularization and keratitis in a feline cornea.

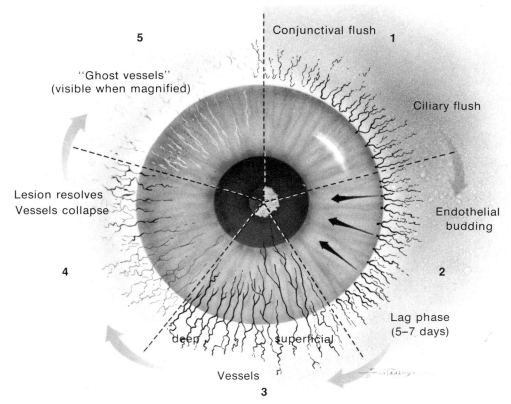

FIGURE 11–19. Sequence of corneal vascularization in a simple injury.

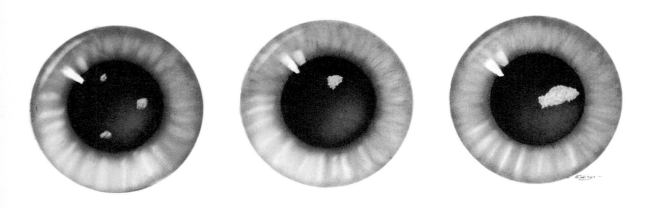

NEBULA   MACULA   LEUKOMA

FIGURE 11–20. Types of corneal scars. Left, Nebula. Center, Macula. Right, Leukoma. If the iris attaches to the leukoma it is called an adherent leukoma.

Corneal vascularization may be either deep or superficial. Depth of the invading vessels indicates depth of the inciting lesion in the cornea.

SCAR FORMATION

When corneal stroma is destroyed, reparation is made by fixed keratocytes and invading fibroblasts and macrophages. Collagen fibrils produced by these cells are not laid down in a regular lattice pattern and do not transmit light. With time, scars may clear optically but often do not do so completely. The tendency to clearing is greater in young animals and also in cattle, sheep, and cats. In dogs and horses, pigmentation of the scarred area often occurs. In dogs, lipid deposition may occur near the scar (Plate IIIC).

The deeper the initial injury, the more dense and permanent the scar and the lesser the tendency for transparency to return. Very superficial stromal injuries are filled in by epithelial facets (see Fig. 11–15). With increasing size, corneal opacities are termed NEBULA, MACULA, and LEUKOMA (Fig. 11–20). Extensive loss of substance with subsequent cicatrization may result in a thin cornea that bulges (Fig. 11–21)—CORNEAL ECTASIA or KERECTASIA.

If the stroma is entirely destroyed and Descemet's membrane is forced outward by the intraocular pressure, the lesion is termed a DESCEMETOCELE (Fig. 11–22). Descemetoceles frequently form after unremitting ulceration, and if untreated, the membrane either ruptures, with escape of aqueous, or becomes surrounded by scar tissue. Descemetoceles do *not* stain with fluorescein. If the cornea ruptures, the escaping aqueous carries the iris forward into the hole. If the iris is incorporated into the healing wound, an ANTERIOR

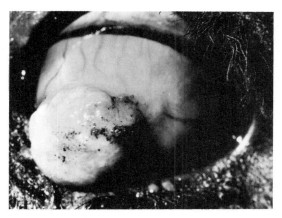

FIGURE 11–21. Kerectasia and corneal granulation after deep ulceration and iris incarceration following an attack of infectious bovine keratoconjunctivitis in a heifer.

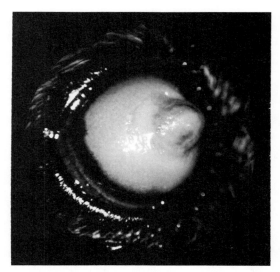

FIGURE 11–22. A descemetocele with corneal edema and vascularization in a Pekingese.

SYNECHIA is formed. (A POSTERIOR SYNECHIA is an adhesion between iris and lens.) If the iris is carried out of the wound, an IRIS PROLAPSE results (Fig. 11–23).

Opacity resulting from uncomplicated corneal stromal wounds can be limited by the careful use of corticosteroids *provided*

1. Infection has been controlled.
2. An epithelial covering, as demonstrated by fluorescein, has been established.
3. The structural integrity of the cornea is not compromised.

Topical corticosteroids (e.g., 0.1% dexamethasone drops, 3–4 times daily) limit opacification by inhibiting fibroplasia, decrease vascularization, reduce pigmentation, and improve final transparency.

Although supervised use of corticosteroids is beneficial in reducing corneal opacification during scar formation, such usage is *contraindicated without an intact epithelium.*

PIGMENTATION

Corneal pigmentation (so-called pigmentary keratitis) is a nonspecific response to corneal inflammation, either severe or mild. Pigment is deposited in the stroma or in the epithelium (Figs. 11–24 and 11–25). Stromal pigment originates from proliferation of normal limbal melanoblasts that migrate into the stroma during inflammation.

Pigment in the corneal epithelium arises from the basal layer, which is of the same embryological origin as the layer that naturally contains pigment in the

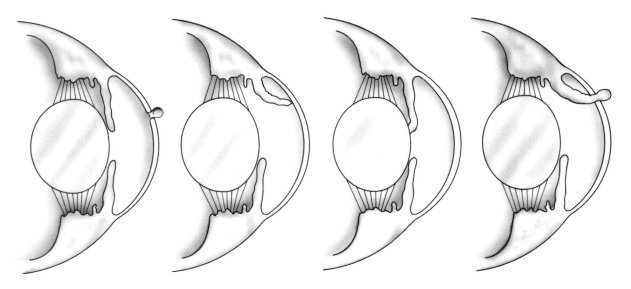

DESCEMETOCELE   ANTERIOR SYNECHIA   POSTERIOR SYNECHIA   IRIS PROLAPSE

FIGURE 11–23. Corneal lesions: descemetocele, anterior synechia, posterior synechia, and iris prolapse.

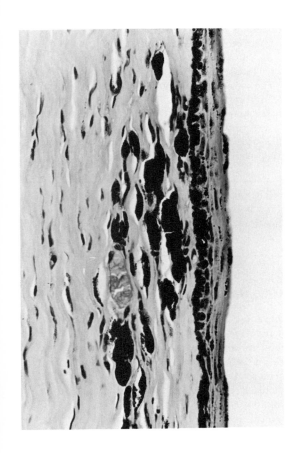

FIGURE 11–24. Corneal stromal pigmentation and vascularization in a canine cornea. Note accumulation of pigment in the basal epithelial and anterior stromal layers.

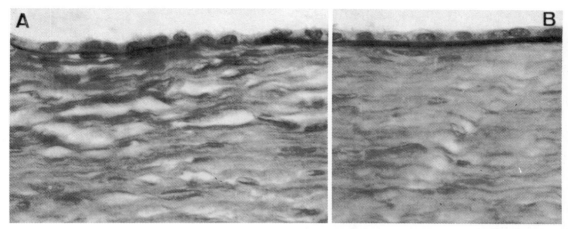

FIGURE 11–25. A, *Section of cornea showing localized thinning and focal absence of Descemet's membrane in a dog with persistent pupillary membrane. B, Section of cornea from normal littermate of A. (From Saunders LZ, Rubin LF: Ophthalmic Pathology of Animals. S Karger AG, Basel, 1975.)*

conjunctiva. Epithelial pigmentation is more common in chronic corneal diseases, especially when continual exposure, irritation, or xerosis (dryness) are present (e.g., distichiasis, trichiasis, irritation from nasal folds, chronic exposure in brachycephalics, keratoconjunctivitis sicca). In these disorders, removal of the stimulus usually prevents progression of the pigmentation. In chronic exposure or lack of precorneal tear film, the corneal epithelium may revert to a simple skin pattern with thickening, rete peg formation, and keratinization. Severe corneal inflammation and vascularization are more commonly associated with greater stromal pigmentation, especially in the dog and horse.

Pigmentation itself is not normally treated unless vision is interfered with. The underlying cause should be eliminated when possible (e.g., control of inflammation in chronic immune-mediated keratoconjunctivitis [Überreiter's], removal of nasal folds, or reconstructive blepharoplasty). Methods used to treat pigmentation include corneal coverage by blepharoplasty, irradiation, and treatment of underlying inflammation with corticosteroids.

Unless pigmentation affects vision, it is not treated directly, but the underlying cause is detected and either eliminated or controlled when possible.

CONGENITAL DISEASES

Congenital disorders of the cornea and sclera are relatively common. With the exception of colobomatous defects (described later), they are discussed only briefly here.

Microcornea

Microcornea can be diagnosed by measuring the horizontal and vertical diameters of the cornea and comparing these with values from the other eye. The condition is usually unilateral and associated with microphthalmia (Chap 2).

Dermoid

See Chapter 8.

Corneal Opacity

Persistent pupillary membranes (PPM) frequently cause corneal opacity in the basenji and occasionally in other animals. Remnants of pupillary membrane extend from the iris collarette to the corneal endothelium (Fig. 11–26) and are associated with defects in the endothelium and Descemet's membrane. A variety of iris defects, cataracts, and uveal colobomata may coexist with the corneal opacity.

Corneal opacity may be hereditary in certain breeds of cattle—e.g., Holstein-Friesian (recessive), Swiss (recessive), and Norwegian red poll in association with hereditary posterior paresis.

Although ocular inflammation during pregnancy can result in corneal opacity at birth, proven examples in clinical situations are rare. Suspected congenital corneal opacity must be distinguished from acquired disorders such as reactions to infectious canine hepatitis vaccination in dogs, anterior synechiae, and the numerous corneal dystrophies.

Colobomatous Defects

Colobomatous defects vary from a small pit, either in the optic disc or in the fundus near the disc, to a

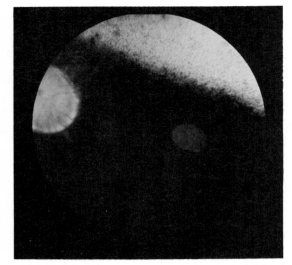

FIGURE 11–26. *Small coloboma in the nontapetal fundus of a horse.*

large outpouching of sclera (scleral ectasia). SCLERAL ECTASIA SYNDROME occurs most commonly in the Collie and Shetland sheepdog. Isolated occurrences of focal ectasia occur sporadically at the posterior pole in numerous dog breeds and occasionally in horses (see Fig. 11–26). COLOBOMATA OF THE POSTERIOR POLE may be seen in basenjis with PPM and in charolais cattle, and ECTASIA OF THE SCLERA in the equatorial region occurs in Californian (Australian [sic]) shepherds.[2]

SCLERAL ECTASIA SYNDROME IN THE COLLIE, BORDER COLLIE, AND SHETLAND SHEEPDOG

Synonyms: collie ectasia syndrome, collie eye anomaly

Etiology

The condition is one of incomplete closure of the embryonic fissure (Chap 2) with simple recessive inheritance of variable expression; it is congenital and nonprogressive.

---

2. The "Australian shepherd" of the US is a misnomer; it is not found in Australia and did not originate there. It is thought to have originated in California. It must be distinguished from the Australian kelpie, Australian cattle dog ("Queensland Blue Heeler" [sic]), border collie, and dingo, which are officially recognized and distinct breeds *unaffected* by scleral ectasia syndrome. The dingo is the world's oldest pure dog breed, having been in existence for 40,000 years prior to the 18th century, and is now a component of the kelpie and Australian cattle dog. The "Australian shepherd" is not recognized by the American Kennel Club, but the breed maintains its own organization that recognizes *functional performance*, as well as appearance, in evaluation.

Clinical Signs (in order of frequency)

1. Chorioretinal dysplasia (Plate III*D*). The affected area lies temporal to the optic disc but is not always continuous with it. Appearance varies from a focal unpigmented zone without choroidal hypoplasia to complete lack of retinal and choroidal pigment. In the latter, the white inner surface of the sclera is visible.

2. Colobomata at the posterior pole or involving the optic disc up to 20 D deep in dogs (Plate III*E*). These colobomata are thin outpocketings of the sclera protruding posteriorly from the posterior pole. When viewed ophthalmoscopically, colobomata appear as whitish excavations into which blood vessels occasionally plunge out of focus.

3. Retinal detachments (in up to 4% of cases).

4. Intraocular hemorrhage.

5. Central corneal opacity.

Other signs—e.g., multiple retinal folds in the inferonasal quadrant, retinoschisis (intraretinal splitting), and neovascularization of the retina—occur with variable frequency. Whether or not retinal vessel tortuosity is a part of the syndrome is a matter of debate. Experience indicates that a diagnosis of scleral ectasia syndrome in a susceptible breed *cannot* be supported on this criterion alone, but tortuosity is frequent in affected animals. The so-called go-normal eye—in which a focal area of lack of pigmentation that may have been called chorioretinal dysplasia in a young dog but that pigments and "disappears" later in life—has received much anectodal discussion in breeding circles but little acceptable study. It is *not* a major feature in diagnosis of scleral ectasia.

The relative frequency of scleral ectasia syndrome in collies and Shetland sheepdogs varies considerably among countries and in different localities of the same countries (Table 11–1), and studies must be interpreted accordingly.

The reason for attempting to identify and remove affected animals from breeding is the incidence of hemorrhage and retinal detachments causing blindness in newborn puppies. Potential pet buyers should be warned to have puppies examined before purchase, especially if the vendor is a pet shop, where affected animals are frequently available.

Indirect ophthalmoscopy is the technique of choice for diagnosis of scleral ectasia syndrome in collies and Shetland sheepdogs.

TABLE 11–1. Frequency of Scleral Ectasia Syndrome

Country	Collie	Shetland Sheepdog
United States	85%	<5–10%
United Kingdom	70%–80%	>80%
Australia	60%–70%	<5–10%

Control

1. Removal of all affected dogs from the breeding program.

2. Examination and certification of all breeding stock at an early age, e.g., 6–8 weeks. Test-crossing may be required with known affected animals for merled animals in which the entire fundus is hypopigmented, depending on the experience of the observer.

3. Programs in which animals with lesser degrees of the syndrome are used for breeding are contraindicated, as there is no evidence that this reduces the incidence of the condition (as would be expected with a recessive gene of variable expressivity). Grading of lesions is also *contraindicated,* as it implies degrees of severity. Unfortunately, the use of these early and differing grading systems, based on histological criteria, for clinical examination, has resulted in much misunderstanding within the breeding community, and it has done much to perpetuate the condition in the collie breed in the US.

4. Significant reductions in frequency have been achieved by adherence to correct examination and breeding procedures, based on accepted Mendelian genetic principles.

> Scleral ectasia syndrome is the most important ocular disorder affecting collies. Because it is hereditary and may cause blindness, every attempt should be made to eliminate it from breeding stock and to educate the general public about the condition.

COLOBOMATA IN THE BASENJI

Colobomata are seen occasionally near the optic disc in basenjis with PPM and sporadically in other animals (Fig. 11–27). These smaller colobomata must be distinguished from albinotic spots by their depth, as determined by direct ophthalmoscopy. The ophthalmoscope is focused onto the top and bottom of the suspected coloboma and the difference in value of the lenses noted. (*Note:* 1 D is approximately 0.3 mm.) The basenji has a slightly depressed surface to the optic disc, and this is not classified as a coloboma when within normal limits.

Colobomata are classified as *typical* (inferior and medial to the optic disc) or *atypical* (other than typical in position).

COLOBOMATA IN CALIFORNIAN ("AUSTRALIAN" [sic]) SHEPHERDS

Colobomata are associated with multiple ocular anomalies—microphthalmia, cataracts, retinal detach-

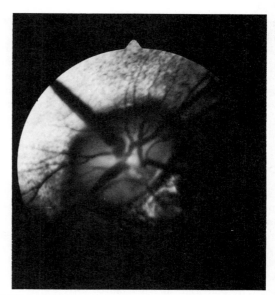

FIGURE 11–27. *Coloboma of the posterior pole, adjacent to the optic disc in a charolais. (Courtesy of Dr. K. C. Barnett.)*

ments, and iridal heterochromia in association with merling of the coat. Colobomata may be present at the posterior pole or may form large ectatic areas in the equatorial regions. The complex of ocular anomalies is inherited as an autosomal recessive trait.

COLOBOMATA IN CHAROLAIS CATTLE

Colobomata of the posterior pole (see Fig. 11–27) occur in charolais in Australia, the United States, and the United Kingdom. The condition is dominant, with complete penetrance in males and with 52% penetrance in females, and of an uncertain mode when transmitted to other breeds. Coloboma in charolais has not been shown to cause blindness, but it has been suggested that the condition should prevent certification of prospective bulls, in order to reduce the affected gene pool within the breed.

NEOPLASIA

Primary neoplasms of the cornea and sclera are rare. In cattle, squamous cell carcinoma (SCC) originates at the limbus and is discussed as a conjunctival neoplasm in Chapter 8. SCCs originating in the conjunctiva frequently invade the cornea and sclera in cattle and, to a lesser extent, in other species in which the primary neoplasm is less common. The sclera is occasionally invaded by melanomas originating in the iris and ciliary body. Ocular lymphosarcoma in dogs often invades the cornea, and one of the first signs may be intracorneal hemorrhage, triangular in shape with the base at the limbus.

Rather than being a site of neoplasia, the sclera is an important barrier preventing spread of intraocular neoplasms to other parts of the body. Thus, malignant neoplasms (e.g., melanoma) often have a good prognosis provided they have not escaped from within the sclera. Neoplasms may leave the eye via the optic nerve, ciliary and vortex veins, and intrascleral nerve canals.

Epibulbar Melanoma

The canine epibulbar melanoma is a specific tumor type, originating from melanocytes in the superficial tissues near the limbus (Fig. 11–28). From there it spreads through the corneal stroma toward the center of the cornea, and it protrudes from the surface or, less frequently, may extend posteriorly and penetrate the sclera and enter the ciliary body. The tumor has a low metastatic potential, and if removed early by cryosurgery, or later by resection and corneoscleral allograft, the prognosis for survival is good. Vision can also frequently be saved. Corneoscleral allografting is described under Surgical Procedures.

ACQUIRED CORNEAL DISEASES

Keratitis

Keratitis is inflammation of the cornea. The term may apply to inflammation of all layers or to inflammation of a specific layer, usually designated by an additional descriptive term.

CLASSIFICATION OF KERATITIS

Keratitis may be classified by etiology, topography, or depth (modified from Duke-Elder and Leigh, 1965). Those based on etiology include

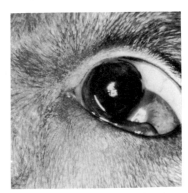

FIGURE 11–28. An epibulbar melanoma in a dog. Note penetration of the cornea by the neoplasm. (Courtesy of Dr. G. A. Severin.)

1. Infectious keratitis of numerous kinds—e.g., due to *Moraxella bovis* in cattle
2. Allergic keratitis—e.g., reactions to infectious canine hepatitis vaccination in dogs
3. Keratitis associated with systemic diseases—e.g., *herpesvirus felis* keratitis in cats
4. Exposure, irritation, desiccation, and neurotrophic disorders
5. Etiology unknown

Because different layers of the cornea may react differently to one agent, and because the cornea has limited patterns of reaction, the same clinical picture may be produced by different types of inflammation. A combination of topographic classification modified by etiological studies is most appropriate for general clinical use (e.g., interstitial keratitis due to *herpesvirus felis* in cats). For this discussion the classification shown in Table 11–2 is used. General reactions such as vascularization, edema, pigmentation, and scar formation or dystrophies are *not* classified as keratitis.

SUPERFICIAL KERATITIS

Superficial Corneal Erosion Syndrome

Synonym: "Boxer ulcer"
Breed Predilection: Boxer, corgi, poodle, samoyed
Clinical Signs
1. Chronic blepharospasm
2. Epiphora
3. Photophobia
4. Lesions usually unilateral

The lesions are due to separation of the corneal epithelium from the stroma, probably because of defective hemidesmosomes attaching the basal layer of the epithelium to the basal lamina (basement membrane). The anterior stromal layers proliferate and become abnormal also. Affected areas are usually 3–4 mm in diameter, have a ragged outline, cause intense pain, and stain with fluorescein (Plate IIIF). Epithelium may accumulate at the edge of the lesion, causing a "rolled-up" appearance, as it cannot attach to the basal lamina.

Superficial corneal erosion syndrome rarely stimulates vascularization, and this is a useful diagnostic feature; however, vascularization may be rapid and marked in the boxer. Vascularization does not aid healing but can result in significant scarring despite later treatment. Acquired superficial corneal erosions are distinguished from superficial corneal erosion syndrome (see the discussion later in this section) for therapeutic purposes.

Treatment
The treatment of choice is superficial keratectomy of the involved area of epithelium and superficial stroma, plus a margin of 2–2.5 mm of normal epithelium. The superficial layers of the stroma only are removed, using an operating microscope. The cornea is covered with a third eyelid flap for 10 days postoperatively. The eye is medicated with broad-spectrum antibiotic drops (e.g.,

TABLE 11–2. Classification of Keratitis by Depth

Superficial	Interstitial	Deep	Ulcerative*
Superficial corneal erosion syndrome	Chronic immune-mediated keratoconjunctivitis syndrome (Überreiter's)	Infectious canine hepatitis keratitis	Descemetocele
Superficial pigmentary keratitis	Neurotrophic keratitis	Malignant catarrhal fever	Iris prolapse
Superficial punctate keratitis	Keratoconjunctivitis sicca	Equine stromal abscess	
Acquired superficial corneal erosions	Herpetic keratitis		
Senile keratopathy	Bullous keratopathy		
	Infectious bovine keratoconjunctivitis		
	Infectious ovine keratoconjunctivitis		
	Infectious caprine keratoconjunctivitis		
	Ovine chlamydial conjunctivitis		
	Mycotic keratitis		
	Feline eosinophilic keratitis		

*Separate because all layers are frequently involved.

Neosporin) 4 times daily for 2 days before surgery and for 10 days after, combined with 1% atropine drops twice a day for the same period. After removal of the flap, topical dexamethasone twice a day is used to reduce scar formation at the keratectomy site—provided the lesion *does not stain* with fluorescein. The lesions rarely recur, and the prognosis is excellent.

Numerous other treatments, including cauterization with tincture of iodine, application of contact lenses, hyperosmotic medications, and multiple punctate keratotomies, have been advocated. Superficial keratectomy is a proven, highly successful method that relieves the patient of much pain when first used and is predictable for the owner; it is much preferable for established cases of this syndrome. Repeat client visits with an unknown outcome are rarely required. Therapeutic bandage lenses have been shown to reduce the rate of healing of corneal epithelial wounds (see also Chap 3).

Acquired Superficial Corneal Erosions

Superficial corneal erosions—apparently following minor trauma and environmental stress such as heat, dry weather, and smog, and which do not heal or which heal temporarily and recur in continuing cycles of pain and epiphora—also occur. They are distinguished from superficial corneal erosion syndrome, in which the lesions do not heal. These erosions are seen in all breeds of dogs and horses and occasionally in cats. A search for an underlying cause is necessary, e.g. ectopic cilia, keratoconjunctivitis sicca, and corneal exposure. The signs are otherwise similar to the erosion syndrome.

Treatment

Although in chronic cases a keratectomy may be required, early erosions can be effectively treated by débridement under topical anesthesia and by cauterization with tincture of iodine, followed by hyperosmotic drops, antibiotics, and atropine. The cornea is examined in 7 days for re-epithelialization. Several repeat treatments may be used, especially in older animals, if scarring is not advancing. The key to success is not to allow the lesion to become chronic.

Corneal Erosions in the Shih-Tzu

In this breed, a deep corneal erosion that progresses to a splitting of the cornea within its lamellae occurs rarely, resulting in much vascularization and scarring. It is treated by deep keratectomy and corneal coverage. Therapy should be attempted by suitably trained and experienced persons only.

Equine Corneal Erosions

Corneal erosions occur less frequently in horses. Because of a high potential for permanent scarring in chronic cases, superficial keratectomy with coverage by either a third eyelid or a conjunctival flap, combined with temporary partial tarsorrhaphy, is the treatment of choice.

Keratoconjunctivitis Sicca

Keratoconjunctivitis sicca is discussed in detail in Chapter 10.

Superficial Pigmentary Keratitis[3]

Breed Predilection: Lhasa Apso, Pekingese, Pug, Boston Terrier

In this condition, pigment production in the epithelium and superficial stroma occurs in association with chronic low-level keratitis (see Fig. 11–25). Vascularization is frequently absent. The most common causes are:

1. Chronic exposure due to prominent globes and a large palpebral fissure (congenital euryblepharon), as seen in brachycephalic breeds
2. Distichiasis
3. Nasal fold trichiasis
4. Subclinical KCS.

---

3. This disorder should not be confused with chronic superficial keratitis—a term inaccurately applied to Überreiter's syndrome and numerous other types of keratitis.

Pigmentation frequently advances to occlude the central cornea and interfere with vision before the owner is aware of its presence. A careful examination with magnification and a focal beam of light is necessary for accurate diagnosis and recording of the extent of the lesion.

Treatment

Treatment is directed at halting progress of the pigmentation and, if necessary, removal of the pigment causing visual impairment. Correction of distichiasis and trichiasis together with reconstructive blepharoplasty usually stops further pigmentation. In young dogs with prominent eyes and early pigmentation, prophylactic reconstructive blepharoplasty is often advisable. Intermittent use of tear replacement solutions is useful during periods of abnormal exposure in order to reduce drying and corneal irritation.

If pigment has already resulted in visual impairment, it can be partially removed (after control of the cause) with superficial radiation with strontium-90 or topical corticosteroids, provided the underlying cause has been corrected.

Senile Keratopathy with Calcium Deposition (Band keratopathy)

This condition occurs in aged dogs and cats, and the etiology is unknown. It is characterized by deposits of calcium and mineral-like material in the epithelium and superficial stroma, often associated with superficial and, less frequently, deep ulceration. It is usually a static condition, and progression is slow, with little tendency to heal. The condition is usually not painful until the later stages.

Treatment is topical application of ethylenediaminetetra-acetic acid (EDTA) drops (1–4%) 4–6 times daily, often for prolonged periods, with topical antibiotics administered intermittently as necessary. In severe cases, surgical repair by keratectomy is useful, but prolonged healing must be expected, and coverage by a conjunctival flap is advisable. If deep ulceration is present, appropriate surgical therapy is indicated. The prognosis is always guarded, but most affected eyes can be saved.

Superficial Punctate Keratitis

This term is applied to superficial defects in the corneal epithelium that do not stain with fluorescein. The affected areas are minute multiple pinpoints, scattered diffusely across the corneal surface (appearing like the surface of an orange skin). The condition, although recognizable, may be induced by numerous insults to the cornea (e.g., chronic exposure during general anesthesia or in brachycephalic breeds; use of topical anesthetics). Superficial punctate keratitis must be differentiated from corneal edema, which produces a different bluish-white appearance of the cornea. No specific treatment can be recommended except to determine and treat the underlying cause.

INTERSTITIAL KERATITIS

Inflammatory disorders affecting the stroma are classified as interstitial keratitis.

Chronic Immune-Mediated Keratoconjunctivitis Sicca

Synonyms: Überreiter's syndrome, pannus, chronic superficial keratitis [sic]. The term "pannus" is to be avoided, as it refers to nonspecific vascularization of avascular tissue, e.g., cartilage. The disease is not restricted to the cornea and is not superficial.

Breed Incidence: German shepherd, greyhound, Siberian husky most commonly. A similar disease occurs in kelpies, Australian cattle dogs, and border collies, but it can be differentiated clinically.

Etiology

The exact etiology of chronic immune-mediated keratoconjunctivitis sicca (CIKS) is unknown. Cell-mediated immunity to corneal and uveal antigens has been demonstrated in affected corneas, but it also occurs in many other chronic corneal inflammatory disorders. Epidemiological evidence suggests the etiological importance of ultraviolet radiation. It has been proposed that ultraviolet radiation alters the antigenicity of tissue in susceptible corneas, resulting in cell-mediated inflammation.

Pathogenesis

In the early stages corneal epithelial cells proliferate and the superficial stroma is infiltrated by plasma cells and lymphocytes (Fig. 11–29A). The epithelium remains intact.

As the disease progresses, melanocytes, histiocytes, and fibrocytes enter, and edema and neovascularization occur (Fig. 11–29B). In the advanced stage, epithelium and anterior stroma are heavily pigmented and vascularized, and the epithelium may become keratinized (Fig 11–29C).

Clinical Signs

1. The syndrome affects the temporal and nasal, inferior and superior corneal quadrants in that order of occurrence and severity.

2. Vascularization and pigmentation occur first at the temporal limbus and gradually move centrally. The other quadrants are gradually affected, and eventually the whole cornea may be involved (Plate IIIG). Small white spots sometimes occur in the clear stroma 1–3 mm ahead of the advancing lesion.

3. Depigmentation and thickening of the external surface of the third eyelid, usually near the margin. This contributes to the inflamed appearance of the eye, but it is rarely of significance except in diagnosis.

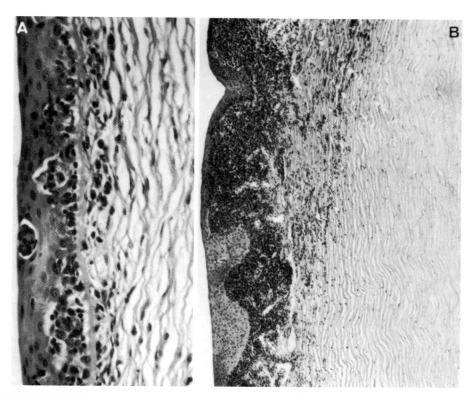

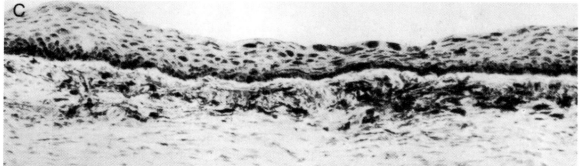

FIGURE 11–29. A, The inferotemporal corneal quadrant of a 5-year-old male German shepherd. The epithelium and anterior stroma are inflamed, characteristic of the advancing edge of the lesion. B, Similar section from a mature female German shepherd with more extensive cellular infiltration of the anterior stroma and early vascularization. The epithelium is beginning to thicken and project into the stroma. C, Biopsy from a 4-year-old female German shepherd with more advanced lesions, including pigmentation of the stroma and epithelium. (From Saunders LZ, Rubin LF: Ophthalmic Pathology of Animals. S Karger AG, Basel, 1975.)

4. Lipid deposits in the corneal stroma adjacent to the advancing edge of the lesions are not uncommon in long-standing cases.

5. The age of onset and breed of the affected animal are of prognostic significance. In animals affected when young (e.g., 1–2 years), the condition usually progresses to severe lesions, whereas animals first affected at a later age (e.g., 4–5 years) develop less severe lesions. Greyhounds show milder lesions and are affected at a younger age (1–2 years).

6. Severity of the disease varies markedly with locality. Animals living at high elevations (e.g., 3000–6000 feet) show more severe lesions that progress to a more advanced state in younger dogs than do those lesions in dogs living at sea level. Lesions in animals living at lower elevations respond more favorably to therapy.

The lesions may be quite advanced before first being noticed by the owner and must affect a large area of the cornea before vision is affected. The epithelium does not stain with fluorescein.

Chronic immune-mediated keratoconjunctivitis sicca (CIKS) is a chronic progressive corneal disorder that *cannot* be cured. It *can be controlled* so that blindness *rarely* occurs.

Diagnosis

Breed and appearance of lesions are usually diagnostic. CIKS must be distinguished from pigmentary keratitis due to chronic irritation, keratitis sicca, and granulation tissue present in vascular healing of chronic corneal stromal wounds.

Treatment

CIKS can be controlled but not permanently cured. It *must* be explained to the owner that life-long therapy is necessary at a level depending on the severity in each patient and the geographical locality. With the exception of areas at high elevation, useful vision can usually be preserved with medical therapy alone. In areas at low elevation, or in mild lesions occurring in middle-aged dogs, the treatment is as follows:

With increasing resistance to treatment, successive steps are used, as outlined here.

Step 1

Topical corticosteroid drops (e.g., 0.1% dexamethasone, 1% prednisolone) 4 times a day for 4 weeks. Application 2 or 3 times daily is usually enough for maintenance. The owner must be advised that if an ocular infection, pain, discharge, or injury occur, the corticosteroid must be discontinued and an immediate consultation sought. Unlike the human eye, mycotic infection, glaucoma, and cataracts are *not* a feature of canine eyes treated long-term with corticosteroids. Improvement in vision usually takes a minimum of 3–4

TABLE 11–3. Chronic Immune-mediated Keratoconjunctivitis Sicca (Überreiter's Syndrome) at High Elevation

Step	Treatment
1	(a) Topical corticosteroids 4–6 times daily. Frequency of application, potency, and concentration of the steroid may be adjusted to response.
2	(a) Subconjunctival injection of corticosteroids, e.g., 3.0 mg of betamethasone acetate and 1.0 mg of betamethasone disodium phosphate.* (This combination was used in preference to other respository agents that may leave visible subconjunctival plaques at the site of injection.)
	(b) Continued treatment with topical corticosteroids as in step 1(a).
3	(a) If no response to step 2 is observed by 30–60 days' beta irradiation (^{90}Sr applicator) is used. Each area of the lesion is irradiated. Up to six slightly overlapping circles may be necessary in a severely affected eye. The irradiated area overlaps the limbus by 2–3 mm. The radiation is applied in 1 dose of from 45 to 75 Gy (4500–7500 R). (This may be administered to each area to cover the entire lesion.) A response is usually evident within 3–6 weeks.
	(b) Subconjunctival corticosteroids as in step 2(a).
	(c) Continued treatment with topical corticosteroids as in step 1(a).
4	(a) Superficial keratectomy of the affected area, up to a maximum of three procedures in severe cases. Every attempt is made to extend the period between keratectomies by intensive medical treatment as above.
	(b) Simultaneous irradiation as in step 3(a).
	(c) Topical antibiotic therapy for 9–12 days until the stroma is covered by epithelium, followed by subconjunctival and topical corticosteroids. Although eventual failure is not uncommon at this stage, useful vision may be extended for years.

From Slatter DH, et al: Überreiter's syndrome (chronic superficial keratitis) in dogs in the Rocky Mountain area—A study of 463 cases. J Sm Anim Pract 18:757, 1977.
*Betavet Soluspan—Schering Corporation, Bloomfield, NJ.

weeks to become apparent. The eyes are re-examined at 4 weeks and frequency of therapy is adjusted as required. At low elevations, topical therapy is usually sufficient for control.

Step 2

Rarely, subconjunctival corticosteroids (preferably short-acting repository preparations of 7–14 days' duration of action) may be necessary in addition to topical therapy.

For treatment of resistant cases, or in localities with high ultraviolet light or at high elevation, the treatment regimen outlined in Table 11–3 is recommended. The prognosis in such cases is shown in Table 11–4. Cyclosporine drops are apparently ineffective in CIKS.

Neurotrophic Keratitis

Neurotrophic keratitis is a form of chronic keratopathy resulting from damage to the sensory (trigeminal)

TABLE 11–4. Guide to Prognosis of Chronic Immune-
mediated Keratoconjunctivitis Sicca
(Überreiter's Syndrome)

Group	Features	Prognosis for Vision (3–5 Years)
1	(a) Early lesions in older dogs (>5 years). Early lesions in young dogs other than German shepherds.	Good
2	(a) Slowly progressive pigmented or vascular lesions, or both, in middle-aged dogs. (b) Pigmented lesions with little vascularity in dogs older than 4 years.	Guarded
3	(a) Rapidly developing lesions in dogs less than 5 years of age. (b) Any dog showing exacerbation while being treated with topical corticosteroids. (c) Dogs that are totally blind at the 1st examination.	Poor

From Slatter DH, et al: Überreiter's syndrome (chronic superficial keratitis in dogs in the Rocky Mountain area—A study of 463 cases. J Sm Anim Pract 18:757, 1977.

innervation of the cornea. It occurs in all species, but it is more common in dogs and cats, especially following orbital trauma. Two forms exist: **NEUROTROPHIC KERATITIS**, which usually responds to treatment, and **NEUROPARALYTIC KERATITIS**, in which severe keratitis and ulceration may cause loss of vision or of the eye. In the early stages, epithelial degeneration and stromal edema occur, but advanced lesions result in desiccation, corneal vascularization, and opacification. Ulceration may progress to perforation.

Treatment

1. Tarsorrhaphy to prevent trauma and desiccation. If there is no response in 2–3 weeks, tarsorrhaphy for up to 6 months may be used.
2. Topical antibiotic therapy.
3. Response to treatment may be poor, and permanent tarsorrhaphy or enucleation may be required.

Herpetic Keratitis

Herpesviruses cause keratitis in cats (in association with upper respiratory tract infections and conjunctivitis) and cattle (infectious bovine rhinotracheitis), and they are a suspected cause in dogs. In the human eye, herpesvirus affects the corneal epithelium or stroma, producing different clinical entities. In cats, severe ulcerative keratitis, geographical (map-like) ulceration, and dendritic keratitis (Fig. 11–30) are the most frequent signs (see Chap 8).

Herpetic keratitis in cats is frequently resistant to treatment, and relapses are common. Idoxuridine, an antiviral agent, must be administered topically every 2 hours in such cases, but by itself it may cause toxic keratopathy. Resistant infections are treated with trifluridine (Viroptic). Surgical removal of the affected tissue by superficial keratectomy is also useful. Topical povidone-iodine (1–4%) drops have been recommended, but their efficacy is unproved. In a minority of cats, the immune-mediated corneal response to the virus may be destructive and painful, and it may be controlled with topical cyclosporine, provided the cornea is kept under skilled observation to detect progression or undesirable side effects.

Continuing infection in human herpetic keratitis and experimental herpetic keratitis in rabbits is associated

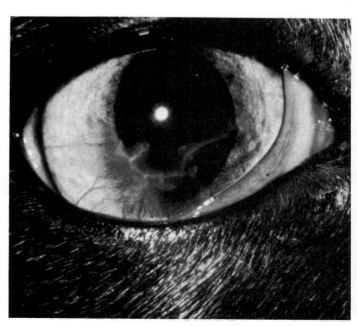

FIGURE 11–30. Right eye of a 2-year-old cat 5 weeks after the onset of upper respiratory disease. Corneal dendrites and vascularization are present. (From Saunders LZ, Rubin LF: Ophthalmic Pathology of Animals. S Karger AG, Basel, 1975.)

with exhaustion of the locally occurring antiproteases alpha$_2$-macroglobulin and alpha$_1$-antitrypsin. This is consistent with clinical observations of a beneficial response in cats with resistant herpetic keratitis when compound ulcer drops containing acetylcysteine are administered. These difficult cases in which severe corneal damage continues may be treated as follows, under the supervision of a veterinary ophthalmologist:

1. Idoxuridine or trifluridine hourly for its antiviral effect. In simple cases, this treatment is all that is usually necessary.

2. Compound ulcer medication 4 times a day for its antibiotic, pain relieving, anticollagenase, and tear replacement properties.

3. Cyclosporine drops twice a day to control damaging immune responses in the cornea.

4. Levamisole systemically 5 mg daily for up to a month, to stimulate nonspecific immunity to *Herpesvirus felis*.

Herpesvirus felis particles (Fig. 11–31) lie quiescent in corneal tissues and the trigeminal ganglion for long periods. Corticosteroids and stress activate such quiescent particles.

Corticosteroids are contraindicated in feline herpetic keratitis and are used with caution in any inflamed feline eye.

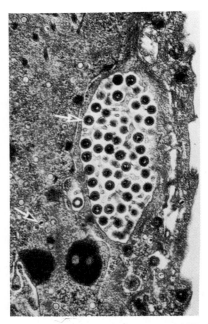

FIGURE 11–31. *Electron micrograph (× 40,000) from the cornea of the cat in Figure 11–30, showing viral particles in an epithelial cell. (From Saunders LZ, Rubin LF: Ophthalmic Pathology of Animals. S Karger AG, Basel, 1975.)*

In infectious bovine rhinotracheitis (IBR), conjunctivitis is more prominent than is keratitis. The presence of an acute infectious upper respiratory tract syndrome, with profuse lacrimal and nasal discharge in a herd, is usually sufficient for differential diagnosis. Peripheral corneal lesions are occasionally present with edema, ulceration, and vascularization. Keratitis due to IBR virus is distinguished from corneal lesions of malignant catarrhal fever (bovine malignant catarrh) and infectious bovine keratoconjunctivitis (see Table 8–9).

Bullous Keratopathy

Bullous keratopathy is a nonspecific response to chronic corneal diseases of numerous kinds. The condition begins as formation of small vesicles in the epithelium that coalesce to form larger bullae. The surrounding epithelium and stroma are edematous and often vascularized, either in response to the bullae or from the underlying corneal disorder.

Differential Diagnosis

Bullous keratopathy must be distinguished from descemetocele, iris prolapse, and epithelial inclusion cysts.

Treatment

1. Treatment of the underlying condition, if known.

2. Surgical removal of the bullae by superficial keratectomy.

3. Coverage with a third eyelid flap.

4. Routine topical treatment with antibiotics, atropine, protease inhibitors, and hyperosmotic solutions if necessary.

Corneal coverage, e.g., temporary tarsorrhaphy or conjunctival flap, or bandage contact lenses may be useful for this condition if they can be retained, e.g., by surgical adhesives. The prognosis for simple bullous keratopathy is good. Extensive bullous keratopathy has a poor prognosis. In complicated cases permanent corneal scar formation is common, and poor response to therapy is frequent.

Infectious Bovine Keratoconjunctivitis (IBK)

Synonyms: Pink eye, New Forest eye (United Kingdom)

Infectious bovine keratoconjunctivitis (IBK) is one of the most common of all diseases of cattle and is of major economic importance in beef- and milk-producing areas throughout the world.

Etiology

Moraxella bovis is considered the most common responsible agent, although attempts to reproduce the disease with the organism are not always successful. Ultraviolet radiation increases the susceptibility of the cornea to infection, and decreases in recorded ambient ultraviolet radiation have been associated with healing of corneal ulcers and decreases in the number of *M.*

bovis organisms isolated during an outbreak. *Moraxella* is transmitted via the crop of the face fly, with transmission apparently minimal in its absence. An undefined genetic influence also affects which animals become infected and reinfected.

Piliated *Moraxella* adhere to the corneal epithelium and produce dermonecrolysins and hemolysins and, together with collagenases from inflammatory cells, cause necrosis of epithelium and stroma (Fig. 11–32). The organisms can enter previously undamaged epithelial cells.

Other organisms, including *Branhamella (Neisseria)* spp, *Listeria monocytogenes, Mycoplasma bovoculi*, and adenoviruses, have been isolated from field outbreaks. Although various mycoplasma, rickettsia, and viruses have been isolated, their relationship, if any, to the etiology and pathogenesis is undetermined.

Clinical Features

In herds with no previous outbreaks, young and older animals are equally severely affected. After the initial occurrence, however, younger animals are more frequently and severely affected. Affected animals possess some immunity that becomes less effective after 1 or 2 years, frequently allowing reinfection. The effectiveness of this immunity depends directly on the severity of the initial disease. Unfortunately, attempts to produce either live or killed vaccines to *M. bovis* have been disappointing. Recent commercial vaccines using pili antigens require further field evaluation before their true value is known. Peak outbreaks are usually in the summer, especially when flies and dusty conditions prevail.

Clinical Signs

1. Keratitis and conjunctivitis, in varying proportions in the early stages; ulcerative keratitis is prominent in most advanced cases.

2. Intense lacrimation and epiphora.

3. Photophobia.

4. Blepharospasm.

5. Central corneal opacity, which enlarges, ulcerates, and becomes yellowish, and finally becomes vascularized around the periphery (see Fig. 11–32).

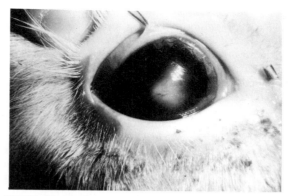

FIGURE 11–33. *Central corneal scar 4 months after the lesion in Figure 11–32, showing dramatic improvement. (Courtesy of Dr. M. Nairn.)*

As ulceration proceeds to deeper corneal layers, descemetocele, penetration, and panophthalmitis may occur. In less severe cases, recovery takes 1–3 weeks, with vascularization and clearing from the limbus toward the center of the cornea. Some residual scar formation occurs (Figs. 11–33, 11–34). The bovine cornea possesses remarkable reparative properties, and many extensively scarred corneas are completely healed a year later. Despite this, severe scarring does remain in a proportion of affected eyes. During the later phases of the disease, the animal is in considerable pain and may be totally blind and have difficulty in walking and in finding food and water. Such animals are often dangerous for farm staff to handle, and extensive weight losses and reduced milk yields may occur.

Treatment and Control

1. If possible, affected animals are segregated to limit spread of the disease and are provided with shade. Attempts to reduce the vector fly population may be instituted, e.g., spraying manure heaps.

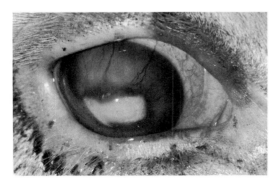

FIGURE 11–32. *The acute phase of IBK, with corneal necrosis and inflammatory cell infiltration and surrounding stromal vascularization.*

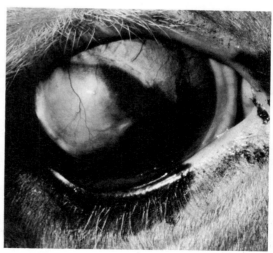

FIGURE 11–34. *Extensive scarring and vascularization after IBK.*

2. A subconjunctival injection of repository penicillin—e.g., 1 million units of a mixture of crystalline, procaine, and benzathine penicillin—is given subconjunctivally. Recent preparations of intramuscular repository tetracycline (20 mg/kg), which penetrates lacrimal fluid, are also useful. Systemically administered oxytetracycline was slightly superior to furazolidone and no treatment in preventing corneal preventing and in allowing affected corneas to heal faster, but recurrences of ulceration were similar (George et al, 1988).

(*Note:* If corneal coverage is provided, some authors recommend the addition of 5–10 mg of a repository corticosteroid such as methylprednisolone to reduce scarring. Although such treatment is contraindicated in other species in the presence of infective ulceration, the remarkable properties of the bovine cornea apparently prevent undesirable sequelae.)

3. Coverage by combined tarsorrhaphy–third eyelid flap. This is probably the most important part of the treatment regimen in severe cases. If chromic gut is used, suture removal is unnecessary, although infection around such sutures can cause problems in a minority of animals.

4. Although elimination of carrier animals (after an outbreak or introduction of new animals) by antibiotic therapy is theoretically desirable, there is no evidence it can be achieved or has any effect on mortality or economic losses.

5. Administration of bacterins containing oil adjuvant to calves between the ages of 21 and 30 days and 6 weeks prior to the onset of the fly season are recommended by vaccine manufacturers. Claims, not yet confirmed by independent scientific observers, are made that the incidence and severity of infection are reduced, but the disease is not eliminated.[4]

Powders and sprays are contraindicated in the treatment of IBK. Such methods provide suitable antibiotic concentrations for short periods only and are irritating. Prolonged antibiotic levels are more suitable. Intravenous sulfonamides result in inhibitory concentrations in tears for short periods, but oral sulphonamides do not. Neither method has achieved wide therapeutic acceptance.

Attempts to produce a vaccine for IBK have met with limited success because of either lack of effect or short-lived immunity. Current attempts to use antigens associated with *M. bovis* pili appear more promising, with seven different serogroups having been identified.[5] Alternative routes of administration have also improved vaccine efficacy, with local subconjunctival injection exposing the antigen to the *mucosa-associated lymphoid system*, allowing greater production of protective IgA. Greater efficacy with a bacterin containing corneadegrading enzyme antigens as well as *M. bovis* pili antigens has also been reported.

Corneal coverage is *an important aspect* of treatment of severe IBK.

Infectious Ovine and Caprine Keratoconjunctivitis

Synonyms: Sheep inclusion conjunctivitis, pink eye, contagious ophthalmia

Infectious ovine keratoconjunctivitis (IOK) and chlamydial conjunctivitis are apparently separate diseases in sheep. IOK is widespread in sheep and has a similar pattern of occurrence to IBK in cattle. Compared with IBK, it causes less severe corneal lesions and, with the exception of widespread outbreaks, interferes less with grazing. The morbidity varies between 10% and 50%, depending on seasonal conditions.

Etiology

Inclusion bodies of *Chlamydia psittaci ovis* (formerly *Colesiota conjunctivae*) have been described, and this organism is probably the primary cause, although other organisms can probably initiate the disease. The clinical picture is complex and is a result of interaction among infecting chlamydia, host resistance factors, and secondary infections caused by opportunistic bacterial pathogens. *Branhamella (Neisseria) catarrhalis* and *Mycoplasma* spp have also been isolated. All breeds of sheep are equally susceptible, although young lambs are more severely affected than adults are. Newly weaned animals are the most susceptible. IOK is spread by dust, flies, long wool and hair, infected secretions, and contact with infected animals. Peak incidence of the disease is in the hot, dusty summer months. There are usually no recurrences until the next summer, and a degree of flock immunity persists for 2–3 years.

Clinical Signs

Clinical signs may occur unilaterally or bilaterally.

1. Lacrimation and epiphora, eventually resulting in a purulent discharge
2. Blepharospasm
3. Conjunctival injection, erythema, and follicle formation
4. Corneal edema and ulceration in severe cases
5. Descemetocele and iris prolapse in rare cases

Purulent discharges occur after 3 or 4 days, and recovery is complete within 10–14 days (a shorter course than IBK).

Diagnosis

Clinical signs are usually diagnostic. Scrapings may be used to confirm the diagnosis. A similar but more severe disease, possibly caused by *Acholeplasma oculusi* (a mycoplasma), occurs in goats, with a course of 3–4 weeks.

---

4. Such claims must be interpreted cautiously, as IBK vaccines have been marketed in previous decades only to be withdrawn when efficacy was demonstrably lacking.

5. Lepper AW, Hermans LR: Characterisation and quantitation of pilus antigens of *Moraxella bovis* by ELISA. Aust Vet J 63:401, 1986; Moore LJ, Rutter JM: Antigenic analysis of fimbrial proteins from *Moraxella bovis*. J Clin Microbiol 25:2063, 1987.

Treatment and Control

1. Isolation of affected animals into a cleaner environment
2. Use of topical preparations, e.g., tetracycline ointment, ethidium bromide, 0.5% ointment or lotion; 1% chloramphenicol

Because the disease is self-limiting and economic losses are low, control of the secondary bacterial infections by topical therapy several times per day is preferable to attempts at microbiological elimination of the organism. This approach will not eliminate the organisms from the flock, and future infections can be expected.

Ovine Chlamydial Conjunctivitis

A similar ocular disease associated with chlamydial polyarthritis is reported in feed-lot lambs. This condition is probably a part of the spectrum of similar diseases (IOK) with differing etiologies but producing similar clinical signs in sheep.

Clinical Signs

1. Epiphora
2. Conjunctival hyperemia
3. Conjunctival follicular hyperplasia
4. Corneal edema, vascularization, and keratitis
5. Enlargement of parotid lymph nodes
6. Polyarthritis
7. Marked weight loss
8. Pyrexia (40–41.5°C)
9. Lameness

Both eyes are affected in about 80% of animals. Morbidity may reach 90%.

Diagnosis

Diagnosis is based upon the following criteria:

1. Clinical signs
2. Demonstration of chlamydial inclusions in conjunctival scrapings (less than 50% of affected animals show inclusions)
3. Serological demonstration of chlamydial antibodies
4. Isolation and culture of *Chlamydia*

In mycoplasma infection, bilateral infection in lambs is less frequent. Chlamydial conjunctivitis is self-limiting as immunity develops. If therapy is indicated, general principles as used for IOK are applicable.

Mycotic Keratitis[6]

Mycotic keratitis with or without ulceration is relatively uncommon and occurs most frequently in horses, especially after injury with objects of vegetable origin. Many species of saprophytic fungi cause human mycotic keratitis, and a similar variety are responsible in animals. The infection is frequently long-standing, it is characterized by bacterial contamination, and it is

6. See also Chap 3.

resistant to treatment with antibiotics. Mycotic keratitis is much more frequent in areas with a humid, subtropical climate, e.g., Florida, northeastern Australia, and is rare in dry climates of the western US. It often follows an injury with vegetable matter, e.g., a scratch from a twig or branch. In cats, *Candida albicans, Drechslera spicifera,* and *Rhinosporidium* spp have been recorded.

Clinical Signs

1. Long-standing resistant keratitis
2. Focal, cloudy, often yellow opacities at the advancing edge of the lesion
3. Striate opacities in the corneal stroma adjacent to the main lesion, which may be edematous and opaque
4. Nonspecific signs of other corneal disorders—blepharospasm, conjunctival and ciliary injection, photophobia, epiphora, and neovascularization

Diagnosis

1. Clinical signs.
2. Culture of corneal scrapings on Saboraud's agar without inhibitors such as chlorhexidine (as the majority of the fungi are saprophytes that do not grow in the presence of inhibitors). The clinician must *ask* most laboratories to use such agar or results will be negative→
3. Cytological examination of KOH scraping preparations. Repeat scraping may be necessary.
4. Histopathological examination of corneal tissues.

Treatment

Numerous drugs are available, but sensitivity of fungi to the different agents varies widely (see Chap 3).

1. Frequent topical treatment with the antimycotic drug of choice (Table 11–5). A nasolacrimal lavage tube assists this therapy.
2. Superficial keratectomy of the lesion and surrounding stromal opacities that may contain fungi, if the lesion is extensive and there is no risk of penetration.
3. Placement of a conjunctival flap to cover the lesion.

From 35 fungal isolates from equine eyes, Moore and associates (1983) found the following susceptibilities—natamycin (97%), nystatin (74%), miconazole (69%), amphotericin (51%), 5-fluorocytosine (49%), and ketaconazole (31%). Such series must be interpreted with caution, as the frequency of different organisms shows geographical variation.

Feline Protozoal Keratitis

Acanthomoeba (formerly *Nosema*) spp cause deep, resistant keratitis in immunosuppressed cats. It has been treated by surgical excision, and more recently by topical propamidine isethionate drops.

Feline Eosinophilic Keratitis

Differential diagnoses: Fungal keratitis, neoplasia, foreign body granuloma, traumatic keratitis with scarring and lipid deposition

TABLE 11-5. Topical Treatment of Mycotic Keratitis

Drug	Preparation	Organisms
Natamycin (Natacyn)	5% suspension every 1–2 hours	*Aspergillus, Fusarium, Cephalosporium* spp
Nystatin	Topical ointment 100,000 units/g Aqueous suspension 200 units/ml Subconjunctival injection of 0.5 ml (100,000 units/ml)	*Candida, Aspergillus* spp
Miconazole	Ophthalmic preparations individually prepared	
Amphotericin B	Aqueous solution 1 mg/ml in 5% dextrose solution (incompatible with saline solution)	*Aspergillus, Candida* spp
Flucytosine	Ophthalmic preparations individually prepared	*Aspergillus, Candida* spp
Ketaconazole	Ophthalmic preparations individually prepared	*Aspergillus, Candida* spp

Feline eosinophilic keratitis occurs as red, infiltrating or raised masses at the limbus, infiltrating the cornea toward the center. The masses ar painless and slowly progressive. Initial involvement is unilateral, but progression can be expected to the other eye if treatment is ineffective. The cause is unknown, but the condition is more common at high elevation, suggesting an association with ultraviolet light. The condition has a guarded prognosis, and lifelong treatment is usually necessary to control the lesions and prevent blindness.

Eosinophilic keratitis is treated with topical dexamethasone or prednisolone 2–4 times a day, depending on response. In resistant cases, systemic megestrol acetate 2.5 mg/kg by mouth may be used with caution (both megestrol and topical steroids may interfere with hepatic function). Azathiaprine may also be required to control the condition.

Miscellaneous Interstitial Keratitis

There are numerous uncommon forms of interstitial keratitis—e.g., due to *Nosema* in cats, *Geotricha* spp and *Leishmania donovani* in dogs—for which the interested reader is referred to reference texts.

DEEP KERATITIS

Infectious Canine Hepatitis

Synonyms: Postvaccinal keratitis, blue eye

Infectious canine hepatitis (ICH) virus (canine adenovirus 1 and 2 [CAV-1, -2]) causes uveitis, but because the major clinical effect is corneal opacity, the condition is discussed with corneal disorders from which it must be distinguished.

In the natural disease, about 20% of infected animals develop uveitis. After vaccination with modified live virus vaccines for CAV-1, a small proportion of dogs develop similar ocular lesions. The proportion is estimated at 1:50,000 to 1:80,000 vaccinations, although the clinician is often confronted with small outbreaks of reactions. Investigations by vaccine producers indicate the reactions are the result of the properties of the virus rather than of any superiority or deficiency of a particular batch or brand of vaccine.

Vaccines produced with CAV-2 are claimed to lack ocular reactions. Such claims are *incorrect*, and although the frequency of reactions is less, the same precautions apply with respect to their use in sight hounds and the warnings to be given to clients. Reactions have been observed with vaccines from different manufacturers.

Pathogenesis[7]

After vaccination, virus particles replicate in the iris and corneal endothelium. Virus replication occurs after 7–10 days and is characterized by a mononuclear infiltrate. This stage is rarely apparent clinically. Antibodies to the viral antigen are formed and specific antigen-antibody complexes form.

Immunologically mediated reactions to the antigen-antibody complexes result in uveitis, temporary or permanent corneal endothelial damage, and increased vascular permeability in the iris vessels. If endothelial damage is temporary, the corneal edema usually resolves in 1–2 weeks, but some animals retain permanent partial or total corneal opacity. Secondary glaucoma may occur if inflammatory cells released during uveitis block the drainage angle (Fig. 11–35). The sight hounds (Afghan, greyhound, saluki, borzoi, and Ibizan) are especially susceptible to postvaccinal ICH reactions with consequent corneal opacity and glaucoma (Figs. 11–36 and 11–37).

Clinical Signs

The clinical signs of ICH and their time of appearance are shown in Figure 11–38.

ICH postvaccinal reaction is a serious disorder with many undesirable sequelae. ICH killed vaccines should be used in Afghans, greyhounds, and other sight hounds.

---

7. Modified from Bistner SI: Ocular manifestations of systemic disease. Vet Clin North Am 3:467, 1973.

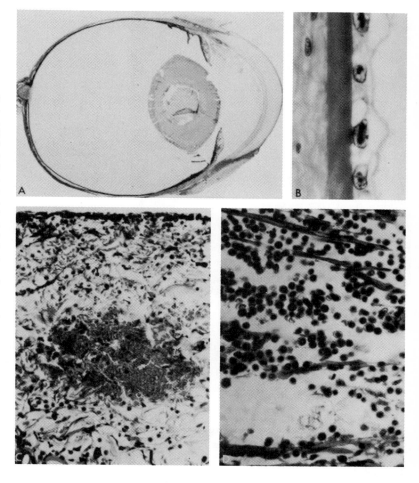

FIGURE 11–35. A, The globe from a case of acute uveitis experimentally induced with canine hepatitis (CAV-1). Note the intense corneal edema and the exudative material in the anterior chamber. B, Endothelial cells from a dog with severe anterior uveitis and corneal edema 8 days after inoculation with CAV-1. Note the large intranuclear inclusion bodies, typical of canine hepatitis, in the degenerating endothelial cells. C, The iris during the acute stage of anterior uveitis following inoculation with CAV-1. A large area of hemorrhage within the iris stroma is evident, as well as a diffuse inflammatory reaction. D, The canine trabecular meshwork taken from a dog with severe anterior uveitis 8 days after inoculation with CAV-1. The trabecular meshwork is densely infiltrated with mononuclear inflammatory cells. (From Bistner SI: Ocular manifestations of systemic disease. Vet Clin North Am 3:467, 1973.)

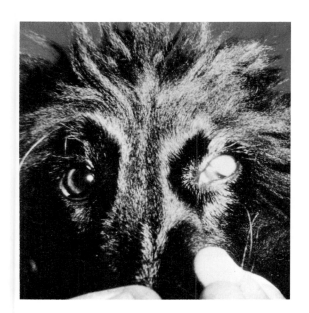

FIGURE 11–36. Persistent postvaccinal ICH corneal edema in an Afghan. (Courtesy of Dr. G. A. Severin.)

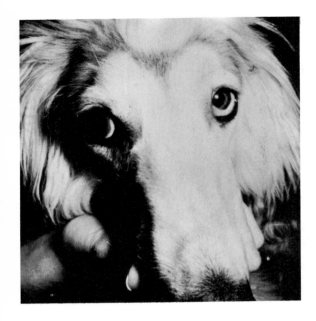

FIGURE 11–37. Glaucoma secondary to ICH in a saluki.

Treatment

1. Topical atropine drops 3–4 times daily during the acute stages.

2. In the acute stages, topical and oral corticosteroids may be used to control uveitis. Frequent re-examinations are advisable.

3. Hyperosmotic topical preparations may be used, although their persistence is transitory.

4. In sight hounds with a higher risk of glaucoma, oral carbonic anhydrase inhibitors are indicated.

If response is not evident in 4–5 weeks, permanent corneal edema is likely. The eye is examined for the onset of glaucoma. Once progressive glaucoma has occurred, several options are available—cyclocryotherapy, intraocular prosthesis, or in hopeless cases only, enucleation.

Because of potential complications and medicolegal implications, patients with ICH vaccine reactions should be referred to a veterinary ophthalmologist as soon as possible.

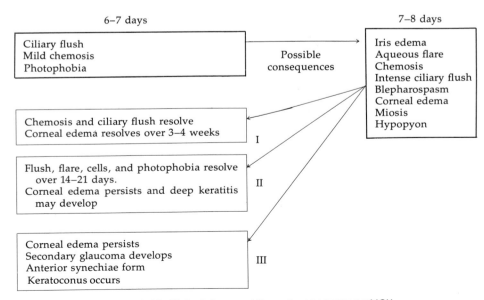

FIGURE 11–38. Clinical signs and time of appearance of ICH.

Malignant Catarrhal Fever (MCF)

Synonym: Bovine malignant catarrh
Etiology: Herpesvirus

All breeds of cattle are susceptible to malignant catarrhal fever (MCF), and the disease occurs in most countries. It usually appears as an isolated case, but the morbidity may reach 50%. Mortality is almost 100%. Outbreaks in herds have been reported.

Clinical and Ocular Signs

There are four forms of the disease:

1. Head and eye form
2. Peracute form
3. Alimentary tract form
4. Mild form

MCF is discussed here because of its corneal signs. The distinctive ocular lesions in an animal with a severe systemic disease are sufficient to assist in diagnosis (Table 11–6). The corneal lesions begin in the center and move toward the limbus. MCF is suspected when nasal, oral, and ocular lesions occur, with persistent pyrexia, enlarged lymph nodes, and encephalitis. The presence of ocular lesions differentiates MCF from rinderpest, mucosal disease–virus diarrhea, infectious stomatitis, and calf diphtheria. IBR is distinguished by its infectious nature, respiratory signs, recovery rate, and predominance of conjunctivitis rather than endophthalmitis. Ocular signs are due to the necrotizing effect of the virus on vascular tissues and vary according to the form of the disease.

Equine Stromal Abscess

After small corneal puncture wounds that allow bacteria to gain entrance to the stroma and then heal over, corneal abscesses may occur. They are not usually associated with large areas of epithelial loss or extensive ulceration. A yellowish corneal opacity usually develops, with ocular discomfort, photophobia, lacrimation, and blepharospasm. Limbal vascularization develops, and associated uveitis.

Treatment

1. Collection of diagnostic samples—scrapings and cultures
2. Frequent topical antibiotics 6–24 times daily, or continuous or intermittent subpalpebral lavage
3. Subconjunctival and systemic antibiotics daily
4. Topical atropine 4 times a day
5. Use of a darkened stall

Corneal scarring is frequent after the infection is controlled.

TABLE 11–6. Ocular Signs of Malignant Catarrhal Fever

Head and Eye Form	Peracute Form	Alimentary Tract Form	Mild Form
Eyelid edema	(Early death)	Mild conjunctivitis	—
Blepharospasm			
Conjunctival erythema			
Ocular discharge			
Nystagmus			
Hypopyon			
Corneal edema and keratitis (spreading centrally)			
Acute severe conjunctivitis			
Anterior uveitis			
Retinitis and optic neuritis (visible histologically)			

ULCERATIVE KERATITIS

Corneal ulceration is a common condition in domestic animals. If treated correctly, many corneal ulcers do not progress and satisfactory results can be achieved.

A CORNEAL ULCER occurs when epithelium and a variable amount of stroma are lost. Such lesions are usually chronic and heal slowly. Small acute ulcers in normal cornea heal rapidly.

Classification

Numerous classification schemes for corneal ulcers have been devised. For clinical purposes the method used in this discussion is shown in Figure 11–39.

Regardless of the initial cause, all ulcers have the potential to progress to endophthalmitis if not treated. The causes of ulceration are *numerous;* the most common are shown in Table 11–7.

In treating corneal ulceration, the most important step is determining the cause and removing it. This is followed by attempts to create an ideal environment for repair of the lesion and to prevent its progression, and by surgical treatment to prevent rupture of the cornea.

In simple traumatic injuries in which a small amount of epithelium is removed, healing is very rapid (see discussion of corneal healing, p 265). Normal corneal epithelium is a very effective barrier against invading bacteria. If the ulcer becomes infected or the epithelium is unable to attach to underlying stroma, healing is delayed, and progression to a deep ulcer and beyond may occur. Progression of the lesion may be limited to a small area of the cornea, or the whole cornea may become affected. In chronic or infected ulcers, proteases

Superficial Ulceration → Deep Ulceration → Descemetocele → Iris Prolapse → Endophthalmitis

FIGURE 11–39. Classification scheme for corneal ulcers.

TABLE 11–7. Causes of Corneal Ulcers

Dog	Cat	Horse	Cow	Sheep
Trauma	Trauma	Trauma	IBK	IOK
Foreign body	Foreign body	Entropion (foals)	Trauma	Entropion
Distichiasis	Herpetic keratitis	Foreign bodies		
Keratitis sicca	Senile keratopathy	Mycotic keratitis		
Entropion		Superficial corneal erosions		
Superficial corneal erosion				
Chronic corneal edema (e.g., glaucoma)				
Tumors of lid margin				
Ectopic cilia				
Hyperadrenocorticism (Cushing's disease)				
Senile keratopathy				
Malicious topical substances				
Dog shampoos and dips				

(enzymes that digest protein) may speed progression of a simple ulcer to rupture and iris prolapse (within 24 hours in some cases). Proteases are produced by healing epithelium and bacteria (Pseudomonas especially), and their action is potentiated by corticosteroids. Corneal dissolution under the influence of proteases is often referred to as melting. Proteases are not important in all corneal ulcers. Ulcers in which they are active have a grayish, gelatinous appearance around the margin, which is distinguished from normal corneal edema found around any penetrating stromal wounds to which tear fluid has access. This differentiation may be difficult in the equine cornea, in which there is greater stromal swelling around ulcers than there is in other species. Corneal ulceration causes secondary uveitis and occasionally hypopyon.

Diagnosis

Clinical signs that elicit suspicion of ulceration are
1. Pain and blepharospasm (often of acute onset)
2. Epiphora
3. Purulent ocular discharge
4. Photophobia

Corneal ulcers are often not clearly visible, even with good lighting. For this reason, all red or painful eyes must be stained with fluorescein and the intraocular with fluorescein, indicating an ulcer, do not risk further damage with a tonometer). Ancillary diagnostic tests (e.g., bacterial culture, corneal scraping for Gram's and Giemsa's staining) are also used, depending on the stage of the ulcer.

Treatment

The phases in treatment of a corneal ulcer are diagrammed in Figure 11–40.

Occasionally it is necessary to institute phases 2 and 3 without knowing the etiology, either because it is obscure or because the structural integrity of the eye must be maintained while awaiting laboratory results. The stage reached by the ulcer determines which specific methods are chosen in phases 2 and 3 (Table 11–8). In addition to the measures outlined, topical atropine therapy (1% twice a day) is used to relieve ciliary spasm and pain due to secondary anterior uveitis and to decrease formation of anterior synechiae from the miotic pupil (as a result of uveitis) to the cornea.

In most cases, no attempt is made to inhibit this secondary uveitis or to remove small amounts of purulent exudate and inflammatory cells (hypopyon) in the anterior chamber, as they aid in resolution of the corneal ulcer. The use of topical vitamin A has been recommended in corneal ulcer treatment in dogs and to aid

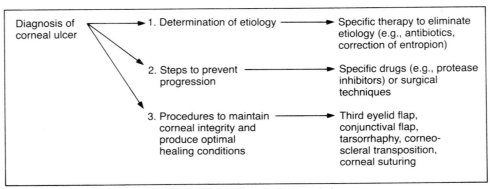

FIGURE 11–40. Treatment of corneal ulcer.

TABLE 11–8. Treatment of Corneal Ulceration

Type of Ulcer	Phase 1	Phase 2	Phase 3
Simple superficial ulcer	Topical antibiotics Correction of lid defects (e.g., entropion, cilia) Topical atropine	Rarely necessary	Rarely necessary
Uncomplicated deep ulcer	Topical antibiotics Topical atropine	Antiprotease agents Débridement	Third eyelid flap Tear replacement
Complicated deep ulcer	Topical, subconjunctival, and systemic antibiotics (subpalpebral lavage) Topical atropine	Antiprotease agents Débridement (surgical, chemical)	Conjunctival or third eyelid flap Tear replacement
Descemetocele	Topical, subconjunctival, and systemic antibiotics (subpalpebral lavage) Topical atropine	Antiprotease agents	Conjunctival or third eyelid flap Tear replacement or corneoscleral transposition Cautious use of surgical adhesives
Iris prolapse	Topical, subconjunctival, and systemic antibiotics (subpalpebral lavage) Topical atropine	Antiprotease agents	Resection or replacement of prolapsed iris Conjunctival or third eyelid flap Suture lacerations Reconstitution of anterior chamber

healing of corneal and scleral wounds, but its efficacy in clinical situations is undetermined. Patients with severe dietary deficiencies may benefit from multivitamin therapy. Although formerly widespread, the use of chemical cautery for treating corneal ulcers has been discontinued in humans and is less popular in veterinary ophthalmology as a result of the ready availability of potent antibiotics. Such chemical cauterants (e.g., liquid phenol, iodine solution) were used to denature protein, enabling them to remove damaged tissue and kill bacteria. Similar and more controlled results with less residual scarring can be achieved by applying basic therapeutic measures—careful surgical débridement, use of antibiotics, and physical coverage of the lesion. Table 11–9 shows a useful medication combining antibiotics, atropine, an antiprotease agent, and a base for topical use in severe ulceration. It is not required in simple ulceration.

Alternatively, artificial tears can be fortified with larger-than-normal concentrations of antibiotics to attain higher corneal concentrations.

Frequency of treatment is decreased from every 1–2 hours for the first few days to 3 or 4 times daily for the next 7–10 days. Other protease inhibitors can also be used (e.g., EDTA, serum; see Chap 3). Serum is thought to act when used topically or subconjunctivally because it contains an alpha$_2$-macroglobulin with anti-

collagenase activity in vitro. The efficacy of serum as the sole anticollagenase agent in limiting the action of collagenase in vivo is debatable.

For uncomplicated corneal ulceration, coverage with one of the various kinds of flaps should be maintained for 7–10 days. During this time topical medications are placed on top of the flap. The flap is removed and the cornea examined if any of the following signs appear during treatment:

1. Purulent discharge
2. Sudden voluminous watery discharge (may indicate corneal rupture)
3. Hemorrhagic discharge
4. Sudden, painful blepharospasm

A small amount of serous discharge from an eye with a conjunctival or third eyelid flap is usual. Such flaps are usually comfortable and do not incite rubbing attempts by the patient.

DESCEMETOCELE (bulging of Descemet's membrane when stroma has been removed) and **IRIS PROLAPSE** are major ocular emergencies requiring immediate intensive treatment. In themselves, these conditions are not indications for enucleation but for correct ophthalmic treatment. The variety of surgical procedures referred to in treatment of corneal ulceration are described at the end of this chapter (for third eyelid flaps, see p 136).

During the healing phase, deep and superficial vascularization occurs, with formation of granulation tissue in the wound bed. Residual scar formation is lessened if corticosteroids are used with care after an epithelial cover has been demonstrated with fluorescein. In these circumstances, the lesion is checked frequently; it should not be covered, and the steroid must be administered in a form (e.g., topical drops) that can readily be discontinued if complications develop. Useful preparations include 0.1% dexamethasone drops and 1% ications may be used provided no infection is present.

TABLE 11–9. Compound Ulcer Drops

Acetylcysteine 20% (Mucomyst)	6 ml
Atropine ophthalmic solution 1%	6 ml
Chloramphenicol succinate 20%	1.2 ml
(or gentamicin 5%)	1.5 ml
Artificial tear solution	sufficient quantity to 25 ml

Modified from Severin GA: Veterinary Ophthalmology Notes, 2nd ed. Ft Collins, CO, 1976.

Corticosteroids are not used without an intact epithelium. Steroids may be used to limit residual scarring after epithelium has covered the defect, during the vascular phase of corneal healing. The place of cyclosporin in this therapy is undetermined.

DEGENERATIVE AND DYSTROPHIC KERATOPATHIES

Focal Corneal Necrosis

Synonyms: Corneal mummification, sequestration, keratitis nigrum
Breed incidence: Persian and occasionally Siamese cats, but it can occur in any breed

The etiology of this disease is unknown, but it usually occurs after chronic ulcerative or inflammatory corneal disease. *Herpes virus felis* is a frequent cause of the initial keratitis, and appropriate steps are taken to treat this infection before treatment of the necrotic process is undertaken. Occasionally the disease is seen with no previous history of corneal disease.

CLINICAL SIGNS

1. A focal, brownish-black corneal lesion (Plate III*H*)
2. Corneal vascularization
3. Epiphora
4. Blepharospasm

The pathogenesis of the lesion is unknown, although the necrotic tissue often fails to stimulate a severe inflammatory reaction. The black material is necrotic cornea, not pigment.

TREATMENT

The necrotic plaque will often detach without the need for surgical intervention. Indications for surgical removal include *persistent pain* and *failure of the material to detach* within a reasonable time, e.g., 3 months. The initiating keratitis must be quiescent, and necrosis must not be extending before keratectomy is performed. Cats with severe pain from the condition should not be subjected to pain, which is often severe, waiting for the necrotic tissue to come off. Prolonged treatment with idoxuridine is indicated if a viral etiology is suspected. The lesion often extends down to Descemet's membrane, and *extreme care* is necessary during removal, which should be performed by a competent ophthalmic microsurgeon. The lesion is covered with a third eyelid flap and treated routinely as a superficial ulcer with antibiotics and atropine.

Corticosteroids may be used to lessen scar formation after 10–14 days *only* if routine fluorescein staining is negative, and *Herpesvirus felis* was not involved in the initial etiology—if in doubt, corticosteroids are omit-

ted. Prolonged protection of the cornea is occasionally necessary before healing occurs. Recurrences after treatment may occur, but results are normally excellent.

> Feline corneal necrosis is a serious corneal disease that must be diagnosed and treated specifically and correctly.

Senile Endothelial Degeneration

Throughout life, the numbers of endothelial cells decrease. In some animals, especially dogs, the numbers fall such that corneal stromal water content is uncontrolled and edema results. Such cell loss can be a function of age alone, or it can be exacerbated by other disease processes, e.g., glaucoma, uveitis. The condition may lead to bullous keratopathy and ulceration or, in less severe cases, to persistent opacity and blindness. Some improvement may occur with hyperosmotic preparations, but definitive therapy is a penetrating corneal allograft (p 301). Chronic corneal edema has been reported in ranch mink (6–11 years of age).

Lipid Keratopathy

Lipid keratopathy refers to deposits—usually cholesterol, cholesterol esters, and triglycerides—in the corneal stroma, causing opacity. Primary lipid keratopathy is deposition in the absence of etiological causes. Secondary lipid keratopathy refers to lipid deposition in association with elevated serum levels of lipid, systemic metabolic hormonal or lipid disturbances, or with chronic keratitis or scleritis. It is relatively rare in dogs, but it is seen both clinically and experimentally.

PRIMARY LIPID KERATOPATHY

Stromal deposits are usually central or isolated from the limbus and may be bilateral or unilateral. In some animals the condition appears familial and may be classified as a dystrophy. The deposits are sometimes progressive and sometimes static and may take a variety of forms, including circles, ovals, and arcs concentric with the limbus. Before a diagnosis of primary keratopathy is made, determination of circulation lipid and thyroid status is made (see later in this chapter). Primary keratopathy often responds to dietary management, but this effect is unreliable, and there may be spontaneous resolution.

SECONDARY LIPID KERATOPATHY

Causes

1. Chronic keratitis and scleritis
2. Hypothyroidism and associated systemic hypercholesterolemia and hypertriglyceridemia

3. Hyperlipoproteinemias of unspecified types

4. In association with chronic corneal scars

In rabbits, the direct source of the deposited cholesterol esters is plasma very low density lipoproteins (TLDL). Phospholipids and triglycerides are metabolized by the keratocytes after uptake of the TLDL, but the amount of cholesterol ester carried by the lipoprotein exceeds the capacity of the cell to remove it, and lipid accumulates in the cornea.

1. Chronic keratitis and scleritis. If progressive lipid keratopathy occurs in the absence of systemic lipid disturbances, low-level inflammation is suspected and corticosteroids (dexamethasone 0.1% 2 or 3 times daily) are applied for prolonged periods. This form is commonly seen in chronic immune-mediated keratoconjunctivitis sicca (Überreiter's syndrome) in dogs. Control of the inflammation will often prevent advancement of the lipid deposits. Dietary therapy is used in addition (see the next section).

2. Hypothyroidism. If hypothyroidism is determined as the cause of systemic lipid disturbances, appropriate replacement therapy is instituted. Dietary therapy is used in addition. This form may be more common in German shepherds.

3. Hyperlipoproteinemia. The range of systemic lipid disturbances in which it is seen is poorly characterized (Figs. 11–41 and 11–42). With overt systemic lipid abnormalities, a whitish deposit extends into the corneal stroma from the limbus. This condition is most frequent in dogs and pet rabbits fed diets containing cholesterol. If the disorder is suspected, serum cholesterol, cholesterol esters, triglycerides, phospholipids, and lipoprotein electrophoretic pattern are determined to characterize the lipid disturbance. Therapy is primarily dietary, in order to reduce serum lipid levels, and antiinflammatory if the lipid is stimulating inflam-

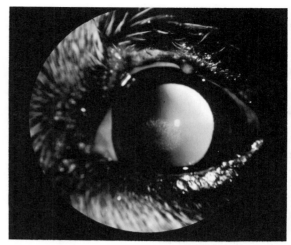

FIGURE 11–42. Secondary lipid keratopathy in a 3-year-old Samoyed with a fasting cholesterol of 400 mg/dl.

mation. Drugs to reduce lipid levels have not been evaluated for this condition in dogs.

4. Chronic corneal scars. Lipid is deposited in previous corneal lesions and scars (Plate IIIC), in either vascularized or nonvascularized areas, and may stimulate further vascularization in previously unaffected areas. Serum lipids are usually within the normal range. This condition is seen most frequently in dogs and horses. Therapy is usually topical corticosteroids to control inflammation caused by the lipid and any residual inflammation which caused the original scar. In dogs, dietary therapy is also used.

Dietary Therapy

1. Reduction of dietary cholesterol and lipids by use of commercial vegetable dog foods, and removal of cheese, milk, and meats from the diet. Commercial dog foods containing meat or bone meal are avoided.

2. Addition of vegetables to the dog's diet, e.g., rice, potatoes.

3. Use of low-cholesterol human foods of vegetable origin, prepared commercially for humans with similar disorder, and available from supermarkets.

Dietary therapy may arrest many instances of lipid keratopathy and, in combination with other methods discussed previously, will sometimes result in absorption of lipid. The aim is prevention of progression, and the owner is advised of this and the long-term nature

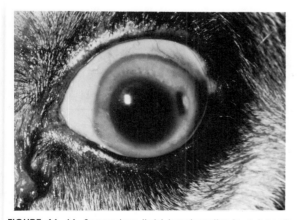

FIGURE 11–41. Secondary lipid keratopathy in a beagle with a total serum lipid in excess of 1000 mg/dl for 12 months. Lipid deposition in this cornea was considerably hastened by deep peripheral vascularization due to a minor corneal ulcer (visible as a white spot at the temporal limbus).

Surgical removal of lipid plaques is *contraindicated*. Keratitis from the keratectomy increases lipid deposition. Similarly, obliteration of limbal feeder vessels increases lipid deposition.

Econqual-cheaper

Maxitrol qid to affected eye
1e/1W
4 ok ✓ TID 2W then BID 2W

of this dietary change. Persistence is necessary with some pampered pets in order to institute a dietary change.

Epithelial Inclusion Cysts

These cysts are a rare, fluid-filled corneal lesion, lined with epithelium but located in the stroma. The cyst appears as an elevation of 3–4 mm on the corneal surface. It is proposed that the cysts are caused by traumatic inclusion of epithelium into the stroma. They are removed by superficial keratectomy (see later in this chapter).

Corneal Dystrophy

Although the terms dystrophy and degeneration are used loosely to refer to a variety of corneal disorders, *dystrophy* implies a developmental and possibly hereditary condition although not always present at birth. Corneal dystrophies may affect the epithelium, stroma, Descemet membrane, or endothelium; they are usually bilateral and may be progressive. Endothelial dystrophies are usually progressive and permanent. Corneal dystrophies are relatively uncommon; details of the more important types are given in Table 11–10. Isolated cases have been described in other breeds. Those forms in which corneal edema occur are treated as for senile endothelial degeneration and bullous keratopathy. Endothelial dystrophy may be treated in selected cases by penetrating corneal graft, but long-term success rates are unreported.

ACQUIRED SCLERAL DISEASES

Acquired disorders of the sclera are uncommon in domestic animals, and a detailed discussion is outside the scope of this book. Because of the inert collagenous nature of the sclera and its relatively poor blood supply, involvement in disease processes is rare.

Episcleritis 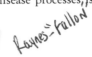 *Raynes-fallon*

Episcleritis is a localized inflammatory disorder affecting conjunctival tissues near the limbus. The lesions may be

1. Nodular (a term borrowed from human ophthalmology, ocular nodular fasciitis, is sometimes applied to these nodules; it is doubtful if the latter condition exists as a separate entity)
2. Diffuse and infiltrative
3. Aggressive and necrotizing, especially in the Airedale

The cause is unknown but is believed to be immunologically mediated. Treatment is by topical and subconjunctival corticosteroid administration and, in severe cases, immunosuppressive agents such as azathia-

prine. Relapses may occur, and the prognosis is guarded.

Scleral Trauma

Trauma to the sclera may result in STAPHYLOMA—a localized ectatic area of sclera or cornea to which a portion of the uveal tract adheres.

Penetrating Wounds

Penetrating wounds are most commonly associated with fights, fixed objects, projectiles, and blunt trauma. The prognosis depends on the extent of damage to the intraocular structures, and careful attempts to perform ophthalmoscopy are advisable. Hyphema, iris prolapse, vitreous hemorrhage or opacity, lens capsule rupture, lens luxation, or retinal detachment in association with either penetrating or perforating scleral wounds indicates a poor prognosis. For simple uncomplicated penetrating wounds, closure and control of postoperative uveitis with corticosteroids and prostaglandin inhibitors is often successful. For more extensive injuries, more sophisticated procedures (e.g., lens removal, vitrectomy, scleral allografting) may be indicated.

Concussive Injuries

Severe concussion causes scleral rupture in the equine eye 1–3 mm from the limbus and concentric with it. These ruptures vary in size from a few millimeters in length to those involving almost the entire circumference, with prolapse of lens, vitreous, iris, and ciliary body. Even extensive scleral ruptures may appear as a small elevation 2–3 mm across, beneath the conjunctiva near the limbus. Less extensive ruptures are treated by suturing with fine nonabsorbable material (e.g., 6/0 nylon) and control of uveitis. The prognosis for extensive ruptures depends on the degree of damage to intraocular structures but is always guarded to poor. Damage to the ciliary body frequently leads to phthisis bulbi.

Penetrating and concussive scleral injuries are major ocular emergencies.

SURGICAL PROCEDURES
Treatment of Corneal Injuries

With penetrating corneal wounds, great care is taken to prevent pressure on the globe in order to avoid the risk of further intraocular damage.

If specialist assistance is not available, a careful examination is made in order to evaluate the extent of intraocular injuries. One of the most common causes for severe endophthalmitis and often secondary glau-

TABLE 11–10. Corneal Dystrophies

Species	Breed	Age of Onset	Clinical Features	References
Dog				
	Afghan hound	—	Superficial ring type	Vainisi and Goldberg, 1984
	Airedale	10 mos	Bilateral progressive axial opacity	Dice, 1974
	Beagle		See Siberian husky	Waring et al, 1977, 1979; Ekins et al, 1980; Roth et al, 1981
	Boston terrier (females)	8 yrs or older	Mild central edema that progresses to total opacity after 2–3 years; epithelial bullae form and rupture in severe cases; endothelium affected; concurrent increase in intraocular pressure occurs in both Boston terriers and Chihuahuas	Severin, 1976; Martin and Dice, 1982
	Cavalier King Charles	2–3 years	Axial, stromal opacities	Slatter, 1980; Crispin and Barnett, 1983
	Chihuahua		See Boston terrier	Dice, 1981; Martin and Dice, 1982
	Collie, rough	most by 2–4 mos	Unilateral and bilateral lipid deposits	Stades and Barnett, 1981
	German shepherd		Central, lipid	Crispin and Barnett, 1983
	Samoyed	6–24 mos	Annular or circular posterior and anterior stromal opacities; opacities are lipid, but serum lipid is normal	
	Shetland sheepdog	Variable	Unilateral and bilateral lipid deposits	Barnett and Stades, 1979
	Siberian husky	6–24 mos	Annular or circular posterior and anterior stromal opacities; opacities are lipid, but serum lipid is normal	Macmillan et al, 1979
Cat				
	Manx	4 mos	Axial stromal haziness and edema, then secondary epithelial involvement	Bistner et al, 1976
Ranch Mink		8–11 yrs	Onset over a month, to total opacity; endothelium affected	Hadlow, 1987

Note: Endothelial dystrophy has also been observed in the boxer, dachshund, and poodle.

If possible, a third eyelid flap is placed over the wound, systemic antibiotic therapy is instituted, and the case is referred to a veterinary ophthalmologist for treatment as soon as possible.

---

coma leading to ENUCLEATION in dogs is unsuspected damage to the lens and its capsule during a perforating corneal injury. If no other intraocular damage is evident, the corneal wound may be sutured. Routine steps to expose and fix the eye are discussed in Chapter 6.

Equipment (see Fig. 6–29)

Magnifying loupe (2× to 4×) (operating microscope preferable)
Lid retractors
Ophthalmic needle holders

Corneal scissors
Iris scissors
Corneal forceps
Cyclodialysis spatula
Anterior chamber irrigating bulb and needle
Fine suture, e.g., 7/0 or 8/0 silk or nylon with swaged needle
Cellulose sponge (WeckCel sponge)
Balanced salt solution (Alcon) for irrigation.
Epinephrine (1:10,000)[8] and dilute heparin may be added to control hemorrhage and fibrin, respectively

CLOSURE OF A CORNEAL WOUND

1. The corneal endothelium is exquisitely sensitive to trauma. It is never touched with instruments or

---

8. Although dilute epinephrine (1:10,000) has been added to irrigating solutions for hemostasis, the risk of inducing cardiac syncope and fibrillation is always present.

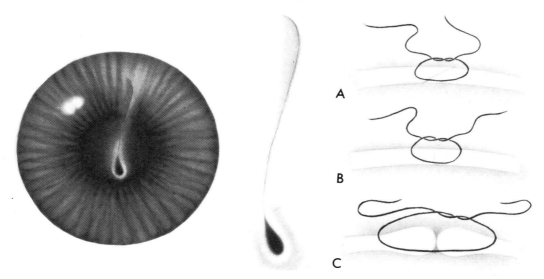

FIGURE 11–43. *Repair of corneal laceration. The diagram illustrates suggested placement of nylon suture material (A) for shelved laceration, (B) for vertical laceration, and (C) for laceration with edematous margins. (From Slatter DH: Cornea and sclera. In Slatter DH [ed]: Textbook of Small Animal Surgery. WB Saunders Co, Philadelphia, 1985. Redrawn from Paton D, Goldberg MF: Management of Ocular Injuries. WB Saunders, Philadelphia, 1976.*

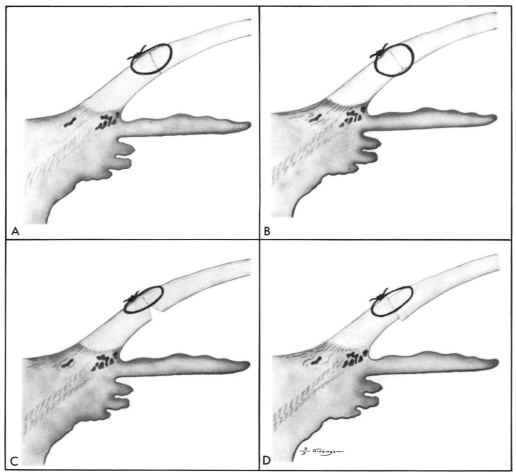

FIGURE 11–44. *A, A correctly placed corneal suture. B, Suture incorrectly penetrates the anterior chamber. C, Suture is too superficial, resulting in poor endothelial closure and persistent edema. D, Bites of the suture have been uneven, resulting in poor apposition of the wound edges. (From Slatter DH: Cornea and Sclera. In Slatter DH [ed]: Textbook of Small Animal Surgery. WB Saunders Co, Philadelphia, 1985. Redrawn from Severin GA: Veterinary Ophthalmology Notes, 2nd ed. Ft Collins, CO, 1976.)*

flushed vigorously. When the edges of a corneal wound are held, the stroma and epithelium only are touched with the forceps.

2. The edges of corneal wounds are not débrided—as much tissue as possible is left in place in order to complete closure.

3. If the wound is fresh, an attempt is made to replace any protruding iris with an iris repositor. If the tissue is damaged, the protruding iris is excised. This process may be assisted if the anterior chamber is reconstituted with sodium hyaluronate. Hemorrhage may be severe if the excision is near the major arterial circle of the iris—electrocautery is advised.

4. Blood and fibrin clots in the anterior chamber are carefully removed with a cyclodialysis spatula or Arruga lens capsule forceps before the wound is closed.

5. Partial-thickness sutures are used in the cornea rather than full-thickness penetrating sutures (Figs. 11–43 and 11–44).

6. The cornea is sutured with simple interrupted sutures about 1 mm apart.

7. After partial closure of the wound, the anterior chamber is *carefully* flushed to remove loose debris.

8. The wound is closed and the anterior chamber reconstituted with balanced salt solution or a small air bubble (Fig. 11–45). In uncomplicated corneal wounds some sutures may be removed in as soon as 7 days.

The prognosis for a corneal wound depends on its initial depth and severity. Lacerations usually have a good prognosis, as do wounds that penetrate the superficial layers only rather than perforating the entire corneal thickness. Perforating wounds usually heal by vascularization, with more scar tissue and opacity. Ruptures of the cornea have a poorer prognosis than do simple lacerations or perforating wounds because of the greater tissue disruption at the wound edge.

Prognosis of Equine Ocular Lacerations

Lacerations involving the cornea alone and sharp lacerations each have a better prognosis than those affecting both the cornea and the sclera or blunt lacerations, respectively.[9]

Descemetocele[10]

A descemetocele is a protrusion of Descemet's membrane through a defect in the corneal epithelium and stroma (see Figs. 5–14, 11–22, and 11–23). It requires urgent repair because of the risk of corneal rupture.

Descemetocele is a surgical emergency.

---

9. Lavach JD, et al: Lacerations of the equine eye: A review of 48 cases. J Am Vet Med Assoc 184:1243, 1984.
10. See also Table 11–7.

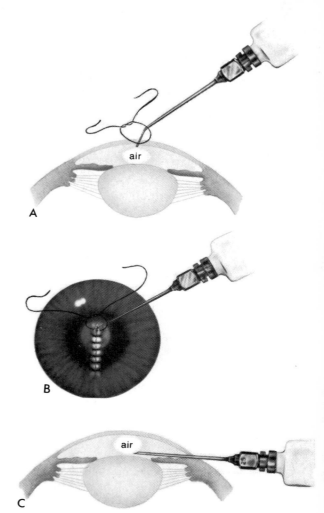

FIGURE 11–45. *Reconstruction of the anterior chamber with a sterile air bubble or balanced salt solution. A and B, A cannula may be placed between the wound edges of (C) via a 25-gauge needle from the limbus. With the sterile air bubble method, care must be taken to use as little air as possible, since, if air gets behind the iris, air-block glaucoma can occur. Balanced salt solution is preferable to air. (Redrawn from Severin GA: Veterinary Ophthalmology Notes, 2nd ed. Ft Collins, CO, 1976.)*

The cause of the corneal lesion is treated and the cornea is given structural support to prevent rupture. Direct suturing is often possible in small descemetoceles but produces corneal distortion (ASTIGMATISM), which is of little significance in dogs and cats. For direct suturing, the surrounding cornea must be strong enough to hold sutures.

THERAPY

Infected or severely damaged ulcer margins are débrided carefully. The defect is closed by direct suturing (Fig. 11–46). As the edges are often edematous, horizontal mattress sutures may be necessary.

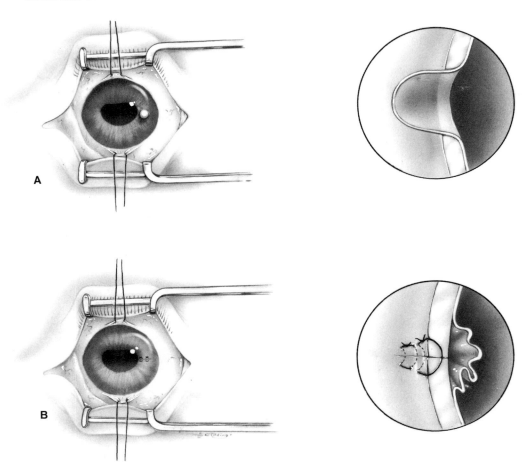

FIGURE 11–46. Direct suturing of a descemetocele. A, A descemetocele prior to direct suturing. A similar method is used for deep ulcers in danger of rupture. B, Horizontal mattress sutures are placed as necessary to close the defect (7/0 or 8/0 nylon is ideal). Descemet's membrane is not penetrated by the suture. The cornea heals with vascularization.

The anterior chamber is reconstituted with an air bubble or balanced salt solution. For simple lacerations and penetrating wounds causing descemetocele, direct suturing is usually the best treatment. If direct closure is not possible, several alternatives are available:

1. PLACEMENT OF A CONJUNCTIVAL FLAP to support the lesion and aid in vascularization. Of the numerous kinds available, a 360° fornix-based flap is the easiest to perform (Figs. 11–47 and 11–48). Further support may be given with a third eyelid flap or temporary tarsorrhaphy. For the occasional operator, a third eyelid flap is easier to perform than is a conjunctival flap, but support is not as secure, and it does not supply fibroblasts to areas of severe corneal destruction.

Structural support can also be achieved by placement of a corneal graft, which is later rejected, or a variety of covering materials, including egg membranes, contact lenses, conjuctiva dissected from the third eyelid and sutured into the defect, and free bulbar and palpebral conjunctival grafts. Recently revived interest in free palpebral conjunctival grafts indicates they may

become vascularized after 10 days, survive, and later become pigmented after 4–6 months. The principle of using a full bridge or 360° graft with intact blood supply is preferable.

2. CORNEOSCLERAL TRANSPOSITION from an adjacent area of normal cornea, to fill substantial defects. Donor tissue is always available with this method, but it is time-consuming and painstaking to perform (Fig. 11–49).

3. INSERTION OF A CORNEAL ALLOGRAFT into the defect to add support. The lesion eventually vascularizes and the button is rejected, but the cornea can often be saved. This method is limited by availability of donor tissue.

4. CONJUNCTIVAL PEDICLE GRAFTING. Such pedicles are a variation on the same principle of the corneoscleral transposition. The steps in placing and securing a bulbar conjunctival pedicle are shown in Fig. 11–50. Such pedicles can be used with minor leakage of aqueous present in the same way as a 360° flap.

Topical antibiotics, atropine, and antiproteases are

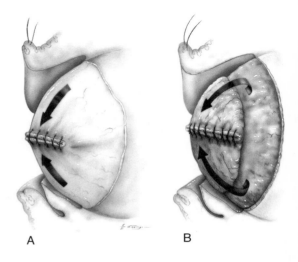

FIGURE 11–47. *Conjunctival flaps. A, Fornix-based flap. B, Limbus-based flap.*

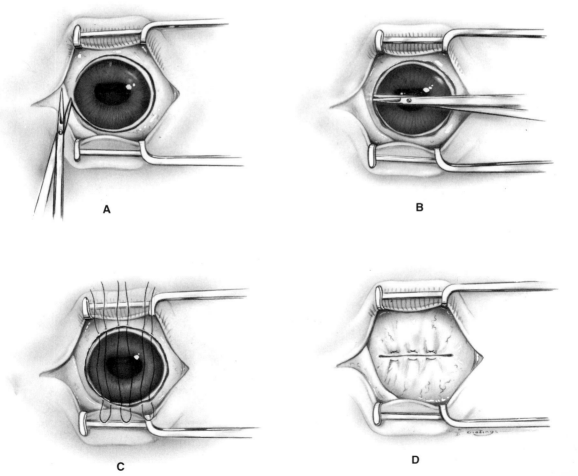

FIGURE 11–48. *Conjunctival flap for descemetocele. A, A fornix-based flap is prepared by dissection around the limbus with strabismus scissors. B, The flap is undermined for 4–5 mm. C, Three or four horizontal mattress sutures of 6/0 silk (to prevent breakage before healing of the corneal lesion) are placed. D, The sutures are tied to cover the cornea entirely.*

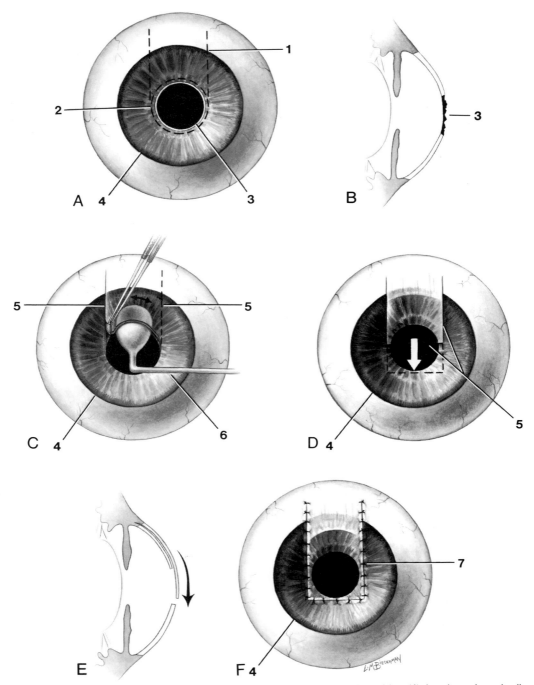

FIGURE 11–49. Corneoscleral transposition (method of Parshall). A, *Line of graft excision (1); borders of surgically excised lesion (2); limits of necrotic tissue (3); limbus (4).* B, *Necrotic tissue (3).* C, *Limbus (4); edge of graft (5); corneal elevator (6).* D, *Limbus (4); end of graft (5).* E, *Graft is moved ventrally to cover defect.* F, *Limbus (4); placement of sutures (7).*

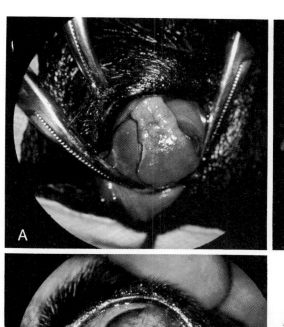

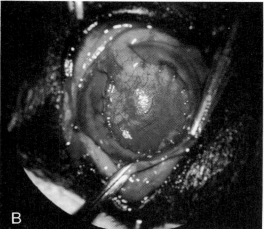

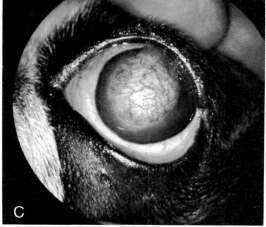

FIGURE 11–50. A, Conjunctival graft placed on the cornea, with the first suture placed in the pedicle midline, dorsal to the ulcer. B, The graft sutured to cover the ulcer (7/0 Vicryl is used). C, A pedicle graft 10 weeks postoperatively. (From Hakanson N, et al: Further comments on conjunctival pedicle grafting in the treatment of corneal ulcers in the dog and cat. J Am Anim Hosp Assoc 24:602, 1988.)

used postoperatively. Severe penetrating wounds of the cornea affected with ulcerative or inflammatory lesions and loss of tissue, e.g., in brachycephalic breeds, often lead to a healed and scarred cornea with loss of the anterior chamber. Iris bombé and secondary glaucoma may result, but the eye may remain painless and cosmetically acceptable.

Removal of Corneal Foreign Bodies

Corneal foreign bodies are removed to limit pain, reduce the risk of infection, and prevent vascularization and scar formation. Small embedded foreign bodies are removed with a needle-shaped instrument called a foreign body spud. In an emergency a 25-gauge needle can be used with a magnifying loupe. Adherent foreign bodies, e.g., flakes of paint, are often found lying in a depression in the corneal epithelium, with the lids passing over them. Such objects may be removed by lifting the edge with an instrument. Objects embedded in the stroma may require an incision in the epithelium over the long axis of the foreign body for removal.

After removal of foreign bodies with the patient under local or general anesthesia, a broad-spectrum topical antibiotic and atropine are administered to limit infection and the effects of secondary uveitis. Corneal epithelial healing is normally rapid, and local anesthetics, which retard epithelial healing, are unnecessary and contraindicated postoperatively. Clumsy attempts to remove a corneal foreign body may result in penetration of the anterior chamber or in corneal damage, causing more severe vascularization and scar formation.

Superficial Keratectomy

Keratectomy is a delicate procedure requiring the correct instruments, magnification, training, and experience.

Keratectomy is removal of the corneal epithelium or stroma. Because the stroma does not regenerate, the number of successive keratectomies that can be performed is limited to two or three, depending on how

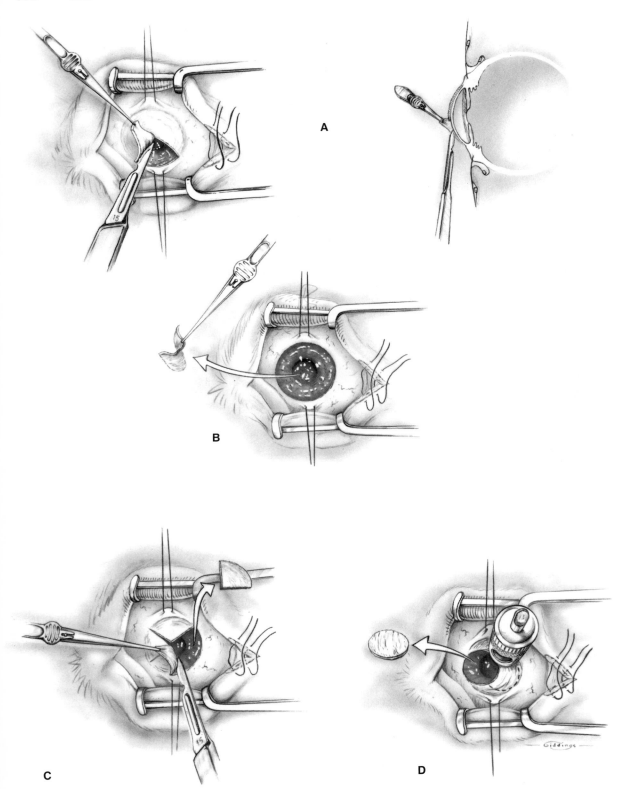

FIGURE 11–51. A and B, Removal of a large lesion en bloc. Canthotomy is used only if required. Although clear at this stage, the cornea soon becomes edematous. C, Division of the cornea into quadrants. D, Outlining the area for removal with a corneal trephine. The canthotomy is closed. (Redrawn from Severin GA: Veterinary Ophthalmology Notes, 2nd ed. Ft Collins, CO, 1976.)

much tissue is removed each time. Thus, keratectomy is of limited use for a pathological process that will continue after the procedure.

INDICATIONS

1. Removal of neoplasms encroaching from the limbus (e.g., SCC in cattle).
2. Treatment of specific keratopathies (e.g., superficial corneal erosion, focal corneal necrosis, epithelial inclusion cysts).
3. Débridement of superficial corneal wounds.
4. Biopsy for diagnostic purposes.

PROCEDURE

Keratectomy may be complete or partial. In complete keratectomy, the area to be removed is outlined with a corneal trephine set to a predetermined depth (0.3–0.4 mm) or by dividing the cornea into segments (Fig. 11–51). The initial incision is made under magnification with a No. 64 Beaver, No. 15 Bard-Parker blade, and dissection is continued with a Martinez corneal elevator. The stroma is removed in sheets to the limbus, where it is cut with corneal scissors or a scalpel. Postoperatively, the cornea is either covered with a third eyelid flap or stained daily with fluorescein to evaluate epithelialization, and topical antibiotics and atropine are applied.

Keratoplasty[11]

Keratoplasty is transplantation of corneal tissue. There are two types of keratoplasties: LAMELLAR (partial thickness) and PENETRATING (full thickness). Because of the "privileged" immunological site of the cornea, corneal transplants have a better survival rate than do transplants in other parts of the body. The indications for their use are infrequent in domestic animals, although successful results can be achieved in dogs, cats, and horses. Meticulous surgical technique and postoperative care are needed for success, and use of the technique is restricted to specialist practices and larger institutions.

REFERENCES

Al-aubaidi JM, et al (1973): Identification and characterization of *Acholeplasma oculusi* from the eyes of goats with keratoconjunctivitis. Cornell Vet 63:117.

Ali Z, Insler MS (1986): A comparison of therapeutic bandage lenses, tarsorrhaphy, and antibiotic and hypertonic saline on corneal epithelial wound healing. Ann Ophthalmol 18:22.

Ashton N, Cook C (1951): Effect of cortisone on healing of corneal wounds. Br J Ophthalmol 35:708.

Barber DM, et al (1986): Microbial flora of the eyes of cattle. Vet Rec 118:204.

Barnett KC, Ogden AL (1972): Ocular colobomata in charolais cattle. Vet Rec 91:592.

Barnett KC, Stades FC (1979): Collie eye anomaly in the Shetland sheepdog in the Netherlands. J Sm Anim Pract 20:321.

Bedford PGC (1982): Collie eye anomaly in the border collie. Vet Rec 111:34.

Befanis PJ, et al (1981): Endothelial repair of the canine cornea. Am J Vet Res 21:113.

Bellhorn RW, Henkind P (1966): Superficial pigmentary keratitis in the dog. J Am Vet Med Assoc 149:173.

Beotista PJ (1979): Infectious bovine keratoconjunctivitis: A review. Br Vet J 135:225.

Bistner SI (1973): Ocular manifestations of systemic disease. Vet Clin North Am 3:467.

Bistner SI, et al (1976): Hereditary corneal dystrophy in the Manx cat: A preliminary report. Invest Ophthalmol 15:15.

Bistner SI, et al (1977): Atlas of Veterinary Ophthalmic Surgery. WB Saunders Co, Philadelphia.

Blogg JR (1970): Collie eye anomaly. Aust Vet J 46:530.

Blogg JR (1983): Corneal oedema after vaccination of dogs with canine adenovirus 2. Aust Vet J 60:284.

Blood DC, et al (1983): Veterinary Medicine, 6th ed. Bailliere Tindall and Cassell, London.

Bogaard AE (1984): Inclusion keratoconjunctivitis ("pink eye"). A proposal for a new name for chlamydial keratoconjunctivitis in sheep and comment on recent clinical trials. Vet Q 6:229.

Bulgin MS, Dubose DA (1982): Pinkeye associated with *Branhamella ovis* infection in dairy goats. Vet Med Small Anim Clin 77:1791.

Buyukmihci N, et al (1977): Encephalitozoon (Nosema) infection of the cornea in a cat. J Am Vet Med Assoc 171:355.

Carrington SD (1983): Lipid keratopathy in a cat. J Sm Anim Pract 24:495.

Catcott EJ (1969): Collie eye panel—summary and conclusion. J Am Vet Med Assoc 155:877.

Chesnokova NB, Maichuk YF (1986): Antiproteases in herpetic keratitis. Metab Pediatr Syst Ophthalmol 9:593.

Cooley PL, Wyman M (1986): Indolent-like corneal ulcers in 3 horses. J Am Vet Med Assoc 188:295.

Cooper BS (1967): Contagious conjunctivokeratitis (C.C.K.) of sheep in New Zealand. New Zealand Vet J 15:79.

Costa ND, Slatter DH (1983): The potency of acetylcysteine in pharmaceutical preparations—Effects of temperature and storage. Aust Vet J 60:195.

Crispin SM (1988) Crystalline corneal dystrophy in the dog. Histochemical and ultrastructural study. Cornea 7:149.

Crispin SM, Barnett KC (1983): Dystrophy, degeneration and infiltration of the canine cornea. J Sm Anim Pract 24:83.

Deas DW (1959): A note on hereditary opacity of the cornea in British Friesian cattle. Vet Rec 71:619.

Dice P (1974): Corneal dystrophy in the Airedale. Proc Am Coll Vet Ophthalmol 5:80.

Dice P (1981): The canine cornea. *In* Gelatt KN (ed): Veterinary Ophthalmology. Lea & Febiger, Philadelphia.

Dice P, Martin CL (1976): Corneal endothelial-epithelial dystrophy in the dog. Proc Am Coll Vet Ophthalmol 7:36.

Dikstein S, Maurice DM (1972): The active control of corneal hydration. Isr J Med Sci 8:1523.

Dohlman C (1971): The function of the corneal epithelium in health and disease. Invest Ophthalmol 10:383.

Duke-Elder S, Leigh AG (1965): System of Ophthalmology, vol 7, part 2, Disease of the Outer Eye. H Kimpton, London.

Ekins MB, et al (1980): Oval lipid corneal opacities in Beagles. Part 2. Natural history over 4 years, and study of tear function. J Am Anim Hosp Assoc 16:601.

Falco M, Barnett KC (1978): The inheritance of ocular colobomata in charolais cattle. Vet Rec 102:102.

---

11. For details of penetrating and lamellar keratoplasty, corneoscleral allografts, corneal preservation, and keratoprosthesis, refer to Slatter DH (1985): Textbook of Small Animal Surgery, vol II, Chap 105, Cornea. WB Saunders Co, Philadelphia, and other reference works.

Fechner PU, Fechner MU (1983): Methylcellulose and lens implantation. Br J Ophthalmol 67:259.

Formston C, et al (1974): Corneal necrosis in the cat. J Sm Anim Pract 15:19.

Gelatt KN, Veith LA (1970): Hereditary multiple ocular anomalies in Australian shepherd [sic] dogs. Vet Med Small Anim Clin 65:39.

George L, et al (1988): Enhancement of infectious bovine keratoconjunctivitis by modified live infectious bovine rhinotracheitis virus vaccine. Am J Vet Res 49:1800.

George L, et al (1988): Topically applied furazolidone or parentally administered oxytetracycline for the treatment of infectious bovine keratoconjunctivitis. J Am Vet Med Assoc 192:1415.

Gibb JA (1975): Colobomata in charolais cattle. Vet Rec 96:253.

Gillette EK, et al (1975): Endothelial repair of radiation damage following beta irradiation. Radiology 116:175.

Glass HW, Gerhardt RR (1984): Transmission of *Moraxella bovis* by regurgitation from the crop of the face fly (Diptera: Muscidae). J Econ Entomol 77:399.

Gwin RL, et al (1982): Decrease in canine corneal endothelial cell density and increase in corneal thickness as functions of age. Invest Ophthalmol Vis Sci 22:267.

Gwin RL, et al (1982): Primary canine corneal endothelial cell dystrophy: Specular microscopic evaluation, diagnosis and therapy. J Am Anim Hosp Assoc 18:471.

Hadlow WJ (1987): Chronic corneal edema in aged ranch mink. Vet Pathol 24:323.

Hakanson N, et al (1987): Conjunctival pedicle grafting in the treatment of corneal ulcers in the dog and cat. J Am Anim Hosp Assoc 23:641.

Hakanson N, et al (1988): Further comments on conjunctival pedicle grafting in the treatment of corneal ulcers in the dog and cat. J Am Anim Hosp Assoc 24:602.

Hammer ME, Burch TG (1984): Viscous corneal protection by sodium hyaluronate, chondroitin sulfate and methylcellulose. Invest Ophthalmol Vis Sci 25:1329.

Hodgson DR, Jacobs KA (1982): Two cases of fusarium keratomycosis in the horse. Vet Rec 110:520.

Hogan MJ, et al (1971): Histology of the Human Eye. WB Saunders Co, Philadelphia.

Hopkins JB, et al (1973): Conjunctivitis associated with chlamydial polyarthritis in lambs. J Am Vet Med Assoc 163:1157.

Hosie BD (1988): Keratoconjunctivitis in a hill sheep flock. Vet Rec 122:40.

Hughes DE, Pugh GW (1970): A five-year study of infectious bovine keratoconjunctivitis in a beef herd. J Am Vet Med Assoc 157:433.

Hughes DE, et al (1965): Ultraviolet radiation and *Moraxella bovis* in the etiology of bovine infectious keratoconjunctivitis. Am J Vet Res 16:1331.

Kaufman HE, Katz JI (1977): Pathology of the corneal endothelium. Invest Ophthalmol Vis Sci 16:265.

Kopecky KE, et al (1986): Infectious bovine keratoconjunctivitis: Contact transmission. Am J Vet Res 47:622.

Knecht CD, et al (1966): Focal degeneration of the cornea in a cat. J Am Vet Med Assoc 149:1192.

Koch SA, et al (1974): Corneal epithelial inclusion cysts in four dogs. J Am Vet Med Assoc 164:1190.

Latimer CA, et al (1983): Azathioprine in the management of fibrous histiocytoma in two dogs. J Am Anim Hosp Assoc 19:155.

Lavach JD, et al (1984): Lacerations of the equine eye: A review of 48 cases. J Am Vet Med Assoc 184:1243.

Lehr C, et al (1985): Serologic and protective characterization of *Moraxella bovis* pili. Cornell Vet 75:484.

Lepper AW, Barton IJ (1987): Infectious bovine keratoconjunctivitis: Seasonal variation in cultural, biochemical and immunoreactive properties of *Moraxella bovis* isolated from the eyes of cattle. Aust Vet J 64:33.

Lepper AW, Hermans LR (1986): Characterisation and quantitation of pilus antigens of *Moraxella bovis* by ELISA. Aust Vet J 63:401.

Macmillan AD, et al (1979): Crystalline corneal opacities in the Siberian husky. J Am Vet Med Assoc 175:829.

Martin CL (1981): Canine epibulbar melanomas and their management. J Am Anim Hosp Assoc 17:83.

Martin CL, Dice PF (1982): Corneal endothelial dystrophy in the dog. J Am Anim Hosp Assoc 18:327.

McCauley EH, et al (1971): Isolation of mycoplasma from goats during an epizootic of keratoconjunctivitis. Am J Vet Res 32:861.

McCormack J, et al (1975): Typical colobomas in charolais cattle. Vet Med Small Anim Clin 70:182.

Mendelsohn AD, et al (1986): Laser photocoagulation of feeder vessels in lipid keratopathy. Ophthalmic Surg 17:502.

Michaelson IC (1975): Proliferation of limbal melanoblasts into the cornea in response to the corneal lesion. Br J Opthalmol 36:657.

Mishima S (1982): Clinical investigations on the corneal endothelium. Am J Ophthalmol 93:1.

Moore CW, et al (1983): Bacterial and fungal isolates from *Equidae* with ulcerative keratitis. J Am Vet Med Assoc 182:600.

Moore LJ, Rutter JM (1987): Antigenic analysis of fimbrial proteins from *Moraxella bovis*. J Clin Microbiol 25:2063.

Morrin LA, et al (1982): Oval lipid opacities in beagles. Ultrastructure of normal beagle cornea. Am J Vet Res 43:443.

Moses RA (1977): Adler's Physiology of the Eye, 6th ed. CV Mosby Co, St Louis.

Myers-Elliot RH, et al (1988): Effect of cyclosporine A on the corneal inflammatory response in herpes simplex virus keratitis. Exp Eye Res 45:281.

Neaderland MH, et al (1987): Healing of experimentally induced corneal ulcers in horses. Am J Vet Res 48:427.

Parshall CJ (1973): Lamellar corneoscleral transposition. J Am Anim Hosp Assoc 9:270.

Paulsen ME et al (1987): Feline eosinophilic keratitis: A review of 15 clinical cases. J Am Anim Hosp Assoc 23:63.

Paulsen ME, et al (1987): Nodular granulomatous episclerokeratitis in dogs: 19 dogs (1973–1985). J Am Vet Med Assoc 190:1581.

Pedersen KB (1973): Excretion of some drugs in bovine tears. Acta Pharmacol et Toxicol 32:455.

Peiffer RL, et al (1977): Tarsconjunctival pedicle grafts for deep cornea: ulceration in the dog and cat. J Am Anim Hosp Assoc 13:387.

Pfister RR (1975): The healing of corneal epithelial abrasions in the rabbit: A scanning electron microscope study. Invest Opthalmol 14:648.

Pitman DR, Reuter R (1988): Isolation of *Branhamella ovis* from conjunctivae of Angora goats. Aust Vet J 65:91.

Prince JN, et al (1960): Anatomy and Histology of the Eye and Orbit in Domestic Animals. Charles C Thomas, Springfield, IL.

Pugh G (1979): Treating infectious bovine keratitis. J Am Vet Med Ass 175:1209.

Pugh GW, et al (1985): Infectious bovine keratoconjunctivitis: Subconjunctival administration of a *Moraxella bovis* pilus preparation enhances immunogenicity. Am J Vet Res 46:811.

Pugh GW, et al (1986): Infectious bovine keratoconjunctivitis: Evidence for genetic modulation of resistance in purebred Hereford cattle. Am J Vet Res 47:885.

Punch PI, Slatter DH (1984): Infectious bovine keratoconjunctivitis—A review. Vet Bull 54:193.

Rebhun WC (1982): Corneal stromal abscesses in the horse. J Am Vet Med Assoc 181:677.

Reddy C, et al (1987): Pathogenesis of experimental lipid keratopathy: Corneal and plasma lipids. Invest Ophthalmol 28:1492.

Roberts SR, et al (1966): The collie ectasia syndrome. Pathology of eye of young and adult dogs. Am J Ophthalmol 62:728.

Roberts SR (1969): The collie eye anomaly. J Am Vet Med Assoc 155:859.

Roberts SR, et al (1972): Dendritic keratitis in a cat. J Am Vet Med Assoc 161:285.

Rogers DG, et al (1987): Pathogenesis of corneal lesions caused by *Moraxella bovis* in gnotobiotic calves. Vet Pathol 24:287.

Rosenbusch RF, Knudtson WU (1980): Bovine mycoplasmal conjunctivitis: Experimental reproduction and characterization of the disease. Cornell Vet 70:307.

Roth AM, et al (1981): Oval corneal opacities in beagles. Part 3.

Histochemical demonstration of stromal lipids without hyperlipidemia. Invest Ophthalmol Vis Sci 21:95.

Saunders LZ, Rubin LF (1975): Ophthalmic Pathology of Animals. S Karger, Basel.

Severin, GA (1976): Veterinary Ophthalmology Notes, 2nd ed. Ft Collins, CO.

Shively JN, Epling GP (1970): FIne structure of the canine eye: Cornea. Am J Vet Res 31:713.

Spangler WL, et al (1981): Oval lipid corneal opacities in beagles. Part 5. Ultrastructure. Vet Pathol 19:150.

Slatter DH (1980): Unpublished data.

Slatter DH, et al (1977): Überreiter's syndrome (chronic superficial keratitis) in dogs in the Rocky Mountain area—A study of 463 cases. J Sm Anim Pract 18:757.

Smith JS, et al (1976): Infiltrative corneal lesions resembling fibrous histiocytoma: Clinical and pathologic findings in 6 dogs and one cat. J Am Vet Med Assoc 169:722.

Spradbrow PB, Marley J (1971): Ovine keratoconjunctivitis: Possible T strain mycoplasms in the conjunctival sac. Aust Vet J 47:116.

Stades FC, Barnett KC (1981): Collie eye anomaly in collies in the Netherlands. Vet Q 3:66.

Stapleton S, Peiffer RL (1979): Specular microscopic observations of the clinically normal canine corneal endothelium.

Startup FC (1988): Corneal necrosis and sequestration in the cat: A review and record of 100 cases. J Sm Anim Pract 29:476.

Sugar J, Chandler JW (1974): Experimental corneal wound strength—Effect of topically applied corticosteroids. Arch Opthalmol 92:248.

Surman PG (1968): Cytology of "pink eye" of sheep, including a reference to trachoma of man, by employing acridine orange and iodine stains and isolation of mycoplasma agents from infected sheep eyes. Aust J Biol Sci 21:447.

Szymanski C (1987): The eye. In Holzworth J (ed): Diseases of the Cat. WB Saunders Co, Philadelphia.

Vainisi S, Goldberg MF (1984): Animal models of inherited human eye disease, 215. In Goldberg MF (ed): Genetic and Metabolic Eye Diseases. Little, Brown, Boston.

Walker KH, et al (1975): Typical colobomata in cattle. Aust Vet Pract 5:25.

Waring GO, et al (1977): Oval corneal opacities in beagles. J Am Anim Hosp Assoc 13:204.

Waring GO, et al (1979): Oval lipid corneal opacities in beagles and crystalline lipid corneal opacities in Siberian huskies. Metab Pediatr Syst Ophthalmol 3:203.

Waring GO, et al (1986): Inheritance of crystalline corneal dystrophy in Siberian huskies. J Am Anim Hosp Assoc 22:655.

Webber JJ, et al (1988): Topical treatment of ovine keratoconjunctivitis. Aust Vet J 65:95.

Wilson WD, et al (1987): Ormetoprim-sulfadimethoxine in cattle: Pharmacokinetics, bioavailability, distribution to the tears, and in vitro activity against *Moraxella bovis*. Am J Vet Res 48:407.

Wijeratne WVS (1975): Coloboma in charolais. Vet Rec 96:139.

Yakely WL, et al (1968): Genetic transmission of an ocular fundus anomaly in collies. J Am Vet Med Assoc 152:457.

Yakely WL (1972): Collie eye anomaly: Decreased prevalence through selective breeding. J Am Vet Med Assoc 161:1103.

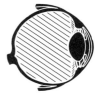

12

Uvea

ANATOMY AND PHYSIOLOGY	**NEOPLASMS**	**MISCELLANEOUS DISORDERS**
PATHOLOGICAL REACTIONS	**UVEITIS**	**SURGICAL PROCEDURES**
CONGENITAL ABNORMALITIES	**INJURIES**	

Uveal diseases are frequent in veterinary practice. An understanding of the structure and function of the uvea contributes to an intelligent approach to handling difficult uveal disorders.

ANATOMY AND PHYSIOLOGY

The eye has three basic layers (Fig. 12–1):
1. Fibrous (outer) layer—the sclera and cornea
2. Vascular (middle) layer—the uvea, or uveal tract

3. Neuroectodermal (inner) layer—the retina and optic nerve

The UVEAL TRACT has three parts: the IRIS, CILIARY BODY, and CHOROID.

Iris

The iris controls the amount of light entering the eye by varying the size of the pupil. Reduction in size of the pupil also increases depth of field for near objects and reduces optical aberrations. To do this the iris has two sets of muscles:

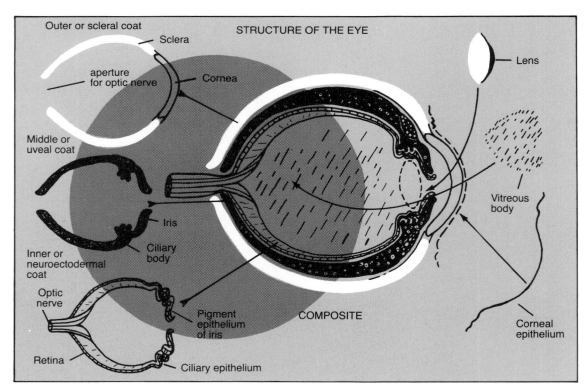

FIGURE 12–1. *The three layers of the eye. (From Fine BS, Yanoff M: Ocular Histology. Harper & Row, New York, 1972.)*

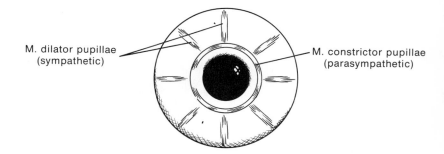

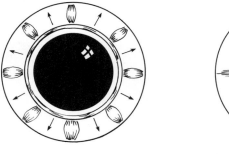

FIGURE 12–2. Control of pupil size. The arrangement of the constrictor fibers varies among domestic species, but the principles are similar.

DILATION
(mydriasis)
Dilators contract: constrictors relax

CONSTRICTION
(miosis)
Constrictors contract: dilators relax

1. M. CONSTRICTOR PUPILLAE—a circular band of muscle fibers concentric with the pupil. These fibers have *parasympathetic* innervation (Fig. 12–2).

2. M. DILATOR PUPILLAE—radially oriented fibers passing from the region near the pupil toward the root of the iris. These fibers have *sympathetic* innervation.

Viewed from the anterior, the iris has two zones: the PUPILLARY ZONE (Figs. 12–3 and 12–4) and the CILIARY ZONE. A variable thickening of the iris anteroposteriorly between these two zones is termed the COLLARETTE. The anterior surface of the iris is covered by a modified layer of stromal cells—the ANTERIOR BORDER LAYER (Fig. 12–5). The remaining parts of the iris are the STROMA and SPHINCTER MUSCLE, the ANTERIOR EPITHELIUM and DILATOR MUSCLE, and the POSTERIOR PIGMENTED EPITHELIUM and PIGMENT RUFF. The posterior pigmented epithelium is continuous with the nonpigmented epithelium covering the ciliary body and eventually with the retina.

The bulk of the iris is stroma, consisting of fibrous connective tissue with bundles of collagen, pigmented and nonpigmented cells, and blood vessels in a mucopolysaccharide matrix (Fig. 12–6). The structure of the iris does not vary with color, variations in hue being due to variations in stromal pigmentation and anterior border layer arrangement (Fig. 12–7).

The TEMPORAL AND NASAL LONG CILIARY ARTERIES enter the iris near its root (see Fig. 12–3) and form the major arterial circle, which may be incomplete. The vascular supply of the iris of domestic animals greatly exceeds that of the human iris, and therefore surgical procedures near the iris root in animals often result in profuse hemorrhage if the major arterial circle is transected.

The dilator pupillae muscle extends as a continuous sheet in front of the anterior epithelium (see Fig. 12–4) and is intimately related to it. The constrictor pupillae muscle is a flat ring of smooth muscle surrounding the pupil in the posterior iris stroma.

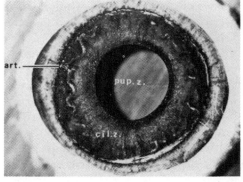

FIGURE 12–3. Canine iris. Note the large posterior ciliary artery on the left as it enters the root of the iris and divides into inferior and superior branches to form the major vascular circle of the iris. pup. z. = pupillary zone; cil. z. = ciliary zone; art. = artery. (From Donovan RH, et al: Histology of the normal collie eye II. Uvea. Ann Ophthalmol 6:1175, 1974.)

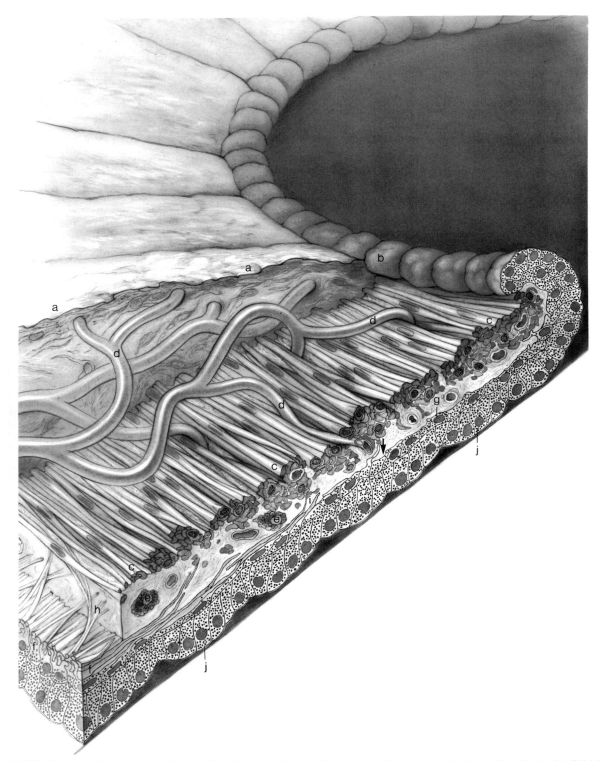

FIGURE 12–4. *Pupillary portion of the iris. The dense, cellular anterior border layer (a) terminates at the pigment ruff (b) in the pupillary margin. The sphincter muscle is at c. The arcades (d) from the minor circle extend toward the pupil and through the sphincter muscle. The sphincter muscle and the iris epithelium are close to each other at the pupillary margin. Capillaries, nerves, melanocytes, and clump cells (e) are found within and around the muscle. The three to five layers of dilator muscle (f) gradually diminish in number until they terminate behind the midportion of the sphincter muscle (arrow), leaving low, cuboidal epithelial cells (g) to form the anterior epithelium to the pupillary margin. Spur-like extensions from the dilator muscle form Michel's spur (h) and Fuchs's spur (i). (These spurs are not commonly described in domestic animals.) The posterior epithelium (j) is formed by columnar cells with basal nuclei. Its apical surface is contiguous with the apical surface of the anterior epithelium. (From Hogan MJ, et al: Histology of the Human Eye. WB Saunders Co, Philadelphia, 1971.)*

306

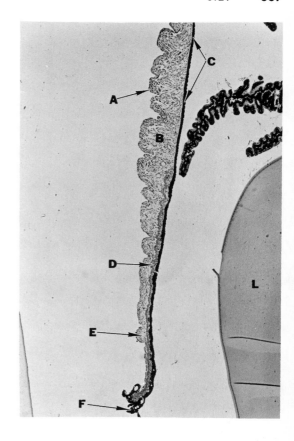

FIGURE 12–5. Structure of the iris. A = anterior border layer; B = stroma; C = posterior epithelium; D = constrictor muscle; E = collarette; F = pigment ruff; L = lens.

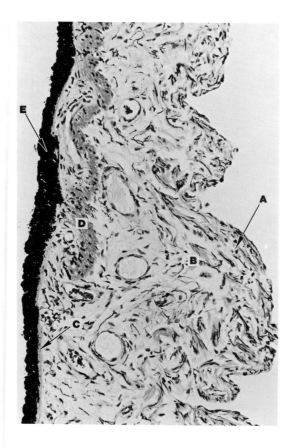

FIGURE 12–6. The canine stroma. A = anterior border layer; B = stroma; C = dilator muscle; D = constrictor muscle; E = posterior epithelium.

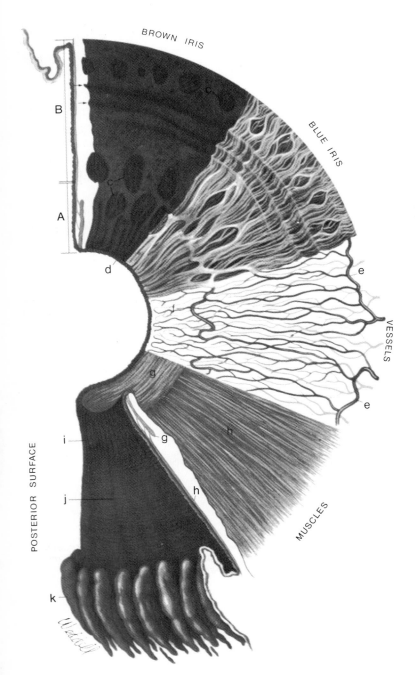

FIGURE 12–7. *Surfaces and layers of the iris. Clockwise from the top: The iris cross-section shows the pupillary (A) and ciliary (B) portions, and the surface view shows a brown iris with its dense, matted anterior border layer. The blue iris surface shows a less dense anterior border layer and more prominent trabeculae. Circular contraction furrows (arrows). Fuchs's crypts (c). Pigment ruff (d). Major arterial circle (e). Radial branches of arteries and veins extend toward the pupillary region. The arteries form the incomplete minor arterial circle (f), from which branches extend toward the pupil, forming capillary arcades. (Note: The incomplete minor arterial circle is variable or absent in many animals.) Circular arrangement of the sphincter muscle (g). Radial processes of the dilator muscle (h). Radial contraction furrows (i). Structure folds of Schwalbe (j). Pars plicata of the ciliary body (k). (From Hogan MJ, et al: Histology of the Human Eye. WB Saunders Co, Philadelphia, 1971.)*

In horses, cattle, sheep, and goats with a horizontally elliptical pupil, black masses suspended from the upper rim of the pupil aid in the control of light entering through the constricted pupil. Depending on their size, these masses are termed either CORPORA NIGRA (e.g., in horses) or GRANULA IRIDICA (e.g., in ruminants). They must be distinguished from pathological masses.

Ciliary Body

The ciliary body lies immediately posterior to the iris. The iris and ciliary body are together referred to as the ANTERIOR UVEA. On its posterior surface, the ciliary body is thrown into numerous folds—the CILIARY PROCESSES (Fig. 12–8). This area of the ciliary body is termed the PARS PLICATA (folded part), and it merges posteriorly into a flat area (PARS PLANA), which joins the retina. The ZONULAR FIBERS, which support the lens, originate from the pars plana and between the ciliary processes (Figs. 12–9 and 12–10).

Viewed in section, the ciliary body is triangular in shape, with one side joining the sclera, one side facing the vitreous body, and the base giving rise to the iris and IRIDOCORNEAL ANGLE (Fig. 12–11). The smooth muscle fibers of the CILIARY MUSCLE (parasympathetic innervation), together with blood vessels, connective tissue, and nerves, occupy a large portion of the ciliary body. The muscle fibers originate near the apex of the triangle and insert into the region of the ciliary cleft and trabecular spaces of the iridocorneal angle.

Contraction of the ciliary muscle causes

1. Relaxation of lens zonules, with change in lens shape and accommodation for near vision

2. Increased drainage of aqueous

Spasm of the ciliary muscle is frequently a cause of pain if the region is inflamed and is the reason that drugs are used to relax the muscle. *Cycloplegics* (e.g., atro-

pine)—drugs that relax the ciliary muscle—frequently also dilate the pupil. Drugs that dilate the pupil but do not relax the ciliary body are known as *mydriatics* (e.g., epinephrine). The ciliary body is covered with two layers of epithelium, the inner layer of which is pigmented and continuous with similar epithelium on the posterior surface of the iris and the pigment epithelium of the retina (Figs. 12–12 and 12–13).

Choroid

The choroid is a thin, pigmented, vascular tissue forming the posterior part of the uvea. It joins the ciliary body anteriorly and lies between the retina and sclera posteriorly. The choroid is extremely vascular, with its capillaries arranged in a single layer on the inner surface to nourish the outer retinal layers (Fig. 12–14). In the horse, with its restricted retinal vasculature, the retina depends to a greater extent on this choroidal supply. The choroidal stroma contains numerous melanocytes, which form a dark optical background to the retina. In all domestic animals except the pig, a reflective layer—the TAPETUM—lies within the inner capillary layer and is penetrated by numerous small capillaries. These capillaries when viewed end on with the ophthalmoscope are termed STARS OF WINSLOW. The arteries and nerves to the anterior parts of the eye pass forward through the choroid. The choroid receives its main arterial supply from

1. SHORT POSTERIOR CILIARY ARTERIES, which penetrate the sclera around the optic nerve

2. LONG POSTERIOR CILIARY ARTERIES, which enter near the optic nerve and branch near the ora ciliaris retinae and lead back into the choroid

3. ANTERIOR CILIARY ARTERIES, which send branches back into the choroid after penetrating the anterior sclera

Histologically the choroid consists of the following layers (see Fig. 12–14):

1. SUPRACHOROIDEA—avascular, pigmented connective tissue lying adjacent to the sclera

2. LARGE VESSEL LAYER—contains numerous melanocytes

3. INTERMEDIATE VESSEL LAYER—contains the tapetum in the superior fundus

4. CHORIOCAPILLARIS—a layer of capillaries adjacent to Bruch's membrane and the retina

In herbivores the tapetum is fibrous in nature (TAPETUM FIBROSUM), whereas in carnivores the cells are polyhedral and contain reflective crystals (TAPETUM CELLULOSUM) (Fig. 12–15A). The tapetum imparts the distinctive color to the fundi of different animals. Fundus color varies with breed, age, and species. The tapetum acts as an amplifying device, reflecting light back through the photoreceptor layer again after its first passage. It is responsible for the shining of animals' eyes in the dark.

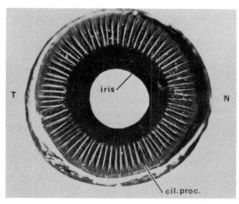

FIGURE 12–8. *Posterior aspect of the canine iris and ciliary body with lens removed. N = nasal; T = temporal; cil. proc. = ciliary processes. The smaller ciliary plicae may be seen between the posterior ends of the processes (× 3). (From Donovan RH, et al: Histology of the normal collie eye II. Uvea. Ann Ophthalmol 6:1175, 1974.)*

Text continued on page 315

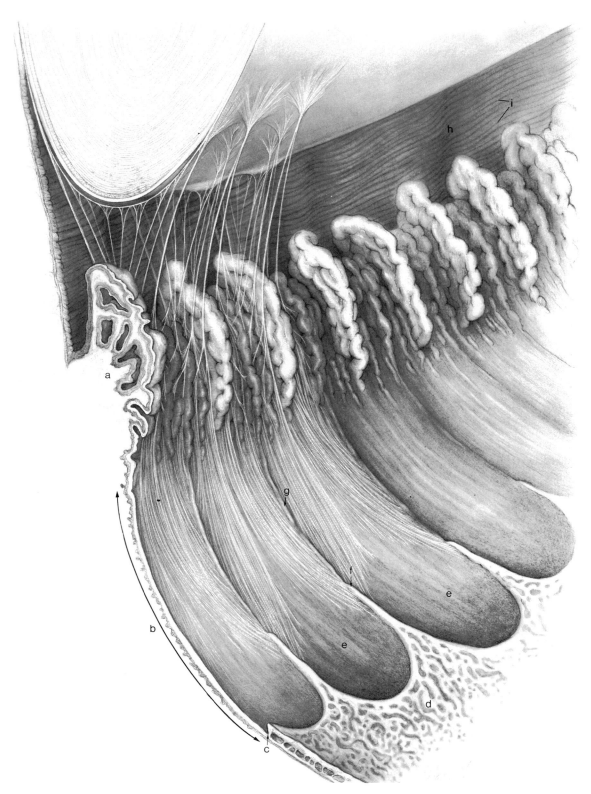

FIGURE 12–9. Posterior aspect of the ciliary body, showing the pars plicata (a) and the pars plana (b). The junction between the ciliary body and the retina is at c, with the retina at d. In primates, this junction is scalloped with bays (e), dentate processes (f), and striae (ora serrata) (g), but in most domestic species it is a straight line (ora ciliaris retinae). [Note: h and i are relevant to the human eye only.] (From Hogan MJ, et al: Histology of the Human Eye. WB Saunders Co, Philadelphia, 1971.)

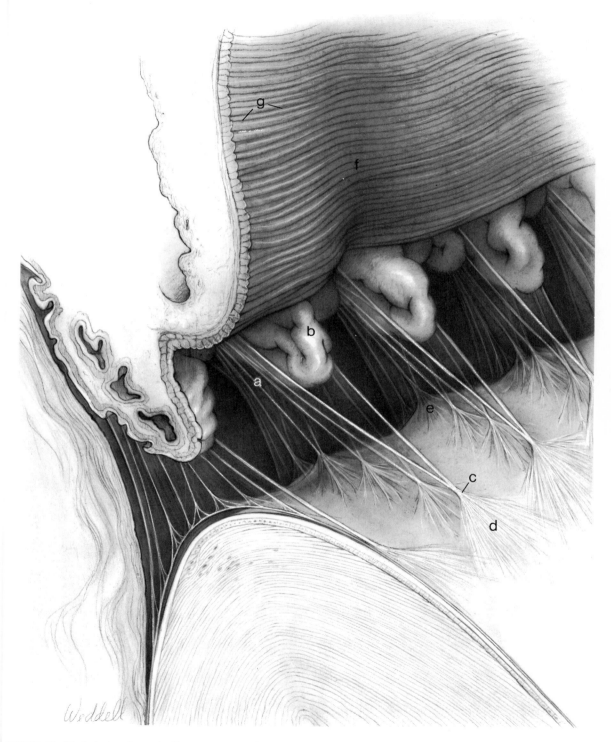

FIGURE 12–10. Anterior view of ciliary processes showing zonules attaching to the lens: a = lens zonules; b = ciliary process; c, d, and e = attachment of zonules to lens capsule; f = radial folds in iris; g = circular folds in iris. (From Hogan MJ, et al: Histology of the Human Eye. WB Saunders Co, Philadelphia, 1971.)

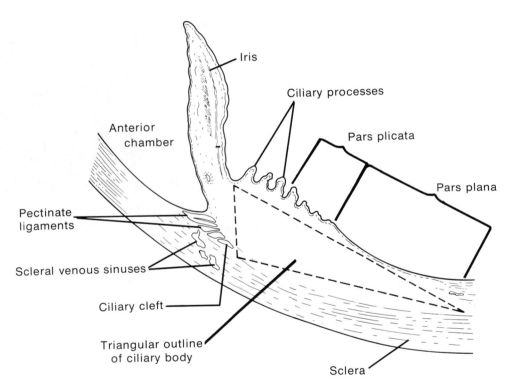

FIGURE 12–11. *Parts of the ciliary body.*

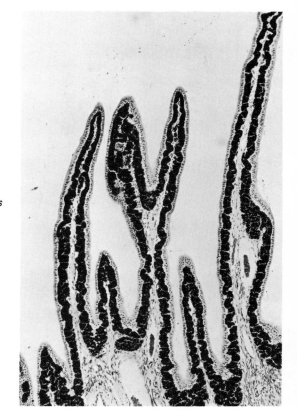

FIGURE 12–12. A canine ciliary process with core of blood vessels and stroma covered by two layers of epithelium.

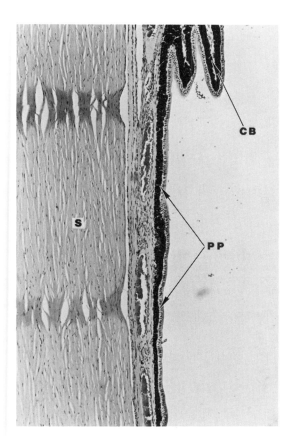

FIGURE 12–13. The ciliary epithelium is continuous with the posterior pigmented epithelium of the iris and the pigment epithelium of the retina. CB = ciliary body; PP = pars plana; S = sclera.

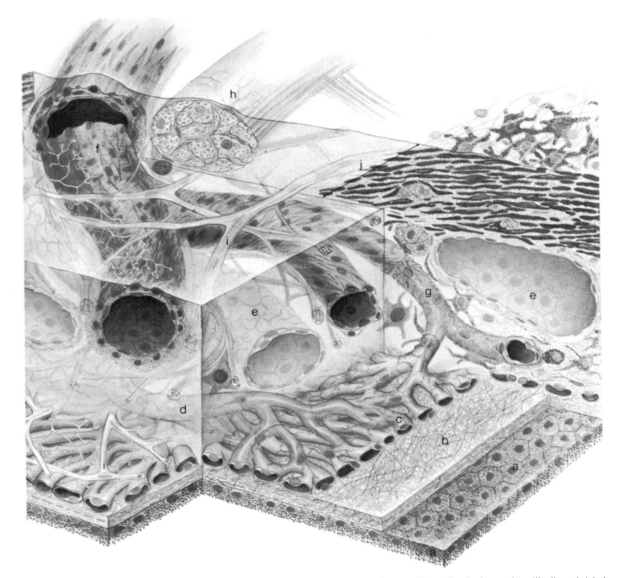

FIGURE 12–14. Choroidal blood supply and innervation and Bruch's membrane. The retinal pigment epithelium (a) is in close contact with Bruch's membrane (b). The choriocapillaris (c) forms an intricate network along the inner choroid. Bruch's membrane is very thin in some domestic species. In the superior portion of the fundus, the tapetum lies between the inner layers of the choriocapillaris and Bruch's membrane. Venules (d) leave the choriocapillaris to join the vortex system (e). The short ciliary artery is shown at f, prior to its branching (g) to form the choriocapillaris. A short ciliary nerve enters the choroid at h and branches into the choroidal stroma (i). The suprachoroidea is at (j). (From Hogan MJ, et al: *Histology of the Human Eye.* WB Saunders Co, Philadelphia, 1971.)

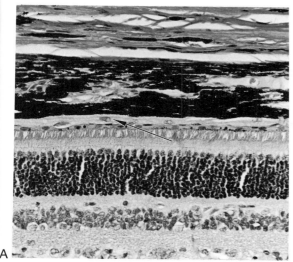

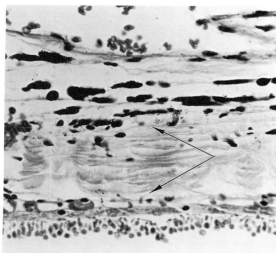

FIGURE 12–15. A, *Tapetum cellulosum (canine) (arrow), located between the choroid and the photoreceptor layer.* B, *Tapetum fibrosum (equine) (arrows). Note the choriocapillaris between the tapetum and the photoreceptor layer.*

PATHOLOGICAL REACTIONS

Definitions

Although the uvea exhibits the same range of reactions as other tissues, inflammation is the most important. The following terms describe inflammation of the various parts of the uveal tract:

UVEITIS	inflammation of the uvea
IRITIS	inflammation of the iris
CHOROIDITIS	inflammation of the choroid
CYCLITIS	inflammation of the ciliary body
IRIDOCYCLITIS	inflammation of the iris and ciliary body

However, because of the continuity of the parts of the uvea, inflammation rarely affects one part alone.

Because they are adjacent, with no major barriers between, the retina and choroid are frequently inflamed together. Consequently, the following terms are preferable:

ANTERIOR UVEITIS	inflammation of iris and ciliary body
POSTERIOR UVEITIS	inflammation of choroid and ciliary body
CHORIORETINITIS	inflammation of choroid and retina with primary focus in the choroid
RETINOCHOROIDITIS	inflammation of the choroid and retina with primary focus in the retina
PANUVEITIS	inflammation of all uveal components

Immune Mechanisms

1. The uvea is an immunologically competent tissue. When antigens in the eye are processed in distant sites, sensitized lymphocytes migrate toward the antigen, enter the uvea, and engage in antibody formation or cell-mediated immune reactions.

2. Subsequent exposure to the same antigen results in an earlier and greater (anamnestic) response. Such recurrent inflammation is readily visible in the eye because of pain, vascular congestion, and increased vascular permeability. In summary, the uvea acts as an accessory lymph node (Fig. 12–16).

3. The uvea is often secondarily inflamed when other parts of the eye are inflamed—e.g., secondary anterior uveitis frequently accompanies keratitis. Such reactions are frequently beneficial in resolution of the primary disease, e.g., production of immune globulins and sensitized lymphocytes. Excessive secondary uveitis may be damaging to the eye.

4. Autoimmune phenomena occur in the uvea. Preceding tissue damage (e.g., previous inflammation) releases tissue-specific uveal antigens normally located out of the path of patrolling lymphocytes (i.e., intracellularly). These antigens involve an immune response in the uvea. It is possible that this is the mechanism involved in recurrent equine uveitis, in which the inciting stimulus (e.g., *Leptospira* spp, *Onchocerca* spp) may vary. Antigens from within the lens capsule, which have been separated from the immune system since before birth, cause a similar response (lens-induced uveitis). Spontaneous uveitis with an unknown autoimmune basis also occurs (e.g., Vogt-Koyanagi-Harada–like syndrome in dogs, exudative uveitis with retinal detachment).

Classification of Uveitis

Uveitis may be classified in numerous ways. A useful pathological classification is

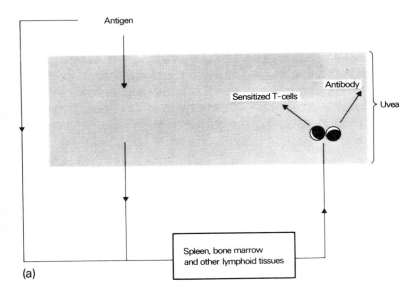

(a)

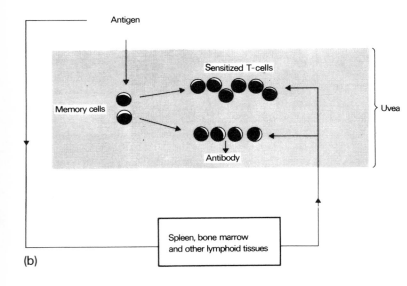

(b)

FIGURE 12–16. *The uvea as a lymph node. a, Intraocular antigen passes into the systemic circulation to stimulate distant lymphoid organs and, after 5–7 days, sensitized lymphocytes and antibodies are present in the uvea. b, Further exposure to the same antigen accelerates activation of residual sensitized lymphocytes (memory cells) within the uvea. In this way the uvea behaves as a regional lymph node. (From Rahi AHS, Garner A: Immunopathology of the Eye. Blackwell, Oxford, 1976.)*

1. Suppurative
2. Nonsuppurative
   a. Nongranulomatous
   b. Granulomatous

Examples for each of these classifications are found in Table 12–1.

Each category may be exogenous or endogenous and may be initiated by numerous stimuli, resulting in one of the following etiological types of uveitis:

1. Infectious uveitis (due to microorganisms)
2. Immune-mediated uveitis (with enhanced immune response)
3. Toxic uveitis
4. Traumatic uveitis
5. Uveitis associated with noninfective systemic diseases
6. Uveitis of unknown etiology

Clinically, no classification is highly successful because the etiology of many cases of noninfectious uveitis remains undetermined despite diagnostic attempts. During inflammation of the uvea, vascular permeability increases, resulting in release of fibrin and inflammatory cells into the anterior chamber—a condition known as HYPOPYON. The iridocorneal angle and posterior chamber may also fill with this exudate. In the early stages of inflammation, increased protein concentration in the aqueous is detectable as AQUEOUS FLARE in a beam of light. The uveal stroma becomes edematous and infiltrated with inflammatory cells appropriate to the type of the inflammation. Inflammatory cells may adhere to the corneal endothelium, in which case they are referred to as KERATIC PRECIPITATES, or KPs.

TABLE 12–1. Examples of Uveitis

Suppurative	Nonsuppurative Nongranulomatous	Nonsuppurative Granulomatous
Listeriosis (Fig. 12–17) Aspergillosis (Fig. 12–18) Blastomycosis	Infectious canine hepatitis (Fig. 12–19)	Tuberculosis (Fig. 12–20) Lens-induced uveitis

One of the most frequent forms of uveitis is the nonsuppurative, nongranulomatous type seen following mild trauma, keratitis, or corneal ulceration.

Sequelae of Uveitis

POSTERIOR SYNECHIAE

Posterior synechiae occur when fibrinous adhesions form between the lens and the iris, with fibrovascular organization occurring later. Formation of synechiae is more likely when aqueous protein content is high. If synechiae form around the entire circumference of the pupil, IRIS BOMBÉ occurs, preventing aqueous flow to the anterior chamber, and secondary glaucoma follows. An irregularly shaped pupil is frequently caused by synechiae. If blood or exudate organizes in the anterior chamber, causing formation of a connective tissue membrane, OCCLUSION OF THE PUPIL occurs.

PERIPHERAL ANTERIOR SYNECHIAE

Adhesions may form between the iris and the trabecular meshwork or between the iris and the cornea. Swelling, iris bombé, and cellular infiltrates may reduce

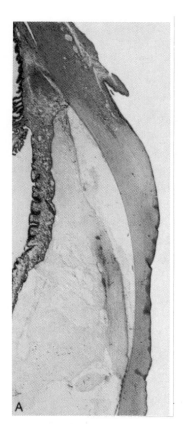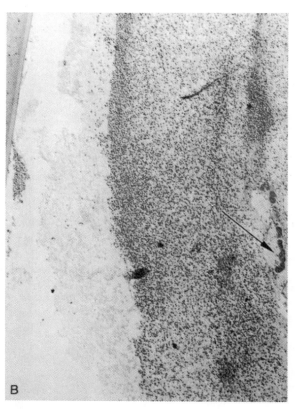

FIGURE 12–17. A, Section from a 5-year-old cow with left facial paralysis involving ear, eyelids, and muzzle. Listeria monocytogenes was isolated from a purulent encephalitis. Corneal ulceration, endothelial sloughing, hypopyon, and a ciliary body abscess are present. B, Higher magnification of the anterior chamber of eye shown in A. Bacterial colonies are present in the purulent exudate, and portions of sloughed corneal endothelium are proliferating in the exudate (arrow). (From Saunders LZ, Rubin LF: Ophthalmic Pathology of Animals. S Karger AG, Basel, 1975.)

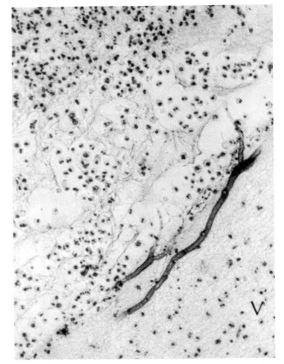

FIGURE 12–18. *Mycotic cyclitis in a turkey. Hyphae of Aspergillus fumigatus are growing in the vitreous (V), causing a heavy outpouring of leukocytes and fibrin from the ciliary body. (From Saunders LZ, Rubin LF: Ophthalmic Pathology of Animals. S Karger AG, Basel, 1975.)*

drainage of aqueous through the iridocorneal angle early in uveitis, but once synechiae have formed, an alternative route for drainage must be provided, as the angle is held closed by the synechiae.

CATARACT

Cataract (opacity of the lens) occurs frequently after uveitis. This is probably caused by altered composition of the aqueous, interfering with lens nutrition. When an animal with a cataract and signs of uveitis is examined, the determination must be made as to which came first—the cataract or the uveitis.

GLAUCOMA

Intraocular pressure is usually *lowered* during uveitis. The passage of aqueous may be reduced by structural alterations occurring during uveitis, such as

1. Blockage of the angle with inflammatory cells and debris
2. Formation of peripheral anterior synechiae (PAS)
3. Cellular infiltration of the drainage angle
4. Pupillary block caused by occlusion of the pupil

In dogs especially, intractable secondary glaucoma following lens-induced uveitis is a frequent entity,

usually seen after penetrating injuries and sometimes after cataract extraction.

RETINAL DETACHMENT

Exudation and cellular infiltration from the choroid may cause retinal detachment.

ATROPHY

The iris and ciliary body atrophy as the stroma is replaced by fibrous tissue. Defects may appear in the iris. Atrophy of areas of the choroid frequently results in atrophy of the overlying retina, which is visible ophthalmoscopically. Severe atrophy of the ciliary body causes **HYPOTONY** (lowered intraocular pressure). In some animals, the color of the iris becomes *darker* after uveitis.

CYCLITIC MEMBRANES

A cyclitic membrane is a band of fibrovascular tissue extending from the ciliary body across the pupil or

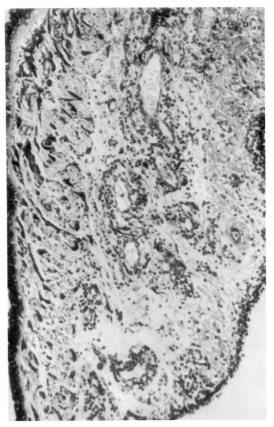

FIGURE 12–19. *Anterior uveitis in infectious canine hepatitis. The iris is edematous and heavily infiltrated with leukocytes, especially around blood vessels. (From Saunders LZ, Rubin LF: Ophthalmic Pathology of Animals. S Karger AG, Basel, 1975.)*

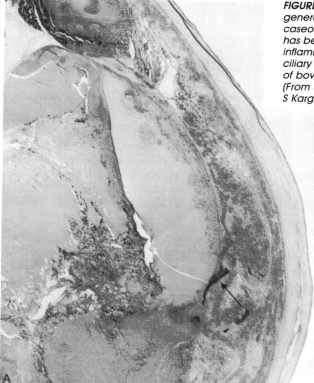

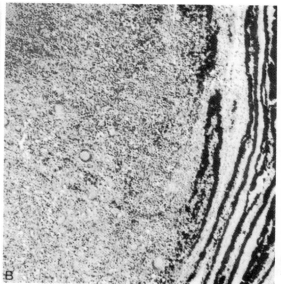

FIGURE 12–20. A, Anterior segment from the eye of a calf with generalized tuberculosis. The anterior chamber is filled with caseous exudate, some of which has calcified (arrow). The iris has been destroyed and the lens damaged by granulomatous inflammation. B, Higher magnification of area at left of A. The ciliary body has been invaded and destroyed. Tubercles typical of bovine tuberculosis are visible within the inflammatory mass. (From Saunders LZ, Rubin LF: Ophthalmic Pathology of Animals. S Karger AG, Basel, 1975.)

across the anterior face of the vitreous. It consists of fibrous tissue and blood vessels and may severely obstruct vision.

Sympathetic Ophthalmia

Sympathetic ophthalmia is a *rare* human condition in which a second eye becomes inflamed after inflammation or damage to the uvea of the opposite eye. It does not occur in domestic animals.

CONGENITAL ABNORMALITIES

Iris Cysts

Iris cysts are bladder-like, fluid-filled structures surrounded by pigmented epithelium, which formed in the posterior pigmented epithelium of the iris. Iris cysts may also occur secondary to inflammation. The cysts either remain attached or break free and float into the anterior chamber, either singly or in groups (Fig. 12–21). In the anterior chamber they may float freely or adhere to the iris or corneal endothelium, occasionally obstructing the visual axis and the pupil.

In the Great Dane, iris cysts are recessively inherited, and large numbers of cysts may be formed and push the root of the iris forward, causing secondary narrow-angle glaucoma. Iris cysts are most often seen in dogs, cats, and horses and may be distinguished from pigmented neoplasms and iris nevi by transillumination.

Removal is indicated in the following circumstances:
1. Presence of large numbers of cysts.

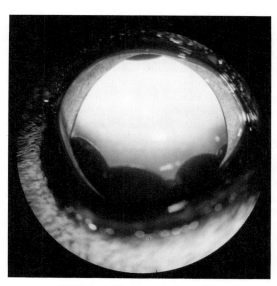

FIGURE 12–21. Iris cysts in a dog.

2. Corneal edema is caused by contact with the endothelium.

3. The pupil is obstructed, impairing vision.

4. Intraocular pressure is elevated, or large numbers of cysts are present, displacing the iris forward.

Cysts are removed by aspiration under microscopic control.

In lightly pigmented irides in horses, cystic areas may be seen in the stroma of the iris at its base. Transillumination distinguishes this type of cyst from a neoplasm.

Abnormalities of the Pupil

Pupillary abnormalities include the following:

POLYCORIA   more than one pupil
CORECTOPIA   eccentrically placed pupil
ANCORIA   no pupil
ANIRIDIA   lack of iris
COLOBOMA   sector defect in iris (discussed later)
DYSCORIA   abnormally shaped pupil

Corectopia is distinguished from a pupil pulled out of shape by an anterior synechia, in which case the pupil is elliptical or teardrop-shaped. Pupillary abnormalities are rarely significant, but they are an important indication of other abnormalities.

Persistent Pupillary Membrane[1]

During development of the eye, the pupillary membrane stretches across the anterior chamber (see Fig. 2–14). Before birth this membrane atrophies, and the space for the pupillary aperture remains. Small remnants of the membrane are frequent in all domestic species, usually attached in the region of the iris collarette, and are of no significance.

In the basenji, persistent pupillary membrane (PPM) occurs as an inherited condition, is more extensive, and may be associated with other ocular defects. Important features of the condition in this breed are

1. PPM is congenital, hereditary, and nonprogressive. The mode of inheritance is recessive but probably not simple mendelian in nature.

2. The remnants may extend across the pupil, to the lens or the cornea, or both.

3. PPM may be associated with corneal opacities (even when the remnants are not attached to the cornea), with colobomata of the optic disc (Fig. 12–22), and with nonprogressive anterior capsular and subcapsular cataracts.

4. All basenji breeding stock should be certified free of the condition after biomicroscopic examination. Animals with minor degrees of PPM may fall within

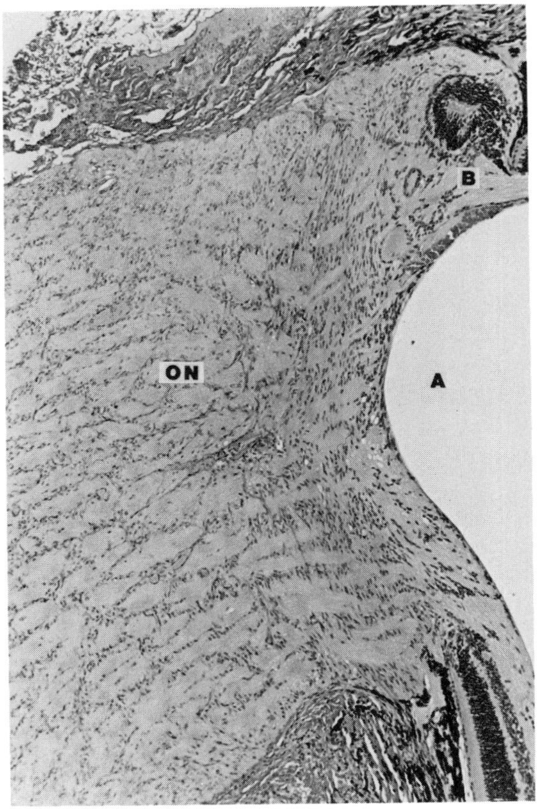

FIGURE 12–22. Coloboma of the optic disc (A) in association with PPM in a basenji. B = retinal dysplasia; ON = optic nerve. (Tissue courtesy of Dr. J. R. Blogg.)

normal limits, and the designation of these animals for breeding depends on the experience of the examiner.

5. Most animals with PPM show no visual deficits.

Biomicroscopy is essential for accurate diagnosis of PPM for certification.

PPM has been recorded in the Afghan hound, American cocker spaniel, American Staffordshire terrier, Australian [sic] shepherd, basenji, beagle, bearded collie, Cardigan Welsh corgi, chow chow, rough or smooth collie, dachshund, Dandie Dinmont terrier, Doberman pinscher, English bulldog, English cocker spaniel, English springer spaniel, golden retriever, Great Pyrenees, greyhound, Irish setter, mastiff, Pembroke corgi, poodle (standard), Portuguese water dog, saluki, Samoyed, miniature and standard schnauzer, Scottish terrier, Shetland sheepdog, Siberian husky, Staffordshire bull terrier, and Tibetan terrier.

Coloboma

A coloboma is a defect in the eye resulting from incomplete closure of the embryonic fissure. TYPICAL

---

1. See also Chap 2.

TABLE 12–2. Breeds Affected by Heterochromia Iridis

Species	Breed	Characteristics
Cat	Siamese	Subalbinism
	Burmese, Abyssinian, Persian	Variable iris hypopigmentation
Dog	Australian cattle dog	Dappling
	Australian [sic] shepherd	Merling
	Boxer	White coat
	Collie	Merling (autosomal dominant)
	Great Dane	Harlequin coat (autosomal dominant)
	Long-haired dachshund	Harlequin coat (autosomal dominant)
	Dalmatian	Dappling (autosomal dominant)
	Malamute	Dappling
	Old English sheepdog	—
	Siberian husky	Dappling (autosomal dominant)
	Weimaraner	Iris hypopigmentation varies
Horse	Pinto, appaloosa, white, and gray horses	Variable heterochromia
Cattle	Hereford, shorthorn	Albinism, subalbinism

COLOBOMATA occur in the inferomedian portion of the iris or choroid, adjacent to the optic disc. Colobomata of the sclera also occur in the scleral ectasia syndrome in collies. Although the embryonic fissure is not involved, the term is also applied to lid defects and to sector defects in the lens.

Disorders of Pigmentation

HETEROCHROMIA IRIDIS

Heterochromia iridis refers to a range of variations of pigmentation of the iris in different species (Fig. 12–23). It is frequently associated with iris hypoplasia and with hypoplasia or aplasia of the tapetum and lack of pigmentation of the nontapetal fundus. For breeds affected with heterochromia iridis and congenital deafness, see Chapter 19.

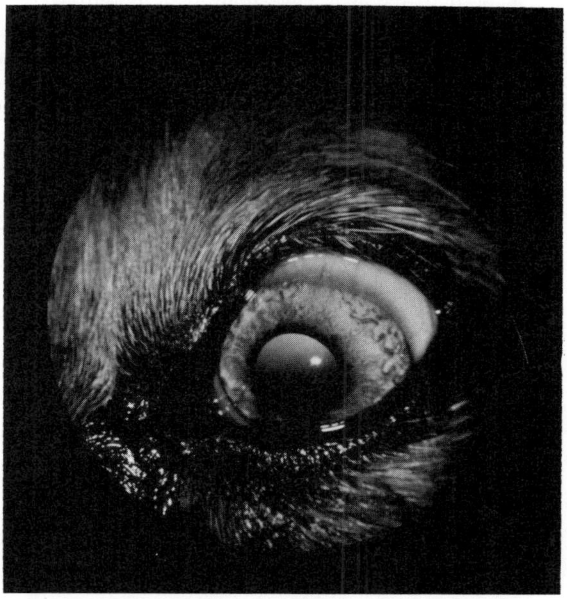

Lay terms for heterochromia include

Wall eye—blue and white iris or part of an iris

China eye—blue iris or part of an iris

Watch eye—blue and yellow-brown iris or part of an iris

Both eyes may be affected, one eye only, or only part of an iris. Heterochromia iridis may be associated with albinism, subalbinism, and variations in coat color (Table 12–2). In dogs, heterochromia is due to incomplete maturation or absence of pigment granules in the iris stroma or anterior pigmented layer. Heterochromia iridis is thought to be due to decreased availability of tyrosine hydrolase, which is necessary for the synthesis of melanin.

$$L\text{-tyrosine} \longrightarrow L\text{-dihydroxyphenylalanine} \longrightarrow$$
melanins
tyrosine
hydrolase

In most species, heterochromia is of no clinical significance. In cattle, ocular albinism has been further subdivided (Table 12–3).

FIGURE 12–23. Heterochromia iridis in a sable and white collie. The iris is blue. The opposite eye showed heterochromia adjacent to the pupillary margin of the iris only.

TABLE 12–3. Ocular Albinism in Cattle

Type of Albinism	Features
Partial	Iris blue and white centrally, brown peripherally; hair color normal
Incomplete	Iris light blue, gray, and white; hair color white; some brown sectors in iris and some colored hair patches; nontapetal fundus is incompletely pigmented, and choroidal vasculature is visible
Complete	Iris very pale blue or white, hair pure white, nontapetal fundus unpigmented; photophobia; variable fundus colobomata and tapetal hypoplasia

IRIS NEVUS (Fig. 12–24)

IRIS NEVI are most commonly observed in cats and dogs. They may consist of focal spots of hyperpigmentation. They must be differentiated from neoplasms that require surgical treatment. Iris nevi do not protrude above the surface of the iris and do not enlarge. Nevi have a low malignant potential and show an increase in number of cells or increased pigmentation of existing cells and must be observed carefully for enlargement, especially in cats, where they may indicate the early stages of diffuse malignant iris melanoma.

WAARDENBURG'S SYNDROME

Waardenburg's syndrome consists of
1. Deafness
2. Heterochromia iridis
3. White coat color

Although this hereditary syndrome occurs most commonly in white, blue-eyed cats, it also occurs in dogs (especially the Australian cattle dog, Great Dane, and Dalmatian), mice, and humans. Not all white, blue-eyed cats are affected. In the cat, the syndrome is inherited as a dominant trait with complete penetrance for the white coat and incomplete penetrance for deafness and blue irides.

NEOPLASMS

The uvea may be affected by both primary and secondary neoplasms.

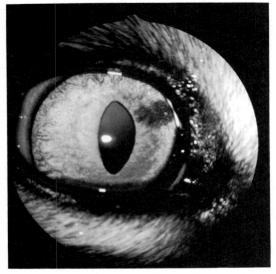

FIGURE 12–24. Iris nevus in a cat. Such lesions are observed regularly for signs of progression.

Intraocular tumors frequently have the clinical signs of glaucoma or chronic, unresponsive uveitis.

Primary Tumors

Classification of primary tumors can be found in Table 12–4. Of these primary types, nevi have been previously discussed; of the remainder, adenoma, adenocarcinoma, and melanoma are the most common.

ADENOCARCINOMA AND ADENOMA

Neoplasms of the ciliary epithelium are occasionally observed in dogs. The lesions usually appear as a single mass protruding from behind the iris into the pupil (Fig. 12–25). The mass may be pigmented or unpigmented, depending on whether it arose from pigmented or unpigmented ciliary epithelium, and must be distinguished from malignant melanoma in the same site. These neoplasms infrequently infiltrate anteriorly into the drainage angle and iris (Fig. 12–26), elevating intraocular pressure. The extent of the lesion may be outlined by transillumination and reflected light from the tapetum. Treatment is either by removal of the tumor and adjacent ciliary body (iridocyclectomy), frequently with replacement of the defect with a scleral graft, or if the tumor is extensive, by enucleation. Provided the tumor remains within the globe, the prognosis is good.

MELANOCYTOMA AND MELANOMA

All uveal melanomas have malignant potential, but many are benign, and they may arise from the iris, ciliary body, or choroid. They are most common in dogs and cats, and less frequent in horses and cattle. Mitotic index is a more useful indicator of behavior and

TABLE 12–4. Classification of Primary Tumors

Melanocytes	Ciliary Epithelium
Acquired	*Congenital*
Iris nevus	Benign medulloepithelioma
Melanocytoma (benign)	Malignant medulloepithelioma
Melanoma (potentially malignant)	Benign teratoid medulloepithelioma
Diffuse iris melanoma (feline)	Malignant teratoid medulloepithelioma
	Acquired
	Nonpigmented
	Adenoma
	Adenocarcinoma
	Pigmented
	Adenoma
	Adenocarcinoma

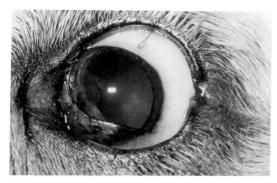

FIGURE 12–25. Adenocarcinoma of the ciliary body in a dog, appearing as a red mass in the pupil.

occur more frequently in the iris and ciliary body (Fig. 12–27) than in the choroid and have a reasonable prognosis if the eye is enucleated before the tumor has penetrated the sclera. Penetration may occur via ciliary arteries, veins, or nerves, by direct extension, or via the optic nerve. In a study of feline ocular melanomas by Patnaik and Mooney (1988), 10 of 16 uveal melanomas had metastases prior to enucleation. Based on three animals only in this same study, feline palpebral melanomas may have a high rate of metastasis.

Clinical Signs

Melanomas usually result in
1. Glaucoma.
2. Uveitis or endophthalmitis due to necrosis of the tumor. Cornea is often opaque.
3. Hyphema.
4. Change in color or visible mass in the iris.

Melanomas often cause secondary glaucoma.

Treatment

1. If the tumor is small or localized, local excision by *iridectomy* or *iridocyclectomy* may be considered. By the time clinical signs are present, many tumors are too large for this.

prognosis in dogs than are the histological criteria used for human ocular melanomas. The potential for metastasis is present, but different studies reveal wide variation in observed rates, making rational generalizations difficult. Prospective studies of staged tumors with long-term follow-up are still required, as retrospective studies on submitted pathological specimens have yielded conflicting data. Intraocular and palpebral melanomas in cats have a greater tendency to metastasize and are more malignant than dermal melanomas, with higher rates of mortality and metastasis. Similarly, ocular melanomas in cats are more malignant than in dogs, with higher rates of mortality and metastasis.

Melanomas in dogs and cats, unlike those in humans,

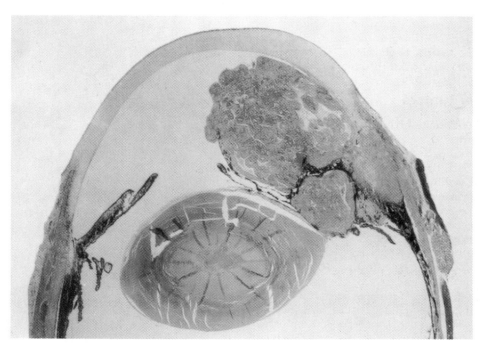

FIGURE 12–26. Adenoma of the ciliary body of a dog, partially filling the anterior chamber and destroying the ciliary body. (From Saunders LZ, Rubin LF: Ophthalmic Pathology of Animals. S Karger AG, Basel, 1975.)

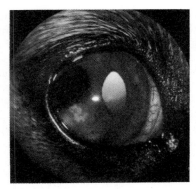

FIGURE 12–27. *Melanocytoma in the iris of a 5-year-old German shepherd presented because of corneal opacity and an unusually shaped pupil.*

2. *Enucleation of the globe* is often mandated by the presence of intractable glaucoma, uveitis, or hyphema. The prognosis after enucleation is good (in a recent compilation from literature reports, 7 of 129 canine uveal melanomas had confirmed metastases). If there is any indication of scleral penetration, *orbital exenteration* is performed in an attempt to remove tumor cells. Frequent postoperative examinations (every 3 months for a year, then annually) are advisable, with special attention given to the submandibular, retropharyngeal, and bronchial lymph nodes. Chemotherapy may be used, although evidence of efficacy is lacking.

PRIMARY FELINE OCULAR SARCOMAS

Primary feline ocular sarcoma may occur with or without a history of trauma to the eye. Clinical signs include chronic uveitis, buphthalmos, and a red eye. Local recurrence or metastasis is common.

Secondary Tumors

With the exception of lymphosarcoma, tumors metastasizing to the uvea are uncommon. Most have been described in the dog and include mammary carcinoma; hemangiosarcoma; thyroid, pancreatic, and renal carcinomas; malignant melanoma of the skin; seminoma; and rhabdomyosarcoma. Any kind of metastasis is possible. It has been suggested that the most frequent instances of metastasis in dogs are those from malignant canine mammary tumors.

LYMPHOSARCOMA[2]

Ocular manifestations of lymphosarcoma occur in the dog, cat, and cow. In the dog, ocular manifestations are clinically similar to uveitis and endophthalmitis and may include infiltration of the iris with swelling,

___

2. See also Chap 19.

hyphema, aqueous flare, retinopathy and retinal detachment, conjunctivitis, keratitis, noninflammatory chemosis, corneal edema with vascularization, keratic precipitates (KPs), intrastromal corneal hemorrhage, miosis, hypotony, ciliary injection, and secondary glaucoma. Approximately 40% of dogs with lymphosarcoma show ocular signs in some form. Histologically, the iris and ciliary body are more frequently affected than is the choroid (Fig. 12–28). Dogs with ocular signs may have a poorer prognosis for long-term remission and response to chemotherapy. Detailed consideration of chemotherapy for lymphosarcoma is beyond the scope of this book; however, animals blinded with lymphosarcoma may recover vision once chemotherapy with one of the standard regimens is commenced (cyclophosphamide-vincristine-prednisolone or doxorubicin regimens).

In cats, similar but less frequent ocular lesions occur in myeloproliferative disease, reticuloendotheliosis, and feline leukemia virus infection. In cattle, ocular lesions in lymphosarcoma are restricted to infiltration of orbital tissues, often resulting in exophthalmos with exposure keratitis. Up to 10% of cattle with lymphosarcoma may have exophthalmos.

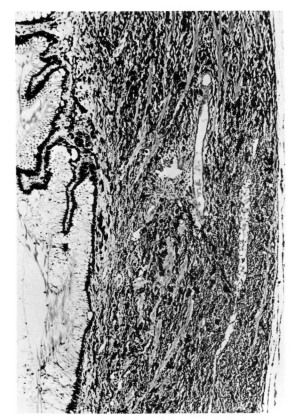

FIGURE 12–28. *Lymphoid cells infiltrating the iris and ciliary body in canine lymphosarcoma.*

Lymphosarcoma should be considered in cattle with exophthalmos.

In poultry, infiltration of the iris and uveal tract with a change in color to bluish gray ("pearly-eye") is seen in Marek's disease and is termed *epidemic blindness*.

UVEITIS

Clinical Signs

The clinical signs of uveitis are similar regardless of etiology and include the following:

1. Photophobia
2. Pain (may be manifested as anorexia or depression)
3. Epiphora
4. Circumcorneal ciliary injection
5. Aqueous flare—very slight milkiness of the aqueous in a light beam, caused by increased protein content
6. KPs—inflammatory cells adherent to the corneal endothelium
7. Miosis
8. Anterior or posterior synechia
9. Swollen or dull appearance to the iris
10. Increased pigmentation of the iris
11. Vitreous haze or opacity
12. Hypopyon (Fig. 12–29) or hyphema
13. Retinal edema, exudate, or detachment
14. Lowered intraocular pressure
15. Resistance to mydriatics

AQUEOUS FLARE is due to increased permeability of vessels in the iris and ciliary body, resulting in release of protein into the aqueous. **KPs** are accumulations of neutrophils and lymphocytes that adhere to the corneal endothelium or, if in large numbers, form a ventral layer called **HYPOPYON**. KPs may be small and scattered (in feline infectious peritonitis) or large and yellow, "mutton fat" KPs (in granulomatous diseases).

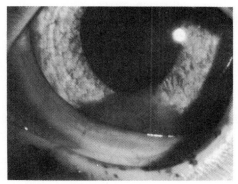

FIGURE 12–29. *Hypopyon in the ventral anterior chamber in uveitis. (Courtesy of Dr. G. A. Severin.)*

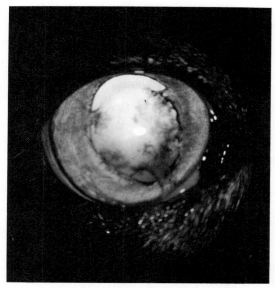

FIGURE 12–30. *Irregularly shaped pupil with anterior capsular pigment deposits and posterior synechiae in chronic uveitis.*

Because of edema the pupil is miotic, but as inflammation subsides, synechiae may form, causing an irregularly shaped pupil (Fig. 12–30) or a scalloped appearance on dilation, with pigment remnants on the anterior lens capsule.

If posterior uveitis is present, the vitreous may become hazy. Inflammation extends to the retina, and retinal edema, exudates, or detachments may be seen.

Diagnosis

The detection of uveitis depends on familiarity with the clinical signs. After a thorough physical examination and history, and classification of the uveitis, specific tests may be performed in an attempt to determine the etiology (e.g., serum titer for *Toxoplasma* spp). Unfortunately, for many cases of uveitis in animals (and humans), the etiology is never determined, and treatment is aimed at control of the inflammation (which may recur) and prevention of further damage and complications to the eye.

Differential diagnosis of the etiology of uveitis often requires specialist assistance, notably when potential zoonotic diseases may be involved.

Anterior uveitis is distinguished from conjunctivitis, superficial keratitis, and glaucoma—other causes of the "red eye" syndrome (Table 12–5).

Once the clinical diagnosis of uveitis has been made, the disorder is subdivided into granulomatous and

TABLE 12–5. Differential Diagnosis of Ocular Inflammations

Factor	Anterior Uveitis	Conjunctivitis	Superficial Keratitis	Glaucoma
Conjunctiva	Not thickened; vessels easily seen	Thick; folded and hyperemic; vessels concealed	Not thickened	Not thickened
Conjunctival vessels	Circumcorneal and straight; not movable with conjunctiva	Superficial, diffuse, and tortuous	Diffuse; vessels form fine network in vicinity of cornea	Diffuse, superficial, and prominent
Secretion or discharge	None	Moderate to copious	Serous to purulent	None
Pain	Moderate	None to slight	Moderate to severe	Severe to acute
Photophobia	Moderate	None	Severe	Slight
Cornea	Clear to steamy	Clear	Clouded to opaque	Steamy
Pupil size	Small, sluggish, irregular, or fixed	Normal	Normal	Dilated, moderate to complete, and fixed
Pupillary light response	Poor	Normal	Normal	Absent
Intraocular pressure	Variable: may be normal, slightly elevated, or diminished	Normal	Normal	Elevated

From Lavignette AM: Differential diagnosis and treatment of anterior uveitis. Vet Clin North Am 3:504, 1973.

nongranulomatous types. Although this division results primarily from the histological classification, the criteria in Table 12–6 have been used as an aid in clinical separation.

From this point, an etiological classification may be attempted. Most granulomatous uveitis is associated with microorganisms or foreign material that stimulates a chronic response by the immune system. Etiological classification of uveitis will place it in one of the following categories:

1. Influence of a microorganism dominant
   a. Exogenous
   b. Endogenous
2. Immune-mediated uveitis
3. Traumatic uveitis
4. Uveitis associated with systemic diseases
5. Toxic uveitis
6. Uveitis of unknown etiology

Influence of a Microorganism Dominant

The causes of uveitis with a predominating exogenous microorganism are summarized (Table 12–7). Uveitis

TABLE 12–6. Classification Criteria for Anterior Uveitis*

Nongranulomatous	Granulomatous
Acute onset	Gradual onset
Short course	Persistent or recurrent
No exudates on lens capsule	Greasy exudate on lens surface
No synechiae	Posterior synechiae

Modified from Magrane WG: Canine Ophthalmology, 3rd ed. Lea & Febiger, Philadelphia, 1977.
*These criteria are useful but not absolute and are interpreted with other clinical signs.

caused by endogenous microorganisms is poorly documented in domestic animals, with the exception of septicemic colibacillosis in neonatal calves and foals. Foci of infection in other parts of the body may cause uveitis (e.g., prostatitis, endometritis, and gingivitis and tooth root abscesses in dogs). Hematology or blood culture may indicate the presence of such foci, which are often recurrent. This type of uveitis may be due to shedding of bacteria into the circulation with a secondary uveitis caused by previously sensitized lymphocytes in the uvea, or it may be due to bacterial toxins released from the primary site.

Blastomycosis and coccidioidomycosis are important causes of uveitis in dogs. If uveitis is present in association with lesions of lungs, bone, lymph nodes, skin, or testicles, or if the animal is located in an endemic area, appropriate serological tests should be performed.

Immune-Mediated Uveitis

The three most common types of immune-mediated uveitis are

1. Primary reaction to an antigen
2. Enhanced reaction because of previous exposure to the antigen
3. Autoimmunity to uveal antigens after some previous insult

VOGT-KOYANAGI-HARADA–LIKE SYNDROME

Synonym: Uveodermatological syndrome

This disorder affects certain breeds more commonly than others—Akita, Old English sheepdog, golden retriever, Siberian husky, and Irish setter. It is a spontaneous autoimmune disease affecting the anterior

TABLE 12–7. Infectious and Parasitic Causes of Uveitis

Disease	Organism(s)	Most Commonly Affected Species
Infectious (Nonparasitic)		
Algae		
Geotrichosis	*Geotricha* spp	Dog
Prototheeosis	*Prototheca* spp	Dog
Bacteria		
Brucellosis	*Brucella canis*	Dog
Colibacillosis	*Escherichia coli*	Cattle, horse
Recurrent equine uveitis	*Streptococcus equi*	Horse
Listeriosis	*Listeria monocytogenes*	Sheep, cattle
Strangles	*Streptococcus equi*	Horse
Thromboembolic meningoencephalitis	*Haemophilus* spp	Cattle
Tuberculosis	*Mycobacterium tuberculosis*	Cattle, cat, dog
Yeasts and Fungi		
Aspergillosis	*Aspergillus* spp	Chickens, turkeys, cat
Blastomycosis	*Blastomyces* spp	Dog, cat
Coccidioidomycosis	*Coccidioides immitis*	Dog
Cryptococcosis	*Cryptococcus* spp	Dog, cat
Histoplasmosis	*Histoplasma capsulatum*	Dog, cat
Pseudoallescheriosis	*Pseudallescheria boydii*	Dog
Viruses		
Infectious canine hepatitis	Canine adenoviruses types 1 and 2 (immune-mediated)	Dog
Feline infectious peritonitis	Coronavirus	Cat
Feline leukemia	Feline leukemia virus (retrovirus)	Cat
Marek's disease	*Herpesvirus*	Chickens, turkeys
Spirochaetes		
Recurrent equine uveitis	*Leptospira pomona* (immune-mediated)	Horse
Leptospirosis	*Leptospira* spp	Dog
Miscellaneous Organisms		
Leishmaniasis	*Leishmania donovani*	Dog
Toxoplasmosis*	*Toxoplasma gondii*	Dog, cat
Parasitic		
Coenurosis	*Taenia multiceps*	Sheep, dog
Echinococcosis	*Echinococcus granulosus*	Horse (rare)
Filarial uveitis	*Angiostrongylus vasorum*	Dog
	Dirofilaria immitis	Dog
	Setaria spp	Horse
Recurrent equine uveitis	*Onchocerca cervicalis*	Horse

*A newly classified organism, *Neosporum caninum*, has been found responsible for some cases of dogs previously diagnosed with *Toxoplasma gondii* infection. The clinical significance is undetermined.

and posterior uvea, frequently resulting in blindness from retinal detachment or glaucoma. In addition, it is associated with often dramatic depigmentation of the mucocutaneous junctions, eyelids, and haircoat. In humans, neurological signs are associated with the syndrome, but these are rare in dogs, with a single instance of head tilt the only claimed reported instance. In some regions the onset of the disease has a definite seasonal incidence, e.g., February to May in Southern California.

Vigorous early anti-inflammatory therapy is often necessary to save vision. Recurrences of the disease can be expected, with the patient being maintained on appropriate medications between recurrences. The im-

mediate assistance of a veterinary ophthalmologist should be sought in the handling of dogs affected with this disease.

LENS-INDUCED UVEITIS

When the lens capsule ruptures or leaks, protein enters the aqueous and is exposed to the immune system of the uvea. This causes both acute and chronic uveitis and frequently endophthalmitis, because the lens proteins are regarded as "foreign"—i.e., they have been separated from the immune system since before birth by the lens capsule. This escape of proteins happens as the result of either (1) penetrating injuries or (2) leakage through the lens capsule.

Penetrating Injuries

These are common in dogs and cats and often progress quickly to endophthalmitis with secondary glaucoma (Fig. 12–31). Bacteria are often inoculated during the injury, resulting in a mixed purulent inflammation with numerous neutrophils. Early lens extraction may offer the greatest chance for saving these eyes, although large case studies are lacking to support this aggressive method of treatment. In older dogs, medical treatment after lens capsule rupture cannot prevent loss of eyes in many patients through uncontrolled inflammation and secondary glaucoma. In young dogs (less than 12 months of age), much of the lens cortex may be resorbed, with less inflammation than in older animals, provided infection is controlled.

Penetrating injury and lens capsule rupture are common causes of uveitis and endophthalmitis in dogs and cats.

Leakage Through the Lens Capsule

This occurs most frequently in the advanced stages of cataract (hypermaturity). The lens capsule becomes permeable and liquefied cortex leaks out, causing uveitis and often secondary glaucoma. Lens-induced uveitis is often present in eyes with cataract presented for unilateral ocular inflammation and discomfort of short duration. Without tonometry and biomicroscopy, this inflammation is not evident, and many such eyes exhibit a dilated pupil—not a miotic pupil, as would be expected in uveitis. In all eyes with cataract, lens-induced uveitis is a hazard that should be anticipated, although it does not always occur. Pre-existing and postoperative lens-induced uveitis are common causes of secondary complications after cataract surgery in dogs, e.g., glaucoma, cyclitic membranes obscuring the pupil. Pre- and postsurgical therapy with topical corticosteroids, often for long periods, may be necessary to control lens-induced uveitis. In contrast, lens-induced uveitis secondary to lens capsule rupture often responds poorly to therapy.

Lens-induced uveitis may go undetected in cataractous eyes if tonometry and biomicroscopic examinations are not performed.

RECURRENT EQUINE UVEITIS

Synonyms: "moon blindness," periodic ophthalmia

History and Geographical Distribution

Recurrent equine uveitis (REU) was recorded by veterinarians attending horses of Alexander the Great.

The disease is worldwide in distribution, although distinct regional differences in frequency occur—it is more common in North America than in Australia, the United Kingdom, or South Africa. The recurrent nature of the disease has long been recognized, and it was thought to be coincident with lunar phases.

Unfortunately, the disease is shrouded in ignorance, folklore, and misconceptions by both horse owners and veterinarians. For example, in parts of Australia the disease is said to be caused by "sand" in the eye, and in Britain it has been stated that the disease has been "bred out," although there is no evidence of heritability. Similar examples occur in other areas. An incidence of up to 12% has been recorded in eastern areas of the United States, and some authors feel it is more prevalent in low-lying areas with high rainfall. There is no age, sex, or breed predilection.

Etiology

There is no single etiology of REU. Hereditary factors, riboflavin deficiency, and *Brucella* infection are rejected former theories. The most commonly held explanation is that this uveitis is caused by a delayed hypersensitivity reaction, with persistence of immunologically sensitized cells causing recurrent cell-bound antibody formation on re-exposure to the antigen. Cell-mediated immunity to uveal antigens has been demonstrated in affected horses. An autoimmune phenomenon in response to damaged uveal tissue has also been proposed, initiated by various noxious stimuli:

1. Postleptospiral uveitis
2. Migrating microfilariae of *Onchocerca cervicalis*
3. *Streptococcus equi* and various unknown stimuli

Postleptospiral Uveitis

One to 2 years after leptospiral infection, ocular lesions can be demonstrated. Lesions and organisms are *not* present in the eye during active infection (similar findings occur in humans, although the interval between the initial infection and the onset of uveitis is greater in horses). Serum titers of greater than 1:4000 have been accepted as evidence of previous infection, although lower titers may also be significant. Considerably higher titers (up to 1:128,000) occur in the aqueous of horses with REU, but high aqueous titers of other immunoglobulins occur in other systemic disorders and after surgical procedures in other parts of the body in horses that have normal protective levels of leptospiral antibodies. IgG synthesis to *Leptospira interrogans* serovar *pomona* has been demonstrated within the eye.

Numerous serological studies have shown widespread exposure (up to 30%) of the equine population to a variety of serotypes of *Leptospira* spp in North America, Britain, Europe, and Australia. Although serological testing is useful in horses with REU, it alone is not diagnostic, as many horses show serological evidence of exposure to *Leptospira* but lack evidence of uveitis.

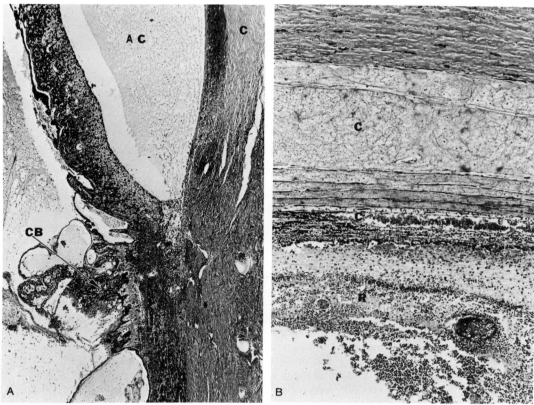

FIGURE 12–31. A, *Chronic lens-induced uveitis after lens capsule rupture in a dog. Macrophages, neutrophils, and lymphocytes are invading the iris, ciliary body, and cornea. AC = anterior chamber; CB = ciliary body; C = cornea. B, Choroiditis and retinitis in lens-induced uveitis (same eye as* A). *C = engorged choroid; R = retina.*

REU is observed 1–2 years after systemic leptospirosis.

Clinical Signs (Fig. 12–32)

ACUTE PHASE

1. Marked blepharospasm
2. Photophobia
3. Lacrimation
4. Pain
5. Protrusion of the third eyelid
6. Scleral injection
7. Aqueous flare (and hypopyon)
8. Miosis
9. Thickened, infiltrated iris
10. Corneal edema and cloudiness
11. Anterior and posterior synechiae
12. Fibrinous clots in anterior chamber
13. Decreased intraocular pressure
14. Depigmented butterfly lesions near optic disc (Fig. 12–33)

In addition to the usual ocular lesions of REU, in onchocerciasis the following may be seen:

1. Focal dermatitis on the head, ventral thorax, and neck
2. Vitiligo—scrotum, lateral canthus, lateral conjunctival limbus (Fig. 12–34)
3. Focal corneal opacities at the lateral limbus
4. Hyperemia and chemosis of the perilimbal temporal conjunctiva

In the acute phase, rapid intensive treatment is mandatory in order to prevent severe complications (e.g., synechiae, cataract, retinal detachment). Acute attacks may last from several days to a week, and most

FIGURE 12–32. *Clinical signs of REU.*

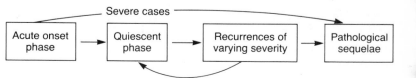

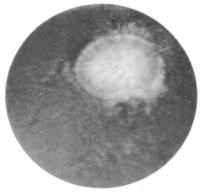

FIGURE 12–33. Depigmented lesions adjacent to the optic disc in REU. Choroidal vasculature is visible posteriorly. (From Rubin LF: Atlas of Veterinary Ophthalmoscopy. Lea & Febiger, Philadelphia, 1974.)

enter the quiescent phase of minimal inflammation to recur at a later date. Histologically, inflammation and altered vascular permeability continue throughout the quiescent period (Fig. 12–35).

QUIESCENT PHASE

During the quiescent phase, inflammation continues but is not apparent clinically. It is during this phase that the effects of previous inflammation are most likely to be seen during clinical examination of apparently normal horses.

1. Pigment on anterior lens capsule (Fig. 12–36)
2. Anterior and posterior synechiae (Fig. 12–37)
3. Cataract (not surgically correctable)
4. Vitreous bands and opacities

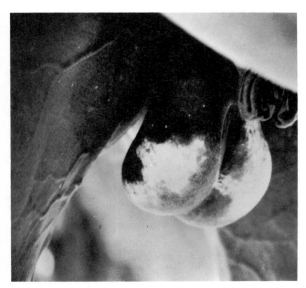

FIGURE 12–34. Scrotal vitiligo (depigmentation surrounded by hyperpigmentation) in REU due to Onchocerca spp. (Courtesy of Dr. L. McMullen.)

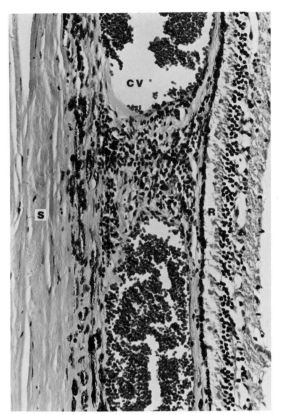

FIGURE 12–35. Choroid affected with REU. A diffuse infiltration with inflammatory cells is present. S = sclera; CV = choroidal vessel; R = retina. (Tissue courtesy of Drs. J. R. Blogg and P. Williamson.)

5. Corneal opacity
6. Retinal detachment
7. Occluded pupil
8. Iris atrophy
9. Phthisis bulbi
10. Partial or complete loss of vision

The presence of inflammatory sequelae in an equine eye indicates the possibility of previous or quiescent REU.

Treatment

1. Place the animal in a dark stall to relieve photophobia.

2. Atropine ointment (1%) twice a day (BID) to relax the ciliary muscle and relieve pain and to reduce synechia formation.

3. Subconjunctival corticosteroids (e.g., 20 mg triamcinolone acetonide). (Note: Methylprednisolone is not recommended for horses because of the unsightly plaques and postinjection irritation it may cause.)

4. Systemic corticosteroids—e.g., dexamethasone 100 mg intramuscularly (IM) daily.

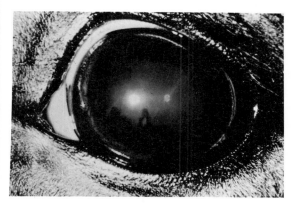

FIGURE 12–36. *Pigment on the anterior lens capsule (at the inferior pupillary border) in a horse during the quiescent phase of REU. (Courtesy of Dr. G. A. Severin.)*

5. Prostaglandin inhibitors to reduce protein leakage into the aqueous in the acute phase.

    a. acetylsalicylic acid 13 g/500 kg daily, per os (PO).

    b. flunixin meglumine (0.2 mg/kg) intravenously (IV) in acute cases.

6. Topical corticosteroids (e.g., 0.1% dexamethasone drops 4 times a day [QID]).

During the quiescent phase, oral aspirin and topical dexamethasone (usually in the ointment form) may be continued for long periods to help prevent recurrence.

Onchocerca Uveitis

Onchocerca cervicalis lives in the ligamentum nuchae of the horse. The microfilariae released by these adults migrate to the skin and ocular region and are transmitted by midges of the genus *Culicoides* and mosquitos. Ocular lesions are associated with the migration of the microfilariae from the ligamentum nuchae to the skin, some entering vessels of the bulbar and palpebral conjunctivae. The microfilariae are most readily found in the conjunctiva adjacent to the temporal limbus and in the corneal stroma adjacent to this area.

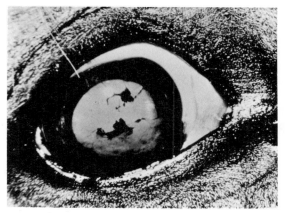

FIGURE 12–37. *Posterior synechia and cataract after REU. (Courtesy of Dr. G. A. Severin.)*

Cello (1971) described the corneal lesions as "superficial subepithelial fluffy or feathery white opacities, 0.5–1.0 mm in diameter, located 1–5 mm from the temporal limbus." The adjacent conjunctiva was hyperemic and chemotic, but biomicroscopic examination was required to demonstrate the corneal lesions.

The ocular lesions of onchocerciasis alone, including conjunctival vitiligo, are insufficient to indicate the presence of microfilariae. Unilateral ocular infestations with microfilariae may also occur.

REU is said either to be caused by the dead microfilariae or to be mediated by immunopathological mechanisms involving IgE. Diethylcarbamazine stimulates IgE antibody responses, and this may account for inflammation following its administration, rather than a reaction by the host to killed microfilariae.

Microfilariae are demonstrated by removing, with the patient under local anesthesia, (a) a small piece of conjunctiva from the affected area, or (b) a piece of skin from the ventral thoracic midline. The tissue is minced with scissors and placed in 5 ml of saline solution at 37°C for 30–50 minutes (e.g., in a small vial in the clinician's pocket). The supernatant is centrifuged and examined for mobile microfilariae. Alternatively, the tissue may be examined in saline solution on a slide immediately after collection. Interpretation of these slides must be made in association with other clinical findings, as many horses without REU have microfilariae.

Microfilaricides must not be used during acute uveitis.

Treatment

1. As for postleptospiral uveitis:

    Darkened stall

    Topical atropine

    Topical, subconjunctival, and systemic corticosteroids

    IV and oral prostaglandin inhibitors

2. After the inflammation has subsided, ivermectin (0.2 mg/kg)[3] may be administered systemically. Alternatively, diethylcarbamazine, 4 mg/kg daily, is administered in the food for 21 days. At the first sign of recurrent inflammation during treatment, corticosteroid therapy is commenced. In endemic areas, prophylactic feeding of diethylcarbamazine and aspirin orally is recommended throughout the season when vectors are present. Aspirin may also be used continuously.

---

3. This recommendation is made based on the study by Herd and Donham (1983), showing high efficacy of ivermectin in treating dermal lesions and microfilariae. They also noted severe dermal inflammation after treatment, and it may be assumed that this will also occur in the eye.

Course

With each subsequent uveitis attack, cumulative damage occurs to the ocular tissues, often resulting in blindness. Vigorous attempts are made to control each episode. Eventual blindness may be caused by corneal opacity, retinitis, retinal detachment, cataract, or optic neuritis.

Toxic Uveitis

Toxicity is an unusual cause of uveitis. Polyethylene glycol poisoning has been associated with anterior uveitis in dogs.

Traumatic Uveitis

Trauma is a common cause of uveitis in domestic animals.

Of the domestic species, the dog and horse are the most susceptible to traumatic uveitis. Examples of trauma that may cause uveitis are
Concussion
Penetrating corneal wounds
Paracentesis of the anterior chamber
Intraocular surgery (e.g., cataract extraction)

CLINICAL SIGNS

Any sign of uveitis (see Fig. 12–35) may be observed, but the most common are
1. Photophobia
2. Blepharospasm and pain
3. Miosis
4. Aqueous flare—may appear yellowish in severe cases
5. Fibrin in anterior chamber
6. Hyphema
7. Corneal edema
8. Ciliary injection
9. Swelling of the iris
10. Injection of the iris vasculature in animals with light-colored irides
11. Pigment deposits on the anterior lens capsule and posterior synechiae
12. Decreased intraocular pressure
The sequelae of traumatic uveitis are similar to those of other causes and require early and vigorous treatment.

In severe ocular trauma, early and vigorous treatment is required in order to prevent permanent ocular lesions.

TREATMENT

The degree of treatment depends on severity.

Mild Uveitis

1. Atropine (1% drops) 3 times daily (TID)
2. Topical corticosteroids (e.g., dexamethasone, 0.1% drops, TID)
3. Subconjunctival corticosteroids (e.g., dexamethasone 1 mg daily, depot betamethasone 3 mg)

Moderate or Severe Uveitis

1. Atropine (1% drops) TID.
2. Topical corticosteroids (dexamethasone 0.1%, 4–6 times daily).
3. Subconjunctival corticosteroids (e.g., triamcinolone 5–10 mg, depot betamethasone 6 mg).
4. Systemic corticosteroids—oral or IV dexamethasone or betamethasone depending on severity. Prednisolone should be avoided in severe uveitis as it is a less potent anti-inflammatory and has marked mineralocorticoid side effects.
5. Prostaglandin inhibitors:
   Aspirin 40 mg/kg daily in divided doses PO (canine dosage). Feline dosage, 40 mg/kg PO every 72 hours.
   Flunixin meglumine 1 mg/kg IV at initial therapy.
   Flurbiprofen topically 6 times daily.
(These drugs cause thrombocytopenia and altered platelet function, and are contraindicated if hyphema is present.) Clients are warned to watch for melena and vomiting (indicating gastrointestinal hemorrhage and gastric ulceration) when patients are receiving corticosteroids and prostaglandin inhibitors concurrently.
6. Systemic antibiotics in appropriate dose. As the blood-aqueous barrier is usually disrupted, most antibiotics will penetrate the eye.

If a wound is present that may be contaminated with bacteria, vigorous antimicrobial therapy—e.g., topical, subconjunctival, systemic, and subpalpebral lavage—may be necessary to prevent infection in the presence of corticosteroids. If corticosteroid therapy is omitted in traumatic uveitis, severe ocular lesions can result if leakage of lens protein has occurred.

Treatment of Uveitis—General Principles

1. MAKE AN ETIOLOGICAL DIAGNOSIS

Concerted attempts are necessary to find a cause for the uveitis. Many attempts will not be successful, but in those that are, specific therapy may be instituted (e.g., control of prostatitis, severe tooth root abscesses, and endometritis). Routine hematology and serum chemistry profiles are useful in indicating the presence of inflammatory disorders and concurrent systemic disease. In endemic areas, appropriate serological tests are indicated, e.g., toxoplasmosis, coccidioidomycosis, blastomycosis, cryptococcosis. Blastomycosis is found most frequently in the Central United States east of the Mississippi River, and coccidioidomycosis is found in Arizona, Nevada, and the Central Valley of California.

2. REMOVE THE INCITING AGENT FROM THE EYE

If bacteria are suspected (e.g., after a penetrating wound), use the appropriate type of antibiotic and route of administration. If the uveitis is lens-induced, anti-inflammatory therapy is indicated.

3. CONTROL INFLAMMATION AND ITS EFFECTS

Corticosteroids

Subconjunctival, topical, and systemic routes may be used. Corticosteroids inhibit cell-mediated immune reactions, decrease antibody production, and stabilize lysosomal membranes, reducing release of intracellular proteolytic enzymes. The following treatment regimens have proved effective:

1. Subconjunctival   dexamethasone—1–2 mg daily
   triamcinolone—10–20 mg once
   depot betamethasone—6 mg
2. Topical   1% prednisolone, 3–4 times a day
   0.1% dexamethasone, 3–4 times a day
3. Systemic   0.1–0.5 mg/kg dexamethasone daily IM (dogs and cats)

Nonsteroidal Anti-Inflammatory Agents

Significant protein leakage from uveal vessels during inflammation is mediated by prostaglandins. Inhibition of prostaglandin production reduces release of protein, decreasing the amount of antibody present to engage in immunological reactions and also decreasing fibrin, which decreases synechiae formation.

Dosages
Dog and Cat
Aspirin 40mg/kg daily in divided doses PO (canine dosage) (feline dosage 40 mg/kg PO every 72 hours)
Flunixin meglumine 1 mg/kg IV at initial therapy
Horse
Aspirin 13 g/50 kg daily PO
Flunixin meglumine 1 mg/kg IV daily
Phenylbutazone 2 g BID PO

Cycloplegics

Cycloplegics are chosen rather than mydriatics, to dilate the pupil, reduce synechiae formation, and relax

the ciliary muscle to lessen pain. If dilatation is insufficient, a complementary mydriatic may be added, e.g., atropine (1%) ointment or drops BID–TID, and 10% phenylephrine drops BID–TID. In horses, higher concentrations of atropine (3–4%) may be required for mydriasis, which may *persist for up to 6 weeks after therapy is discontinued.*

Atropine is used to control the pain of SECONDARY ANTERIOR UVEITIS occurring with corneal ulceration. This uveitis is usually *beneficial,* and corticosteroid therapy is contraindicated because of the risk of interference with treatment of the corneal ulcer and enhancement of collagenase activity.

Immunosuppressive Agents

Azathioprine may be used orally in nonresponsive uveitis, concurrent with laboratory evaluation for systemic side effects. A dose rate of 2 mg/kg/day for 4–7 days then gradual reduction based on clinical signs has been used.

4. RELIEVE PAIN

Atropine relaxes the ciliary muscle. The animal may be placed in the dark to reduce reflex parasympathetic stimulation of the iris and ciliary body. In severe pain, systemic analgesics, e.g., pethidine (Demerol), oxymorphone, may be used.

Uveitis in Systemic Disorders

The uvea is involved in numerous systemic disorders (see Table 12–1). As such diseases usually affect other parts of the eye in addition to the uvea, they will be discussed in Chapter 19.

INJURIES

Common uveal injuries include
1. IRIS PROLAPSE—protrusion of a portion of the iris through a corneal or scleral perforation.
2. HYPHEMA—hemorrhage into the anterior chamber.
3. STAPHYLOMA—a weakened or protruding lesion in the cornea or sclera into which a portion of the uvea protrudes from the inside. The uvea usually adheres to the cornea or sclera.
4. CONCUSSION—after traumatic injuries to the eye.
5. IRIDODIALYSIS—tearing of the iris from the ciliary body at its root. This condition is uncommon in animals.

Iris prolapse and hyphema are discussed here in greater detail.

Iris Prolapse

Iris prolapse is a common sequel to penetrating corneal wounds or ruptured corneal ulcers. The iris is carried forward into the corneal defect by escaping aqueous. Emergency treatment of such lesions is described in Chapter 21. When the iris passes through such a corneal defect, its vascular supply is usually compromised, resulting in venous congestion and edema. This changes the appearance of the protruding mass, so that it frequently looks like a blob of mucus adhering to the cornea.

SIGNS

1. The color of the prolapsed portion becomes lighter than the remaining iris.
2. The protruding iris tissue forms a mound on the cornea.
3. The tissue has a gelatinous mucoid appearance and frequently attracts adhering strands of conjunctival mucus.
4. The pupil is eccentric, as a result of traction of the protruding iris tissue.
5. The corneal wound is often obscured by the edematous iris tissue.

Protrusion of the ciliary body occurs most frequently in horses as a result of scleral rupture behind the limbus following blunt trauma.

TREATMENT

If the corneal wound is small, an iris prolapse may be treated temporarily with a third eyelid flap and topical and systemic antibiotics until specialized assistance is available. In larger wounds requiring immediate repair, an attempt is made to replace the iris with an iris spatula before suturing the cornea. If this is not possible, the protruding piece may be carefully excised with the use of an electrosurgical unit. The cornea is then sutured and the anterior chamber reconstituted with a sterile air bubble. *Caution:* If the major arterial circle of the iris is transected, profuse intraocular hemorrhage can result.

Hyphema

The emergency treatment of hyphema is discussed in Chapter 20.

ETIOLOGY

Hyphema may be idiopathic or may result from many factors including

1. Trauma
2. Fragility of vessel walls, especially those formed in the process of neovascularization in chronic inflammation and chronic glaucoma
3. Clotting disorders, platelet disturbances, and blood dyscrasias
4. Neovascularization of the iris or retina (e.g., scleral ectasia syndrome in collies and Shetland sheepdogs)
5. Highly vascularized tumors
6. Severe uveitis
7. Retinal dysplasia with rupture of vessels (e.g., in Bedlington terriers)
8. Systemic disease (e.g., tropical canine pancytopenia)
9. Severe pressure around the neck, as from choking, or increased intrathoracic pressure in severe traumatic compression and dystocia
10. Chronic glaucoma (poor prognosis)
11. Several months after cataract surgery in dogs, probably due to neovascularization and subsequent rupture

Erythrocytes released into the anterior chamber undergo phagocytosis by the cells lining the trabecular meshwork. The surface of the iris provides fibrinolysin, which aids in resolving clots in the anterior chamber. The sequelae of hyphema are of more clinical significance to the eye than is the hemorrhage itself (Fig. 12–38).

TREATMENT

Most hyphemas are small and resorb spontaneously in a few days.

The treatment of hyphema is controversial because of conflicting experimental results with different drug regimens in different species. Although different methods are used, the aims are to

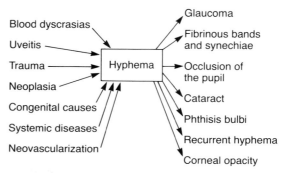

FIGURE 12–38. *Causes and effects of hyphema. (Modified from Blogg JR: The Eye in Veterinary Practice. Philadelphia, WB Saunders Co, 1980.)*

1. Identify the cause
2. Prevent recurrent bleeding
3. Control uveitis
4. Limit the sequelae of uveitis

Surgical attempts to remove clots from the anterior chamber are contraindicated.

The following treatment is recommended:

1. Prevent further trauma by immediate and enforced cage or stall rest.

2. Administer corticosteroid drops (dexamethasone 0.1%, prednisolone 1%) TID. Subconjunctival corticosteroids may also be used. Nonsteroidal anti-inflammatory agents are not used because of their effects on platelets and blood clotting.

Mild Hyphema

3. Administer pilocarpine drops (1%) TID and dilate the pupil every 2nd day with phenylephrine (10%) to prevent synechiae formation. Avoid atropine in mild hyphema because of the risk of glaucoma.

Severe Hyphema

4. Atropine drops (1%) TID to relieve the pain of uveitis (see no. 5).

5. Monitor intraocular pressure BID.

6. Administer systemic corticosteroids (e.g., prednisolone or dexamethasone) in appropriate systemic dosages.

7. If glaucoma is incipient, administer carbonic anhydrase inhibitors PO.

If recurrent hyphema occurs, a complete laboratory examination including complete blood count, platelets, and clotting parameters is indicated. In the absence of specific indications, use of vitamins C and K is not advised, nor are such treatments as proteolytic enzymes or carbonic anhydrase inhibitors.

MISCELLANEOUS DISORDERS

Iris Atrophy

Several types of iris atrophy occur, as discussed here.

ATROPHY ASSOCIATED WITH IRIS HYPOPLASIA

In congenital iris hypoplasia in color-dilute, albinotic, and subalbinotic animals, iris atrophy may progress, leaving large spaces in the iris.

PRIMARY IRIS ATROPHY

A slowly progressive iris atrophy in previously normal adults occurs in dogs and cats. Spaces and holes develop in the iris and are especially visible in light reflected from the tapetum. The condition is seen in Siamese cats, miniature schnauzers, poodles, and Chihuahuas especially. There is no convincing evidence that primary iris atrophy can cause glaucoma, as it does in humans.

SENILE IRIS ATROPHY

Senile iris atrophy occurs in older animals of all species and is characterized by irregular pupillary margins, spaces in the iris, and sluggish or absent pupillary reflexes. The condition must be distinguished from secondary iris atrophy. It is common in poodles and chihuahuas and is significant in the evaluation of cataractous or visually impaired patients (Fig. 12–39).

SECONDARY IRIS ATROPHY

Atrophy of the iris may follow
1. Chronic glaucoma
2. Chronic recurrent uveitis
3. Severe ocular trauma

SURGICAL PROCEDURES

Surgical procedures for primary diseases of the iris are rarely performed even in specialty practice. Examples include:

1. IRIDECTOMY (removal of part of the iris)—for focal circumscribed melanomas of the iris.

2. IRIDOCYCLECTOMY (removal of a portion of iris and ciliary body)—for neoplasms of the ciliary body. Many neoplasms are too advanced at presentation for this procedure, but in the early stages the technique,

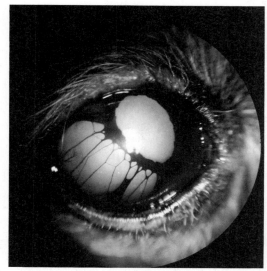

FIGURE 12–39. Advanced iris atrophy in a poodle with diabetic cataract. (Courtesy of Dr. C. Martin.)

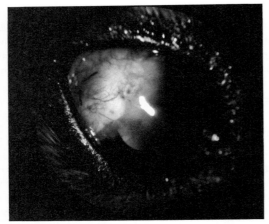

FIGURE 12–40. Replacement of a scleral defect, after iridocyclectomy for a ciliary body neoplasm, with a corneoscleral allograft (4 weeks postoperatively). The graft has been vascularized, and the rejection reaction has been controlled with topical corticosteroids.

although demanding, allows removal of affected tissue and salvage of the eye and vision. For larger neoplasms infiltrating the sclera, the scleral defect may be replaced with an autogenous graft (Fig. 12–40).

3. SPHINCTEROTOMY (incision of the sphincter)—performed occasionally during cataract surgery. The sphincter is cut in one or more places if mydriasis is poor, to allow access to the lens and to reduce the chance of a small pupil postoperatively. Since the advent of nonsteroidal anti-inflammatory agents the technique is rarely necessary.

The use of iridectomy and iridencleisis for canine glaucoma has been superseded by correctly applied cyclocryotherapy (see Chap 13).

REFERENCES

Acland GC, et al (1980): Diffuse iris melanoma in cats. J Am Vet Med Assoc 176:52.

Barnett KC, Knight GC (1969): Persistent pupillary membrane and associated defects in the basenji. Vet Rec 85:242.

Barron CM, et al (1963): Intraocular tumors in animals. III. Secondary intraocular tumors. Am J Vet Res 24:835.

Baszler T, et al (1988): Disseminated pseudallerescheriasis in a dog. Vet Pathol 25:95.

Bellhorn RW, Henkind P (1970): Intraocular malignant melanoma in domestic cats. J Sm Anim Pract 10:631.

Bergsma DR, Brown KS (1971): White fur, blue eyes and deafness in the domestic cat. J Hered 62:171.

Bertroy RW, et al (1988): Intraocular melanoma with multiple metastases in a cat. J Am Vet Med Assoc 192:87.

Bistner SI (1974): Medullo-epithelioma of the iris and ciliary body in a horse. Cornell Vet 64:588.

Bistner SI, et al (1972): A review of persistent pupillary membrane in the basenji dog. J Am Anim Hosp Assoc 7:143.

Bussanich MN, et al (1982): Granulomatous uveitis and dermal depigmentation in dogs. J Am Anim Hosp Assoc 18:131.

Bussanich MN, et al (1987): Canine uveal melanomas: Series and literature review. J Am Anim Hosp Assoc 23:415.

Buyukmihci N (1982): Ocular lesions of blastomycosis in the dog. J Am Vet Med Assoc 180:426.

Campbell KL, et al (1986): Generalized leukoderma and poliosis following uveitis in a dog. J Am Anim Hosp Assoc 22:121.

Cello RM (1971): Ocular onchocerciasis in the horse. Equine Vet J 3:148.

Cook CS, et al (1983): Equine recurrent uveitis. Equine Vet J Supp 2:57.

Cottrell BD, Barnett KC (1987): Harada's disease in the Japanese Akita. J Sm Anim Pract 28:517.

Diters R, et al (1983): Primary ocular melanoma in dogs. Vet Pathol 20:379.

Donovan RH, et al (1974): Histology of the normal collie eye II. Uvea. Ann Ophthalmol 6:1175.

Dubey JP, et al (1988): Newly recognized fatal protozoan disease of dogs. J Am Vet Med Assoc 192:1269.

Fischer CA (1971): Lens-induced uveitis in dogs. J Am Anim Hosp Assoc 8:39.

Fox LE (1987): Reversal of ethylene glycol–induced toxicosis in a dog. J Am Vet Med Assoc 191:1433.

Gelatt KN, et al (1969): Ocular anomalies of incomplete albino cattle: Ophthalmoscopic examination. Am J Vet Res 30:1313.

Green WR (1986): Uveal tract. *In* Spencer WH (ed): Ophthalmic Pathology, 3rd ed, vol 3. WB Saunders Co, Philadelphia.

Gwin RM, et al (1980): Idiopathic uveitis and exudative retinal detachment in the dog. J Am Anim Hosp Assoc 18:163.

Gwin RM, et al (1981): Multiple ocular defects associated with partial albinism and deafness in the dog. J Am Anim Hosp Assoc 17:401.

Gwin RM, et al (1988): Anterior uveitis: Diagnosis and treatment. Semin Vet Med Surg 3:33.

Halliwell RH, Hines MT (1985): Studies on equine recurrent uveitis. I. Levels of immunoglobulin and albumin in the aqueous humor of horses with and without intraocular disease. Curr Eye Res 4:1023.

Halliwell RE, et al (1985): Studies on equine recurrent uveitis. II. The role of infection with *Leptospira interrogans* serovar *pomona*. Curr Eye Res 4:1033.

Hamilton HB, et al (1984): Pulmonary squamous cell carcinoma with intraocular metastasis in a cat. J Am Vet Med Assoc 185:307.

Herd RP, Donham JC (1983): Efficacy of ivermectin against *Onchocerca cervicalis* microfilarial dermatitis in horses. Am J Vet Res 44:1102.

Hoganesch H, et al (1987): Seminoma with metastases in the eyes and the brain in a dog. Vet Pathol 24:278.

Huston K, et al (1968): Heterochromia iridis in dairy cattle. J Dairy Sci 51:1101.

Kern TJ, et al (1985): Uveitis associated with poliosis and vitiligo in six dogs. J Am Vet Med Assoc 187:408.

Krohne SDG, et al (1987): Ocular involvement in canine lymphosarcoma—A retrospective study of 94 cases. 18th Ann Sci Proc, Am Coll Vet Ophth, Fort Worth.

Leipold HW, Huston K (1966): A herd of glass-eyed albino cattle. J Hered 57:179.

Leipold HW, Huston K (1968): Incomplete albinism and heterochromia iridis in Herefords. J Hered 59:2.

Leipold HW, Huston K (1969): Dominant incomplete albinism of cattle. J Hered 59:222.

Matthews AG, Handscombe MC (1983): Uveitis in the horse: A review of the aetiological and immunological aspects of the disease. Equine Vet J Supp 2:61.

Matthews AG, et al (1987): Serological study of leptospiral infections and endogenous uveitis among horses and ponies in the United Kingdom. Equine Vet J 19:125.

Meincke JE (1966): Reticuloendothelial malignancies with intraocular involvement in the cat. J Am Vet Med Assoc 148:157.

Moran CT, James ER (1987): Equine ocular pathology ascribed to *Onchocerca cervicalis* infection: A reexamination. Trop Med Parasitol 38:287.

Ohrstrom A (1972): Treatment of traumatic hyphema with corticosteroids and mydriatics. Acta Ophthalmol 50:549.

Patnaik AK, Mooney S (1988): Feline melanoma: A comparative study of ocular, oral and dermal neoplasms. Vet Pathol 25:105.

Peiffer RL (1983): Ciliary body epithelial tumors in the dog and cat: A report of 13 cases. J Sm Anim Pract 24:347.

Pomorski Z, et al (1984): Demonstration of the participation of autoagressive processes in the pathogenesis of equine recurrent uveitis. Pol Arch Weter 24:155.

Rahi AHS, Garner A (1976): Immunopathology of the Eye. Blackwell, Oxford.

Rebhun WC (1979): Diagnosis and treatment of equine uveitis. J Am Vet Med Assoc 175:803.

Roberts SR (1963): Fundic lesions in equine periodic ophthalmia. Am J Ophthalmol 55:1049.

Roberts SR, Bistner SI (1968): Persistent pupillary membrane in basenji dogs. J Am Vet Med Assoc 153:533.

Rubin LF (1966): Cysts of the equine iris. J Am Vet Med Assoc 149:151.

Rubin LF, Gelatt KN (1968): Spontaneous resorption of the cataractous lens in dogs. J Am Vet Med Assoc 152:139.

Ryan AM, Diters RW (1984): Clinical and pathologic features of canine ocular melanomas. J Am Vet Med Assoc 184:60.

Saunders LZ, Barron CN (1958): Primary pigmented intraocular tumors in animals. Cancer Res 18:234.

Schaffer EM, Funke K (1985): Primary intraocular melanomas in dogs and cats. Tierarztl Prax 13:343.

Schmidt GM, et al (1982): Equine ocular onchocerciasis: Histopathologic study. Am J Vet Res 43:1371.

Shively JN, Phemister RD (1968): Fine structure of the iris of dogs manifesting heterochromia iridis. Am J Ophthalmol 66:1152.

Sillerud CL, et al (1987): Serologic correlation of suspected *Leptospira interrogans* serovar *pomona*–induced uveitis in a group of horses. J Am Vet Med Assoc 191:1576.

Slatter DH, Hawkins CD (1982): Prevalence of leptospiral titres in normal horses. Aust Vet J 59:84.

Slatter DH, et al (1976): Ocular manifestations of myeloproliferative disease in a cat. Aust Vet J 50:164.

Strande A, et al (1988): Persistent pupillary membrane and congenital cataract in a litter of English cocker spaniels. J Sm Anim Pract 29:257.

Trucksa RC, et al (1985): Intraocular canine melanocytic neoplasms. J Am Anim Hosp Assoc 21:85.

Twigg GI, et al (1971): Occurrence of leptospirosis in thoroughbred horses. Equine Vet J 2:52.

Wilcock BP, Peiffer RL (1986): Morphology and behavior of primary ocular melanomas in 91 dogs. Vet Pathol 23:418.

Wilcock BP, Peiffer RL (1987): The pathology of lens-induced uveitis in dogs. Vet Pathol 24:549.

Williams RD, et al (1971): Experimental chronic uveitis. Invest Ophthalmol 10:948.

Zimmerman LE, et al (1976): Malignant intraocular teratoid medulloepithelioma in three dogs. Vet Pathol 13:343.

13

Glaucoma

AQUEOUS PRODUCTION AND	PATHOGENESIS	TREATMENT
DRAINAGE	CLASSIFICATION	FELINE GLAUCOMA
DIAGNOSTIC METHODS	CLINICAL SIGNS	

Glaucoma is defined as a series of pathological conditions with clinical manifestations varying with the elevation in intraocular pressure and its consequences (modified from Duke-Elder and Jay, 1969).

AQUEOUS PRODUCTION AND DRAINAGE[1]

Aqueous is free of cells and protein and is produced by active secretion and ultrafiltration at the epithelium covering the ciliary body. Its composition is controlled by the filtering action of blood vessel walls in the ciliary body and by junctions between cells in the ciliary epithelium. The volume of aqueous produced is affected by mean arterial pressure; a lower pressure results in less aqueous. Carbonic anhydrase is associated with aqueous production; although the exact mechanism is not understood, inhibition of this enzyme reduces aqueous production.

Inhibition of carbonic anhydrase decreases aqueous production *unrelated* to diuretic properties of the drug.

Aqueous passes into the **POSTERIOR CHAMBER** and through the pupil into the **ANTERIOR CHAMBER** (Fig. 13–1*B*). From the anterior chamber the aqueous passes between the **PECTINATE LIGAMENTS** and enters the **CILIARY CLEFT**, which contains the **TRABECULAR MESHWORK**. Aqueous filters through the meshwork to enter the vessels of the **SCLERAL VENOUS PLEXUS** and re-enters the venous system (see Fig. 13–25*A*). Because of temperature differences between the iris and the cornea, thermal convection currents are set up in the

anterior chamber. These currents, which are occasionally visible when cells and particulate matter circulate in them, may produce specific patterns of cellular deposits on the corneal endothelium during inflammation. During passage of the aqueous through the anterior chamber, changes in chemical composition of the aqueous occur owing to diffusional exchange and metabolism of surrounding ocular tissues. In the anterior chamber, values approximate plasma values (Table 13–1).

Numerous mechanisms have been proposed to account for the formation of aqueous—e.g., redox pump, bicarbonate transport, Na- and K-activated ATPase, and pinocytosis.

Causes of Variations in Aqueous Production

DIURNAL VARIATION

Intraocular pressures are slightly higher during the day than at night in all species investigated. The exact mechanism of this cyclical change is unknown, but it is probably a combination of hormonal, neurogenic, and metabolic influences.

TABLE 13–1. Average Steady-State Composition of Rabbit Aqueous
(Expressed as fraction of plasma concentrations)

Constituent	Posterior Chamber	Anterior Chamber
Chloride	0.88	0.94
Hydrogen ion	0.70	0.84
Bicarbonate	1.70	1.35
Ascorbate	57.0	44.0
Protein	0.007	0.009

Reproduced by permission from Kolker AE, Hetherington J: Becker-Shaffer's Diagnosis and Therapy of the Glaucomas, 5th ed. St Louis, 1983, The CV Mosby Co.

---

1. See also Chap 2.

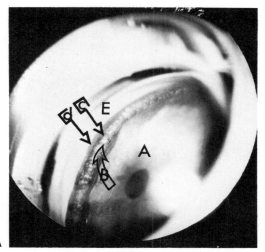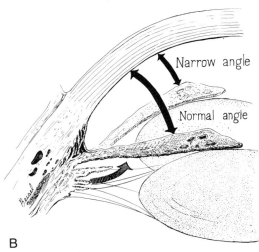

A   **B**

FIGURE 13–1. *A, Goniosopic view of the iridocorneal or drainage angle, showing iris (A), pectinate ligament with white trabecular zone posteriorly (B), deep pigmented zone (c), superficial pigmented zone (d), and cornea (E). B, The narrow angle that may cause closed-angle glaucoma because of apposition over the outflow channels and resultant peripheral anterior synechiae. (From Martin CL, Wyman M: Primary glaucoma in the dog. Vet Clin North Am 8:257, 1978.)*

AGE

In humans, aqueous production and intraocular pressure decline after 60 years of age. In both humans and animals, the ease with which aqueous leaves the eye (aqueous outflow facility) declines with age, and therefore, for intraocular pressure to decline, aqueous production must fall at a correspondingly greater rate.

BLOOD PRESSURE

Disorders that are associated with lower mean arterial pressure result in lower intraocular pressure, e.g., hypoadrenocorticism, dehydration, and hypovolemic and cardiogenic shock. Ligation of a carotid artery reduces intraocular pressure on the same side.

DRUGS

Carbonic anhydrase inhibitors cause up to a 50% decrease in aqueous production at maximal effective dosage; further increases in dosage have no further inhibitory effect. Topical administration of epinephrine lowers aqueous secretion in dogs. (In humans this effect is additive to that produced by carbonic anhydrase inhibitors.) Anesthetics and tranquilizers cause intraocular pressure to fall, with the exception of ketamine in cats, which causes large temporary increases in intraocular pressure, believed to be due to spasm of the extraocular muscles.

OCULAR INFLAMMATION

Both spontaneous and surgically induced inflammation lower aqueous production and intraocular pressure.

A profound fall in intraocular pressure is an *important diagnostic clue* to the presence of intraocular inflammation, especially uveitis. The relationship among aqueous production, aqueous outflow facility, and intraocular pressure is shown in Figure 13–2.

DIAGNOSTIC METHODS

Measurement of Intraocular Pressure

Measurement and normal values for intraocular pressure are discussed in Chapter 5. The reader is referred to this discussion before proceeding with this chapter. Despite its disadvantages, the most economical and technically applicable instrument in general veterinary practice is the Schiøtz tonometer with the *human* calibration tables (veterinary tables do not agree as well with applanation methods and are not reliable).

The ability to perform diagnostic Schiøtz tonometry is essential to every veterinarian engaged in small animal practice.

A useful rule is that *all red eyes not affected with a purulent or infectious condition should be stained with fluorescein and examined, and if the results are negative, the intraocular pressure should be determined.* The occurrence of important or even catastrophic errors in diagnosis may thus be minimized.

Measurement of Outflow Facility

Outflow facility is measured by tonography, in which a known mass is placed on the globe and the reduction

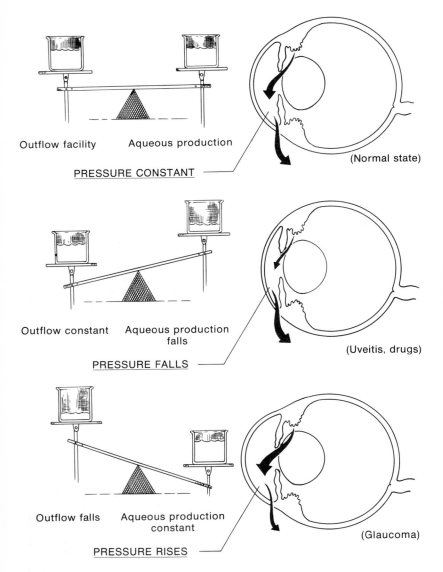

Outflow facility   Aqueous production

PRESSURE CONSTANT

(Normal state)

Outflow constant   Aqueous production falls

PRESSURE FALLS

(Uveitis, drugs)

Outflow falls   Aqueous production constant

PRESSURE RISES

(Glaucoma)

FIGURE 13–2. Common alterations in aqueous production and outflow facility and their effects on intraocular pressure.

in intraocular pressure is measured over several minutes. This is related to experimentally determined values for aqueous outflow facility (liter/minute/mmHg pressure gradient). Normal values for beagles vary up to a maximum of 0.22, whereas in glaucomatous dogs values reach a maximum of 0.09. Equipment for tonography is unavailable in general practice or even in most referral centers and veterinary eye clinics. Because of the expense of the equipment, lack of patient cooperation, and relatively little use of the technique by veterinary ophthalmologists, tonography remains a research tool and is not an integral part of management of the glaucomatous patient.

Gonioscopy

Gonioscopy is used to examine the iridocorneal angle and is discussed in detail in Chapter 5. Gonioscopy allows the differentiation of OPEN-ANGLE and CLOSED-ANGLE types of glaucoma; measurement of the degree of obstruction of the iridocorneal angle in such conditions as goniodysgenesis (mesodermal dysgenesis), intraocular neoplasms, and foreign bodies; and evaluation of therapeutic methods. Accurate gonioscopy is useful in managing glaucoma patients, especially for evaluating the contralateral eye, but as it requires considerable practice to recognize the many normal variations, gonioscopy is practiced almost exclusively by veterinary ophthalmologists. Examples of gonioscopic findings are shown in Figures 13–3 to 13–9.

Provocative Tests

A provocative test identifies patients with a latent tendency to glaucoma but that have normal intraocular pressure at examination. Although a variety of such

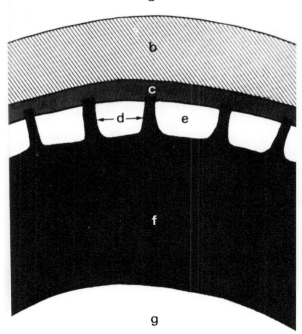

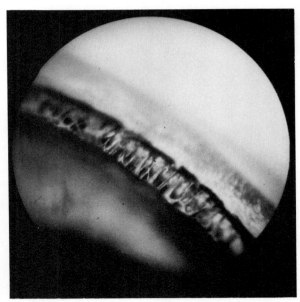

FIGURE 13–3. Gonioscopic view of the normal iridocorneal angle, showing (a) cornea, (b) superficial pigment zone, (c) deep pigment zone, (d) pectinate ligaments, (e) ciliary cleft containing trabecular meshwork, (f) iris, and (g) pupil. (From Bedford PGC: Gonioscopy in the dog. J Sm Anim Pract 18:615, 1977.)

FIGURE 13–5. A normal open angle with a deeply pigmented insertion of the pectinate ligaments. (From Bedford PGC: Gonioscopy in the dog. J Sm Anim Pract 18:615, 1977.)

tests are used in humans, the administration of water has been the only one to be evaluated in dogs. When water is given orally, intraocular pressure increases.

In a dog predisposed to glaucoma, pressure elevation caused by a standard dose of water is greater. The

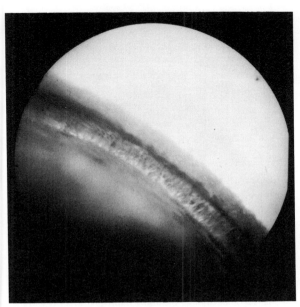

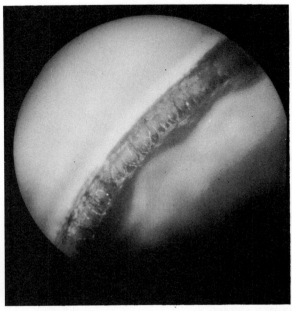

FIGURE 13–4. Normal canine iridocorneal angle. (From Bedford PGC: Gonioscopy in the dog. J Sm Anim Pract 18:615, 1977.)

FIGURE 13–6. A normal open angle with no pigmentation. The white band of the scleral shelf is visible superiorly. (From Bedford PGC: Gonioscopy in the dog. J Sm Anim Pract 18:615, 1977.)

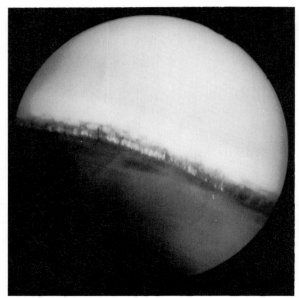

FIGURE 13–7. A narrow but open angle in a normotensive 10-year-old English cocker spaniel. (From Bedford PGC: Gonioscopy in the dog. J Sm Anim Pract 18:615, 1977.)

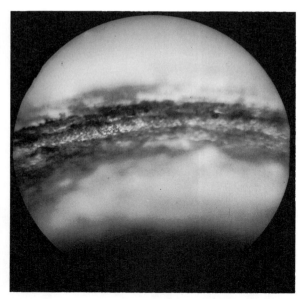

FIGURE 13–8. Complete obstruction of the ciliary cleft by sheets of mesodermal tissue in a 6-year-old basset hound. Aqueous outflow facility is severely decreased. The angle is not narrowed but is obstructed, and intraocular pressure is not yet elevated. (From Bedford PGC: Gonioscopy in the dog. J Sm Anim Pract 18:615, 1977.)

magnitude of this increase helps identify dogs with a latent tendency to glaucoma. Normal beagles given 50 ml/kg of water orally showed increases in intraocular pressure of from 3.1 to 8.6 mmHg over the succeeding 90 minutes, compared with increases of from 7.3 to 10.9 mmHg in glaucomatous beagles. Provocative testing is *not* widely used clinically.

PATHOGENESIS

The effects of increased intraocular pressure on ocular tissues are similar regardless of the cause of the elevation. It is essential to consider whether the lesions and clinical signs observed are *associated with the etiology* of the increased pressure or *result from it*. A discussion of the general effects of increased intraocular pressure is followed by consideration of the different *mechanisms* that cause increased intraocular pressure.

Effects of Increased Intraocular Pressure

In chronic glaucoma, most ocular tissues are affected. Vision is most affected by lesions in the optic nerve and retina.

OPTIC NERVE

The optic nerve is dramatically and *irreversibly* affected at the optic disc, which becomes "excavated" or

"cupped." Initially, tissues anterior to the lamina cribrosa appear *compressed*. This is caused by *interruption of normal posterior axoplasmic flow* in the cell processes that make up the optic nerve. This flow is normally from

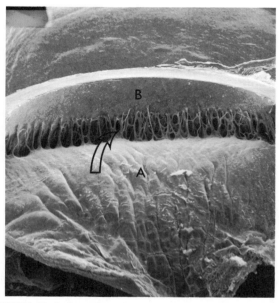

FIGURE 13–9. Scanning electron micrograph of a canine iridocorneal angle. A = iris; B = cornea; arrow = pectinate ligament. (From Martin CL, Wyman M: Primary glaucoma in the dog. Vet Clin North Am 8:257, 1978.)

the ganglion cell body within the ganglion cell layer of the retina toward the dendrites of the cell processes in the lateral geniculate body. Eventually these fibers atrophy, and pressure forces the lamina cribrosa outward (Fig. 13–10). Secondary wallerian degeneration of the ascending fibers of the optic nerve follows (Figs. 13–11 and 13–12). Cupping of the optic disc can be seen ophthalmoscopically (Fig. 13–13).

RETINA

Elevation of intraocular pressure decreases blood flow into the eye, causing ischemia. As the pulse pressure (systolic pressure − intraocular pressure) falls, ischemia occurs. This ischemia can be demonstrated functionally by depressed electroretinograms. The retinal ganglion cell is least likely to recover from even brief periods of ischemia. Early in the course of glaucoma, the nerve fiber and ganglion cell layers begin to degenerate and may be completely absent on histological sections. In advanced chronic glaucoma, the outer layers of the

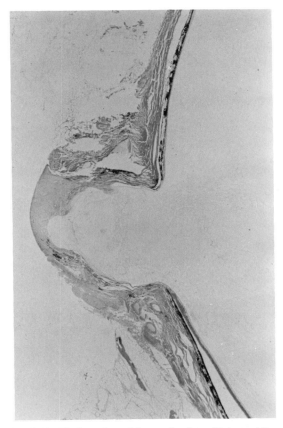

FIGURE 13–10. *Cupping of the optic disc with loss of tissue anterior to the lamina cribrosa, which is bowing outward (left side of the photomicrograph). Cupping is due to a form of degeneration in the optic nerve known as Schnabel's cavernous optic neuropathy. (Tissue courtesy of Dr. Stuart Young.)*

retina also disappear, and the whole retina is replaced by a glial scar (Fig. 13–14). Ophthalmoscopically this is seen as increased tapetal reflectivity as in any other severe retinal atrophy; the condition is irreversible.

UVEA

With acute elevations of intraocular pressure (between 40 and 50 mmHg in dogs), the **CONSTRICTOR PUPILLAE MUSCLE** becomes paralyzed, resulting in pupillary dilatation. With long-standing elevations, the muscle and iris stroma atrophy, and the ciliary body and processes atrophy, owing to decreased blood supply because of the high intraocular pressure (Fig. 13–15).

Atrophy of the ciliary body and reduced aqueous production are noteworthy, as they explain the balance between increased intraocular pressure and scleral stretching and buphthalmos in advanced chronic glaucoma in some dogs. In these eyes aqueous production is decreased, the eye stretches no further, and the condition becomes tolerable to the animal despite advanced pathological changes and unsightly appearance. Iris atrophy is visible clinically as spaces, giving a lace-like appearance, especially with light reflected from the tapetum (retroillumination; Fig. 13–16). Iris atrophy is *not* a cause of glaucoma as it is in humans.

LENS

Cataract frequently occurs in chronic glaucoma, often in association with lens luxation or subluxation. Glaucoma and lens luxation together require determination of whether luxation was the *cause* or *result* of glaucoma. As the sclera stretches with increased intraocular pressure, lens zonules break and the lens luxates. Similarly, primary cataract formation is frequently followed by lens luxation and glaucoma. Thus the combination of glaucoma, cataract, and lens luxation (Fig. 13–17) in any particular eye may occur through several mechanisms. Any of these three disorders may have been the primary insult.

Lens luxation in a glaucomatous eye does not necessarily mean it was the inciting cause of the glaucoma. The luxation may have resulted from the glaucoma.

CORNEA

In acute glaucoma, interference with function of the corneal endothelium by high intraocular pressure and disturbance of the balance between hydrating and dehydrating forces in the corneal stroma cause corneal edema. Epithelial edema also occurs, and epithelial bullae may form in chronic glaucoma. In chronic edema

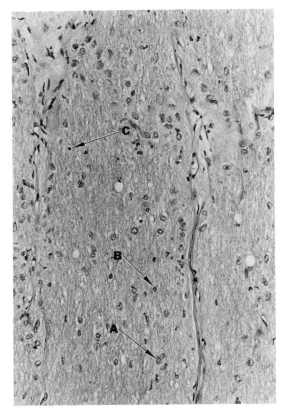

FIGURE 13–11. Normal canine optic nerve (longitudinal section). A = astrocyte; B = oligodendrocyte; C = microglia.

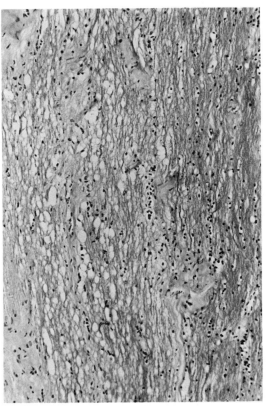

FIGURE 13–12. Wallerian degeneration of a canine optic nerve in chronic glaucoma. Demyelination and gliosis are present.

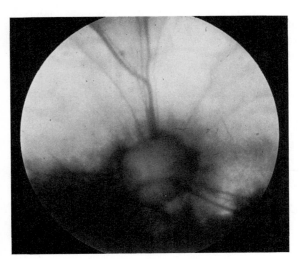

FIGURE 13–13. Direct ophthalmoscopic view of optic disc cupping. Most retinal vessels disappear at the disc edge, and the center of the disc is in focus below the level of the retinal surface. (Courtesy of Dr. G. A. Severin.)

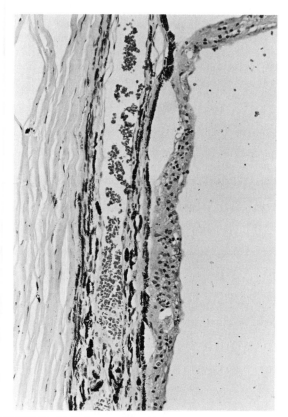

FIGURE 13–14. Retina replaced by a glial scar in advanced glaucoma.

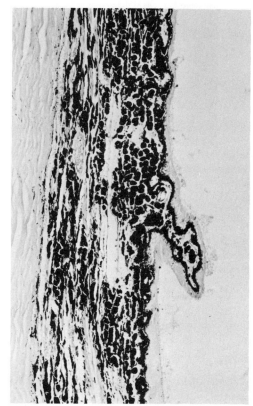

FIGURE 13–15. Atrophy of the ciliary processes and ciliary body in advanced glaucoma. (Compare with Fig. 12–12.)

FIGURE 13–16. Iris atrophy in chronic glaucoma must be distinguished from primary iris atrophy.

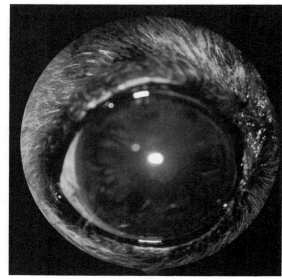

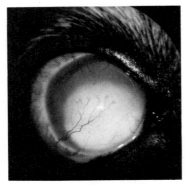

FIGURE 13–17. *Chronic glaucoma, cataract, lens luxation, and keratitis in a poodle—a diagnostic challenge (see Chap. 14).*

due to glaucoma, both superficial and deep vascularization and pigmentation frequently occur (Fig. 13–18). The presence of this vascularization makes clinical differentiation between glaucoma and uveitis even more crucial if the eye is to be saved. Both glaucoma and uveitis may also be present, and consultation with an veterinary ophthalmologist in diagnosis and therapy of glaucoma and uveitis is recommended.

SCLERA

In chronic glaucoma, the sclera stretches and the eye enlarges (buphthalmos) (Figs. 13–19 and 13–20). This *stretching is irreversible,* even if intraocular pressure is later reduced to normal. Not all eyes with glaucoma undergo stretching. By the time buphthalmos has occurred, vision is usually lost, although the presence of pain is variable.

Mechanisms That Increase Intraocular Pressure

GONIODYSGENESIS

In goniodysgenesis (mesodermal dysgenesis)—as seen in the basset hound, Bouvier des Flandres, American and English cocker spaniel, Norwegian elkhound, Siberian husky, dachshund, miniature poodle, Welsh terrier, wire-haired fox terrier, and Chihuahua—sheets of tissue obstruct the drainage angle *to a variable degree* from birth (Figs. 13–21 and 13–22). Intraocular pressure does not increase until later life. With increasing age, collagenous cores of the pectinate ligaments and tissues traversing the ciliary cleft *thicken,* as with other collagenous tissues in the eye, and this restricts the space between ligaments for aqueous to flow through on its way to the scleral venous plexus.

In addition to variation in degree of mesodermal obstruction, the amount of the angle affected varies; some eyes have only 20–30° of the circumference

obstructed while others have 360° affected. This variation accounts for differences in or lack of expression of glaucoma in later life. Increases in pressure are thought to be due to combinations of angle closure and pupillary block phenomena and possibly uveitis further compromising aqueous drainage to the partially obstructed angle (which is still *open* by definition) and whose aqueous outflow facility is decreasing with age. Goniodysgenesis is bilateral.

OBSTRUCTION OF IRIDOCORNEAL ANGLE

In addition to sheets of tissue obstructing the open angle, neoplastic cells (especially melanocytes), macrophages filled with lens debris after capsule rupture (phacolytic glaucoma), and inflammatory cells and tissue may obstruct the iridocorneal angle. Few cases of glaucoma in these categories are free of pupillary block or angle closure by peripheral iris in later stages. With inflammation, peripheral anterior synechiae form, causing narrowing of the angle with each subsequent attack. Intraocular melanoma and inflammation due to lens capsule ruptu.? by penetrating injuries are common causes of secondary glaucoma in dogs and, to a lesser extent, in cats (Figs. 13–23 and 13–24).

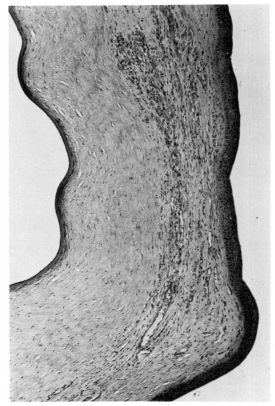

FIGURE 13–18. *Corneal vascularization in the anterior corneal stroma (right side of illustration) in chronic glaucoma.*

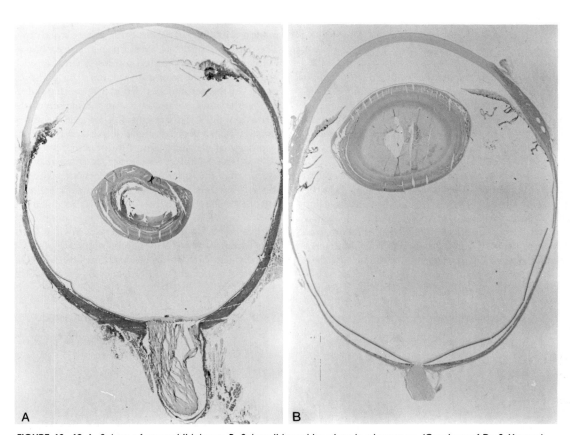

FIGURE 13–19. A, *Sclera of normal thickness.* B, *Sclera thinned by chronic glaucoma. (Courtesy of Dr. S. Young.)*

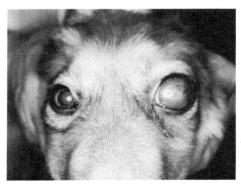

FIGURE 13–20. Gross buphthalmos in chronic untreated glaucoma. (Courtesy of Dr. G. A. Severin.)

PUPILLARY BLOCK

In pupillary block, resistance to aqueous flow from the posterior chamber to the anterior chamber is increased. Aqueous accumulates in the posterior chamber and pushes the root of the iris forward, causing angle closure (see Fig. 13–27). A shallow anterior chamber, increased contact between the iris and the lens, or a large lens may all cause pupillary blockage—e.g., swollen (intumescent) lens in mature cataract. With inflammation, posterior synechiae may form between the posterior surface of the iris and the lens, causing pupillary blockage. The degree of pupillary block may increase with each episode of recurrent inflammation (e.g., due to uveitis). If the iris is totally bound to the lens throughout its circumference, an IRIS BOMBÉ (ballooned iris) develops as aqueous pushes the iris forward.

Pupillary blockage and angle closure were formerly accepted as the main causes of glaucoma in domestic animals, especially dogs, but it is now known that congenital angle anomalies are also responsible. Uveitis is also a factor, but so far poorly defined.

LENS LUXATION AND SUBLUXATION

Lens luxation and subluxation cause glaucoma, especially in the wire-haired and smooth fox terriers, Sealyham, Manchester, and Cairn terriers, miniature schnauzer, and miniature poodle. In these breeds the condition is inherited, usually in a recessive manner. The lens zonules break in early life, usually after 12 months and often in *apparent* response to minor trauma. The lens may subluxate (remain in the fossa but out of normal position) or luxate completely into the vitreous or anterior chamber or forward into the plane of the pupil. If the lens moves forward, pupillary blockage and angle closure usually occur, together with the formation of peripheral anterior synechiae and glaucoma. In cats, because of the deeper anterior chamber, pupillary block and angle closure are less frequent. When the lens luxates posteriorly, nothing may happen except that the anterior chamber becomes deeper and the iris is thus unsupported and moves tremulously (IRIDODONESIS) when the eye moves. Secondary, low-level uveitis due to lens movement is often an early sign of impending lens subluxation in dogs. At this time intraocular pressure may be *reduced*.

Many eyes with posterior lens luxation have increased pressure when examined. This may be accounted for by

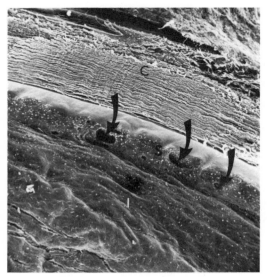

FIGURE 13–21. Sheets of mesodermal tissue obstructing access by aqueous to the ciliary cleft. Compare with the normal angle in Figure 13–9. Note the flow holes (arrows). C = cornea; I = iris; S = sclera. (From Martin CL, Wyman M: Primary glaucoma in the dog. Vet Clin North Am 8:257, 1978.)

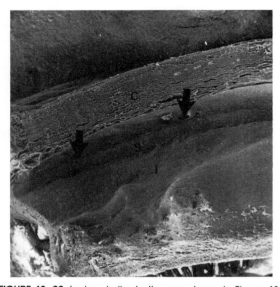

FIGURE 13–22. Lesion similar to the one shown in Figure 13–21, but with more extensive obstruction. I = iris; C = cut cornea; S = sclera. Arrows delineate sheet with pores. (From Martin CL, Wyman M: Primary glaucoma in the dog. Vet Clin North Am 8:257, 1978.)

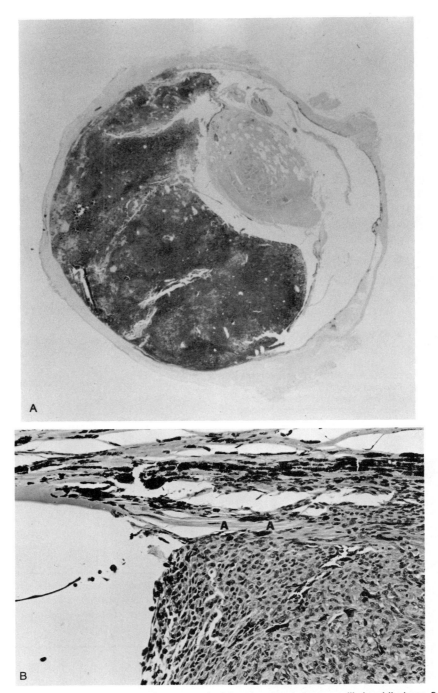

FIGURE 13–23. *A, Intraocular melanoma in a dog, presented for chronic glaucoma with buphthalmos. B, Neoplastic cells have infiltrated the drainage angle (A), which is collapsed.*

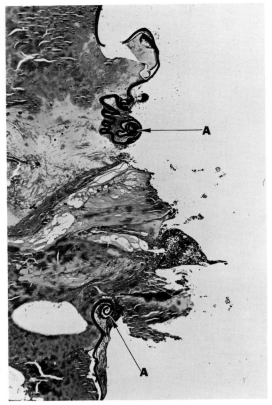

FIGURE 13–24. Lens capsule rupture (A) and retraction after a penetrating injury to the eye of a 5-year-old miniature schnauzer. Endophthalmitis and angle closure occurred, resulting in severe intractable glaucoma requiring enucleation.

1. Earlier anterior luxation having caused pupillary block or angle closure
2. Movement of the lens having caused pupillary block, angle closure, or inflammation

Luxated lenses must be either removed or placed into the vitreous.

Relative Frequency of Etiology of Glaucoma

In the basset hound and cocker spaniel, goniodysgenesis is the most common cause of glaucoma in areas where these breeds are popular (e.g., United Kingdom, United States). In the beagle, an open-angle glaucoma associated with secondary lens luxation occurs in research colonies and to a much lesser extent in the general population in parts of the United States. Goniodysgenesis is common in susceptible breeds, but lens luxation and endophthalmitis due to penetrating injuries are also frequent causes of glaucoma.

Histological studies on canine eyes enucleated for chronic glaucoma indicate that penetrating injuries with lens capsule rupture and severe endophthalmitis are a common cause of glaucoma (see Fig. 13–24). The lesions of the initial penetrating corneal wound (e.g., cat's claw) are often difficult to distinguish from corneal edema and vascularization due to chronic glaucoma. In cats, in which glaucoma is much less common than in dogs, chronic endophthalmitis of various causes frequently results in glaucoma, but the etiology of apparent feline primary glaucoma is poorly understood. Recent reports indicate chronic low-level uveitis may be an important cause.

CLASSIFICATION

Glaucoma is classified by numerous methods, although the most consistently useful is based on the state of the iridocorneal angle, i.e., whether it is open, narrow, or closed (see later in this section). As other methods are frequently referred to and compound classifications are sometimes used (e.g., secondary open-angle glaucoma), commonly used terms are briefly defined here. Correct classification is essential to choosing appropriate therapy (Tables 13–2 and 13–3).

Definitions

PRIMARY GLAUCOMA—unassociated with other ocular disease or actual cause unknown
SECONDARY GLAUCOMA—increases in intraocular pressure due to pre-existing or concomitant diseases
CONGENITAL GLAUCOMA—present at or soon after birth; rare in domestic animals

State of the Drainage Angle[2]

Figures 13–25, 13–26, and 13–27 illustrate aqueous flow in the normal eye and in open- and closed-angle glaucoma, respectively. In open- and closed-angle glaucoma, the subclassifications in Table 13–3 may be made.

Pupillary blockage refers to increased resistance to passage of aqueous from the posterior to the anterior chamber through the pupil (Fig. 13–28).

Frequently, a given case of glaucoma has several contributing factors, making simple classification into any one category difficult. Because of the wide variety of causes of glaucoma, accurate evaluation of medical and surgical treatments depends on correct diagnosis and classification.

---

2. *Note:* This refers to the *angle* itself, and not the patency of the trabecular meshwork and ciliary cleft.

TABLE 13–2. Classification of Canine Glaucoma

I. Open-angle glaucoma: Normal, wide angle on gonioscopy

  A. Primary: No observable predisposing factors, angle normal on gonioscopy, bilateral, breed predisposition

  B. Secondary: Normal angle obstructed by aqueous contents or elevated episcleral venous pressure interferes with aqueous drainage

    1. Inflammation—White blood count and fibrin obstruct outflow
    2. Hyphema—Erythrocytes and fibrin obstruct outflow
    3. Pigment—Deposition or proliferation obstructs outflow
    4. Lipids in anterior chamber obstruct outflow
    5. Anterior luxated lens—May obstruct angle or create pupil block
    6. Elevated episcleral venous pressure—Arteriovenous fistula, orbital lesion, or increased blood pressure (rare)

II. Closed-angle glaucoma: Angle is collapsed or covered with peripheral iris or connective tissue

  A. Primary

    1. Congenital: Goniodysgenesis—maldeveloped angle covered with mesodermal tissue; usually bilateral; age of glaucoma onset varies
    2. Acquired: Closure associated with abnormal anterior chamber conformation
      a. Forward displacement of lens presumably due to slack zonules; creates a relative pupillary blockage from increased adhesive forces between lens and iris
      b. Shallow anterior chamber with small anterior segment; pupillary block may occur that results in peripheral anterior synechiae
      c. Plateau iris—Iris plane is flat, but peripheral iris has a recess adjacent to angle, which is susceptible to angle closure with pupillary blockage

  B. Secondary: Acquired lesions precipitate closure of previously normal angle; also, angle conformations under II (A) have an increased susceptibility to pupillary blockage

    1. Associated with pupillary block
      a. Intumescent lens
      b. Posterior synechiae, iris bombé
      c. Subluxated lens, luxated lens
      d. Aphakic vitreous herniation
      e. Increased volume in vitreous compartment, i.e., accumulation of aqueous, swelling of vitreous
    2. No pupillary block
      a. Neoplasia with invasion of angle and/or pushing iris forward or thickening of iris
      b. Inflammation with peripheral anterior synechiae
      c. Subluxated lens pushing iris base forward
      d. Epithelial downgrowth—Perforating corneal wound with epithelium proliferating over angle

From Martin CL, Vestre WA: Glaucoma. *In* Slatter DH (ed): Textbook of Small Animal Surgery, p 1573. WB Saunders Co, Philadelphia, 1985.

CLINICAL SIGNS

Glaucoma is one of the most frequently misdiagnosed eye conditions. *Failure to recognize the disease early* in its course may prevent effective treatment; it is *essential* that clinicians be thoroughly familiar with the signs of glaucoma.

The clinical signs of glaucoma are summarized in Figure 13–29. The signs present in a particular case depend on the duration and intensity of the pressure elevation (Table 13–4) and its cause.

Corneal Edema

Owing to interference with endothelial function, water enters the corneal stroma in greater amounts, forcing the collagen fibers apart and causing opacity. Profound edema and opacity are most common in the early stages of glaucoma or when pressure increases are dramatic. Edema may also be present with other, nonglaucomatous conditions, such as penetrating injury, keratitis, corneal ulceration, uveitis, and endothelial dystrophy. Corneal edema must be distinguished from corneal scars and opacities.

TABLE 13–3. Subclassifications of Glaucoma

Open Angle	Closed Angle
A. Primary (goniodysgenesis or mesodermal dysgenesis)	A. With pupillary block
B. Secondary	1. Primary
1. Inflammation, especially uveitis and secondary glaucoma	2. Secondary
	a. Lens intumescence (advanced cataract)
2. Phacoanaphylactic uveitis	b. Iris bombé with posterior synechiae
3. Tumors	c. Lens subluxation
	B. Without pupillary block
	1. Peripheral anterior synechiae
	2. Tumors
	3. Inflammation

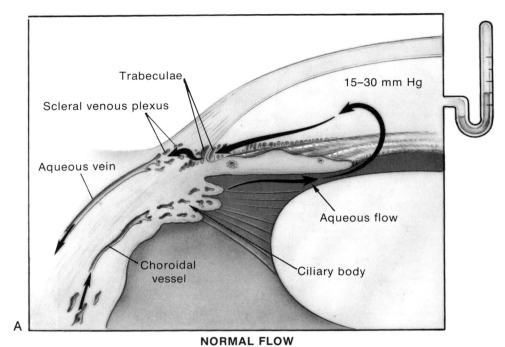

Trabeculae

Scleral venous plexus

15–30 mm Hg

Aqueous vein

Aqueous flow

Choroidal
vessel

Ciliary body

A

NORMAL FLOW

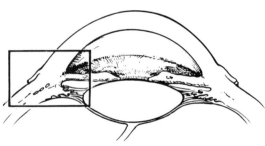

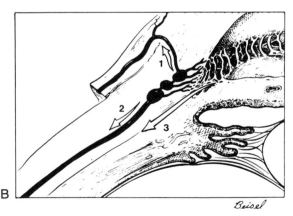

B

Beisel

FIGURE 13–25. A, *Pathway of normal aqueous production and drainage.* B, *The routes of aqueous drainage from the canine iridocorneal angle. Aqueous taken up by the venous system in the angle may drain anteriorly to the episceral and conjunctival veins (1), posteriorly into the vortex venous system (2), or through the ciliary muscle interstitium to the suprachoroid and diffuse through the sclera (uveoscleral flow, 3). (B from Martin CL, Vestre WA: Glaucoma. In Slatter DL [ed]: Textbook of Small Animal Surgery. WB Saunders Co, Philadelphia, 1985.)*

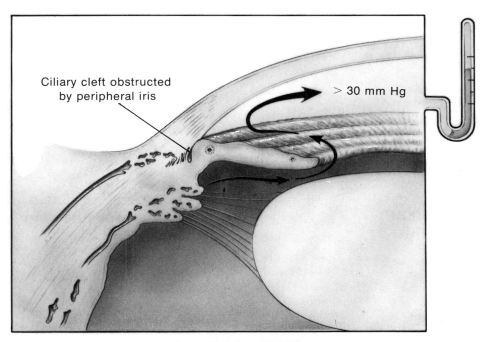

CLOSED-ANGLE GLAUCOMA

FIGURE 13–26. Open-angle glaucoma due to trabecular obstruction. The angle itself is normal.

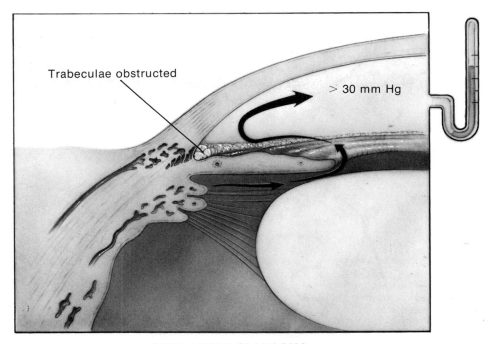

OPEN-ANGLE GLAUCOMA

FIGURE 13–27. Closed-angle glaucoma. The peripheral iris prevents access by the aqueous to the ciliary cleft and drainage network.

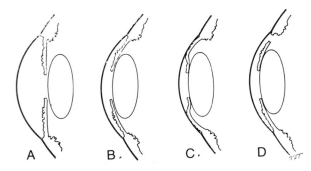

FIGURE 13–28. Pathogenesis of pupillary blockage in closed-angle glaucoma. A, The iris in a normal eye with a deep anterior chamber. B, The iris in an eye with a shallow anterior chamber. The iris is compressed against the lens by the iris sphincter. C, The iris when pupillary blockage becomes complete. An iris bombé is present with occlusion of the angle by the root of the iris. D, Relief of pupillary blockage by peripheral iridectomy. (Reproduced by permission from Duke-Elder, Sir Stewart, editor: System of Ophthalmology. Section III. Glaucoma and Hypotony [by Duke-Elder, Sir Stewart, and Jay, Barrie]. St Louis, 1969, The CV Mosby Co.)

Pain, Blepharospasm, and Altered Behavior

In ACUTE glaucoma, the dog often rubs the affected eye with a paw or along the carpet. Pressure to the affected eye through the upper lid or to the surrounding area may cause severe pain. If the condition is not treated, severe pain and blepharospasm may diminish and be replaced by signs of chronic lower-level pain—timidity (e.g., hiding under furniture), anorexia, and less playful or friendly behavior. Occasional patients become aggressive.

> Glaucoma is usually an extremely painful condition, especially in its early stages.

Fixed Dilated Pupil
(see Fig. 13–17)

As intraocular pressure increases, the pupillary constrictor muscle is paralyzed and the pupil dilates. Mydriasis is not an invariable sign of glaucoma—miosis may be present in some of the pupillary block types,

CLINICAL SIGNS OF GLAUCOMA

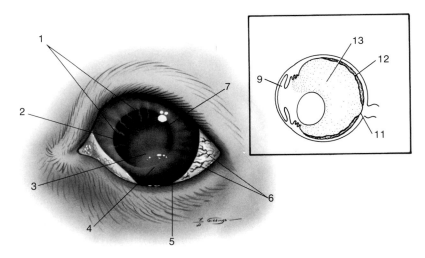

1. Descemet's streaks (advanced cases)
2. Aphakic crescent
3. Luxated lens (some cases)
4. Corneal edema
5. Iris atrophy
6. Enlarged episcleral vessels
7. Fixed, dilated pupil
8. Increased intraocular pressure
9. Shallow anterior chamber
10. Partial or complete vision loss
11. Cupping of the optic disc
12. Retinal atrophy and vascular attenuation
13. Buphthalmos
14. Ocular pain
15. Loss of corneal sensitivity

FIGURE 13–29. Clinical signs of glaucoma.

TABLE 13–4. Clinical Signs of Glaucoma

Early	Moderate or Subacute	Advanced or Chronic
Pain	Pain	Pain (variable)
Corneal edema	Corneal edema	Corneal vascularization and pigmentation
Blepharospasm	Blepharospasm	Lack of corneal aphakic crescent
Cataract (see Fig. 13–17)	Blindness	Lens opacity (see Fig. 13–17)
	Leukokoria	
Anorexia	Anorexia	Anorexia
Depression	Depression	Depression, timidity, or aggression
Fixed, dilated pupil	Fixed, dilated pupil	Fixed, dilated pupil
Episcleral engorgement (with conjunctival erythema)	Episcleral engorgement (with conjunctival erythema)	Episcleral engorgement
Increased intraocular pressure	Increased intraocular pressure	Increased intraocular pressure (variable)
Shallow anterior chamber (if visible)	Shallow anterior chamber	Shallow anterior chamber
Impaired vision	Impaired vision	Impaired vision
Lens luxation (variable)	Lens luxation (variable)	Lens luxation (variable)
	Descemet's streaks (variable)	Descemet's streaks (variable)
Direct pupillary reflex abolished	Direct pupillary reflex abolished	Direct pupillary reflex abolished
		Iris atrophy
		Retinal and optic atrophy

but these are less common. In these latter cases, a careful examination is necessary to distinguish glaucoma from uveitis (both may be present). The dilated pupil is present in most cases of glaucoma, and direct and consensual reflexes are abolished. The longer glaucoma remains unresolved, the greater the chance of formation of peripheral anterior synechiae that may permanently block the drainage angle by fixing the peripheral iris in position. The size of the pupil is *not* correlated with aqueous outflow facility.

A dilated pupil with increased tapetal reflectivity and pain may be one of the first signs noticed by the owner ("the eye looks different").

A dilated, unresponsive pupil may be due to other diseases besides glaucoma (e.g., progressive retinal degeneration, optic atrophy) and is not diagnostic by itself.

Engorged Episcleral Vessels
(Fig. 13–30)

Engorgement of episcleral veins is one of the more common signs of increased intraocular pressure. Conjunctival capillaries may also be engorged, but usually to a lesser degree. The two may be distinguished by

| Conjunctival capillary erythema | Conjunctiva is pink, individual vessel not prominent |
| Episcleral vein engorgement | Large individual vessels visible, passing over a conjunctiva that is usually white |

Conjunctival engorgement is more frequently associated with uveitis in which the ciliary vasculature is engorged. Episcleral engorgement arises because the increased intraocular pressure reduces flow through the ciliary body to the vortex veins, and the increased flow passes forward via anastomosing episcleral veins at the limbus.

Increased Intraocular Pressure

Pressures above 30 mmHg with clinical signs are sufficient for a presumptive diagnosis. Care is necessary to distinguish patients with higher pressure and no acute signs—this condition is called OCULAR HYPERTENSION, usually results in lesions in the longer term, and is more frequent in small breeds, e.g., Chihuahua and Yorkshire, Australian, and Sydney silky terriers.

In the absence of a Schiøtz tonometer, a *rough guide* can be obtained by palpation through the upper lid. In

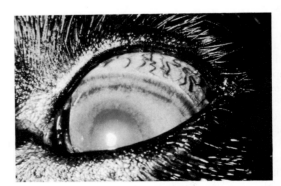

FIGURE 13–30. Episcleral venous engorgement in chronic canine glaucoma. Note the large red vessels on a white scleral background. Perilimbal vascularization is also present. (Courtesy of Dr. G. A. Severin.)

most cases of glaucoma, pressure is 40 mmHg or more. Increased intraocular pressure decreases blood supply to the retina. The longer the pressure is increased, the less the chance that vision can be retrieved; after 24 hours, the effects are usually irreversible. Although vision is often lost before the condition is noticed by the owner, *prompt treatment* often saves the eye and vision.

Owners must be counseled on the appearance of early glaucoma so that the remaining eye can be treated early when it eventually gets glaucoma.

Frequent measurement of intraocular pressure is an integral part of diagnosis and treatment of the glaucoma patient.

Shallow Anterior Chamber

Depth of the anterior chamber (distance between cornea and iris) is evaluated with an oblique focal source of light or by biomicroscopy. Decreased depth is correlated with narrowness of the drainage angle and is a useful diagnostic sign. Note that in *posterior* lens luxation the anterior chamber may be much deeper, but that intraocular pressure is usually not increased.

Impaired Vision

Vision is lost early in the affected eye if the pressure elevation is great. Preservation of vision depends on rapid reduction of pressure. Loss of vision in the first eye is rarely noticed by the owner if the other eye is normal, but it can be demonstrated by the "cotton test" (Chap 5). A black patch can sometimes be placed over the normal eye to reveal the deficit in the affected eye.

Optic Disc Cupping
(see Fig. 13–13)

In chronic glaucoma when the ocular media are clear, cupping of the optic disc is sometimes visible ophthalmoscopically. It indicates irreversible damage to the optic nerve head. In acute glaucoma the ocular media are rarely transparent enough to see the disc. The retinal vessels disappear over the edge of the crater-like depression, out of focus. In the normal dog eye, the surface of the disc is in focus from 0 to −3 diopters (D). If the lens is luxated, a +7 or +8 lens is used. The depth of the depression is the difference between the "in focus" values for the rim and those for the bottom of the cup.

For example, if these values are −2 and −5, respectively, the difference is 3 D and the depth of the depression is 0.9 mm (1 D = 0.3 mm).

Retinal and Optic Atrophy
(see Fig. 13–14)

In advanced glaucoma, profound retinal atrophy with increased tapetal reflectivity occurs, together with attenuation or complete loss of retinal vessels, atrophy of the pigment epithelium in the nontapetal fundus, and optic atrophy (grayish-white appearance). These findings are also present in advanced progressive retinal degeneration (progressive retinal atrophy). In progressive retinal degeneration the other signs of glaucoma are lacking, the disease is usually bilateral, and differential diagnosis may be determined by the breed of dog and lack of other clinical signs of glaucoma. Ophthalmoscopically visible retinal and optic nerve lesions are irreversible.

Buphthalmos and Descemet's Streaks (Fig. 13–31)

As intraocular pressure increases, the sclera and cornea stretch and enlarge (buphthalmos), especially in younger animals. This propensity of the sclera to stretch varies with breed and with individuals. In severe cases in animals with highly elastic globes, the eye may enlarge considerably and become quite unsightly. The change is *irreversible* even if the pressure is later reduced, although a variety of surgical procedures are available to restore a cosmetically acceptable appearance.

By the time severe stretching has occurred, atrophy of the ciliary body may have reduced the intraocular pressure to normal and pain may be less. As the cornea stretches, linear ruptures in Descemet's membrane, called DESCEMET'S STREAKS, may occur.

Iris Atrophy (see Fig. 13–16)

In advanced glaucoma, the iris stroma becomes atrophic and may appear lacy or moth-eaten, especially

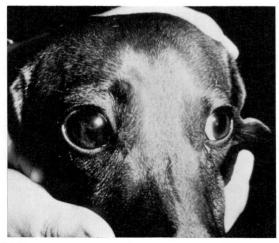

FIGURE 13–31. Descemet's streaks in chronic glaucoma. (Courtesy of Dr. G. A. Severin.)

when viewed with light reflected from the tapetum. Iris atrophy secondary to glaucoma is differentiated from primary iris atrophy, such as that seen in aged miniature schnauzers and Siamese cats.

Lens Luxation (Fig. 13–32; see also Fig. 13–17)

Lens luxation in glaucoma may be either PRIMARY or SECONDARY. In secondary luxation, lens zonules break as the globe enlarges, and the lens may be displaced anteriorly, posteriorly, or in the plane of the iris (either superiorly or inferiorly). BREED PREDISPOSITION and the presence of VITREOUS STRANDS and RUPTURED ZONULES in the pupil assist diagnosis of primary lens luxation. Primary lens luxation may also cause glaucoma.

Primary hereditary lens luxation followed by glaucoma has been discussed (Chap 16). Lens luxation may be recognized by any one of the following signs:

1. Presence of the lens *in front of* the iris (anterior luxation).
2. Presence of an *aphakic crescent* in the pupil (most frequent in subluxation).
3. Movement of the iris (*iridodonesis*).
4. *Deep anterior chamber.*
5. *Vitreous strands* and *ruptured zonules* in the pupil.

The fundus is viewed directly through the aphakic crescent—the region between the edge of the lens and the pupillary border of the iris. After luxation, the lens frequently but not invariably becomes cataractous. If a luxated lens enters the anterior chamber and touches the corneal endothelium, an area of corneal opacity may appear. This opacity is frequently permanent, even if the lens is later removed. A glaucomatous eye with a luxated, cataractous lens may have reached this state by one of several means:

1. cataract → lens intumescence → glaucoma → buphthalmos → lens luxation
2. lens luxation → glaucoma → cataract
3. glaucoma (variety of etiologies) → buphthalmos → lens luxation → cataract

The recognition of how the final state was reached is important in determining which combination of therapeutic methods is required.

Ocular Hypertension

Ocular hypertension is measurable elevated intraocular pressure in the absence of other clinical signs. In small breeds, manual palpation as an indication of intraocular pressure is inaccurate. The condition occurs infrequently in small-breed dogs—Chihuahua, Yorkshire terrier, Sydney silky terrier, Australian terrier. Ocular hypertension may persist for long periods without apparent clinical signs, but when signs do appear, such as pain or retinal atrophy, the condition is treated as for any other glaucoma. In the early stages, the use of topical medications, e.g., echothiophate iodide 0.25% twice a day (BID), timolol maleate 0.5% BID, is appropriate. During such early therapy, frequent pressure measurements are necessary.

TREATMENT

Glaucoma is treated by a veterinary ophthalmologist, after initial diagnosis and emergency therapy by the family veterinarian.

Canine Glaucoma

Three important points in treating glaucoma are

1. Correct choice of treatment depends on understanding the pathogenesis in the particular patient and the state of the iridocorneal angle.
2. Treatment of acute glaucoma is an *emergency* if vision or the eye is to be saved.
3. Primary glaucoma is a *bilateral* disease. The remaining eye requires prophylactic treatment for life, in addition to continuing treatment for the affected eye.

Needle paracentesis is contraindicated in the treatment of glaucoma.

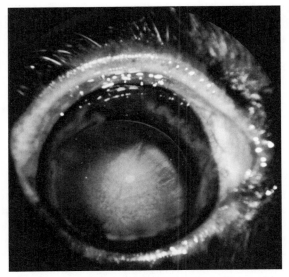

FIGURE 13–32. Primary anterior lens luxation with secondary glaucoma in a wire-haired fox terrier. Note corneal edema due to endothelial damage. (Courtesy of Dr. C. L. Martin.)

Immediate and Long-Term Management

EMERGENCY TREATMENT OF ACUTE GLAUCOMA

Early reduction of intraocular pressure is essential to prevent permanent damage. Although initial response may be dramatic, *definitive treatment must follow* in order to prevent recurrence. Veterinarians must be aware that medical therapy of glaucoma in animals, unlike that in the human eye, is restricted to short-term control of pressure and is *not effective* in the long term, except in very specific circumstances.

In almost all cases, topical atropine is contraindicated in glaucoma.

The following regimen may be used for initial reduction of intraocular pressure:

1. Mannitol (1.0–1.5 g/kg intravenously)—7.5 ml/kg of 20% solution over 15–20 minutes. Reduction in pressure is rapid but temporary.

2. Acetazolamide (Diamox) (5–10 mg/kg intravenously).

3. Pilocarpine (2.0% drops)—1 drop every 5 minutes for 30 minutes, then 2 or 3 times hourly for 3–4 hours until pressure is reduced. *Note:* Miotics should not be used if pupillary block is present. Caution is necessary in patients with cardiac disorders. Heart rate is monitored for bradycardia during initial therapy.

4. Oral glycerin 2 ml/kg is less effective and slower acting, but it is useful for owner administration. To limit vomiting, the dose is divided into 3 and given chilled; it may be mixed with food. Glycerin may cause nausea and vomiting but is a useful drug:

a. For use between emergency treatment and definitive treatment, and

b. During long-term management, as an emergency medication for use by the owner to treat sudden attacks of glaucoma, immediately prior to seeking professional assistance.

LONG-TERM MANAGEMENT OF GLAUCOMA

Long-term effective treatment of glaucoma involves correctly performed cyclocryotherapy or intraocular prosthesis insertion.

In most cases, definitive control for glaucoma is surgical, occasionally supplemented by additional medication. Certain types of glaucoma (e.g., phacolytic, postinflammatory) may be treated medically first; if medical treatments fail, surgical methods may then be used. Glaucoma following primary lens luxation frequently responds well to medical therapy, provided the lens is posterior to the iris.

Principles of Glaucoma Treatment

By the time many canine patients are seen for glaucoma, peripheral anterior synechiae have formed, and results of evaluation of the iridocorneal angle by gonioscopy can be predicted. If possible, the evaluation is performed for diagnostic purposes and to evaluate the angle of the contralateral eye.

The three basic principles of glaucoma treatment are

1. *Early reduction of intraocular pressure* (see "Emergency Treatment of Acute Glaucoma," earlier in this chapter)

2. *Reduction of aqueous production* by one of the following means:

a. Oral carbonic anhydrase inhibitors, e.g.,
Dichlorphenamide, 2 mg/kg, 3 times a day (TID) by mouth (PO)
Ethoxzolamide, 5 mg/kg, 2–3 times a day PO
Acetazolamide, 5–10 mg/kg, 2–3 times a day PO (*not* recommended because of emesis)

b. Sympathomimetic agents—1% epinephrine, or dipivalyl epinephrine 3–4 times a day

c. Sympatholytic agents—timolol maleate 0.5% BID

d. Surgical methods
Cyclocryotherapy—the effectiveness of this method has changed the therapy of glaucoma
Intraocular prosthesis insertion—the method of choice for blind, buphthalmic globes

3. *Increasing aqueous drainage,* using one of the following:

a. Parasympathomimetic agents—pilocarpine 2% 3–4 times a day

b. Cholinesterase inhibitors—echothiophate, demecarium bromide BID

c. Sympathomimetics—epinephrine may also function in this way

d. Surgical methods
Iridectomy (increases drainage between posterior and anterior chambers in pupillary block)
Iridencleisis, trephination, cyclodialysis, iridectomy, and sclerotomy
Lens removal in primary lens luxation

A variety of combinations of medical and surgical therapy may be used. The choice depends on the cause and stage of glaucoma and the experience of the clinician. Unfortunately, many of the advocated techniques are unsupported by follow-up studies and in this author's experience cannot be recommended. Cyclocryotherapy when correctly performed with liquid nitrogen as the cryogen is reliable both for blind eyes and in early cases for retaining vision.

The reason for lack of efficacy of long-term medical

therapy in dog eyes compared with the human eye is twofold:

1. The majority of canine glaucoma is of the narrow-angle type, often associated with goniodysgenesis, whereas most human glaucoma is of the slow-onset, open-angle type, similar to that seen experimentally in the beagle.

2. The cholinergic supply to the filtration mechanism of the dog is sparse, although supply to the ciliary body may account for some altered tension of inserting fibers from the ciliary to the filtration mechanism. Thus, some effect of cholinergic drugs may be expected, and this is consistent with clinical observations at least in early glaucoma and short-term therapy.

Owners must be clearly advised that medical therapy, with which many are familiar from their own experience as humans, is rarely curative or even efficacious in animals. This difference can be a significant impediment to owners' understanding of the therapy of their pet's glaucoma and must be explained.

Surgical Techniques

Surgical therapy is required for long-term control of glaucoma.

The following types of glaucoma may be effectively managed by surgical means:

NARROW-ANGLE GLAUCOMA WITH GONIODYSGENESIS[3]

After initial lowering of intraocular pressure, cyclocryotherapy is used to decrease aqueous formation. The combined technique of trephination-iridectomy (Bedford, 1977) is no longer the treatment of choice owing to a lower long-term success rate than cyclocryotherapy, of about 60%.

Cyclocryotherapy

Controlled application of intense cold to the sclera overlying the ciliary body causes necrosis and reduced aqueous production (Fig. 13–33). When carefully ap-

---

3. Attempts to use different types of intraocular implants as a conduit for aqueous to the subconjunctival space in glaucomatous canine eyes have been unsuccessful by numerous investigators over many years. The implant is rapidly obstructed with fibrous tissue. Until such implants are *proved* effective and economical, they are experimental and are contraindicated in clinical patients.

---

plied, the technique can also be used in eyes with acute glaucoma, with some chance of saving vision. Although phthisis bulbi after cyclocryotherapy is possible, it is very unusual in the hands of an experienced surgeon.

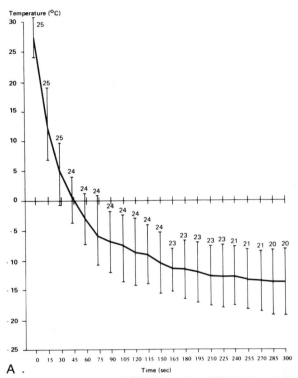

A.

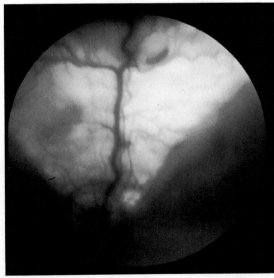

B

FIGURE 13–33. *A, Typical cooling curve of average ciliary body temperature (°C ± 1 SD) for 25 eyes cannulated with a 24-gauge thermocouple and frozen using a 2.5-mm diameter cryoprobe tip with nitrous oxide as the cryogen. Numbers above each point indicate total number of eyes measured. (From Martin CL, Vestre WA: Glaucoma. In Slatter DL [ed]: Textbook of Small Animal Surgery. WB Saunders Co, Philadelphia, 1985.) B, Retinal detachment associated with extensive cyclocryotherapy. (Courtesy of Dr. W. L. Vestre.)*

Adverse Effects

The incidence of adverse reactions to cyclocryotherapy can be minimized and resolution accelerated by careful application of the cryogen, preoperative use of systemic flunixin meglumine, and postoperative use of subconjunctival corticosteroid. Adverse effects include retinal detachments (usually resolves in the *untreated normal eye* within 10–20 days), chemosis and conjunctival inflammation (7–10 days), transient increase in intraocular pressure (1–3 days), and uveitis (7–10 days). The base of the iris may be frozen at the same time as cyclocryotherapy is performed, causing iris atrophy, posterior synechiae, pupillary distortion, and liberation of pigment into the anterior and posterior chambers. This pigment may be later deposited on the anterior lens capsule.

In certain breeds—cocker spaniel, Siberian husky, Norwegian elkhound, chow chow—more aggressive therapy with greater ciliary body destruction is required in order to ensure long-term pressure control.

Technique

1. The patient is anesthetized and treated with flunixin meglumine (0.5 mg/kg) intravenously to limit postoperative discomfort and secondary retinal detachment.

2. A cryoprobe cooled by liquid nitrogen (Fig. 13–34) is applied 5 mm behind the limbus, at three or four sites, and cryogen is applied until the ice ball advances to the limbus. The peripheral cornea is not frozen.

3. A subconjunctival injection of 10 mg (0.25 ml) of triamcinolone acetonide is given on the side of the globe opposite to the area of cryotherapy.

4. The eye is treated postoperatively with an antibiotic-steroid ointment for 7 days, and the owner is advised that postoperative chemosis will resolve in 4–6 days.

5. Intraocular pressure is monitored after 1 and 6 months.

6. Prophylactic treatment of the contralateral eye with miotics is commenced. Prophylaxis with echothiophate iodide in the contralateral unaffected eye significantly extends the interval to development of glaucoma in that eye in predisposed breeds.

Liquid nitrogen cryotherapy yields superior and more reliable results than those of nitrous oxide cryotherapy, which can be unreliable.

For chronic glaucoma when buphthalmos is already present, see "Absolute Glaucoma," later in this chapter.

PRIMARY LENS LUXATION

Primary lens luxation is bilateral and usually hereditary.

In glaucoma with lens luxation (see Fig. 13–17), the treatment of choice depends on duration of the condition (and consequent damage to the angle) and position of the lens. Regardless of the lens location, if glaucoma has been present for some time and peripheral anterior synechiae have formed, cyclocryotherapy is indicated for normal-sized eyes, and intraocular prosthesis for enlarged globes.

If lens luxation is acute and the lens has luxated posteriorly, the eye is treated medically to reduce pressure and with miotics to ensure that the lens does not enter the anterior chamber. Many animals tolerate a lens in the vitreous for long periods without recurrences of glaucoma, provided medications are continued. If the lens is opaque (cataractous) and interferes with vision in the vitreous, it may be removed by

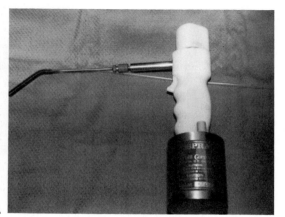
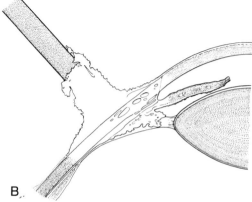

FIGURE 13–34. *A, Liquid nitrogen cryotherapy unit. B, Cryoprobe cooled by liquid nitrogen, positioned 5 mm posterior to the limbus and adjacent to the ciliary body. (B from Roberts SM, et al: Cyclocryotherapy. Part I: Evaluation of a liquid nitrogen system. J Am Anim Hosp Assoc 20:823, 1984.)*

intracapsular extraction, although the prognosis is guarded even in skilled hands.

If the lens has luxated into the pupil or anterior chamber, two surgical methods of treatment are available, provided anterior synechiae and permanent drainage angle damage are not yet present.

1. The lens may be removed by intracapsular extraction. This is the preferable method (see Chap 14).

2. The lens may be "couched" or reclined. In "couching," the pupil is dilated temporarily, the lens is placed into the vitreous, and medical treatment is continued thereafter. "Couching," or reclination, is an ancient technique adapted from human ophthalmology for use in older animal patients when anesthesia or costs are a factor. Superior visual results can be obtained by lens extraction.

GLAUCOMA SECONDARY TO UVEITIS

Glaucoma is a frequent complication of uveitis, resulting from blockage of the drainage angle by inflammatory cells, swollen iris tissues, or lenticular debris (if the lens capsule has been ruptured by a penetrating foreign body). Initially the intraocular pressure is reduced with osmotic agents and carbonic anhydrase inhibitors (*note:* avoid miotics or mydriatics) and the uveitis treated intensively with subconjunctival steroids (e.g., 3–6 mg depot betamethasone) and systemic steroids.

Once the inflammation has been reduced, gonioscopy is performed, and if the angle is undamaged, medical therapy is slowly reduced. If peripheral anterior and posterior synechiae are present and pressure does not fall, cyclocryotherapy is indicated once the uveitis is controlled. With lens capsule rupture and severe phacoanaphylactic uveitis, once the pressure is elevated the prognosis is poor. If the eye is treated before glaucoma occurs and uveitis is controlled, the prognosis is better.

Secondary glaucoma following infectious canine hepatitis vaccination reactions (with *both* canine adenovirus 1 and 2) is not uncommon in the Afghan hound, greyhound, and other sight hounds. (Statements that this applies to all hounds are unproved, but care should be exercised.)

Once uveitis is controlled, and if the pressure does not fall in response to medical therapy, glaucoma secondary to uveitis can be treated with either cyclocryotherapy or intraocular prosthesis insertion.

GLAUCOMA SECONDARY TO INTRAOCULAR NEOPLASIA

Melanoma of the iris or ciliary body is a relatively frequent cause of secondary glaucoma in dogs. In most cases, enucleation, with or without an orbital prosthesis at the owner's discretion, is the treatment of choice, but in early cases iridocyclectomy (removal of a portion of the iris and ciliary body) is successful in treating circumscribed tumors. By the time glaucoma is present, the tumor is usually too advanced for this type of therapy.

ABSOLUTE GLAUCOMA

Absolute glaucoma is the end stage of chronic, increased intraocular pressure with buphthalmos, severe degenerative changes in most ocular tissue, blindness, and pain (Fig. 13–35). Unfortunately, this stage is common in dogs and is due to

1. Failure of the owner to observe the condition early

2. Incorrect or inadequate early diagnosis or treatment

3. Poor response of the patient to medical or surgical treatment

If buphthalmos is left untreated, eventual corneal degeneration and ulceration with rupture may be expected, with enucleation inevitable. This results from central corneal anesthesia, lagophthalmos and drying, degenerative keratitis, and trauma from exposure. The time interval to eventual rupture is unpredictable, and a minority of patients achieve a stable, painless, although unsightly state.

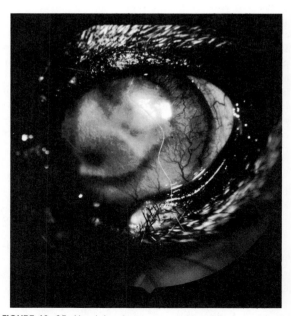

FIGURE 13–35. *Absolute glaucoma and buphthalmos in a 5-month-old German shepherd, after penetration of the lens capsule. The condition was not treated until glaucoma occurred, and the eye was lost.*

Absolute glaucoma may be very painful and debilitating. The patient's comfort is the paramount consideration in the treatment of this stage of the disease.

There are three possible methods of treatment:

Cyclocryotherapy

This technique results in improvement only if there is sufficient ciliary body left to be damaged by the technique and reduce aqueous production. If buphthalmos is present, the eye will *not* shrink after cyclocryotherapy, and an intraocular prosthesis is cosmetically more acceptable.

Intraocular Prosthesis

The globe is eviscerated by removing the internal contents through a limbal incision, leaving a scleral and corneal shell. After hemorrhage is controlled, a silicone prosthesis (see Fig. 18–37)[4] is inserted. As most owners greatly prefer to retain the eye, this method is very useful. Postoperative complications are minimal, and long-term therapy is usually not required.

The enlarged globe shrinks to the size of the prosthesis over 3–4 weeks postoperatively. During this time the cornea may vascularize and appear red. This eventually resolves, and the cornea assumes its final gray or black color. The degree of pigmentation is impossible to predict, and owners are made aware of this prior to surgery. Overt endophthalmitis due to microorganisms and neoplasia are *contraindications* to prosthesis insertion. Prostheses may also be used after severe injury, when phthisis bulbi is beginning, to preserve a cosmetically acceptable eye.

A high percentage of success may be expected with intraocular prosthesis insertion by an experienced surgeon. The failure rate of 10% (Koch, 1981) is unacceptable, and more recent studies have shown a lower rate of complications.

Prostheses should not be inserted into eyes when

1. Melanoma (extracted tissue should be examined histologically) is present.
2. Panophthalmitis is present.
3. After penetrating injury, except after prolonged antibiotic therapy.
4. Ulcerative keratitis or degenerative epithelial conditions are present.
5. Patients have foci of bacterial infections, e.g., severe untreated dental disorders.

Ocular contents removed for prosthesis insertion should be examined histologically for the presence of neoplasia.

Technique

1. The horizontal corneal diameter of the *contralateral normal eye* is measured and recorded prior to induction of anesthesia.
2. With the patient under general anesthesia and routine preparation, the globe is fixed at the limbus with curved hemostats and incised parallel to the limbus beneath a fornix-based conjunctival flap (Fig. 13–36A).
3. The uvea and retina are removed by dissection between the choroid and the inner scleral surface (Fig. 13–36B).
4. The globe is temporarily packed with a surgical sponge in order to control hemorrhage.
5. A prosthesis is chosen based on the size of the contralateral normal eye—corneal diameter plus 1 mm; e.g., if the diameter is 16 mm, use a 17-mm prosthesis. The prosthesis is inserted with a prosthesis inserter (Fig. 13–36C). Sodium penicillin solution (250,000 units) is placed around the prosthesis after insertion.
6. The sclera is sutured with interrupted absorbable sutures with the knot tied on top of the conjunctival flap. The flap seals the incision and prevents leakage of blood postoperatively (Fig. 13–36D).
7. The eye is medicated with topical antibiotics for 14 days postoperatively. If inflammation has been significant prior to prosthesis insertion, systemic antibiotics may also be indicated.

Note that this prosthesis differs from the EXTRAOCULAR porcelain type with painted pupil used to cover a shrunken eye with phthisis bulbi (see Chap 18).

Enucleation

Once an eye has been thoroughly evaluated and a diagnosis of absolute glaucoma with pain has been made, the owner may decide to have the eye removed. This is *rarely* necessary unless neoplasia or intractable infection is suspected because intraocular prosthesis insertion is such a successful procedure with a relatively trouble-free postoperative course. The same kind of pain relief and change in personality is associated with prosthesis insertion as was a feature of enucleation for chronic glaucoma before the technique for prosthesis insertion was perfected.

If enucleation is elected by the owner, the alternative of insertion of an INTRAORBITAL prosthesis is available for its vastly superior postoperative appearance (see Chap 18).

---

4. The use of nonsterile, industrial silicone preparations is contraindicated.

---

1. **For the protection of the patient and the veterinarian, *all* enucleated eyes must**

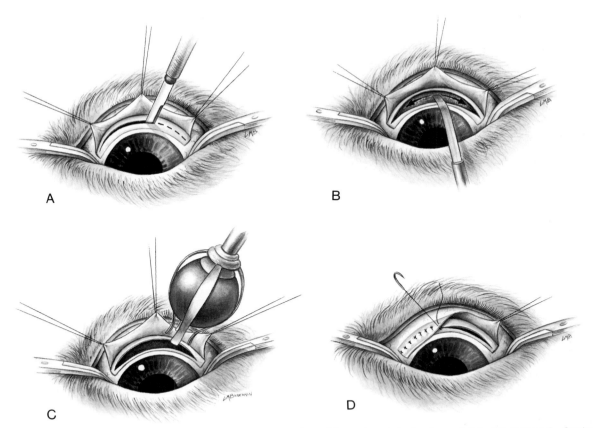

FIGURE 13–36. A, A fornix-based conjunctival flap is prepared, and the sclera is incised parallel to the limbus. B, Ocular contents are removed by dissection between the choroid and the inner scleral layers. C, A suitable prosthesis is inserted with a prosthesis inserter. Penicillin solution is placed around the prosthesis. D, The sclera is closed with interrupted, absorbable McLean's sutures that also appose the conjunctival flap over the scleral incision.

be examined by an experienced ophthalmic pathology laboratory.

2. For most patients with glaucoma, enucleation is not a substitute for specific diagnosis and treatment; it is an admission that diagnosis, therapy, or client counseling has failed, and it is usually chosen for the economic convenience of the owner.

FELINE GLAUCOMA

The general principles of etiology apply also to feline glaucoma, which is much less common than it is in dogs. Primary feline glaucoma may be much more insidious in onset, often apparently does not cause pain, and may result in extreme buphthalmos. By the time the patient is presented, the etiology may be difficult to determine. It is important to note that insidious stretching of the globe and rupture of lens zonules may give a false appearance of primary lens luxation. Cyclo-

cryotherapy must be quite aggressive if used, and liquid nitrogen is recommended as the cryogen to limit treatment failures. Intraocular prostheses are equally applicable as in dogs.

REFERENCES

Barrie KP, et al (1980): Effect of iridocryothermy in the normal dog. Am J Vet Res 41:51.

Bedford PGC (1973): A practical method of gonioscopy and goniophotography in the dog and cat. J Sm Anim Pract 14:601.

Bedford PGC (1975): The etiology of primary glaucoma in the dog. J Sm Anim Pract 16:217.

Bedford PGC (1977): Gonioscopy in the dog. J Sm Anim Pract 18:615.

Bedford PGC (1977): The surgical treatment of canine glaucoma. J Sm Anim Pract 18:713.

Bedford PGC (1978): A gonioscopic study of the iridocorneal angle in the English and American breeds of cocker spaniel and the basset hound. J Sm Anim Pract 18:631.

Bertoy RW, et al (1988): Intraocular melanoma with multiple metastases in a cat. J Am Vet Med Assoc 192:87.

Brightman AH (1980): Pharmacologic management of glaucoma in the dog. J Am Vet Med Assoc 177:326.

Brightman AH, et al (1982): Cryosurgery for the treatment of canine glaucoma. J Am Anim Hosp Assoc 18:319.

Cottrell B, Barnett KC (1988): Primary glaucoma in the Welsh springer spaniel. J Sm Anim Pract 29:185.

Duke-Elder S, Jay B (1969): System of Ophthalmology, vol 9, Diseases of the lens and vitreous: Glaucoma and hypotony. H Kimpton, London.

Fischer CA (1972): Lens-induced uveitis in dogs. J Am Anim Hosp Assoc 8:39.

Formston C (1945): Observations on subluxation and luxation of the crystalline lens in the dog. J Comp Pathol 55:168.

Gelatt KN (1972): Familial glaucoma in the beagle dog. J Am Anim Hosp Assoc 8:23.

Gelatt KN, Gum GG (1981): Inheritance of primary glaucoma in the beagle. Am J Vet Res 42:1691.

Gelatt KN, Ladds PW (1971): Gonioscopy in dogs and cats with glaucoma and ocular tumors. J Sm Anim Pract 12:105.

Gelatt KN, et al (1976): Consecutive water provocative tests in normal and glaucomatous beagles. Am J Vet Res 37:269.

Gelatt KN, et al (1977): Tonography in the normal and glaucomatous beagle. Am J Vet Res 38:51.

Gelatt KN, et al (1979): Ocular hypotensive effects of carbonic anhydrase inhibitors in normotensive and glaucomatous beagles. Am J Vet Res 40:334.

Gelatt KN, et al (1983): Dose response of topical pilocarpine-epinephrine combinations in normotensive and glaucomatous beagles. Am J Vet Res 44:2018.

Gelatt KN, et al (1984): Dose response of topical carbamyl–choline chloride (carbachol) in normotensive and glaucomatous beagles. Am J Vet Res 45:547.

Gelatt KN, et al (1987): Evaluation of the Krupin-Denver valve implant in normotensive and glaucomatous beagles. J Am Vet Med Assoc 191:1404.

Gwin RM, et al (1977): The effect of topical pilocarpine on intraocular pressure on pupil size in normotensive and glaucomatous beagles. Invest Ophthalmol Vis Sci 16:1143.

Gwin RM, et al (1978): Effects of topical L-epinephrine and dipivalyl epinephrine on intraocular pressure and pupil size in the normotensive and glaucomatous beagle. Am J Vet Res 39:83.

Gwin RM, et al (1979): Adrenergic and cholinergic innervation of the anterior segment of the normal and glaucomatous dog. Invest Ophthalmol 18:674.

Koch SA (1981): Intraocular prosthesis in the dog and cat: The failures. J Am Vet Med Assoc 179:883.

Kolker AE, Hetherington J (eds) (1983): Becker-Shaffer's Diagnosis and Therapy of the Glaucomas, 5th ed. CV Mosby Co, St Louis.

van der Linde-Sipman JS (1987): Dysplasia of the pectinate ligament and primary glaucoma in the Bouvier des Flandres dog. Vet Pathol 24:201.

Lovekin LG (1971): Water provocative test for glaucoma: Range of normal tonometric responses for the canine eye. Am J Vet Res 32:1179.

Lovekin LG, Bellhorn RW (1968): Clinicopathologic changes in primary glaucoma in the cocker spaniel. Am J Vet Res 29:379.

Magrane WG, et al (1977): Intraocular prosthesis in the dog. J Am Anim Hosp Assoc 13:481.

Martin CL (1969): Gonioscopy and anatomical correlations of the drainage angle of the dog. J Sm Anim Pract 10:171.

Martin CL (1975): Scanning electron microscopic examination of selected canine iridocorneal angle anomalies. J Am Anim Hosp Assoc 11:300.

Martin CL, Vestre WA (1985): Glaucoma. In Slatter DH (ed): Textbook of Small Animal Surgery. WB Saunders Co, Philadelphia.

Martin CL, Wyman M (1968): Glaucoma in the basset hound. Am J Vet Res 29:379.

Martin CL, Wyman M (1978): Primary glaucoma in the dog. Vet Clin North Am 8:257.

McLaughlin SA, et al (1987): Intraocular findings in three dogs and one cat with chronic glaucoma. J Am Vet Med Assoc 191:1443.

Peiffer RL, Gelatt KN (1980): Aqueous humor outflow in beagles with inherited glaucoma: Gross and light microscopic observations of the iridocorneal angle. Am J Vet Res 41:861.

Peiffer RL, et al (1980): Aqueous humor outflow in beagles with inherited glaucoma: Constant pressure perfusion. Am J Vet Res 41:1808.

Radius RL, Bade B (1981): Pressure-induced optic nerve axonal transport interruption in cat eyes. Arch Ophthalmol 99:2163.

Roberts SM, et al (1984): Cyclocryotherapy, part I. Evaluation of a liquid nitrogen system. J Am Hosp Assoc 20:823.

Roberts SM, et al (1984): Cyclocryotherapy, part II. Clinical comparison of liquid nitrogen and nitrous oxide cryotherapy on glaucomatous eyes. J Am Anim Hosp Assoc 20:828.

Slater MR, Erb HN (1986): Effects of risk factors and prophylactic treatment on primary glaucoma in the dog. J Am Vet Med Assoc 188:1028.

Spencer WH (ed) (1985): Ophthalmic Pathology, vol 3. WB Saunders Co, Philadelphia.

Vainisi SJ (1973): The diagnosis and therapy of glaucoma. Vet Clin North Am 3:453.

Vestre WA, Brightman AH (1983): The effects of cyclocryotherapy on the clinically normal canine eye. Am J Vet Res 44:187.

Vestre WA, Brightman AH (1983): Ciliary body temperatures during cyclocryotherapy in the clinically normal dog. Am J Vet Res 44:135.

14

Lens

ANATOMY AND PHYSIOLOGY	CONGENITAL ANOMALIES	LENS LUXATION
PATHOLOGICAL REACTIONS	CATARACT	

ANATOMY AND PHYSIOLOGY

Development of the lens is described in Chapter 2. The lens is a transparent, avascular, biconvex body, with the anterior surface being flatter or less curved than the posterior surface. The centers of the surfaces are called the ANTERIOR and POSTERIOR POLES. The rounded circumference is the EQUATOR, which has numerous irregularities where zonular fibers attach (Fig. 14–1).

The lens is supported at the equator by the LENS ZONULES or suspensory ligaments—collagenous fibers that attach to the ciliary body (see Figs. 12–9 and 12–10). Alterations of tension in these fibers change the curvature of the lens' surfaces and thus its optical power—the phenomenon of ACCOMMODATION. During accommodation, contraction of the ciliary muscle relaxes the zonules, the natural elasticity of the lens capsule causes the lens to become more spherical, the optical power increases, and the optical system is accommodated to view *near* objects. Accommodative

mechanisms in domestic animals are poorly developed, as is the ciliary muscle.

The cornea is the most important refracting surface in the eye, accounting for the majority of the optical power. The lens accounts for the remainder and is a fine adjustment for objects at different distances.

The lens consists of the CAPSULE (Fig. 14–2), ANTERIOR EPITHELIUM, LENS CELLS, and AMORPHOUS CEMENT SUBSTANCE. It is divided into two general regions: the CORTEX (outer areas near the capsule) and the NUCLEUS (central areas). As the lens *grows throughout life,* layers of fibers are produced in the equatorial area and are laid down on top of each other, forcing older fibers toward the lens center. These successive layers are visible clinically by biomicroscopy. They are termed the ADULT, FETAL, and EMBRYONAL NUCLEI, respectively (Fig. 14–3).

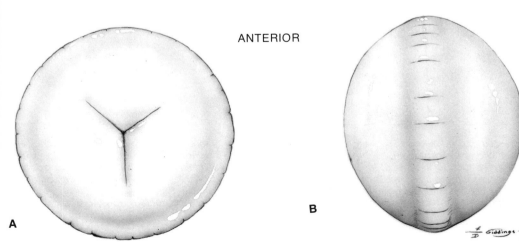

ANTERIOR

POSTERIOR

A

B

FIGURE 14–1. Canine lens anatomy A, Anterior view showing the upright *anterior* Y suture and equatorial margin. B, *Lateral view of the poles and equator. Note the greater curvature of the posterior surface.*

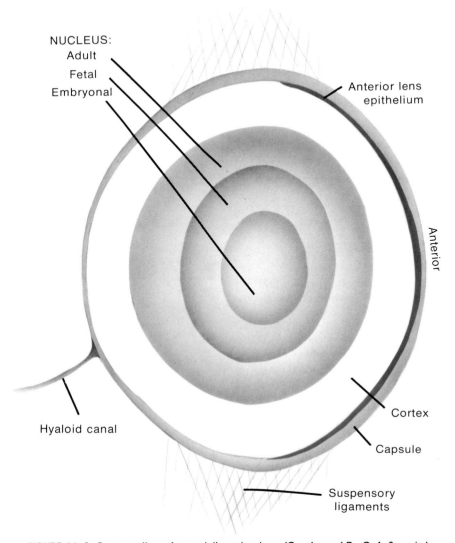

NUCLEUS:
Adult
Fetal
Embryonal

Anterior lens
epithelium

Anterior

Hyaloid canal

Cortex

Capsule

Suspensory
ligaments

FIGURE 14–2. Cross-section of an adult canine lens. (Courtesy of Dr. G. A. Severin.)

FIGURE 14–3. Embryonal and adult lenses, showing sutures and arrangement of lens cells. A, The embryonal nucleus. The anterior Y suture is at a and the posterior at b. The lens cells are wide, shaded bands. Cells attaching to tips of Y sutures at one pole of the lens attach to the fork of the Y at the opposite pole. B, Adult lens cortex. The anterior and posterior organization of the sutures is more complex. Lens cells arising from the tip of a branch of the suture insert farther anteriorly or posteriorly into a fork at the posterior pole. This arrangement conserves the shape of the lens. This drawing shows the suture lying in a single plane for pictorial reasons, but it extends through the cortex and nucleus down to the Y sutures in the embryonal nucleus.

The exact shape of the adult sutures varies in domestic species, but in young animals especially, the Y shape of the embryonal nucleus predominates and must be distinguished clinically from pathological lens opacities (cataract).

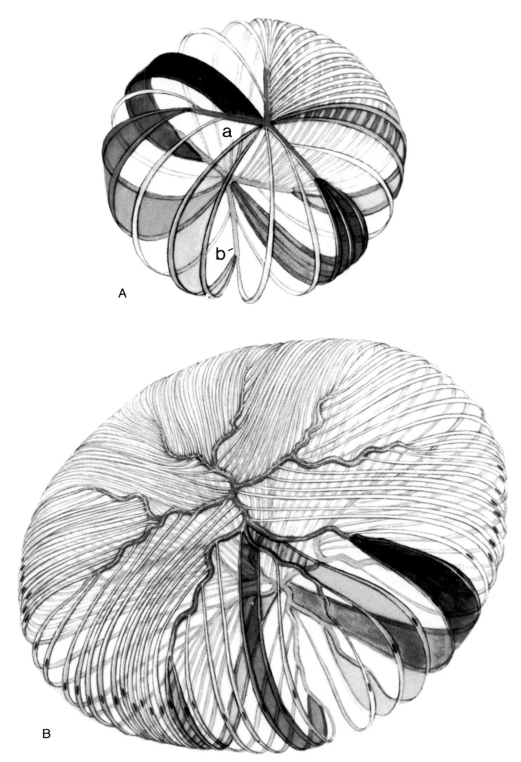

A

B

FIGURE 14–3 See legend on opposite page

Illustration continued on following page

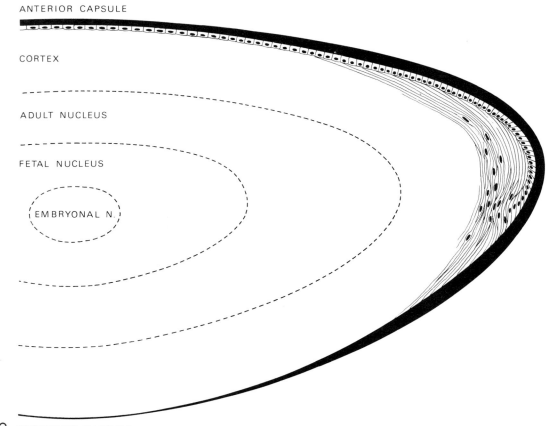

ANTERIOR CAPSULE

CORTEX

ADULT NUCLEUS

FETAL NUCLEUS

EMBRYONAL N.

C POSTERIOR CAPSULE

FIGURE 14–3 Continued C, *The adult lens, showing the nuclear zones, epithelium, and capsule. The thickness of the lens capsule in various zones is shown. (From Hogan MJ, et al: Histology of the Human Eye. WB Saunders Co, Philadelphia, 1971.)*

Lens Components

CAPSULE

The capsule is a transparent, *elastic* envelope surrounding the lens. It is the lamina propria, or basement membrane, of the inverted epithelium that forms the lens fibers, and it is composed of collagen fibers and complex carbohydrates. The capsule regulates lens shape by its elasticity and provides insertion for zonular fibers. The capsule is impermeable to large molecules (e.g., albumin, globulin) but allows water and electrolytes to pass. Because of its elasticity, penetration of the lens capsule results in retraction of the edges (see Fig. 13–24).

LENS EPITHELIUM

Cuboidal epithelial cells lie beneath the anterior capsule and columnar cells lie beneath the equator. New lens fibers are formed by the epithelium near the equator. Because of mitotic activity in this area, these cells are susceptible to toxic and pathological influences, which may become apparent as equatorial opacities. The lens epithelium is important in transport of cations through the lens capsule.

LENS CELLS AND CEMENT SUBSTANCE

Lens cells make up the substance of the cortex and are arranged in interdigitating layers held together by cement (Fig. 14–4). The older cells (NUCLEUS) are denser and less transparent than the younger cells (CORTEX) laid down around them. The lens is supported by zonules and vitreous and sits in a depression in the vitreous called the HYALOID FOSSA. Collagen fibers from the vitreous insert into the posterior lens capsule, firmly attaching the two. In humans this attachment becomes weaker with age and can be broken mechanically or with alpha chymotrypsin (a process known as zonulysis, as zonules are digested), so that the lens and capsule are removed without withdrawing vitreous. In domestic animals the attachment is much stronger, and attempts to remove the posterior lens capsule also cause loss of vitreous.

Metabolism and Composition

The lens requires oxygen and metabolites for maintenance and continued production of lens cells and for maintenance of capsule elasticity and lens transparency. Most of the oxygen required comes from the aqueous,

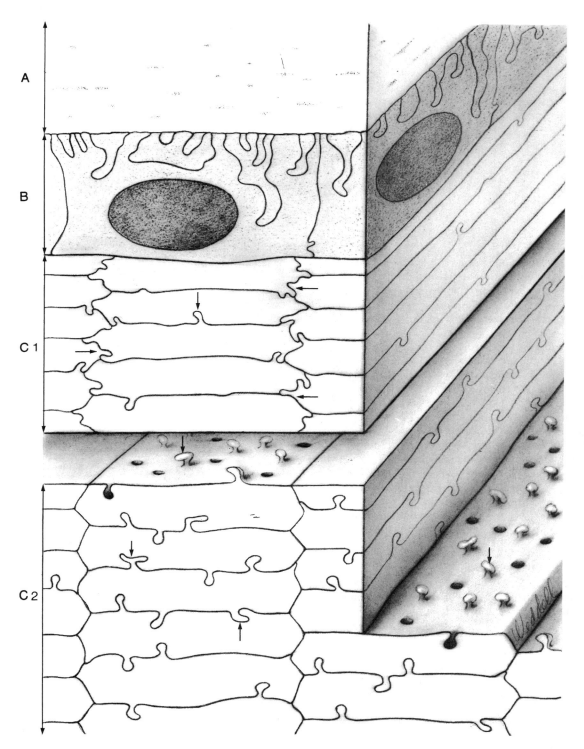

FIGURE 14–4. The lens, showing interrelation of the capsule and underlying lens cells. The capsule (A) shows inclusion of fine filamentous material. The anterior lens epithelium (B) shows interdigitation of its basal surface with adjacent cells. The superficial cells of the cortex show the hexagonal shape and interdigitations at their hexagonal ends as well as along their edges (C₁) (arrows). The deeper cortical cells (C₂) also show a tongue-and-groove type of interdigitation along their long sides (arrows), but the interlocking is absent at the short ends. (From Hogan MJ, et al: Histology of the Human Eye. WB Saunders Co, Philadelphia, 1971.)

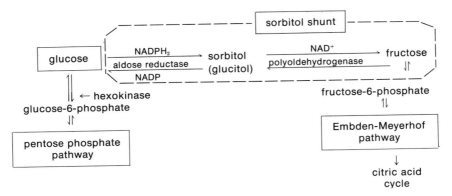

FIGURE 14–5. Metabolism of glucose.

although the amount required is small and is consumed by cortical cells and anterior epithelium. Metabolism of glucose provides most of the energy required by the lens. Glucose enters by diffusion from the aqueous and by assisted transport. Most of the glucose is broken down anaerobically to lactic acid via the Embden-Meyerhof pathway, although some aerobic glycolysis occurs via the citric acid cycle. The hexose-monophosphate shunt also oxidizes hexoses directly. Conversion of glucose to fructose via the sorbitol pathway is significant (Fig. 14–5).

The lens is high in protein (35%) and water (65%) and low in minerals. The proportion of proteins present varies with species, age, and size of the lens. A typical bovine lens has proteins in the proportions shown in Table 14–1.

The insoluble albuminoids are formed from alpha crystallins and increase during cataract formation. Mucoproteins come from the lens capsule and nucleoproteins from the epithelium and equatorial lens cells.

Because the lens is avascular, lens metabolism is precarious and depends on constant composition of the aqueous. Disturbances in composition affect lens metabolism.

TABLE 14–1. Protein Composition of the Bovine Lens

	Type of Protein		Percentage
Primary lens proteins	Insoluble albuminoid		12.50
	Alpha crystallin	} Soluble proteins	31.70
	Beta crystallin		53.40
	Gamma crystallin		1.50
	Mucoprotein		0.80
	Nucleoprotein		0.07

From Krause AC: Chemistry of the lens: Nature of lenticular proteins. Am J Ophthalmol 17:502–514, 1934. Published with permission from The American Journal of Ophthalmology. Copyright by The Ophthalmic Publishing Company.

Aging

With age, more lens cells are produced at the equator, forcing older cells toward the nucleus. These gradually becomes denser and harder as the cells become more tightly packed. The lens slowly grows in size throughout life. In dogs, after about 6 years of age this increased nuclear density causes a grayish-blue haze (**NUCLEAR SCLEROSIS**) (Fig. 14–6). This haze is probably associated with increased insoluble proteins and decreased soluble crystallins (gamma crystallin).

PATHOLOGICAL REACTIONS

Because the lens is avascular, confined within a capsule, and suspended in aqueous, the range of pathological reactions exhibited by it is small. The complicated metabolism of the lens is aimed at preservation of transparency, and many insults may upset it, causing degeneration and opacification. Most lens reactions fall within the following groups:

1. Release of lens material within the eye
2. Changes in position of the lens
3. Loss of transparency

For a detailed discussion of properties of different parts of the lens, reference to standard texts on ophthalmic pathology is recommended.

Release of Lens Material

After injury, the subcapsular lens epithelium is the only part of the lens to show limited reparative activity. Once the capsule is perforated, the hole usually remains and aqueous enters. Lens fibers imbibe fluid, swell, and become opaque within a few hours. Small holes in the anterior polar region may heal with residual opacity in dogs. Usually the swollen lens material undergoes proteolytic digestion, exposing further lens substance to attack and finally rendering the lens opaque and swollen (intumescent).

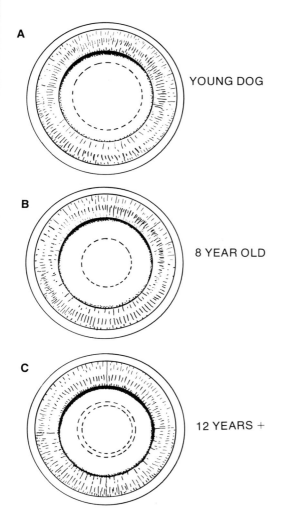

A   YOUNG DOG

B   8 YEAR OLD

C   12 YEARS +

FIGURE 14–6. Aging of the canine lens. A, Lens of a young dog, showing a relatively large nucleus and indistinct corticonuclear junction. B, Lens of an 8-year-old dog, showing distinct corticonuclear junction and nuclear sclerosis. C, After about 12 years of age, a nuclear sclerotic ring develops in the cortex of the lens. (These changes are best observed in light reflected from the tapetum.) (Courtesy of Dr. G. A. Severin.)

Nuclear and cortical material from the lens may reach the aqueous either by liquefying and passing through the capsule or by rupture of the capsule.

This may cause

1. A humoral and cell-mediated immune reaction to this released protein by the uvea, with SEVERE UVEITIS and its sequelae. (Lens proteins are separated from the immune system before birth and are regarded as foreign. These antigens—especially the alpha crystallins—are organ-specific rather than species-specific and cross species lines.) Reaction to released material is less severe in younger animals.

2. Ingestion of lens material by macrophages, which become enlarged and obstruct the drainage angle (phacolytic glaucoma).

Changes in Position

Alterations in lens position are called LUXATION (*complete* dislocation from the hyaloid fossa) and SUBLUXATION (*partial* removal from the hyaloid fossa). Changes in lens position frequently interfere with passage of aqueous, resulting in glaucoma (see Chap 13).

Loss of Transparency

Cataract is a focal or diffuse lens opacity.

Regardless of the etiology, morphological cellular changes in the lens are similar in different kinds of cataracts. As described by Hogan and Zimmerman:[1]

Once lens changes begin they may assume many clinical forms such as spokes, fissures, lamellar separation, dot and wedge-shaped opacities, rosettes, etc. Histologically, the process is not so varied. . . . The initial change in the cortical lens cells during cataract formation is acidification. This is probably due to accumulation of products of a slowed or altered metabolism. The fibers lose fluid, shrink, and fluid collects in resulting clefts or vacuoles. . . .

Coagulation of proteins in the cells then occurs, and true [permanent] lens opacities form. The clinical picture is determined by the nature and position of these opacities. They seldom appear simultaneously throughout the whole lens cortex. Sometimes they remain stationary for a long time, and interfere little with vision. At other times, when they are associated with considerable imbibition of fluid into the cortex, complete opacification may be rapid. Degeneration of all the cortical cells then may occur, with rapid liquefaction of the fibers. [The nucleus is the last to liquefy and may settle to the bottom of the lens capsule in MORGAGNIAN CATARACT.] Microscopically the fibers become edematous and the cell walls disintegrate. Vacuoles form which coalesce to form larger spaces; eventually the fibers break down into morgagnian globules.

As lens fragments disintegrate, the intercellular fluid becomes albuminous and takes a pale pink stain. If the lens epithelium has proliferated beneath the posterior capsule, the contents often are retained . . . [and malformed fibers appear at the posterior pole. Dystrophic calcification of the degenerate lens may occur, but complete liquefaction is frequently observed.]

Disintegration of the cortex proceeds much more rapidly than does autolysis of the sclerotic nucleus. In these hypermature cataracts, the nuclear remains may be freely movable in the milky cortical fluid in which they are suspended. Such cataracts typically appear shrunken because varying amounts of the liquid cortex are absorbed. Rarely, all of the lens tissue may escape, even though the capsule remains intact.

As the hypermature lens cortex escapes through the capsule into the posterior chamber it provokes a macrophagic response. The flow of aqueous carries both the cells

---

1. Hogan MC, Zimmerman LE: Ophthalmic Pathology. WB Saunders Co, Philadelphia, 1962.

SEQUENCE OF CATARACT DEVELOPMENT

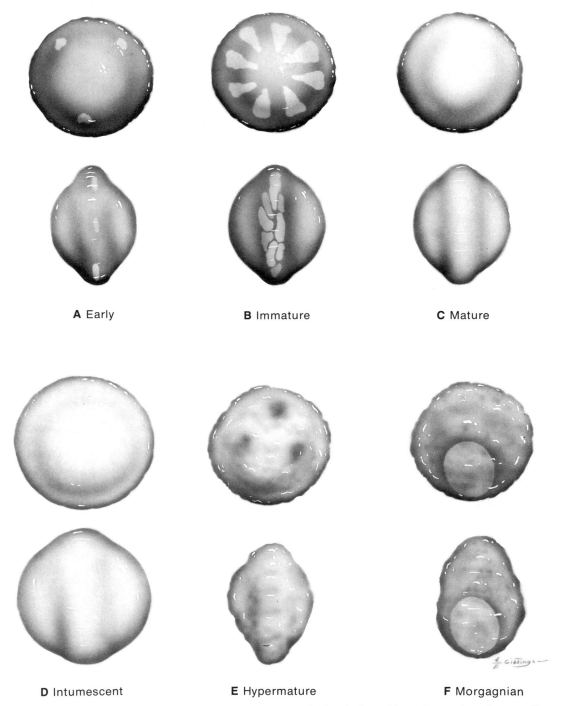

A Early   **B** Immature   **C** Mature

D Intumescent   **E** Hypermature   **F** Morgagnian

FIGURE 14–7. Sequence of cataract development. A, Early opacity (beginning of immature cataract)—opacities are variable in position. B, Immature cataract—opacities progress. C, Mature cataract—may progress to D, E, or F. D, Intumescent (swollen) cataract. E, Hypermature cataract (cortex liquefies and may leak, causing uveitis). F, Morgagnian cataract—cortex liquefies, and nucleus sinks.

and the free cortical fluid into the anterior chamber. [Here the cells may obstruct the drainage angle, causing PHA-COLYTIC GLAUCOMA.]

The sequential steps in the development of cataract are illustrated in Figure 14–7.

Biochemistry of Cataract

Lens biochemistry is complex, as are the many different causes of cataract. With the exception of diabetic, galactosemic, and experimental cataracts, the exact biochemical disorders are imperfectly understood in most spontaneous cataracts in domestic animals. Noxious influences affecting any of the following lens functions may result in opacity:

1. Lens nutrition
2. Energy metabolism
3. Protein metabolism
4. Osmotic balance

This accounts for the large number of factors that may cause cataract (e.g., genetic, nutritional, toxic, radiation, microbiological or infectious, parasitic, and senile). A brief discussion of two spontaneous forms of cataract—diabetic and galactosemic—that occur in animals demonstrates the principles and complexity of the biochemistry of cataract.

DIABETIC CATARACT (Fig. 14–8)

The pathways of energy metabolism in the lens have been summarized previously (see Fig. 14–5). The sorbitol pathway becomes active in hyperglycemia. Hexokinase is saturated in hyperglycemia, and more glucose enters the sorbitol pathway. Sorbitol accumulates in the lens, irreversibly changing the configuration of alpha crystallin, halting the monophosphate shunt and amino acid and protein synthesis, and causing the initial lesion in diabetic cataract.

GALACTOSEMIC CATARACT[2]

Galactosemic cataracts occur spontaneously in young macropods (kangaroos, wallabies, wallaroos, and related species, e.g., cuscus) that are fed cow's milk, which is high in galactose and lactose (unlike doe's milk) (Fig. 14–9). Adult macropods are deficient in galactokinase and galactose-1-phosphate uridyl transferase.

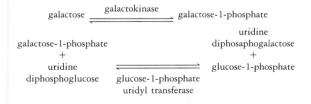

---

2. Cataracts in captive wallabies have also been caused by toxoplasmosis. This disease should be included in the differential diagnosis.

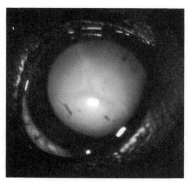

FIGURE 14–8. Mature diabetic cataract. Note the clefts in the region of the sutures.

In the absence of these enzymes, galactose and galactose-1-phospate accumulate and are converted to dulcitol by aldose reductase. Like the other sugar alcohols, dulcitol stays within the cell, accumulates, and draws fluid into the cells, with effects similar to those of sorbitol.

CONGENITAL ANOMALIES

Congenital anomalies of the lens are rarely seen in clinical practice (congenital cataract is discussed later). They include the following:

APHAKIA—absence of lens (rare).

MICROPHAKIA—small lens, usually associated with other ocular malformations.

SPHEROPHAKIA—spherically shaped lens.

LENTICONUS—protrusion of the lens capsule anteriorly or posteriorly at the pole. Posterior lenticonus may occur with persistent hyaloid artery and persistent hyperplastic primary vitreous. The lens capsule may rupture, releasing lens material into the vitreous.

COLOBOMA—notching of the lens equator in the typical or atypical position, associated with similar defects in the ciliary body and zonules.

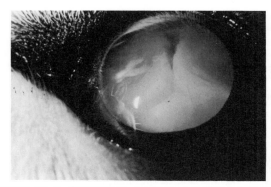

FIGURE 14–9. Cataract in a young kangaroo that had been fed cow's milk.

CATARACT

The term CATARACT comprises a common group of ocular disorders manifested by lens opacities of varying sizes and shapes and varying in etiology and rate of progression.

Classification

Because of the variable nature and appearance of cataracts, numerous methods of classification are commonly used (Table 14–2). For this reason, and because changes between classification systems are often made within a single discussion of cataract, familiarity with the different systems is necessary.

Cataract refers to a group of lens disorders
of varying age of onset, speed and extent of
progression, appearance, and etiology.

A particular cataract may be described according to features cited in Table 14–2. Stage of development, position within the lens, and time of development are the most commonly used categories. The terms used in various classifications are described more fully in the following paragraphs.

STAGE OF DEVELOPMENT[3]

INCIPIENT (see Fig. 14–7A)—Early opacity with sight unaffected. In older animals, nuclear sclerosis may be difficult to distinguish from incipient cataract.

---

3. Modified from Severin GA: Diseases of the lens. *In* Home Study Course in Ophthalmology. American Animal Hospital Association, Mishawaka, IN, 1974.

TABLE 14–2. Summary of Cataract Classification

Feature	Subclassification of Terms
Stage of development	Incipient, immature, mature, hypermature, morgagnian
Position within the lens	Anterior subcapsular, posterior subcapsular, peripheral cortical, posterior cortical, equatorial, nuclear, lamellar (zonular), posterior polar, axial
Time of development	Embryonal, congenital, developmental, juvenile, senile, acquired
Appearance	Brunescent (cataract nigra), cerulean, coronary, corolliform, cuneiform, cupiliform, discoid, floriform, fusiform, membranous, punctate, pyramidal, spear, stellate, sutural, spindle
Etiology or pathogenesis	Secondary, traumatic aftercataract, radiation, diabetic, galactosemic, electric, toxic, complicated, reduplication
Consistency	Fluid, soft, hard

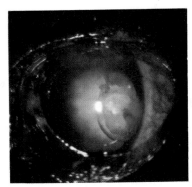

FIGURE 14–10. *A morgagnian cataract in which the lens cortex has liquefied (and in this case has been resorbed) and the nucleus remains. Lens-induced uveitis is also present as indicated by injection of ciliary vessels.*

IMMATURE (see Fig. 14–7B)—Opacity is more marked but still incomplete, and the fundus may be partially obscured ophthalmoscopically. Sight is affected, and the lens may begin to swell. Pupillary block glaucoma may occur because of lens enlargement. Visual difficulty begins if the condition is bilateral.

MATURE (see Figs. 14–7C and 14–8)—The lens is totally opaque, and the fundus can no longer be examined ophthalmoscopically. Some "water clefts" may appear, often along suture lines or in a radial spoke-like fashion. If mature cataracts are bilateral, the animal is blind. This is the ideal stage for surgical cataract removal, prior to the onset of lens-induced uveitis.

INTUMESCENCE (see Fig. 14–7D)—The lens begins to swell. Not all cataracts go through this stage. With swelling the eye is susceptible to secondary angle-closure glaucoma and leakage of lens proteins, causing lens-induced uveitis.

HYPERMATURE (Fig. 14–10; see also Fig. 14–7E)—In hypermaturity some lenses begin to liquefy, and occasionally some vision may return (lens resorption). The nucleus liquefies last and may sink to the bottom of a lens whose cortex has liquefied (MORGAGNIAN CATARACT). In some dogs the liquefied cortex leaks out slowly, causing uveitis. The nucleus may remain with a shrunken capsule around it after the cortex has escaped.

Miosis, hypotony, photophobia, and vascular injection are signs of uveitis in an eye with cataract.

POSITION IN THE LENS

Positions of the different types of cataract are shown in Figure 14–11.

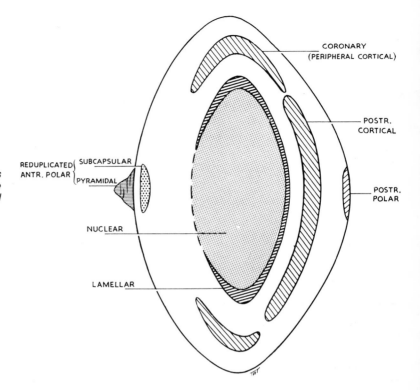

FIGURE 14-11. *Classification of cataracts according to their position within the lens. (From Trevor-Roper PD: The Eye and Its Disorders. Blackwell, Oxford, 1974.)*

TIME OF DEVELOPMENT

EMBRYONAL—due to prenatal influences.

CONGENITAL—present at birth and often nonprogressive.

DEVELOPMENTAL—occurring at any time before the adult state is reached (cf. juvenile).

JUVENILE—a imprecise term, to be avoided in scientific discussion, that has no commonly accepted definition. Severin (1974) restricts the term to cataracts in animals less than 6 years of age.

SENILE—occurring in aged animals and usually preceded by nuclear sclerosis.

ACQUIRED—any noncongenital cataract.

APPEARANCE

Discussion of terms used to describe the multitude of sizes and shapes of cataract is beyond the scope of this book. The terms are used to accurately describe cataracts that may form a discrete syndrome in a particular breed of animal and as such are readily recognizable.

ETIOLOGY AND PATHOGENESIS

AFTERCATARACT—pieces of lens capsule or an opaque posterior capsule remaining after extracapsular cataract extraction.

COMPLICATED—cataracts occurring in the presence of other ocular diseases (e.g., penetrating corneal wound or uveitis).

DIABETIC, GALACTOSEMIC, HOMOCYSTINE—cataracts caused by the metabolic disturbance or disease referred to.

ELECTRIC—cataract caused by large flows of electric current, as in electrocution of animals or people.

REDUPLICATION—a capsular opacity in which a second layer of epithelium covers a defect in the capsule. This type is rarely described in animals but does occur.

RADIATION—cataract caused by radiation, usually used in radiotherapy.

SECONDARY—cataracts due to other ocular diseases (Fig. 14-12).

TOXIC—cataract caused by toxins, e.g., naphthalene, diosophenol in dogs, hygromycin in sows.

TRAUMATIC—cataracts due to direct or indirect trauma (Fig. 14-13).

CONSISTENCY

Whether the lens is soft, hard, or fluid determines the kind of surgical technique employed. Soft or fluid cataracts are more frequent in young animals.

Inheritance of Cataract

Inheritance of cataract has been reported in many different breeds and species (Table 14-3). Caution is necessary in applying findings from one observer in one

TABLE 14–3. Cataract Syndromes

Species	Breed	Inheritance	Age of Onset	Features	Reference
Dog	Afghan hound	Recessive	4½–24 months	Equatorial and cortical vacuoles; progressive	Roberts and Helper, 1972; Barnett, 1976, 1978
	American cocker spaniel	Recessive	Congenital	Anterior and posterior cortical	Yakely et al, 1971, 1978
	American cocker spaniel	Nonhereditary	Congenital	Cortical lamellar	Yakely et al, 1971
	Australian terrier	?	3–6 years	Cortical striae and clefts	Slatter, 1976
	Beagle	Nonhereditary	21–26 weeks	Posterior plaque, anterior capsular, posterior polar, nonprogressive	Heywood, 1971b; Hirth et al, 1974
	Boston terrier	Recessive	8 weeks	Radiating lines and white sutural flecks; mature by about 12 months	Barnett, 1972, 1978
	Cavalier King Charles spaniel	—	Congenital	Lenticonus, cataracts, and microphthalmia	Narfstrom and Dubielzig, 1984
	Chesapeake Bay retriever	Dominant with incomplete penetrance	6 months–6 years	Cortical-posterior axial and equatorial, variable progression	Gelatt et al, 1979
	English cocker spaniel	?	Congenital	Bilateral anterior capsular	Barnett, 1972, 1978
	German shepherd	Nonhereditary	—	Bilateral nuclear and anterior capsular opacities	Høst and Sveinson, 1936
	German shepherd	Dominant	Congenital	—	von Hippel, 1930
	Golden retriever	Dominant with incomplete penetrance	Congenital	Triangular, posterior, subcapsular; slowly progressive	Gelatt, 1972; Rubin, 1974; Barnett, 1972
	Labrador retriever	Dominant with incomplete penetrance	Congenital	Posterior polar, cortical, progressive	Barnett, 1972
	Miniature poodle	?	2–6 years	Cortical striae and clefts (radial)	Roberts, 1973
	Miniature schnauzer	Recessive	Congenital	Equitorial and posterior subcapsular	Gelatt et al, 1983a,b; Rubin et al, 1969
	Old English sheepdog	Recessive (?)	7 months–2 years	Nuclear and cortical	Koch, 1972; Barnett, 1978
	Pointer	?	Congenital	—	von Hippel, 1930
	Springer spaniel	Nonhereditary	Congenital	—	von Hippel, 1930
	Staffordshire bull terrier	Recessive	1 year	White sutural flecks	Barnett, 1972, 1978
	Standard poodle	Recessive	Soon after birth	Equatorial and cortical	Barnett, 1985; Rubin and Flowers, 1972
	West Highland white terrier	Recessive	Congenital	Nuclear	Narfstrom, 1981
Cat	Various	?	—	Cataracts relatively uncommon	Peiffer and Gelatt, 1974
Cattle	Friesian	Probably nonhereditary	Congenital	Bilateral spherical nuclear cataract, nonprogressive	Ashton et al, 1977
	Holstein-Friesian	Recessive	Congenital	—	Detlefson and Yapp, 1920
	Jersey	Dominant	Congenital	—	Carter, 1960
	Jersey	Recessive	Congenital	—	
	White shorthorn	Dominant (?)	Congenital	Associated with multiple ocular anomalies	Leipold et al, 1971
	All breeds	Infectious	Congenital	Materal infection with MD–BVD* during pregnancy; cortical cataract	Bistner et al, 1970
Horse	Belgian	Dominant	Congenital	—	Eriksson, 1955
	Morgan horse	—	Congenital	Nuclear	Beach and Irby, 1985; Beach et al, 1984
	Thoroughbred	Dominant	Congenital	—	
	Various	—	Congenital	—	Gelatt et al, 1974

*Mucosal disease–bovine virus diarrhea.

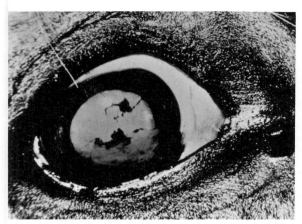

FIGURE 14–12. Cataract in a horse with recurrent equine uveitis. (Courtesy of Dr. G. A. Severin.)

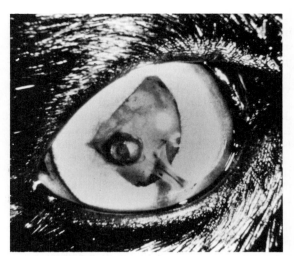

FIGURE 14–13. Cataract in a cat caused by an air rifle pellet. (Courtesy of Dr. G. A. Severin.)

area to different populations of animals in differing geographical locations. Also, cataracts may be inherited in several different ways in the same breed. Although the tendency to cataract is very often hereditary within breeds, no definite statement can be made to this effect without evidence of transmission between generations. This caution does not alter the general advice that animals with cataracts of uncertain status are unsuitable for breeding.

Congenital cataracts are not necessarily hereditary.

Examination of the Lens[4]

Lens examination is part of a complete ophthalmic examination. The pupil is dilated to adequately evaluate the lens; if this is not done, peripheral cortical changes and capsular opacities near the equator may be overlooked. Topical tropicamide (1%) administered immediately after the initial examination and repeated once in 5–10 minutes produces adequate mydriasis in most patients in 20 minutes.

Routine evaluation can be adequately performed with a focal examining light and binocular loupe. Biomicroscopic examination reveals lens changes that may go unnoticed. The iris is examined for ABNORMAL MOTION and the anterior chamber for DEPTH. The iris moves freely over the anterior lens surface and depends on the lens for position. Change in size of the pupil is the only normal movement of the iris. If the zonules deteriorate or pull free from the lens, rapid eye movement causes the lens to oscillate in the patellar fossa. This oscillation causes iris vibration (IRIDODONESIS).

Iridodonesis is the first sign of impending lens displacement and becomes more evident as the lens continues to loosen from the zonules. Initially the vitreous may swell, forcing the lens forward and resulting in a shallow anterior chamber. Anterior chamber depth is best evaluated by observing the eye from the side rather than from the front. If the lens is displaced, iris position is altered accordingly.

Increased lens movement causes the vitreous touching the lens to separate from the deeper vitreous, allowing more movement of the lens. Eventually the damaged vitreous liquefies and is replaced by aqueous. This process of liquefaction of the vitreous is referred to as SYNERESIS. Posterior displacement causes a deep anterior chamber, with the iris appearing flat or concave. Syneresis may continue until most of the vitreous disappears. When this occurs, the lens may settle toward the retina and disappear from the pupil.

Anterior displacement of the lens without passing through the pupil causes a shallow anterior chamber and increased convexity to the anterior iris surface. If the pupil dilates, the lens may luxate through the pupil into the anterior chamber. This may be partial or complete. Luxation into the anterior chamber results in corneal edema at the point where the lens touches the corneal endothelium, and the iris is concave at the point where the posterior surface of the lens touches the iris.

When the cornea is cloudy there are two methods to determine the lens position.

1. A focal light source is directed across the eye at the limbus to transilluminate the luxated lens. Light is trapped internally in the lens, producing a visible reflex arc of light at the equator opposite the light source.

2. The lens will fluoresce in ultraviolet light (Wood's lamp).

If the lens subluxates in the equatorial plane, the iris

---

4. Modified from Severin GA: Diseases of the lens. In Home Study Course in Ophthalmology. American Animal Hospital Association, Mishawaka, IN, 1974.

is convex at the point where it touches the lens and flat in the area of dislocation. The edge of the lens is visible in the pupil. The area of the pupil where the lens is missing is called an APHAKIC CRESCENT. In incomplete equatorial subluxation the aphakic crescent may not be visible until the pupil is dilated.

Variation in lens size also affects the iris and the depth of the anterior chamber. Swelling of the lens in early cataract formation causes a shallow anterior chamber and a convex iris surface, *without* iridodonesis.

If the lens is small, the anterior chamber is deep and the iris flat. A small lens cannot be differentiated from posterior displacement until the pupil is dilated. Whenever there is a possibility of a small lens, the iris is carefully examined for uveitis. In congenital microphakia the iris is normal. An absorbing cataract can produce chronic uveitis.

Visual loss depends on the location and severity of the cataract. Cataracts on the visual axis interfere with vision through a small pupil but have minimal effect with a dilated pupil. Because of this, owners of patients with centrally located cataracts observe that the patient sees better under diminished light conditions (cloudy days, evenings, or inside buildings) than it does in bright sunshine. In diminished light the pupil dilates, and the patient sees around the cataract. The severity of the lens opacity determines the effect on vision—small vacuoles and opacities have minor effects. When the lens is diffusely opaque, sight is reduced.

The patient's vision should correlate with the fundus detail observed ophthalmoscopically by the examiner. Therefore, cataract patients having significant visual loss but in whose eyes fundic detail can be seen ophthalmoscopically must have additional pathological conditions in the retina or optic pathways.

Biomicroscopic examination by an experienced observer is essential before statements of cataract-free status can be made for breeding purposes.

Signs and Symptoms

Most animals with cataract are presented because the owner noted a change in behavior due to failing vision or total blindness (e.g., bumping into objects in familiar surroundings, timidity or change in personality, inability to catch a ball) or a change in appearance of the eye itself (e.g., a white appearance that is worse at night when the pupil is dilated). Often, some degree of vision is maintained until the advanced stages of maturity of bilateral cataracts. With the exception of traumatic and secondary cataracts, the second eye usually becomes cataractous.

Owners often ask how long it will take for the cataract to become mature in the other eye and for total

blindness to occur. With the exception of diabetic cataracts, which may progress rapidly to maturity (e.g., in 2–4 weeks), this is most difficult to predict. It is also important to determine from the owner whether there has been any history of poor night vision during cataract development. This *may* indicate that the cataract is secondary to progressive retinal degeneration, if the fundus cannot be adequately examined. A history of poor day vision occurs with axial cataracts; the pupil becomes miotic in bright light, restricting light entrance through the small pupil to the opaque area of the lens.

If the owner is considering cataract extraction when the cataract becomes mature, an ophthalmoscopic examination of one or both eyes by a veterinary ophthalmologist early in the course of cataract may prevent the need for electroretinographic examination for retinal disease prior to surgery.

Congenital Cataracts[5]

Congenital cataracts begin during fetal life, are present at birth, and may be stationary or progressive. When they are extensive enough to be seen, they are generally noticed in calves and colts before 2 weeks of age and in small animals by 8–12 weeks of age. They may be inherited, secondary to other ocular developmental abnormality, or the result of maternal influences.

It is important to breeders to determine whether genetic factors are involved. Fortunately, the majority are not inherited. A thorough history is needed to better determine inheritance.

When questioning the breeder, ask

1. Were previous litters normal?
2. How many of the litter were affected?
3. What was the survival rate of the litter?
4. Were the parents normal?
5. Have cataracts been diagnosed in the bloodline?
6. Was the dam ill during pregnancy?
7. What was the dam's diet?
8. Was the dam given drugs during pregnancy?
9. Did the dam have access to chemicals?

A thorough ocular and physical examination should be performed. The presence of other conditions (ocular or general physical) reduces the probability of inherited cataracts. If a genetic cause cannot be eliminated, rebreeding of the parents may be necessary in order to determine whether a genetic influence is involved.

Congenital cataracts are observed secondary to or

---

5. Modified from Severin GA: Diseases of the lens. *In* Home Study Course in Ophthalmology. American Animal Hospital Association, Mishawaka, IN, 1974.

associated with other ocular developmental abnormalities, such as:

1. Persistent pupillary membrane
2. Persistent hyaloid artery
3. Microphthalmia
4. Multiple ocular abnormalities

PERSISTENT PUPILLARY MEMBRANE is inherited in the basenji, and therefore, cataracts secondary to this condition are as important genetically as those directly inherited. Persistent pupillary membrane may result in cataracts or corneal endothelial dystrophy, or both. Stationary anterior capsular cataracts develop if a strand of membrane adheres to the lens. The strand may or may not absorb before maturity; in either case, it will leave a permanent capsular opacity that seldom interferes with vision. Adhesion of a strand of pupillary membrane to the corneal endothelium results in permanent corneal endothelial dystrophy, which is more likely to interfere with vision. Strands are not clinically significant if both ends attach to the iris or if one end is free in the anterior chamber. Surgical removal of pupillary strands that do not spontaneously absorb is not recommended because of the stationary character of the cataract and corneal lesions. If the lens opacity is large enough to disturb vision, topical 1% atropine applied every 2–3 days will dilate the pupil and help vision. Retinal damage from chronic dilatation of the pupil has not been reported.

PERSISTENT HYALOID ARTERY (or remnants of it) may be seen in the vitreous without lens abnormalities. When the lens is involved, cataracts of the posterior capsule or cortex, or both, result. The most common lesion resulting from a nonvascular remnant is a small, stationary posterior polar cataract involving the capsule and sometimes the subcapsular cortex. The degree of visual interference depends on the size of the opacity. The hyaloid artery may persist as

1. A single blood vessel attached to the posterior pole of the lens.
2. An artery with a capsular, vascular tunic and posterior polar cataract.
3. A vascularized area in the posterior axial cortex. Cortical vascularization will appear as a dark area.

Congenital cataracts disturb vision, but topical 1% atropine applied every 2–3 days may result in intraocular hemorrhage from the hyaloid artery and cannot be recommended.

Most cataracts in foals are congenital. Occasionally a foal's history suggests an acquired cataract, but the cataract has probably been present since birth and is now becoming clinically visible. Inheritance should be considered in foals with congenital or acquired cataracts. In experimental animals, including cats and monkeys, reduction of light stimuli reaching central visual pathways during the period of light susceptibility—namely, from the time the eyelids open to approximately 12 weeks of age—can result in severe neurophysiological anomalies. Experimental evidence indicates that lack of adequate light or pattern stimulation (visual stimulation to the central nervous system) produces irreversible functional and structural abnormalities in the lateral geniculate nuclei and visual cortex.

AMBLYOPIA can develop in very young animals with dense congenital cataracts, corneal opacities, or lid occlusion. In considering whether an animal with congenital cataracts is a candidate for cataract surgery, the phenomenon of amblyopia must be recognized. Additionally, third eyelid flaps or tarsorrhaphies placed over the globe of young animals (for 3–12 weeks) may, depending on the length of time the cornea is occluded, predispose to amblyopia.

Acquired Cataracts[6]

Acquired cataracts may appear between 1 and 6 years of age. They generally affect the cortex first and the nucleus later, but they can be found in both areas simultaneously. They may be hereditary, nutritional, inflammatory, toxic, or secondary to radiation. Inheritance is a major cause and has been proposed in the Afghan, beagle, Boston terrier, Chesapeake Bay retriever, cocker spaniel, German shepherd, golden retriever, Labrador retriever, miniature schnauzer, Old English sheepdog, pointer, toy and miniature poodles, Sealyham terrier, Staffordshire bull terrier, wire-haired fox terrier, and other breeds. Hereditary cataracts can be either recessive or dominant genetic traits. Genetic modes have been proposed for several breeds, but additional studies are required to determine the exact mode of inheritance for a particular clinical cataract.

Determining the genetics of a particular cataract in one breed does not exclude another genetic factor from causing a different type of cataract in the same breed. There is evidence that both dominant and recessive cataracts are present in the golden retriever. Because of the effect inherited cataract can have on the breeding value of a bloodline, there is a tendency for the veterinary profession to call acquired cataracts hereditary before breeding studies can be evaluated. This position has a damaging effect on dogs with acquired cataract from nongenetic causes, but it prevents further dissemination of genetic factors until they can be determined. Patients with bilateral acquired cataracts should not be bred if the eye is normal in all other respects. If there is evidence that the cataract is secondary to some nonhereditary cause, the preceding restriction is not necessary. Careful examination of young animals with acquired cataracts often demonstrates changes at 6–8 weeks of age, but clinical signs may not become evident until as late as 6 years of age.

PROGRESSION (Table 14–4)

Most animals develop cataract by 4 months to 3 years of age. In some dogs slit-lamp examination at an

6. Modified from Severin GA: Diseases of the lens. *In* Home Study Course in Ophthalmology. American Animal Hospital Association, Mishawaka, IN, 1974.

TABLE 14–4. Cataract Prognosis Based on Position

Position	Prognosis
Anterior capsular polar	Usually nonprogressive
Anterior cortical	Variable progression
Equatorial	Usually progressive
Nuclear	Usually static or reduce in size
Posterior cortical	Variable progression
Posterior capsular and axial	Usually nonprogressive

Modified from Gelatt KN et al: Biometry and clinical characteristics of congenital cataracts and microphthalmia in the miniature schnauzer. J Am Vet Med Assoc 183:99, 1983.

early age reveals changes before they can be seen by other methods. Common sites for initial development are at the equator, in anterior and posterior subcapsular areas, and along Y sutures. Opacities progress through the cortex, and concurrent nuclear involvement occurs.

1. EQUATORIAL OPACITIES begin with vacuolation, followed by opacity. Opacities in the anterior and posterior cortices progress toward the axis of the lens like spokes in a wheel. Eventually the cortex is uniformly opaque.

2. ANTERIOR AND POSTERIOR SUBCAPSULAR OPACITIES generally start near the poles and spread outward to involve the adjacent cortical layers next. The lens may remain clear at the equator, even with dense opacity of the central lens, when the origin is near the poles.

3. POSTERIOR Y SUTURE CATARACTS may develop very slowly and not interfere with vision for many years.

In some dogs cataract development is rapid, and the entire lens is opaque within months of onset. It is impossible to predict accurately the rate of cataract development. Acquired cataracts progress to eventual maturation of the opacity. This may take months or as long as several years. Some animals develop lens capsule leakage, and the cataract resorbs. Other cataracts remain as stable mature lesions without change. If resorption is going to occur, it generally becomes evident within a year of examination. Signs of resorption are

1. Deepening of the anterior chamber
2. Decrease in lens diameter and thickness
3. Corrugation of the anterior capsule

As the lens becomes small, vision can be aided with mydriatics (1% atropine every 2–3 days). Complete resorption allows vision comparable with that occurring after successful surgical lens removal. Lens-induced uveitis may occur and is treated as described in Chapter 13. Lens removal is not performed in the presence of uveitis or resorption.

Senile Cataracts [7]

Senile cataracts are part of the aging process and occur in all species of domestic animals. They are of

7. Modified from Severin GA: Diseases of the lens. *In* Home Study Course in Ophthalmology. American Animal Hospital Association, Mishawaka, IN, 1974.

greatest clinical importance in the dog, after which come the horse, the cat, and last, cattle. They are preceded by nuclear sclerosis and can begin in the cortex or nucleus. A typical senile cortical cataract begins in the deep equatorial layers with opaque streaks extending toward the axis like spokes of a wheel. Opacification continues until clear areas are present only at the Y suture lines of the cortex. The clear areas are referred to as water clefts and give the lens a segmented appearance. With continuing opacification, the water clefts become thinner and eventually disappear. When the lens is uniformly opaque, the cataract is mature (see Fig. 14–7C). Cortical and nuclear opacification occur at the same time.

The mature cataract continues to lose fluid and decrease in size. It may remain firm for several years before showing hypermaturity—signs of becoming shrunken and dehydrated (see Fig. 14–7E) or of sinking of the nucleus (see Fig. 14–7F) (morgagnian cataract). Shrinking can separate the lens from its attachments and cause luxation. Sight returns in the morgagnian cataract, similar to the return of sight in resorption of a juvenile cataract, provided ocular damage caused by lens-induced uveitis is not severe. Elderly patients, past the age at which cataract extraction is advisable, usually tolerate the low levels of uveitis, controlled by topical dexamethasone (1–2 times a day), for prolonged periods quite comfortably.

Diabetic Cataracts

Most animals with diabetes mellitus eventually develop cataract, despite administration of insulin, and owners should be advised of this when beginning insulin therapy. With more accurate diabetic control the onset may occur later. The onset of diabetic cataracts may be particularly rapid, as short as a few days, and they frequently have marked "water cleft" formation. Dogs with diabetes do not develop diabetic retinopathy unless maintained on insulin for many years, and then it is doubtful whether it is significant. All potential cataract patients are *screened* for elevated tear glucose with urine test paper prior to administration of mydriatics and topical anesthetics (false-negative results may occur but not strong false-positive results). All clinically affected diabetics require a complete hematological, biochemical, and thoracic radiographic evaluation before the decision to remove a cataract is made.

In general, diabetic patients are good cataract surgical candidates provided they have been on *stable insulin control* for at least 3 months and are free of major complications of diabetes such as ketoacidosis and liver or renal failure. This is necessary as drugs administered before and during surgery may later disturb this control and cause glycosuria, and it is necessary to continue insulin at the preoperative dose until requirements stabilize again.

Any dog 3 years of age or older with a rapidly developing cataract is screened for diabetes mellitus.

Complicated and Traumatic Cataracts[8]

Cataract may occur following ocular injury or inflammation of adjacent structures or develop in the course of systemic diseases. The course is variable; the cataract may improve with time, become stationary, or progress to maturity. Anterior uveitis is the most common cause of complicated cataracts in all species and is the most common cause of acquired blindness in the horse (see Fig. 14–12). An attack of uveitis usually results in minor posterior synechiae and capsular changes. If uveitis does not recur, lenticular change is minimal. If uveitis recurs, total cataracts may result. The feline lens with complicated cataracts remains functional longer than does either the equine or the canine lens.

Miscellaneous Cataracts

1. Orphan kangaroos and wallabies and other macropods develop galactosemic cataracts when fed cow's milk containing galactose and lactose (see Fig. 14–9). This occurs because these animals are ruminants and lack the necessary enzymes to metabolize glucose. During the monogastric phase of forestomach development, galactose and lactose are absorbed. The problem can be avoided by feeding proprietary milk substitutes lacking galactose and lactose, such as those designed for human infants with galactosemia. These cataracts are usually *not amenable* to surgical correction by lens extraction, as the primary vitreous is also opaque.

Warning: Some *commercially available* macropod milk replacement preparations contain lactose and galactose and are unsuitable for use in these species.

Orphan wallabies and kangaroos must not be fed cow's milk.

2. Spontaneous cataracts have been observed in turkeys and in chickens with avian encephalomyelitis and Marek's disease.

---

8. Modified from Severin GA: Diseases of the lens. *In* Home Study Course in Ophthalmology. American Animal Hospital Association, Mishawaka, IN, 1974.

3. Radiation may cause cataracts by affecting dividing cells in the equatorial area. Therapeutic doses of beta radiation do not usually penetrate sufficiently to cause opacities in domestic animals. However, if prolonged diagnostic studies are undertaken around the head or radiotherapy is used in this area, the eyes should be protected with lead shields. The risk of cataract is relatively small and is acceptable for alpha and gamma radiation used for therapeutic purposes. Older animals with the types of neoplastic lesions requiring such therapy seem to be more resistant to radiation-induced cataract than are younger animals. Other complications of radiation including keratitis sicca, chronic conjunctivitis, and keratopathy must still be considered.

4. Numerous species of fish throughout the world are affected by different species of trematode larvae that enter the lens and cause cataract (Fig. 14–14). As the fish is an integral part of the life cycle and is usually eaten by a bird in the next phase, presumably the blindness increases the likelihood of the fish's being caught and eaten by a bird. Reports from Canada indicate little visual disturbance from even extensive trematode infestation of the lens.

5. Nutritional cataracts occur in fish raised in trout hatcheries with poorly formulated rations.

6. Cataracts in pups fed bitch replacement milk
    Synonym: "Esbilac" cataracts

These cataracts occur with a number of commercial bitch replacement milks and are significant for diagnosis. They do not progress to maturity and do not

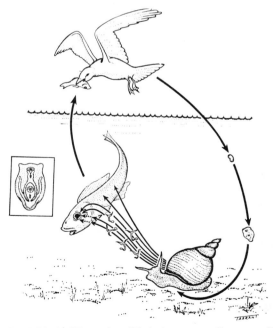

FIGURE 14–14. *Life cycle of* Diplostomum spathaceum. *The inset shows a metacercaria, which enters the lens. (From Ashton, N et al: Trematode cataract in fresh water fish. J Sm Anim Pract 10:471, 1969.)*

interfere with vision. The opacities are located in the equatorial and posterior subcapsular regions. The cause is unknown. Different batches of milk from the same manufacturer may cause different effects, and the production of cataracts is not consistent, although the appearance of the opacities is characteristic. Similar cataracts have been observed in wolf cubs.

Treatment

In the early stages of cataract, especially when the opacity lies on the visual axis, vision can be improved by use of a mydriatic when required. Because of its shorter duration of action, homatropine (2%) is preferable to atropine and may be used 1–2 times daily as necessary.

With monotonous regularity, various unproven agents have been suggested to resolve cataract, such as selenium (Poulos, 1966), orgotein (Cobble and Lynd, 1977), *Actinomyces bovis* extract (Ivy et al, 1959), and most recently "zinc ascorbate." These have *all* been shown to lack therapeutic effect; in addition, the use of subconjunctival and intraocular orgotein causes numerous secondary complications. Most recently with zinc ascorbate, studies showed an increased incidence of cataract in control *treated* normal animals. The apparent improvement from these medications probably resulted from their use during spontaneous lens resorption or from inadequate evaluation of the lens by unqualified observers, including animal owners and breeders.

In my experience, some animals being treated with these medications have nuclear sclerosis and normal vision at the onset of treatment, guaranteeing excellent results at the first and subsequent examinations. Medical therapy for cataracts currently has no place in the regimens presented by informed and responsible veterinarians.

Medical therapy for cataracts is ineffective, delays effective therapy, and decreases the chance of success of therapy by allowing the unsupervised and untreated progression of lens-induced uveitis.

Surgical removal is the only effective treatment for mature cataracts.

SURGICAL CORRECTION

Four methods of surgical correction are commonly used (Fig. 14–15):

1. DISCISSION—opening of the anterior lens capsule and aspiration of the liquid contents from within the capsule (so-called endocapsular extraction) by careful flushing via a two-way needle (O'Gawa's cannula). This method is restricted to young animals with liquid cataracts.

2. EXTRACAPSULAR EXTRACTION—removal of the anterior lens capsule, nucleus, and cortex. The posterior lens capsule, which is attached to the vitreous, remains intact. This is the most commonly used method.

3. PHACOEMULSIFICATION—ultrasonic shattering and removal by irrigation and aspiration. This is a variant method used either after complete removal of the anterior lens capsule or through an incision in the lens capsule, with later removal of the capsule. The method has not achieved widespread usage because of the cost of equipment and the success rate, which is similar to a correctly performed, standard extracapsular extraction by an experienced surgeon on a properly evaluated patient.

In the 1970s, up to 50% of human cataract extractions were performed with phacoemulsification, but this rate has fallen to less than 20%. The long-term success rate with cataracts removed by phacoemulsification is similar to that with extracapsular extraction. Complications include hyphema, retinal detachment, glaucoma, uveitis, posterior capsular opacification, and synechiae. The technique has the advantages of requiring a smaller incision and allowing more complete removal of lens cortical material. Phacoemulsification and extracapsular cataract extraction cause similar endothelial cell loss. Endothelial cell loss in phacoemulsification can be decreased by the use of viscoelastic substances (sodium hyaluronate, methylcellulose) in the anterior chamber or by endocapsular phacoemulsification.

4. INTRACAPSULAR EXTRACTION—removal of the entire lens, including anterior and posterior capsules. This method, although commonly used in humans, is restricted to the removal of luxated lenses in domestic animals, because it results in loss of vitreous, retinal detachment, and a generally unsuccessful outcome when used on unluxated lenses. The results after primary lens luxation in dogs can be excellent.

Postoperative Function and Optical Correction

After cataract extraction, animals do not usually require optical correction; a good surgical result with minimal postoperative inflammation is more critical. Dogs do not have the same degree of visual acuity that humans do and can usually function normally without correction. Intraocular lenses of approximately 30-D power are now available for use in dogs. Complications of their use include uveitis, implant displacement, and secondary glaucoma, and these are similar to those of the surgical technique itself.

The aim of cataract extraction is to give a blind animal vision to allow it to live a relatively normal life without running into things or being intimidated by

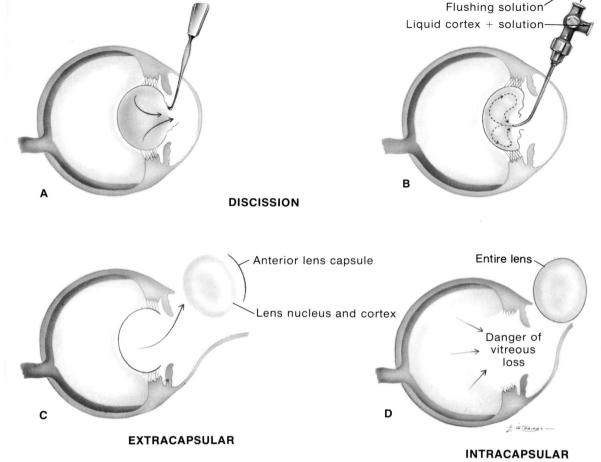

FIGURE 14–15. *Methods of lens removal. A, Discission—rupture of lens capsule. B, Discission—aspiration of contents via two-way cannula. C, Extracapsular extraction. D, Intracapsular extraction.*

stairs and other obstacles. If this aim is achieved, the procedure has been successful.

The optical reasons for adequate vision being achieved without supplementary lenses are as follows:

1. Accommodation in the normal animal is poorly developed, and therefore, absence of the lens has relatively little effect.

2. The lens represents only a portion of the total optical power of the eye—the cornea provides more of the optical power.

3. The dog has no fovea and a poorly defined macular area.

Most dogs and horses have acceptably good vision after surgery, provided the other complications are controlled. Anecdotal reports of improved vision in aphakic dogs after intraocular lens implantation indicate that lens implantation may become an additional alternative for canine cataract extraction, subject to confirmation by publication of controlled studies. Near vision in these animals is improved.

Case Selection

Not all animals with cataract are suitable for surgery. The following prerequisites are fulfilled before recommending cataract extraction:

1. The owner must be prepared to sustain the expense and inconvenience of preoperative and postoperative treatment and return visits. The importance of a cooperative, enthusiastic owner cannot be overemphasized—willingness to pay the bill is not enough.

2. The affected eye should have a significant visual deficit. The recommendation that *both* eyes should be blind is not currently accepted as a reason for delay; waiting for maturity of the other lens often results in lens-induced uveitis and a poorer prognosis in the first eye.

3. Any incipient lens-induced uveitis—indicated by ciliary injection, hypotony, miosis, change in iris color, or resistance to mydriasis—must first be controlled by topical corticosteroids under the supervision of the

person who will perform the surgery. The incidence of short- and long-term complications is greater when uveitis is present preoperatively.

4. The fundus is examined by the surgeon early in the disease, or electroretinography is performed to ensure that progressive retinal degeneration (PRD; progressive retinal atrophy [PRA]) is not present. As PRD can occur in any breed, this evaluation is routine in bilaterally affected dogs when the fundus cannot be examined. The speed of pupil contraction in response to light is *not* a reliable indicator of the presence or absence of PRD. The owner is carefully questioned about the relative onset of visual difficulty, cataract, and nyctalopia.

5. There should be no other ocular pathological process present. The eye must be examined by a person experienced in veterinary ophthalmic diagnosis.

6. The patient must be amenable to intensive handling, as frequent topical medications are required in both the pre- and the postoperative periods. An excitable dog that cannot be handled and medicated is usually an unsuitable candidate. During initial preoperative topical therapy is the ideal time for the owner to make this evaluation.

7. The patient should be in good general health, and the following tests are performed prior to surgery if the patient is over 6 years of age:

　　a. Complete blood count and serum chemistry profile.

　　b. Thoracic radiographs in two views.

All animals with rapidly progressing cataracts are evaluated and, if necessary, treated for diabetes mellitus and stabilized prior to cataract surgery. Once a patient has fulfilled these criteria, cataract removal may be considered.

Surgical Methods

The veterinary literature for over 75 years has been replete with reports of poor results of cataract extraction in animals. In 1969, this was finally disproved by Magrane, who, in a series of 429 cases, demonstrated that with accurate and detailed case selection and a meticulous approach to operative technique and postoperative treatment, a success rate of over 90% can be achieved in dogs. The success rate has also been related to the experience of the surgeon.

Once pre-existing uveitis has been controlled and retinal function determined, cataract extraction is performed unilaterally. Numerous studies have shown a higher success rate on unilateral extractions than on bilateral extractions. It is rare that both lenses are at the same stage of cataract at the same time, and even in these patients, unilateral extraction is recommended, with the second procedure planned after 3 months.

Poor past results have been due to

1. Failure to understand the differences between the human and the canine eyes, both anatomically and pathologically.

2. Use of an inappropriate operative technique—intracapsular extraction, the procedure once used most often in humans, gives a much lower success rate in animals, except when used for removal of luxated lenses.

3. Failure to identify and control pre- and postoperative uveitis.

4. Failure to treat intensively after surgery.

5. Poor selection of cases.

6. Inadequate surgical exposure of the operative area.

7. Poor mydriasis, now resolved by preoperative administration of nonsteroidal anti-inflammatory agents and corticosteroids.

8. Inadequate control of the patient postoperatively.

In experienced hands, using a proved and practiced technique for animals, cataract extraction gives a high success rate in properly selected cases.

Detailed descriptions and discussion of cataract extraction are beyond the scope of this text. The interested reader is referred to more specialized texts and original literature. The three most common methods of extracapsular extraction—via limbal incision, scleral groove beneath the conjunctival flap, and discission—are illustrated in Figures 14–16, 14–17, and 14–18. The technique for phacoemulsification is similar to that for discission (Fig. 14–18).

Text continued on page 389

FIGURE 14–16. *Extracapsular cataract extraction via limbal incision. A, A canthotomy is performed and the lids are retracted with sutures of 4/0 silk. Two fixation sutures of 6/0 silk are placed. A method that does not place pressure on the globe is used, e.g., Vierheller's speculum. B, A limbal incision is made. C, The incision is extended with left and right corneal scissors. D, A suture with a porcelain bead attached is preplaced at the 12 o'clock position. Alternatively, two preplaced sutures may be used for manipulation of the cornea. These sutures are used to prevent instrument damage to the endothelium (7/0 silk, Vicryl, or Dexon is suitable). E, The anterior lens capsule is grasped with lens capsule forceps, and the edge of the capsule is incised. The capsule is removed.*

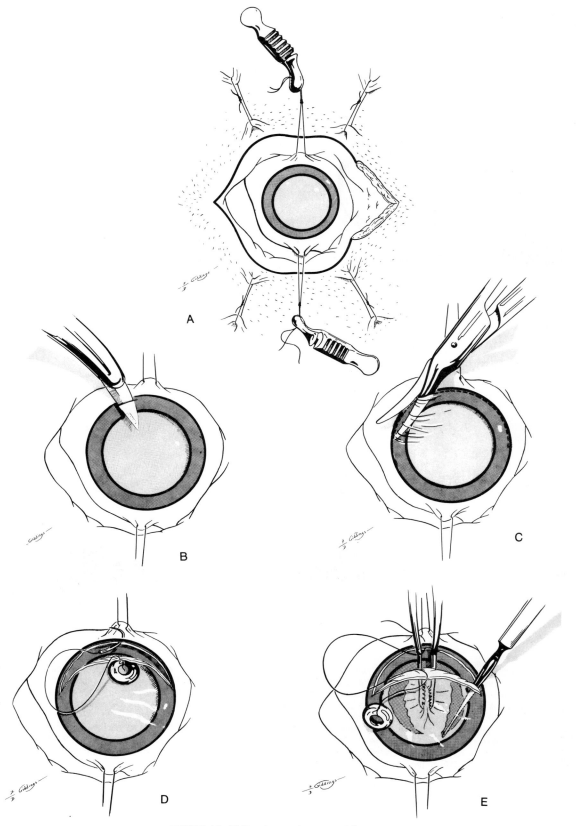

FIGURE 14–16 *See legend on opposite page*

Illustration continued on following page

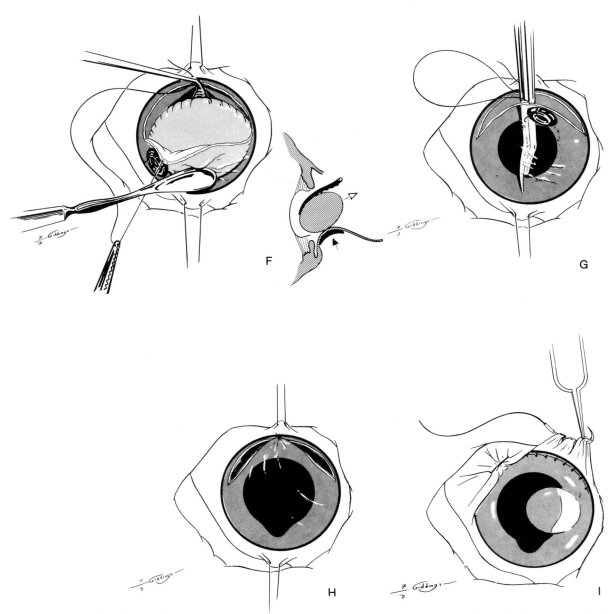

FIGURE 14–16 Continued F, *An irrigator is placed between the lens cortex and the posterior capsule, and the cortex is gently irrigated forward with balanced salt solution. A lens loop is placed behind the lens to remove it. Alternatively, the lens may be removed by careful pressure from the ventral limbus, without placing a loop or irrigator in the eye. Care is taken to avoid the corneal endothelium. G, A sphincterotomy may be performed at the 6 o'clock position if miosis occurs. Alternatively, an iridectomy may be performed if necessary, at the 12 o'clock position, with electrocautery. H, The preplaced suture(s) is tied and the incision closed with simple interrupted sutures at 1-mm intervals under magnification. I, A modified conjunctival flap is positioned with 6/0 silk, and the anterior chamber is reconstructed with an air bubble. Preplaced McLean's sutures may be used to position the flap over the corneal wound and seal it. (Modified from Severin GA: Veterinary Ophthalmology Notes, 2nd ed. Ft Collins, CO, 1976.)*

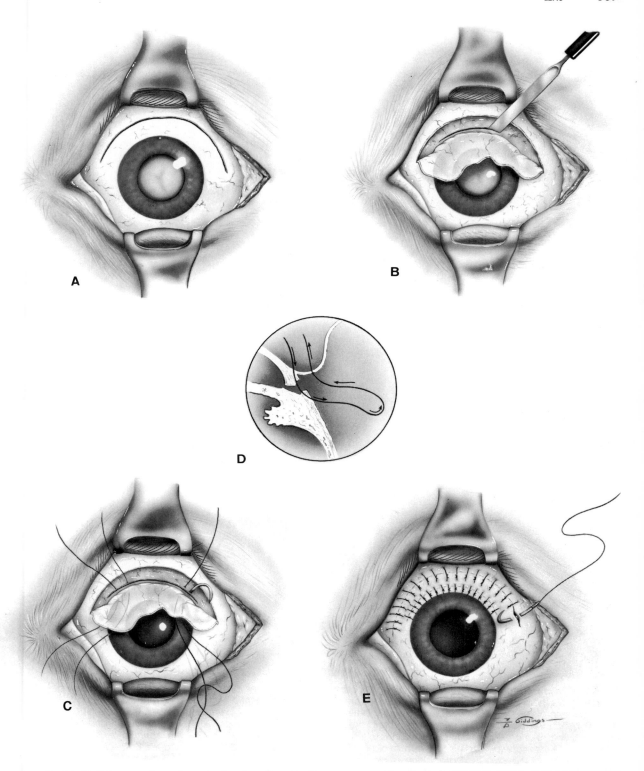

FIGURE 14–17. Extracapsular cataract extraction via scleral groove and limbus-based conjunctival flap. A, The conjunctiva is incised 4–5 mm from the limbus. B, A limbus-based conjunctival flap is formed. C, A scleral groove is prepared 1 mm behind the limbus with an electrosurgical unit, down to one half the thickness of the sclera. Two to four sutures are preplaced. D, Preplaced McLean's suture. E, Sutures are placed to one side, and the anterior chamber is entered as was shown in Figure 14–16. The incision is similarly lengthened. Prepared sutures of 7/0 or 8/0 Vicryl, Dexon, or silk are tied, and additional sutures are placed as necessary. An air bubble is placed in the anterior chamber, and the conjunctival flap is closed with a continuous suture.

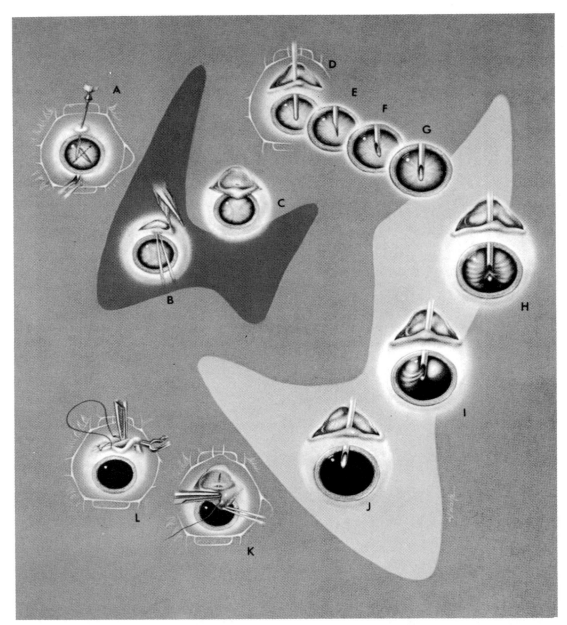

FIGURE 14–18. *Discission and aspiration of soft cataracts. A, The anterior lens capsule is opened with a cystitome or knife-needle. B, A limbus-based conjunctival flap is prepared. C, A small puncture is made 1–2 mm from the limbus. D, An O'Gawa cannula or 19-gauge needle is inserted, bevel edge down, into the anterior chamber. E, F, and G, The needle is rotated with the bevel held anteriorly to protect the posterior lens capsule and vitreous during aspiration. H, I, and J, Balanced salt solution is carefully pumped in and aspirated (simultaneously if an O'Gawa cannula is used) to remove remnants of lens material. Care is taken to avoid damaging the corneal endothelium and iris. K, The incision is closed with 6/0 Vicryl. L, The conjunctival incision is closed with a simple continuous suture of 6/0 Vicryl. The technique for phacoemulsification is similar. (From Scheie HG, Albert DM: Textbook of Ophthalmology, 9th ed. WB Saunders Co, Philadelphia, 1977.)*

LENS LUXATION

Luxation is displacement of the lens from the hyaloid fossa (see Chap 13). Subluxation is partial displacement of the lens from the hyaloid fossa. Luxation is usually caused by complete disruption of the lens zonule, whereas in subluxation some zonules usually remain intact. Primary lens luxation is most commonly seen in dogs. The lens may luxate anteriorly, posteriorly, or in the vertical plane of the lens (Figs. 14–19 and 14–20).

Etiology

1. **CONGENITAL**—seen in multiple ocular anomalies, rare in clinical practice.

2. **TRAUMATIC**—trauma violent enough to cause lens luxation usually causes other severe ocular lesions (e.g., hyphema, retinal detachment, scleral rupture).

3. **SECONDARY LUXATION**

a. Intraocular tumors—as a tumor enlarges, it may displace the lens, creating a luxation or subluxation.

b. Glaucoma—when the globe enlarges in chronic glaucoma, the zonules may break and the lens luxates.

c. Cataract—if a cataractous lens swells (*intumescence*), the zonules may break.

4. **HEREDITARY**—due to weakened lens zonules that rupture early in life (up to 5 years of age). This is the most common form of lens luxation and is seen as an inherited condition in wire-haired fox terriers, Sealyham, Manchester, Cairn, Jack Russell, Tibetan, and miniature bull terriers, and miniature schnauzers. It is also common in poodles, but the hereditary nature is unconfirmed. Electron microscopic studies in the Tibetan terrier have shown that the insertions of the lens zonules into the lens capsule are abnormal.

Luxation may follow minor trauma, which ruptures the weakened zonules. However, trauma is usually *not* the primary etiology.

Clinical Signs and Diagnosis

Clinical signs of lens luxation are

1. Abnormal motion of the iris (iridodonesis) when the eye is moved, because the iris is no longer resting on the lens.

2. Increased or decreased depth of the anterior chamber (see Figs. 14–19A, B, and 14–20).

3. Presence of an aphakic crescent (aphakic—without a lens) (Fig. 14–21; see also Fig. 13–17).

4. Increased intraocular pressure, especially in anterior luxations.

5. Corneal edema resulting from the lens touching the endothelium if an anterior luxation has been present.

6. Traumatic uveitis manifested by ciliary vessel

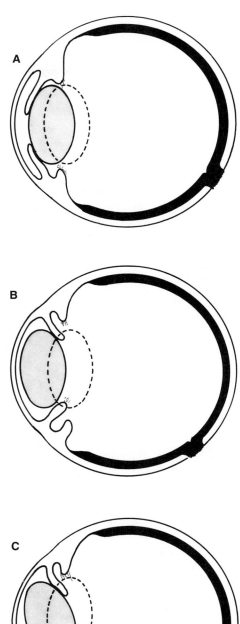

FIGURE 14–19. A, *Anterior lens luxation with anterior displacement of the iris (and possible pupillary blockage of aqueous passage). Anterior chamber is shallow. B, Luxation into the anterior chamber, which appears deep. Endothelial damage causes corneal edema where the lens capsule touches it. C, Subluxation of the lens through the pupil. (Courtesy of Dr. G. A. Severin.)*

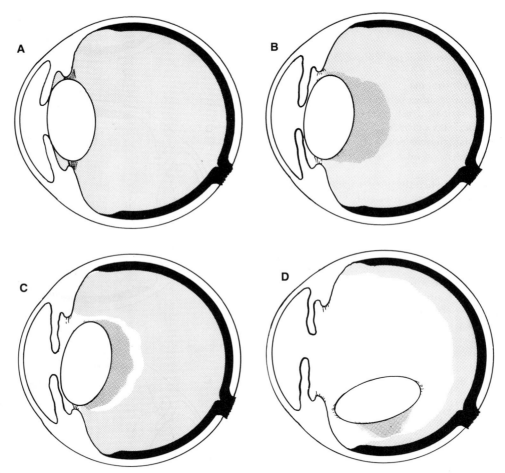

FIGURE 14–20. Posterior lens luxation and vitreous syneresis. A, Normal lens position. B, Zonules are ruptured but lens is held in place by the vitreous. C, Early liquefaction of the vitreous, allowing more lens movement. D, Lens motion accelerates syneresis, and the lens may sink vertically. (Courtesy of Dr. G. A. Severin.)

A

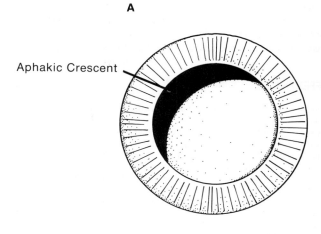

Aphakic Crescent

FIGURE 14–21. Mechanism of aphakic crescent formation. (Courtesy of Dr. G. A. Severin.)

B

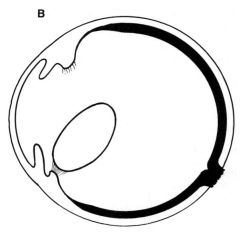

engorgement, pain, and blepharospasm. This may be one of the first signs of impending luxation. At a more advanced stage, increased pressure caused by an anterior luxation may be balanced by the decreased pressure due to this traumatic uveitis, resulting in a normal pressure with signs of both uveitis and lens luxation present.

7. Liquefaction of the vitreous (syneresis). Mobile collagenous strands from the vitreous framework may be visible through the pupil in the anterior vitreous or protruding into the anterior chamber.

Luxated lenses frequently become cataractous (see Fig. 13–17). The possible pathways by which a cataractous luxated lens may occur in an eye with elevated

intraocular pressure are discussed more fully in Chapter 13. Briefly, these mechanisms are shown in Figure 14–22.

Treatment[9]

In anterior luxations, the lens may be either
a. Removed by intracapsular extraction or
b. Replaced in the vitreous (*reclination*) and *permanent* miotic therapy instituted. If chronic glaucoma is present and peripheral anterior synechiae have formed, glau-

---

9. See also Chap 13.

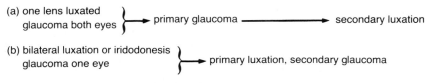

FIGURE 14–22. Possible mechanisms for lens luxation. (Modified from Severin GA: Veterinary Ophthalmology Notes, 2nd ed. Fort Collins, CO, 1976.)

coma will persist after lens removal, unless other steps are taken to provide aqueous outflow. In this situation, intraocular prosthesis insertion is preferable, with lens recession and cryotherapy a less preferable alternative.

REFERENCES

Aguirre G, Bistner SI (1973): Posterior lenticonus in the dog. Cornell Vet 63:455.

Alpar JJ (1987): Use of healon in different cataract surgery techniques: Endothelial cell count study. Ophthalmic Surg 18:529.

Anderson AC, Shultz FT (1958): Inherited (congenital) cataract in the dog. Am J Pathol 34:965.

Ashton N (1979): Ocular toxoplasmosis in Wallabies (*Macropus rufogriseus*). Am J Ophthalmol 88:322.

Ashton N, et al (1969): Trematode cataract in freshwater fish. J Sm Anim Pract 10:471.

Ashton N, et al (1977): Congenital nuclear cataracts in cattle. Vet Rec 100:505.

Barnett KC (1972): Types of cataract in the dog. J Am Anim Hosp Assoc 8:2.

Barnett KC (1976): Comparative aspects of canine hereditary eye disease. Adv Vet Sci Comp Med 20:39.

Barnett KC (1978): Hereditary cataract in the dog. J Sm Anim Pract 19:109.

Barnett KC (1980): Cataract in the golden retriever. Vet Rec 111:315.

Barnett KC (1980): Hereditary cataract in the Welsh springer spaniel. J Sm Anim Pract 21:621.

Barnett KC (1985): Hereditary cataract in the standard poodle. Vet Rec 117:15.

Barnett KC (1986): Hereditary in the German shepherd dog. J Sm Anim Pract 27:387.

Beach J, Irby N (1985): Inherited nuclear cataracts in the Morgan horse. J Hered 76:371.

Beach J, et al (1984): Congenital nuclear cataracts in the Morgan horse. J Am Vet Med Assoc 184:1363.

Bistner SI, et al (1970): The ocular lesions of bovine viral diarrhea—mucosal disease. Path Vet 7:272.

Bouillon DR, Curtis MA (1987): Diplostomiasis (Trematoda: Strigeidae) in Arctic charr (Salvelinus alpinus) from Charr lake, northern Labrador. J Wildl Dis 23:502.

Brainard J, et al (1982): Evaluation of superoxide dismutase (orgotein) in medical treatment of canine cataract. Arch Ophthalmol 100:1832.

Brightman AH, et al (1981): Effect of aspirin on aqueous protein values in the dog. J Am Vet Med Assoc 178:572.

Buschmann W, et al (1987): Microsurgical treatment of lens capsule perforations. Part I: Experimental research. Ophthalmic Surg 18:731.

Carter AH (1960): An inherited blindness (cataract) in cattle. Proc New Zealand Soc Anim Prod 20:108.

Cobble RS, Lynd FT (1977): Preliminary observations on orgotein treatment of canine cataract. Mod Vet Pract 58:1009.

Curtis RC (1983): Aetiopathological aspects of inherited lens dislocation in the Tibetan terrier. J Comp Pathol 93:151.

Curtis RC, Barnett KC (1983): Primary lens luxation in the miniature bull terrier. Vet Rec 112:328.

Curtis RC, et al (1983): Clinical and pathological observations concerning the aetiology of primary lens luxation in the dog. Vet Rec 112:238.

Davies RB, et al (1973): Diplostomiasis in North Park, Colorado. J Wildl Dis 9:362.

Detlefson JA, Yapp WW (1920): The inheritance of congenital cataract in cattle. Am Natural 54:277. Cited by Ashton et al, 1977.

DeVolt HM (1944): Lamellar cataracts in chickens. Poult Sci 23:346.

Duke-Elder S, Jay B (1969): System of Ophthalmology, vol 9,
Diseases of the lens and vitreous: Glaucoma and hypotony. H Kimpton, London.

Eriksson K (1955): Hereditary aniridia with secondary cataract in horses. Nord Vet Med 7:773.

Flowers AI, et al (1958): Cataracts: A new flock problem in chickens. Poult Sci 37:420.

Gelatt KN (1971): Cataracts in cattle. J Am Vet Med Assoc 159:195.

Gelatt KN (1972): Cataracts in the golden retriever dog. Vet Med Small Anim Clin 67:1113.

Gelatt KN, Rubin LF (1969): Delayed postoperative staphylomas in dogs. J Am Vet Med Assoc 154:283.

Gelatt KN, et al (1974): Aspiration of congenital and soft cataracts in foals and young horses. J Am Vet Med Assoc 165:611.

Gelatt KC, et al (1979): Cataracts in Chesapeake Bay retrievers. J Am Vet Med Assoc 175:1176.

Gelatt KN, et al (1983a): Biometry and clinical characteristics of congenital cataracts and microphthalmia in the miniature schnauzer. J Am Vet Med Assoc 183:99.

Gelatt KN, et al (1983b): Inheritance of congenital cataracts and microphthalmia in the miniature schnauzer. Am J Vet Res 44:1130.

Gwin RM, et al (1983): Effects of phacoemulsification and extracapsular lens removal on cornea thickness and endothelial cell density in the dog. Invest Ophthalmol Vis Sci 24:227.

Heywood R (1971a): Drug-induced lenticular lesions in the dog. Br Vet J 127:301.

Heywood R (1971b): Juvenile cataracts in the beagle dog. J Sm Anim Pract 12:171.

Hirth RS, et al (1974): Anterior capsular opacities (spurious cataracts) in beagle dogs. Vet Pathol 11:181.

Hogan MJ, et al (1971): Histology of the Human Eye. WB Saunders Co, Philadelphia.

Høst P, Sveinson S (1936): Arvelig Kataract hos hunder Norsk Vet Tidskr 48:244. (Cited by Roberts and Helper, 1972.)

Ivy AC, et al (1959): Therapeutic improvement of canine cataract. Vet Med 54:205.

Knight GC (1960): Canine intraocular surgery. Vet Rec 72:644.

Knight GC (1962): The indications and technique for lens extraction in the dog. Vet Rec 74:1065.

Koch SA (1967): Probable non-hereditary congenital cataracts in dogs. J Am Vet Med Assoc 150:1374.

Koch SA (1972): Cataracts in interrelated Old English sheepdogs. J Am Vet Med Assoc 160:299.

Lavach JD, Severin GA (1977): Posterior lenticonus and lenticonus internum in a dog. J Am Anim Hosp Assoc 13:685.

Lawson DD (1969): Luxation of the crystalline lens in the dog. Trans Ophthalmol Soc UK 59:259.

Leipold HW, et al (1971): Multiple ocular anomalies and hydrocephalus in grade beef shorthorn cattle. Am J Vet Res 32:1019.

Lynd FT, McDonald MD (1978): The treatment of senile cataracts in dogs by the intraocular injection of superoxide dismutase. J Vet Pharmacol Ther 1:85.

Magrane WG (1961): Cataract extraction: An evaluation of 104 cases. J Sm Anim Pract 1:163.

Magrane WG (1969): Cataract extraction: A follow-up study (429 cases). J Sm Anim Pract 10:545.

Martin CL (1978): Zonular defects in the dog. A clinical and scanning electron microscopic study. J Am Anim Hosp Assoc 14:571.

Martin CL, Chambreau T (1982): Cataract production in experimentally orphaned puppies fed a commercial replacement for bitch's milk. J Am Anim Hosp Assoc 18:115.

Martin CL, Leipold HW (1974): Aphakia and multiple ocular defects in Saint Bernard puppies. Vet Med 69:448.

Martin CL, et al (1972): Formation of temporary cataracts in dogs given a disophenol preparation. J Am Vet Med Assoc 161:294.

Miller TR, et al (1987): Phacofragmentation and aspiration for cataract extraction in dogs: 56 cases (1980–1984). J Am Vet Med Assoc 190:1577.

Murphy JM, et al (1980): Sequelae of extracapsular lens extraction in the normal dog. J Am Anim Hosp Assoc 16:17.

Narfstrom K (1981): Cataract in the West Highland white terrier. J Sm Anim Pract 22:467.

Narfstrom K, Dubielzig R (1984): Posterior lenticonus, cataracts and microphthalmia: Congenital ocular defects in the Cavalier King Charles spaniel. J Sm Anim Pract 25:669.

Nassise MP, et al (1986): Response of the canine corneal endothelium to intraocular irrigation. Proc Am Coll Vet Ophthalmol 16:16.

Norton JH (1980): Cataracts in sows. Aust Vet J 56:408.

Oosterhuis JA, Jeltes IG (1975): Cataract extraction in the dog. Ophthalmologica 171:296.

Oz HH, et al (1986): Bilateral cataract surgery in a Suffolk ewe. Vet Rec 118:512.

Paulsen ME (1986): The effect of lens-induced uveitis on the success of extracapsular cataract extraction—A retrospective study of 65 lens removals in the dog. J Am Anim Hosp Assoc 22:49.

Peiffer RL, Gelatt KN (1974): Cataracts in the cat. Feline Pract 4:34.

Peiffer RL, Weintraub BA (1979): Clinical and histopathologic effects of lensectomy and anterior vitrectomy in the canine eye. J Am Anim Hosp Assoc 15:421.

Playter RF (1977): The development and maturation of a cataract. J Am Anim Hosp Assoc 13:317.

Poulos P (1966): Selenium-tocopherol treatment of senile lenticular sclerosis in dogs (four case reports). Vet Med 61:986.

Rahi AHS, Garner A (1976): Immunopathology of the Eye. Blackwell, Oxford.

Rigdon RH (1959): Cataracts in chickens with lymphomatosis. Am J Vet Res 20:467.

Rigdon RH, et al (1959): Spontaneous cataracts in turkeys. Am J Vet Res 20:961.

Riis RC, Rumsey G (1974): Cataract in trout. Proc Am Coll Vet Ophthalmol, 16:65.

Roberts SR (1973): Hereditary cataracts. Vet Clin North Am 3:433.

Roberts SR, Helper LC (1972): Cataracts in Afghan hounds. J Am Vet Med Assoc 160:427.

Rooks RL, et al (1985): Extracapsular cataract extractions: An analysis of 240 operations in dogs. J Am Vet Med Assoc 190:1580.

Rubin LF (1974): Cataract in golden retrievers. J Am Vet Med Assoc 165:457.

Rubin LF, Flowers RD (1972): Inherited cataract in a family of standard poodles. J Am Vet Med Assoc 161:207.

Rubin LF, Gelatt KN (1968): Spontaneous resorption of cataractous lenses in dogs. J Am Vet Med Assoc 152:139.

Rubin LF, et al (1969): Hereditary cataracts in miniature schnauzers. J Am Vet Med Assoc 154:1456.

Sanford SE, Dukes TW (1978): Acquired bilateral cortical cataracts in mature sows. J Am Vet Med Assoc 173:852.

Severin GA (1974): Diseases of the lens. In Home Study Course in Ophthalmology. American Animal Hospital Association, Mishawaka, IN.

Slatter DH (1976): Unpublished data.

Slatter DH (1985): Ophthalmology, Proceedings No. 74. Postgraduate Committee in Veterinary Science, University of Sydney, Australia.

Slatter DH, et al (1980): Cataracts and depressed galactose-1-phosphate uridyl transferase deficiency in a cuscus (Phalanger maculatus). Aust Vet J 56:141.

Slatter DH, et al (1983): Hereditary cataracts in canaries. J Am Vet Med Assoc 183:872.

Startup FC (1967): Cataract surgery in the dog. J Sm Anim Pract 8:667.

Stephens T (1975): Nutrition of orphan marsupials. Aust Vet J 51:453.

Stephens T, et al (1974): Deficiency of two enzymes of galactose metabolism in kangaroos. Nature 248:524.

Sweating RA (1974): Investigations into natural and experimental infections of freshwater fish by the common eyefluke Diplostomum spathaceum. Parasitology 69:291.

Vierheller RC (1957): Canine cataract surgery. Vet Med 52:487.

von Hippel E (1930): Embryologische Untersuchungen über vererbung angeborener Katarakte über Schichstar des Hundes sowie über eine besondere Form von Kapselkatarakt. Graefes Arch Ophthalmol 124:300. (Cited by Koch, 1972.)

Wills MB, et al (1979): Genetic aspects of lens luxation in the Tibetan terrier. Vet Rec 104:409.

Yakely WL (1978): A study of heritability of cataracts in the American cocker spaniel. J Am Vet Med Assoc 172:814.

Yakely WL, Filby RH (1971): Selenium in the lens of the dog. J Am Vet Med Assoc 158:1561.

Yakely WL, et al (1971): Familial cataracts in the American cocker spaniel. J Am Anim Hosp Assoc 7:127.

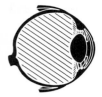

15

Vitreous

ANATOMY AND PHYSIOLOGY
PATHOLOGICAL REACTIONS
ABNORMALITIES AND DISORDERS
    OF THE VITREOUS
SURGICAL PROCEDURES

ANATOMY AND PHYSIOLOGY

The vitreous body occupies about three quarters of the volume of the eye (Fig. 15–1). During development, PRIMARY, SECONDARY, and TERTIARY VITREOUS are formed and laid down (Fig. 15–2) (see also Chap 2). The hyaloid artery, which nourishes the lens during development, atrophies before or soon after birth (Fig. 15–3). For further discussion of vitreous development and the hyaloid vasculature, see Chapter 2.

In the adult eye, the vitreous body has numerous attachments (Fig. 15–4). The vitreous body has the following components:

1. ANTERIOR HYALOID (anterior to the ora ciliaris retinae).

2. POSTERIOR HYALOID (posterior to the ora ciliaris retinae).

3. CORTEX (covering the entire vitreous).

    a. VITREOUS BASE (attachment posterior to the ciliary body; see Fig. 15–4).

    b. PERIPAPILLARY VITREOUS (adjacent to the optic disc).

4. CENTRAL VITREOUS, including CLOQUET'S CANAL. (Cloquet's canal is visible with the biomicroscope.)

Vitreous is a complex gel consisting of

1. Water (99%)

2. Collagen fibrils as a skeleton for the gel (Fig. 15–5)

3. Cells ("hyalocytes")

4. Mucopolysaccharides

Collagen fibrils form a meshwork internal to the retina (the vitreous cortex) and intermingle with the fibers of the internal limiting membrane of the retina. A potential space exists between the vitreous and the inner surface of the retina. Blood and exudates may accumulate in this space if the vitreous and retina

separate, as in SUBHYALOID HEMORRHAGES (see Fig. 16–29C).

Collagen fibrils are present in greater concentrations at the vitreous bases and around the optic disc, where attachment is the strongest. The insertion of these fibrils into the posterior lens capsule from the anterior vitreous face is especially significant in dogs. Removal of the posterior lens capsule, as in intracapsular cataract extraction, results in loss of vitreous unless this attach-

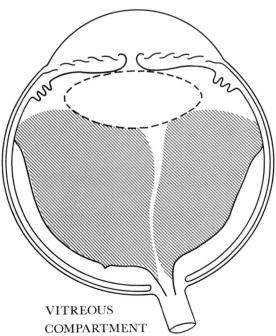

VITREOUS
COMPARTMENT

FIGURE 15–1. The vitreous body (shaded area) occupies the posterior compartment of the eye. (From Fine BS, Yanoff M: Ocular Histology. Harper & Row, New York, 1972.)

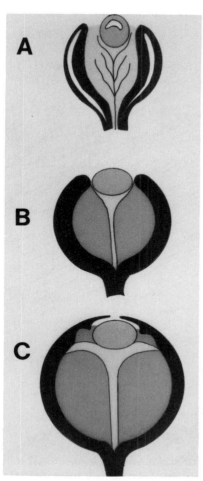

FIGURE 15–2. Stages of vitreous development. A, Primary vitreous and hyaloid vessels. B, Secondary vitreous laid down around the primary vitreous; this becomes the hyaloid canal. C, Tertiary vitreous (lens zonules or ligaments) at the lens periphery. (Courtesy of Dr. G. A. Severin.)

FIGURE 15–4. Relations and attachments of the vitreous body: (1) attachment of orbiculoanterior zonular fibers, (2) attachment of orbiculoposterior zonular fibers, (3) attachment of anterior vitreous face to posterior lens capsule, (4) anterior extremity of Cloquet's canal, (5) anterior-most attachment of vitreous base to mid pars plana, (6) region of vitreous "base," (7) region of diminishing adherence of vitreous base to retinal surface, (8) vitreous-retinal attachment, (9) vitreous-retinal attachment at margin of fovea centralis (absent in domestic animals), (10) attachment of posterior vitreous around optic disc, (11) posterior extremity of Cloquet's canal, (12) cortical vitreous, (13) central vitreous. Density of lines indicates approximate relative degrees of strength of attachment. (From Fine BS, Yanoff M: Ocular Histology. Harper & Row, New York, 1972.)

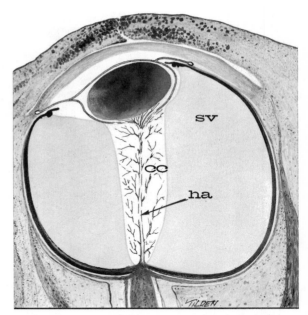

FIGURE 15–3. Early atrophy of the hyaloid vessels. Hyaloid artery (ha) is still attached to the lens and optic disc but is beginning to atrophy. sv = secondary vitreous; cc = Cloquet's (hyaloid) canal. (From Tolentino FI, et al: Vitreoretinal Disorders. WB Saunders Co, Philadelphia, 1976.)

ment has already been broken, e.g., in LENS LUXATION.

The lens sits in a depression in the anterior face of the vitreous—the PATELLAR FOSSA.

Hyalocytes are numerous within the vitreous and are more numerous near the cortex. The functions of these

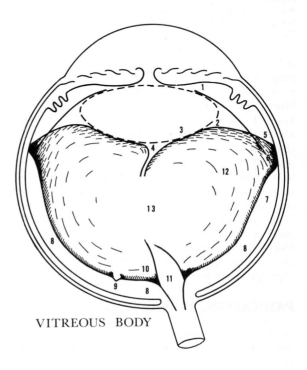

VITREOUS BODY

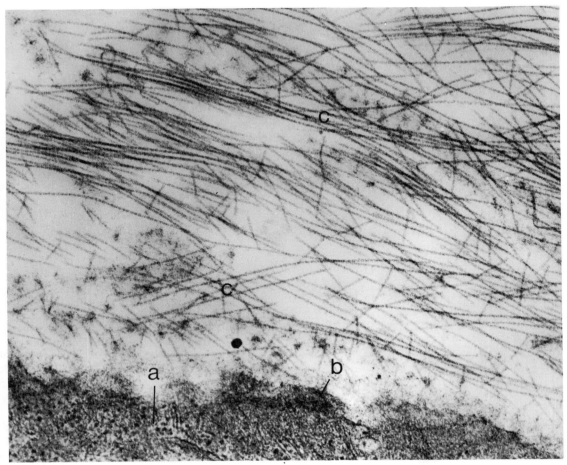

FIGURE 15–5. *The vitreous base near the peripheral retina. The Müller cells (a) have a basement membrane (b) that forms the inner limiting membrane of the retina. The collagen fibrils (c) of the vitreous base form a meshwork internal to the retina. These fibrils join the internal limiting membrane. (From Hogan MJ, et al: Histology of the Human Eye. WB Saunders Co, Philadelphia, 1971.)*

cells are unclear, but they may possess secretory and phagocytic capability as well as potential for reversion to a primitive fibroblast able to form scar tissue. Mucopolysaccharides containing a high proportion of hyaluronic acid are intimately related to the collagen fibrils and hyalocytes and are present in higher concentration where hyalocytes are common. Hyaluronic acid provides the viscoelasticity of the vitreous body.

With the exception of collagens and hyaluronic acid, aqueous and vitreous are similar in composition, with free movement of many substances between them. Water turnover in the vitreous is high (total replacement every 10–15 minutes according to Kinsey et al, 1942). The principles that govern entry of substances, including drugs, from the circulation to the aqueous apply generally to the vitreous also.

PATHOLOGICAL REACTIONS

Because of its simple structure and lack of vascular and lymphatic supply, the range of reactions of vitreous is limited to

1. *Liquefaction.* Because of its high water content, the vitreous may liquefy (*syneresis*) in response to many stimuli (e.g., infection, trauma, senile changes). After liquefaction, the vitreous separates from the retina, encouraging retinal detachment from the underlying pigment epithelium.

2. *Cicatrization.* After inflammation of surrounding tissues or infection, scar tissue may form in the vitreous. These vitreous bands may contract and detach the retina—a "traction detachment," which is relatively uncommon in animals.

3. *Vascularization.* The vitreous has no blood supply, but blood vessels may grow into it (*neovascularization*) from an inflamed or malformed retina. These vessels often are incomplete or fragile and are one source of vitreous hemorrhages, e.g., in the scleral ectasia syndrome in collies.

4. *Infection and inflammation.* Because of its lack of vasculature in the vitreous, inflammation per se does not occur as it does in other tissues. The vitreous is frequently involved in inflammatory disorders of surrounding tissues (e.g., chorioretinitis, optic neuritis,

uveitis). Opacification, hemorrhages, syneresis, and cellular exudates are frequently seen.

Infection of the vitreous by a variety of microorganisms is common and is seen in penetrating injuries, systemic bacteremias, and fungal infections. After the initial infection, the surrounding vitreous liquefies and the infection spreads rapidly. Infections of the vitreous are associated with endophthalmitis (inflammation of all tissues of the eye except the sclera) and often progress to vitreous abscessation. Almost invariably the retina is destroyed in severe vitreous infections. By the time most animal patients are examined, ocular function is usually destroyed.

ABNORMALITIES AND DISORDERS OF THE VITREOUS

Persistent Hyaloid Artery

After birth, the hyaloid artery atrophies after a variable period in different species:

Dog—3 weeks (no longer patent by 17 days)

Cat—8 weeks

Foal—first few days

Calf—4–8 weeks (80% of adults have large remnants)

Sheep—30% in the 1–3-year-old age group have remnants

Persistent hyaloid artery appears ophthalmoscopically, end-on, as a red or white spot anterior to the optic disc, extending a variable distance into the vitreous. In some cases it extends to the lens and must be differentiated from PERSISTENT HYPERPLASTIC PRIMARY VITREOUS (PHPV) and PERSISTENT TUNICA VASCULOSA LENTIS with hemorrhage into the lens itself. The small area of attachment to the posterior lens capsule (actually to the anterior vitreous face) is visible and is known as MITTENDORF'S DOT. In normal rats, the hyaloid artery may bleed into the vitreous during atrophy.

Persistent hyaloid artery must be differentiated from

1. Posterior capsular and subcapsular cataracts—by accurate localization of the opacity. In the golden retriever and Labrador retriever, Mittendorf's dot is differentiated from a cataract by its smaller size. The cataract is much larger and usually has a triangular shape. Mittendorf's dot usually has the anterior remnant of the hyaloid artery attached as a small white "tail," visible biomicroscopically.

2. Normal lens sutures (especially in cattle and horses)—by familiarity with the normal appearance.

3. Vitreous bands—by linear appearance, usually away from Cloquet's canal, and the presence of other signs of injury or inflammation, e.g., syneresis.

4. PHPV—by the more extensive nature of the opacity and by breed incidence.

5. Persistent tunica vasculosa lentis—by the presence of a net-like opacity, especially over the posterior lens capsule.

Persistent hyaloid artery is of more importance in differential diagnosis than as a cause of detrimental visual effects.

Persistent Hyperplastic Primary Vitreous (Fig. 15–6)

This developmental disorder is spontaneous in most dog breeds, and hereditary in the Doberman pinscher, as an autosomal incomplete dominant with variable expression. PHPV in the Doberman has been reported from several countries, including the United States, but is most common in the Netherlands. It also occurs in the Staffordshire bull terrier in the United Kingdom.

There is apparent proliferation of the primary vitreous (see Chap 2) rather than atrophy and failure of the hyaloid artery and tunica vasculosa lentis to atrophy. PHPV is present in young puppies but may not be noticed until later life.

Clinically, PHPV appears as a white or fibrovascular plaque in the posterior pupil near the posterior lens capsule and anterior vitreous. Vessel ingrowth and frank hemorrhage into the vitreous and lens substance, calcium deposits, posterior lenticonus, microphakia, lens colobomata, intralental pigmentation, progressive cataracts, and elongated ciliary processes may also be present.

In the Doberman, a mature cataract has usually developed by 5–6 years of age. The cataract can be removed by either extracapsular extraction or combined intracapsular extraction and anterior vitrectomy, but the prognosis is guarded.

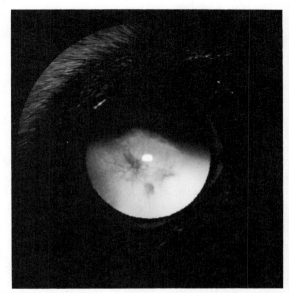

FIGURE 15–6. PHPV in a golden retriever. Note the fibrovascular opacity with patent vessels near the posterior lens capsule.

Vitreous Hemorrhages

Vitreous hemorrhages occur commonly in
1. Ocular trauma
2. Retinitis and retinochoroiditis, e.g., feline infectious peritonitis, blastomycosis, cryptococcosis, coccidioidomycosis
3. Severe posterior uveitis, e.g., Vogt-Koyanagi-Harada–like syndrome, posterior uveitis with effusive retinal detachment in dogs
4. Clotting disorders, e.g., drug-induced or spontaneous thrombocytopenia, autoimmune thrombocytopenia, and occasionally von Willebrand's disease
5. Hypertensive retinopathy in dogs and cats
6. Scleral ectasia syndrome in collies

Whether vitreous hemorrhages resorb depends on the associated pathological changes in adjacent tissues and on the location of the hemorrhage within the vitreous body. Resorption is infrequent in scleral ectasia syndrome, as neovascularization of the vitreous near the retina has occurred with rupture of some of the vessels. In hypertensive retinopathy, resorption may occur if the hypertension is controlled. In retinitis, retinochoroiditis, ocular trauma, and posterior uveitis, resorption is more likely, provided the underlying inflammation and vascular damage resolve. Conservative treatment is recommended with recent hemorrhages.

Vitreous Opacities

Synonym: "Floaters"

Small vitreous opacities are relatively frequent in all species, especially in aged animals. They are distinguished from
Synchysis scintillans
Asteroid hyalosis
Vitreous hemorrhage
Hyaloid artery remnants
Traction bands
Retinal detachment
Vitreous "haze" due to retinitis or optic neuritis

Increased numbers of vitreous floaters may occur after intraocular inflammation, especially in horses. A focal light source with a binocular loupe or direct ophthalmoscope is adequate to demonstrate vitreous opacities. Vitreous haze is common in inflammatory disorders of the posterior globe, and its disappearance is a valuable indicator of the adequacy of treatment. Reduction of this haze often improves vision.

Asteroid Hyalosis

Former synonym: Asteroid hyalitis

Asteroid hyalosis is a degenerative disorder of dogs and horses in which numerous, small, refractile bodies of a calcium-lipid complex occur scattered through the vitreous (Fig. 15–7). Vision is not affected. Asteroid

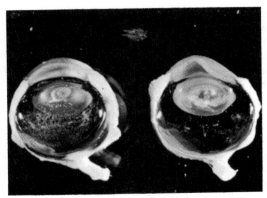

FIGURE 15–7. *Numerous asteroid bodies in the right eye of a 10-year-old Manchester terrier. (From Rubin LF: Atlas of Veterinary Ophthalmoscopy. Lea & Febiger, Philadelphia, 1974.)*

hyalosis occurs spontaneously in older animals and also in association with chronic inflammatory and degenerative ocular disorders.

The condition is distinguished from SYNCHISIS SCINTILLANS because in asteroid hyalosis the refractile bodies move with movement of the head or globe and are *fixed* in position in the vitreous. In synchisis scintillans, the bodies move within the vitreous, which is liquified (VITREOUS SYNERESIS). The opacities in asteroid hyalosis are visible with the ophthalmoscope and may prevent examination of the fundus.

Synchysis Scintillans

In synchysis scintillans, syneresis of the vitreous occurs, and numerous small, yellowish opacities settle in the ventral vitreous. If the head is moved, the particles can be distributed throughout the vitreous, but they eventually settle again. Synchysis scintillans may occur with retinal detachment in horses and retinal degeneration in dogs. The opacities are believed to be cholesterol. In asteroid hyalosis the bodies are attached to the collagen framework of the vitreous, but in synchysis scintillans the crystals are free in a liquefied vitreous. The condition occurs much less frequently than does asteroid hyalosis; it is associated with other ocular disorders; and it is not treated.

Vitreous Mass

DIFFERENTIAL DIAGNOSIS

A mass in the vitreous may be
Retinal detachment
Cataractous or normal, luxated lens
Intraocular neoplasm
Hemorrhage (acute or chronic)
Foreign body
PHPV

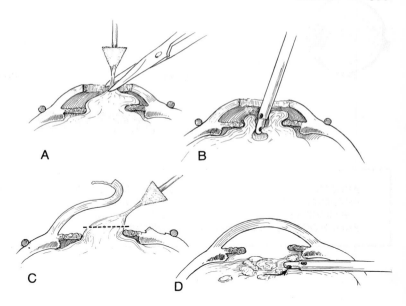

FIGURE 15–8. *Four basic techniques for performing vitrectomy. Choice of technique depends on the individual requirements of the injured eye and the availability of instrumentation. A, The Kasner technique of performing a vitrectomy with cellulose sponge through a trephined corneal defect prior to keratoplasty. B, Vitrectomy performed with a vitreous suction cutter through a corneal laceration. C, Kasner's technique for vitrectomy performed through a large limbal incision after previous repair of a corneal laceration. D, Lensectomy and vitrectomy performed with a vitreous suction cutter introduced through the pars plana. (From Deutsch TA, Feller DB: Paton and Goldberg's Management of Ocular Injuries. WB Saunders Co, Philadelphia, 1985.)*

Persistent hyaloid artery

Traction band or fibrous tissue

Vitreous abscess or endophthalmitis

Parasites (e.g., *Dirofilaria immitis, Toxocara canis* larvae in dogs)

SURGICAL PROCEDURES

Vitrectomy

Vitrectomy is removal of a portion of the vitreous body. The use of vitrectomy in domestic animals is restricted to experienced ophthalmic surgeons in the treatment of ocular injuries and occasionally during intraocular operative procedures. The incidence of postoperative complications is relatively high. Because of the intimate association among the collagen framework of the vitreous body, the lens capsule, and the inner limiting membrane of the retina, removal of large amounts of vitreous carries a significant risk of postoperative retinal detachment. An intact vitreous body maintains retinal attachment.

Careful removal of smaller amounts of vitreous, as in lens removal after luxation, is less dangerous and rarely results in complications (Fig. 15–8). After lens luxation, syneresis is usually present. When syneresis or loss of vitreous is anticipated, use of hyperosmotic agents is advised to reduce the size of vitreous body and subsequent loss.

Numerous sophisticated devices (*vitrectors*) for controlled removal of vitreous are available. In emergency situations, simple manual methods using cellulose sponge and scissors are most commonly used (see Fig. 15–8A–C). When vitreous is removed, it must not remain either between wound edges, as it interferes with wound healing, or in the anterior chamber, as glaucoma may result.

Vitreous Replacement

If larger amounts of vitreous are removed, the physical deficit must be replaced. Many different substances have been used for this, but balanced salt solution and air are the most common temporary replacements. After vitreous is removed, it is replaced by aqueous.

REFERENCES

Duddy JA, et al (1983): Hyaloid patency in neonatal beagles. Am J Vet Res 44:2344.

Fine BS, Yanoff M (1972): Ocular Histology. Harper & Row, New York.

Hogan MJ, et al (1971): Histology of the Human Eye. WB Saunders Co, Philadelphia.

Kinsey VE, et al (1942): Water movement and eye. Arch Ophthalmol 27:242.

Leon A, et al (1986): Hereditary persistent hyperplastic primary vitreous in the Staffordshire bull terrier. J Am Anim Hosp Assoc 22:765.

Peiffer RL, Weintraub BA (1979): Clinical and histopathologic effects of lensectomy and anterior vitrectomy in the canine eye. J Am Anim Hosp Assoc 15:421.

Rubin LF (1963): Asteroid hyalosis in the dog. Am J Vet Res 24:1256.

Rubin LF (1974): Atlas of Veterinary Ophthalmoscopy. Lea & Febiger, Philadelphia.

Saunders LZ, Rubin LF (1974): Ophthalmic Pathology of Animals. S Karger, Basel.

Stades FC (1980): Persistent hyperplastic tunica vasculosa lentis and persistent hyperplastic primary vitreous in Doberman pinschers: Pathological aspects. J Am Anim Hosp Assoc 16:791.

Stades FC (1980): Persistent hyperplastic tunica vasculosa lentis and persistent hyperplastic primary vitreous in Doberman pinschers: Techniques and results of surgery. J Am Anim Hosp Assoc 16:393.

Stades FC (1980): Persistent hyperplastic tunica vasculosa lentis and persistent hyperplastic primary vitreous (PHTVL/PHPV) in 90 closely related Doberman pinschers: Clinical aspects. J Am Anim Hosp Assoc 16:739.

Tolentino FI, et al (1965): Biomicroscopy of the vitreous in collie dogs with vitreous abnormalities. Arch Ophthalmol 73:700.

Tolentino FI, et al (1976): Vitreoretinal Disorders. WB Saunders Co, Philadelphia.

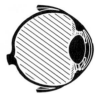

16

Retina

ANATOMY	OPHTHALMOSCOPIC	RETINOPATHY
PHYSIOLOGY AND	VARIATIONS	RETINITIS
BIOCHEMISTRY	CONGENITAL RETINAL	SYSTEMIC DISORDERS
PATHOLOGICAL MECHANISMS	DISORDERS	RETINAL DETACHMENT

The retina is primarily responsible for vision. A knowledge of its function and disorders affecting it is necessary to understand visual disturbances. The retina has been uniquely studied with the ophthalmoscope to show intense details of pathological processes during life and to correlate clinical findings with histopathological studies. This frequently allows specific, accurate diagnosis to the cellular layer involved, during clinical examination.

The retina and optic nerve are derivatives of the forebrain and share similar morphological and physiological characteristics. The retina is connected to the visual cortex by the optic nerve via the optic chiasm, optic tracts, and lateral geniculate body. The photoreceptors of the retina are a complex layer of specialized cells—the RODS and CONES—which contain photopigments that produce chemical energy on exposure to light. This energy is converted to electrical energy, which is transmitted to the visual cortex for interpretation. In domestic animals, some interpretation is known to occur at subcortical levels, since removal of the cortex does not cause complete blindness.

The RETINAL PIGMENT EPITHELIUM furnishes metabolites to receptors and removes the outer ends of the external segments of the photoreceptors, as they are continually produced by the photoreceptors. In cats, dogs, primates, and humans, the two eyes are oriented for binocular vision. This is achieved by the position of the eyes at the front of the head and by the crossing of the axons derived from the ganglion cells of the nasal portions of the retinae at the optic chiasm. Axons from the temporal areas do not cross. In this way, impulses arising from an object seen on the left (in the left visual field), although seen by both eyes, end up in the right optic tract and pass to the right visual cortex. In horses

and cattle, the eyes are positioned more laterally on the head, and more crossing over is necessary in the chiasm.

ANATOMY

The retina consists of a three-neuron sensory unit (Fig. 16-1 and Table 16-1). There are ten layers from the outside toward the center of the vitreous (Fig. 16-2A and B).

Externally the retina is in contact with Bruch's membrane (a much less concrete structure in animals than in humans) and the choriocapillaris. Internally it adjoins the vitreous.

The PIGMENT EPITHELIUM (layer 1) is the outermost layer of the retina. It is pigmented in the nontapetal part of the fundus in domestic animals and gives a homogeneous brown color to this area. It is normally unpigmented in the tapetal fundus and cannot be seen clinically. This allows light to reach the tapetum and

TABLE 16-1. The Three-Neuron Sensory Unit of the Retina

Layer	Neuron
1. Pigment epithelium	
2. Photoreceptor layer (rods and cones)	
3. External limiting membrane	Neuron I
4. Outer nuclear layer	
5. Outer plexiform layer	
6. Inner nuclear layer	Neuron II
7. Inner plexiform layer	
8. Ganglion cell layer	
9. Optic nerve fiber layer	Neuron III
10. Internal limiting membrane	

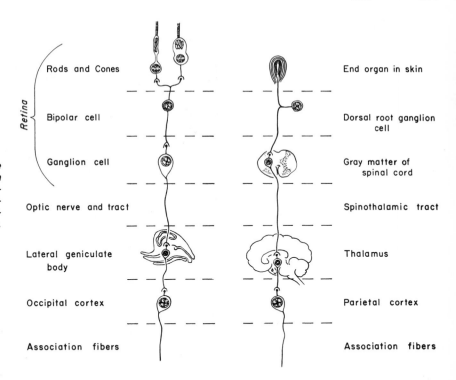

FIGURE 16-1. Comparison of the visual neuronal organization with that of the general sensory system. (From Cogan DG: Neurology of the Visual System. Courtesy of Charles C Thomas, Publisher, Springfield, IL, 1966.)

Figure labels (left):
Rods and Cones
Bipolar cell
Ganglion cell
Optic nerve and tract
Lateral geniculate body
Occipital cortex
Association fibers

Retina

Figure labels (right):
End organ in skin
Dorsal root ganglion cell
Gray matter of spinal cord
Spinothalamic tract
Thalamus
Parietal cortex
Association fibers

be reflected back through the photoreceptor layer, thus allowing the tapetum to act as an amplifier (Fig. 16–3).

Normal function of the pigment epithelium is essential to retinal integrity and function.

The outer limbs of the photoreceptors are embedded in the pigment epithelium (Fig. 16–4). Rod discs are continually synthesized and move from the base of the rod toward the pigment epithelium, at which point they are engulfed by it. The pigment epithelium is intimately associated with biochemical events occurring in the photoreceptors during response to light.

The PHOTORECEPTOR LAYER (layer 2) is composed of outer limbs of rods and cones, which contain the visual pigments within discs that are stacked like a pile of coins (Fig. 16–4). The EXTERNAL LIMITING MEMBRANE (layer 3) is formed by terminal bars joining the cell membranes of rods, cones, and Müller cells. The Müller cell, extending from the external limiting membrane to the internal limiting membrane, is the structural "skeleton" of the retina. It also performs important metabolic functions. Small cell processes pass between the outer limbs of rods and cones (Fig. 16–5). The Müller cell is the largest cell in the retina and extends across nine of the retinal layers, with its nucleus located in the inner nuclear layer. The OUTER NUCLEAR LAYER (layer 4) consists of nuclei of rods and cones and connecting fibers that join the cell to the inner segments

of photoreceptors at the external limiting membrane. The OUTER PLEXIFORM LAYER (layer 5) is composed of axonal extensions of photoreceptors enclosed in cytoplasm of Müller cells. In the inner areas of the plexiform layer, ends of photoreceptors dilate to form SYNAPTIC EXPANSIONS, which connect with bipolar cells.

The INNER NUCLEAR LAYER (layer 6) contains four types of nuclei: (1) bipolar cells, (2) Müller cells, (3) horizontal cells, and (4) amacrine cells. Bipolar cells connect with photoreceptor cells in the outer plexiform layer. Horizontal and amacrine cells are lateral communicating cells. The INNER PLEXIFORM LAYER (layer 7) consists of axons of bipolar, horizontal, and amacrine cells and dendrites of ganglion cells. Numerous synapses occur in the inner plexiform layer between bipolar and ganglion cells, as well as laterally between horizontal and amacrine cells and between bipolar and ganglion cells. These lateral connections between cells coordinate and integrate retinal function.

The GANGLION CELL LAYER (layer 8) consists of cell bodies of large ganglion cells and their dendrites, which connect with the axons of bipolar cells in the preceding inner plexiform layer. The ganglion cell layer is usually one cell thick. Axons of ganglion cells form nerve fiber bundles, which make up the NERVE FIBER LAYER (layer 9), and pass parallel to the retinal surface, to the OPTIC DISC and LAMINA CRIBROSA, at which point they are myelinated to form optic nerve fibers.

These axons next connect in the LATERAL GENICULATE BODY. The innermost layer, the INTERNAL LIMITING MEMBRANE (layer 10), is a basement membrane to which the inner ends of the Müller cells are closely attached.

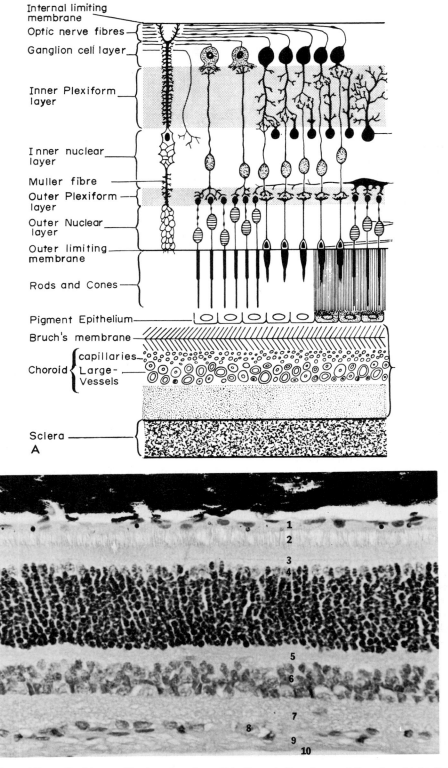

FIGURE 16–2. A, Plan of the retinal layers. The tapetum lies within the capillary layer of the choroid (in the nontapetal area of the fundus only). (From Trevor-Roper PD: The Eye and Its Disorders, 2nd ed. Blackwell, Oxford, 1974.) B, Retinal layers of the dog: 1 = pigment epithelium; 2 = photoreceptor layer; 3 = external limiting membrane; 4 = external nuclear layer; 5 = external plexiform layer; 6 = inner nuclear layer; 7 = inner plexiform layer; 8 = ganglion cell layer; 9 = optic nerve fiber layer; 10 = internal limiting membrane.

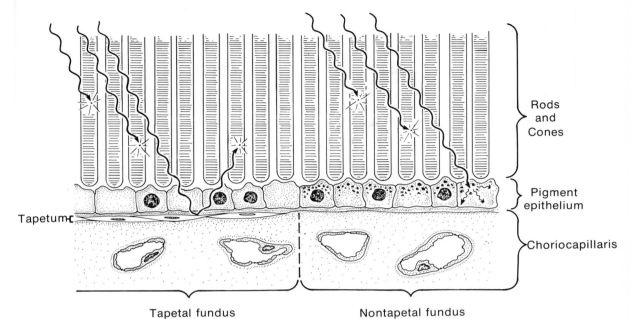

FIGURE 16–3. Function of the tapetum.

Knowledge of retinal structure (Table 16–2) helps explain the clinical appearance and pathogenesis of retinopathies (pathological processes involving the retina), which will be discussed later.

Nuclei of axons in the optic nerve lie in the ganglion cell layer of the retina.

With the exception of birds, domestic animals have no fovea—the small, cone-rich avascular area of the primate retina that is responsible for fine visual discrimination. The peripheral retina in the dog has a higher concentration of rods, and an area temporal to the optic

TABLE 16–2. Summary of Retinal Structure

Layer	Constituents
1. Pigment epithelium	Pigment epithelial cells
2. Photoreceptor layer	Inner and outer limbs of photoreceptors; processes of Müller's cells
3. External limiting membrane	Terminal bars joining rods, cones, and Müller's cells
4. Outer nuclear layer	Connecting fibers, nuclei, and axons of rods and cones
5. Outer plexiform layer	Axons of rods, cones, and horizontal cells
6. Inner nuclear layer	Nuclei of bipolar, Müller's, horizontal, and amacrine cells
7. Inner plexiform layer	Axons of bipolar and amacrine cells
8. Ganglion cell layer	Cell bodies of ganglion cells and their dendrites
9. Nerve fiber layer	Axons of ganglion cells
10. Internal limiting membrane	Basement membrane and footplates of Müller's cells

disc (sometimes called **AREA CENTRALIS**) has a higher cone concentration.

Retinae of domestic animals are classified by their vasculature (Table 16–3). The outer layers are supplied by vessels in the choroid, whereas inner layers are supplied by retinal vessels and their associated capillary network. In horses, retinal vasculature is poorly developed, and the retina depends more on choroidal supply; thus, the consequences of interruption to choroidal supply by trauma or anemia are more serious for the retina. The avian fundus is modified by the presence of a **PECTEN**—a pigmented vascular structure protruding into the vitreous from the retina (Fig. 16–6A and B). The avian retina is usually avascular, and the pecten may have a nutritional role. Unlike in the primate system, retinal vessels of domestic animals arise from the ciliary system and penetrate the sclera in a circle around the optic disc. There is no central retinal artery.

PHYSIOLOGY AND BIOCHEMISTRY

The complete series of events that occurs after light falls on the photoreceptors and results in an impulse in the optic nerve is incompletely understood, although considerable information about various parts of the process are known. The exact relationship between these visual processes and the generation of the electroretinogram (ERG) is even less well understood, although this does not detract from the diagnostic value of electroretinography.

The retina is the most metabolically active tissue in the body, as indicated by its high oxygen consumption. Interruption of either choroidal or retinal vasculature

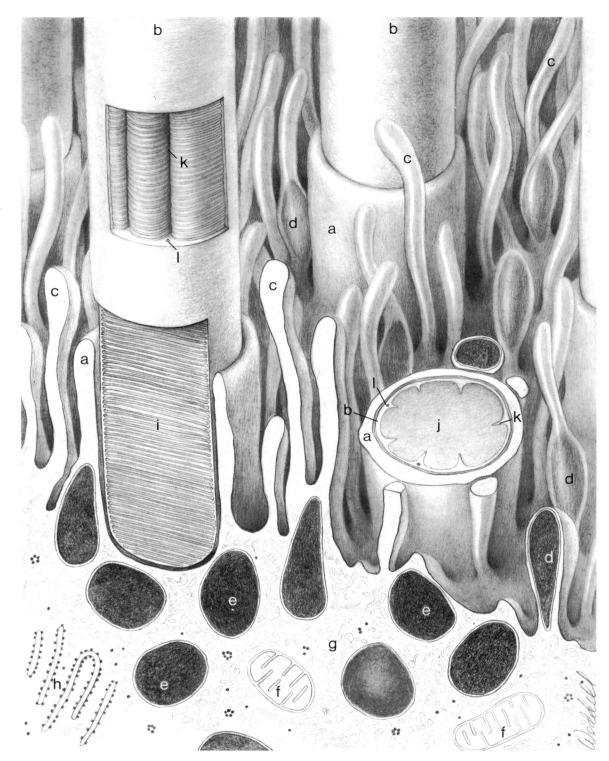

FIGURE 16–4. Relationship between the outer segments of the rods and the pigment epithelium. Thick sheaths (a) of the pigment epithelium enclose the external portions of rod outer segments (b). Numerous finger-like processes (c) occur between the photoreceptors and contain pigment granules (d). The apical portion of the pigment epithelial layer is seen at the bottom. It contains numerous pigment granules (e), mitochondria (f), a well-developed, smooth-surfaced endoplasmic reticulum (g), a poorly developed, rough-surfaced endoplasmic reticulum (h), and scattered free ribosomes. The stacks of rod outer segment discs are shown at i and j, with scalloping at the periphery of the discs (k). Microtubules originating in the basal body of the rod cilium extend externally into the outer segment (l). (From Hogan MJ, et al: Histology of the Human Eye. WB Saunders Co, Philadelphia, 1971.)

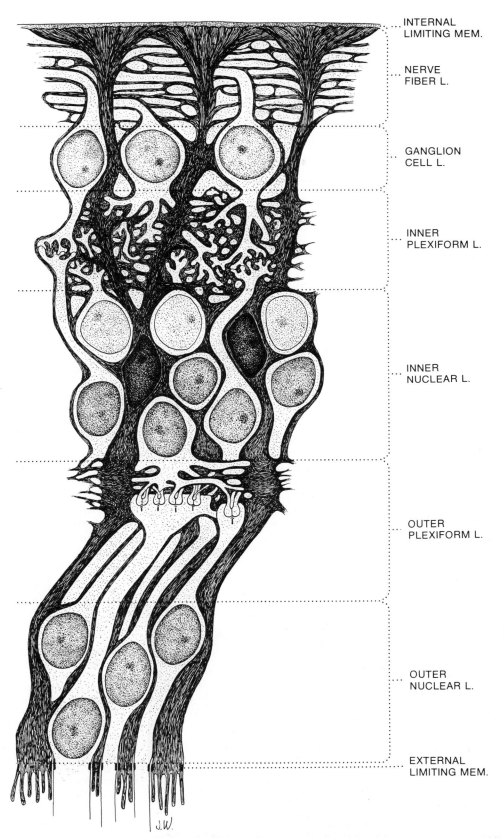

INTERNAL
LIMITING MEM.

NERVE
FIBER L.

GANGLION
CELL L.

INNER
PLEXIFORM L.

INNER
NUCLEAR L.

OUTER
PLEXIFORM L.

OUTER
NUCLEAR L.

EXTERNAL
LIMITING MEM.

FIGURE 16–5. *Structure of the Müller cell in nine of the ten retinal layers. (From Hogan MJ, et al: Histology of the Human Eye. WB Saunders Co, Philadelphia, 1971.)*

TABLE 16–3. Classification of Retinal Vascular Patterns

Type	Features	Examples
Holangiotic	The whole retina receives a direct blood supply, either from a central artery or from cilioretinal arteries that emerge as a single trunk or as several branches from or around the optic disc	Dog, cat, sheep, cow, goat, rat, primates, mouse
Merangiotic	Part of the retina is supplied with vessels	Rabbit
Paurangiotic	The vessels are minute and extend only a short distance from the disc	Horse, guinea pig
Anangiotic	Retina is devoid of blood vessels	Beaver, chinchilla, porcupine, armadillo, sloth, bat

Leber T: Die Circulations und Ernahrungs verhaltnisse des Auges. *In* Von Graetes A, Saemisch T (eds.): Handbuch der gesameten Augenheilkunde, vol 2, 2nd ed. Engelmann, Leipzig, 1903.

quickly results in ischemia and severe, irreversible loss of function, despite reserves of glycogen within Müller cells. (The clinical consequence is that retinal detachment must be treated early to avoid loss of function. Unfortunately, this is rarely possible in animals.) The blood-retina barrier is formed by the capillary endothelial cells and their basement membrane, and this barrier limits the passage of substances into the retina. There is little extracellular space in the retina, and transport of solutes from capillaries occurs via Müller cells and astrocytes.

Rods and Cones

Outer limbs of rods and cones contain photopigments that are sensitive to light and change when illuminated by it. Because rods and cones have differing functions (Table 16–4), the pigments in each are different, and they also vary among species. Rods are much more sensitive than cones and function in low illumination (**SCOTOPIC VISION**), for example, at night. They are incapable of fine visual discrimination and are located in larger numbers in the peripheral retina. Some nocturnal animals have pure rod retinae with no cones.

Cones are less sensitive and function predominantly at high levels of illumination (**PHOTOPIC VISION**).

Although cones, like rods, are present throughout the retina, they are present in greater concentration in a central area temporal to the optic disc. Cones give greater visual discrimination than do rods, and in some species they contain pigments for color vision.

Some of the difference in sensitivity between rods and cones is accounted for by **RETINAL SUMMATION**. For instance, in the cat retina there are approximately 130 million photoreceptors but only 1 million axons in the optic nerve. Some axons have more than one photoreceptor connected to them. By converging large numbers of photoreceptors in a particular area onto a single bipolar cell, and by converging several bipolar cells onto a ganglion cell, amplification occurs at the expense of fine discrimination. Maximum visual discrimination and minimal sensitivity occur when one photoreceptor is connected to one bipolar cell and then to one ganglion cell (Figs. 16–7 and 16–8).

Whether or not domestic animals have color vision is not clear-cut. All of the common domestic species have both rods and cones, but this may merely reflect adaptation for vision in high and low light levels. Stimulation experiments show different electroretinographic responses, as well as impulses in the optic nerve for different-colored lights. On the basis of objective and subjective experiments, it is probable that dogs

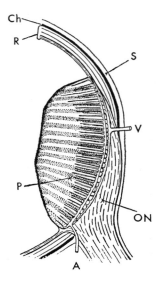

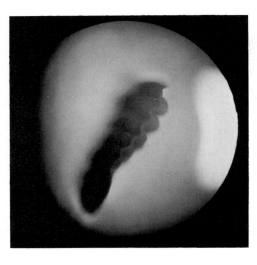

FIGURE 16–6. A, Structure of the pecten, showing its relationship to the entrance of the optic nerve and its vascular connections. A = supplying artery, which sends a branch to each fold; Ch = choroid; ON = optic nerve; P = pecten; R = retina; S = sclera; V = efferent vein, which receives a branch from each angle of the fold. (Reproduced by permission from Duke-Elder S: System of Ophthalmology, Vol 1. St. Louis, 1958, The CV Mosby Co.) B, Ophthalmoscopic view of the fundus of a barn owl (Strix flammea).

RODS   **CONES**

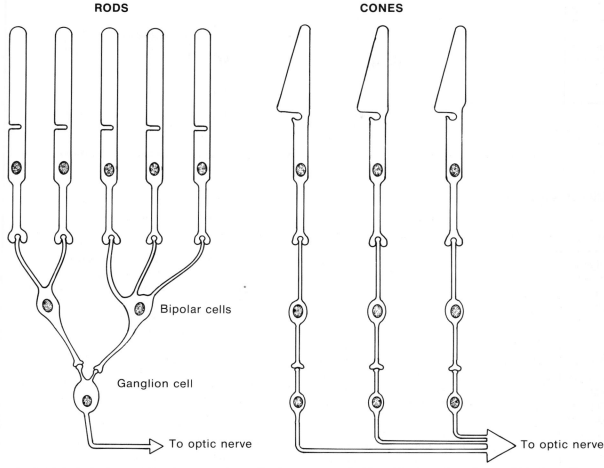

Bipolar cells

Ganglion cell

To optic nerve   To optic nerve

FIGURE 16–7. Retinal summation: Large numbers of rods are connected to a bipolar cell, and several bipolar cells are connected to a ganglion cell.

FIGURE 16–8. Retinas of diurnal and nocturnal animals of two related species. The different ratios of visual-cell types call for different relative numbers of the various conductive-cell types, leading to varying degrees of summation in the optic nerve fibers and producing characteristic differences in the relative thickness of the retinal layers. (Reproduced by permission from Duke-Elder S: System of Ophthalmology, Vol 1. St. Louis, 1958, The CV Mosby Co. Drawing by Gordon Walls.)

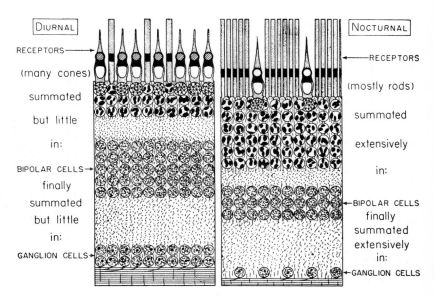

TABLE 16–4. Comparison of Photoreceptor Function

Rod	Cone
High sensitivity	Low sensitivity
Low visual discrimination	High visual discrimination
No color differentiation	Color differentiation
Predominate in peripheral retinal areas	Predominate in central retinal areas

and cats have some color vision, although whether it modifies behavior is uncertain. Cattle and sheep are probably colorblind. Birds possess a highly developed color sense, as well as fine visual discrimination.

Visual Pigments

Substances that absorb parts of the visible spectrum are termed *pigments.* Their color is due to the wavelengths they reflect, not to what they absorb. Visual pigments in the photoreceptors absorb a range of wavelengths, with each pigment having a peak absorption at a particular wavelength. This peak is known as the absorption maximum (λ), or lambda max (Fig. 16–9).

Visual pigment molecules consist of a *carotenoid portion* (derivative of vitamin A) combined with a protein, or *opsin* (Fig. 16–10). There are four visual pigments thought to account for light absorption in animals: (1) rhodopsin, (2) iodopsin, (3) porphyropsin, and (4) cyanopsin, and all are combinations of rod and cone opsins with the carotenoids *retinal$_1$* and *retinal$_2$.*

Because rhodopsin ("visual purple"), which consists of retinal$_1$ and rod opsin, is the pigment about which most is known, it is used as the example of photopigments, all of which are believed to have similar properties.

Photochemistry

Vitamin A may be modified at one of three sites, which are shown in Figure 16–11. If the end group at

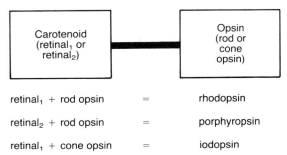

retinal$_1$ + rod opsin	=	rhodopsin
retinal$_2$ + rod opsin	=	porphyropsin
retinal$_1$ + cone opsin	=	iodopsin

FIGURE 16–10. *General structure of a photopigment molecule.*

A in Figure 16–11 is an alcohol, the compound formed is *retinol;* if the end group is an aldehyde, the compound formed is *retinal.* If the side chain of retinol or retinal is *straight,* the compound is called *all-trans* (referring to the spatial variation of molecular orientation known as *cis-trans* isomerism). If the side chain is twisted at *B* (carbon atom No. 11 of the main chain), the compound is called 11-*cis* retinal or 11-*cis* retinol. If the C–C bond at *C* is saturated, the compound is designated retinal$_2$ or retinol$_2$. Most vertebrate retinae contain 11-*cis* retinal$_1$.

When a photon of light strikes a rhodopsin molecule containing 11-*cis* retinal$_1$, it forms unstable *prelumirhodopsin* and enters a series of reactions resulting in the more stable all-*trans* retinal$_1$ plus opsin (Fig. 16–12). Alternatively, once the all-*trans* retinal$_1$ is free of opsin, it can be isomerized back to the 11-*cis* retinal$_1$ to reform rhodopsin (Fig. 16–13), or it can be reduced to all-*trans* retinol and become esterified. The esters are stored in the pigment epithelium until required for dark adaptation. After all-*trans* ester has been de-esterified, oxidized, and isomerized, it is available for spontaneous regeneration of rhodopsin in the dark.

Vitamin A in the eye turns over very slowly with other body stores of vitamin A, and only a small proportion of ingested vitamin A reaches the eye.

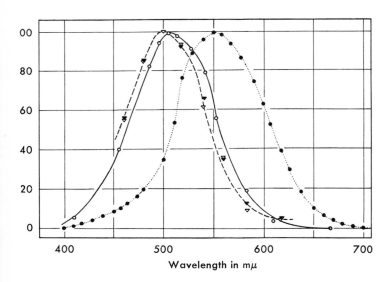

FIGURE 16–9. *Visibility curves and absorption spectrum of rhodopsin.* Broken line and triangles: *Absorption spectrum of rhodopsin.* Open circles and continuous line: *Relative effectiveness of spectrum at lowest intensities.* Filled circles and dotted line: *Effectiveness of spectrum at high intensities of illumination.* (From Moses RA: Adler's Physiology of the Eye, 5th ed. WB Saunders Co, Philadelphia, 1970. Modified from Hecht.)

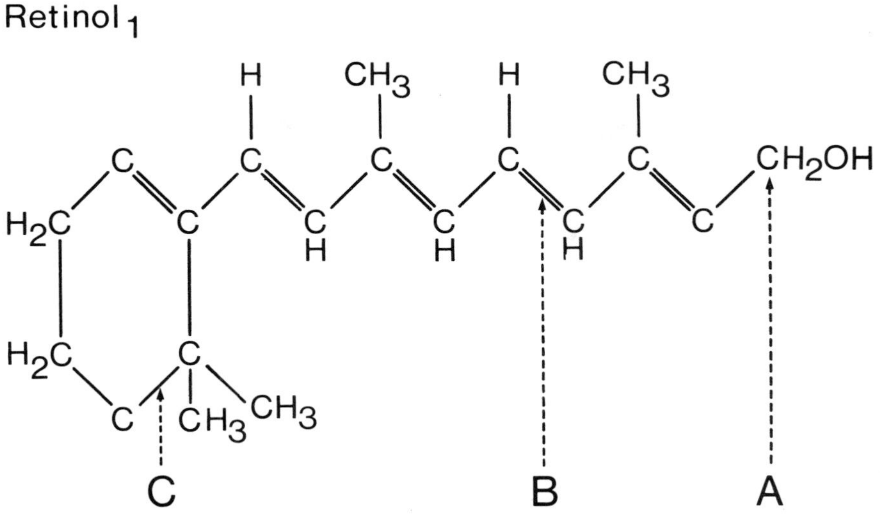

Retinol₁

FIGURE 16–11. The structure of vitamin A. The A, B, and C sites are areas in which structural changes important in photoreception are made. (From Hogan MJ, et al: Histology of the Human Eye. WB Saunders Co, Philadelphia, 1971.)

FIGURE 16–12. Intermediates in bleaching and regeneration of rhodopsin: Wavy arrows indicate photoreactions; straight arrows indicate thermal ("dark") reactions. Interrelationships of pararhodopsin with final products of bleaching are poorly understood. (From Wald G: Molecular basis of visual excitation. Science 162:230, 1968. © Nobel Foundation 1968.)

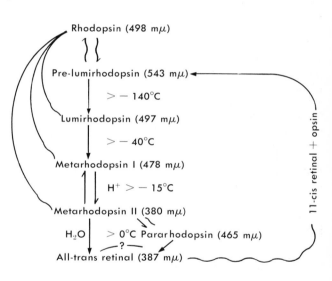

Rhodopsin (498 mμ)

Pre-lumirhodopsin (543 mμ)

$> - 140°C$

Lumirhodopsin (497 mμ)

$> - 40°C$

Metarhodopsin I (478 mμ)

$H^+ > - 15°C$

Metarhodopsin II (380 mμ)

H_2O | $> 0°C$ Pararhodopsin (465 mμ)

$- ? -$

All-trans retinal (387 mμ)

11-cis retinal + opsin

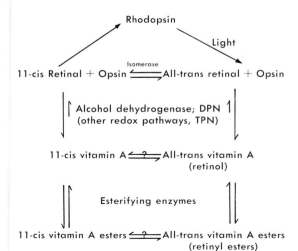

Rhodopsin

Light

11-cis Retinal + Opsin ⇌ (Isomerase) All-trans retinal + Opsin

Alcohol dehydrogenase; DPN (other redox pathways, TPN)

11-cis vitamin A ⇌ —?— All-trans vitamin A (retinol)

Esterifying enzymes

11-cis vitamin A esters ⇌ —?— All-trans vitamin A esters (retinyl esters)

FIGURE 16–13. All-trans retinal may be isomerized to reform rhodopsin, or it may be reduced to all-trans retinol. Following esterification it can be stored in the retinal pigment epithelium until needed for dark adaptation. (From Wald G: Molecular basis of visual excitation. Science, 162:230, 1968. © Nobel Foundation 1968.)

Vitamin A deficiency does not affect the eye until other body stores are depleted.

Vitamin A deficiency causes night blindness (NYCTALOPIA), retinal optic atrophy, and convulsions in cattle, and microphthalmia and nyctalopia in the offspring of deficient sows.

Administration of vitamin A has no therapeutic value for progressive degenerative retinal diseases in dogs that are not deficient in it and does not improve visual function in normal animals.

The first electrical event after exposure to light is the EARLY RECEPTOR POTENTIAL, which may be due to isomerization of all-*trans* retinal. How this is amplified and propagated to the optic nerve is unknown.

Dark Adaptation

Dark adaptation is the transition of the retina from the light-adapted (photopic) to the dark-adapted (scotopic) state—sensitivity increases about 100,000 times. *Visual acuity* is greatest in the photopic state, whereas *sensitivity* is maximal in the scotopic state. Maximal sensitivity is reached after 30–40 minutes, depending on the light level before adaptation began. In making the transition from light to dark, the brighter the pre-existing light level, the longer it takes the eye to reach maximal sensitivity, presumably because rhodopsin stores are lower after exposure to bright light and have to be reconstituted from stores in the pigment epithelium.

Dark adaptation in domestic animals is measured by (1) an increase in amplitude of the ERG with dark adaptation (Fig. 16–14) and (2) a decrease in the stimulus required to produce a given ERG amplitude in the dark with adaptation.

Electroretinography

The ERG is the electrical response recorded when the retina is stimulated by light (Fig. 16–15). It is used primarily to assess retinal function (assuming that pathways from the retina to the visual cortex are intact) in animals affected with visual disorders. Even in the presence of a corneal opacity or cataract, sufficient light reaches the retina to cause a response provided that the retina is functional. Electroretinography is useful in the following circumstances:

1. Routine preoperative evaluation of retinal function before cataract extraction, which is necessary because of the common concurrence of progressive retinal degeneration (PRD) or progressive retinal atrophy (PRA) with simultaneous cataract. If the opposite fundus can be seen ophthalmoscopically, the test is unnecessary.

2. Diagnosis of retinal disorders in which no ophthalmoscopic abnormalities are evident, for example, early PRD, hemeralopia in Alaskan malamutes.

3. Differentiation of photoreceptor abnormalities—for example, rod-cone dystrophy in Norwegian elkhounds, cone dysfunction in Alaskan malamutes.

4. Investigation of unexplained visual loss in which retinal lesions are not visible, for example, sudden acquired retinal degeneration in dogs.

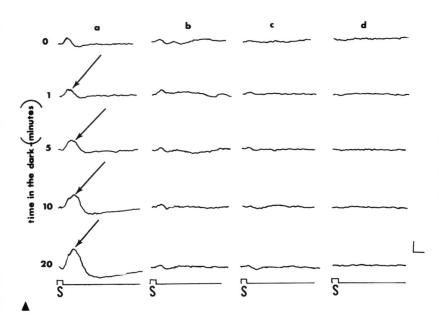

FIGURE 16–14. Increasing amplitude of the b-wave (arrow) in response to flashes of light during dark adaptation in a normal canine. (From Aguirre GD, Rubin LF: The early diagnosis of rod dysplasia in the Norwegian elkhound. J Am Vet Med Assoc 159:429, 1971.)

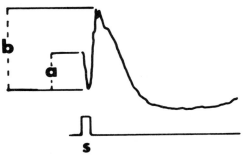

FIGURE 16–15. ERG of a normal dark-adapted canine in response to a 1/50-second white light flash. The downward deflection (a) is the a wave, which is followed by an upward (positive) deflection (b), the b wave. (From Rubin LF: Atlas of Veterinary Ophthalmoscopy. Lea & Febiger, Philadelphia, 1974.)

Electroretinography is a summed response and cannot detect focal retinal lesions.

Parameters that are measured in electroretinography include (1) a and b wave amplitude to red, blue, and white light (Fig. 16–18); (2) a and b wave latency (Figs. 16–16 and 16–17) to red, blue, and white light; and (3) flicker fusion frequency (Fig. 16–18).

Flicker fusion frequency is the frequency of stimulation beyond which individual ERG responses are not recorded, and it depends on whether the rods or cones are functioning under the prevailing levels of illumination. Although attempts have been made to relate different parts of the ERG wave to different structures within the retina (e.g., the a wave to the rods and cones, the b wave to the inner nuclear layer, and the c wave to the pigment epithelium), such attempts are an oversimplification of a complex process that is incompletely understood. For clinical purposes, the ERG is best considered a mass response of the entire retina to light; for definitive determination of defects in specific layers, electron microscopy is required. Rod and cone defects can be differentiated by electroretinography.

The ERG is a test of retinal function, not of vision.

Large focal lesions within the retina, for example, focal scars, may not affect the ERG.

Disadvantages of electroretinography include the expense of the equipment required (Fig. 16–19), the specialized training required for operation of the equipment and interpretation of the results, and the time required to perform the procedure. Electroretinography remains a valuable diagnostic tool for the veterinary ophthalmologist. A summary of electroretinographic alterations in various ocular disorders is given in Table 16–5.

PATHOLOGICAL MECHANISMS

Only mechanisms relevant to common retinal disorders, or those that can be seen ophthalmoscopically, are considered here. For more detailed discussion, readers are referred to standard texts of ophthalmic pathology.

Ischemia

The retina has a high metabolic rate and precarious bipartite blood supply from the choriocapillaris and the retinal vasculature, and it is particularly susceptible to interruptions in blood supply. After hypoxia begins, death of retinal cells follows rapidly, intra- and extracellular edema occurs, neural elements disintegrate, and atrophy and gliosis of the retina result. Many disease processes (e.g., inflammation, retinal detachment, increased intraocular pressure, decreased orbital circulation following trauma) may result in decreased circulation and tissue hypoxia.

FIGURE 16–16. ERG parameters. (From Howard DR, et al: J Am Anim Hosp Assoc 9:219, 1973.)

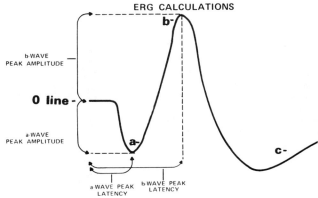

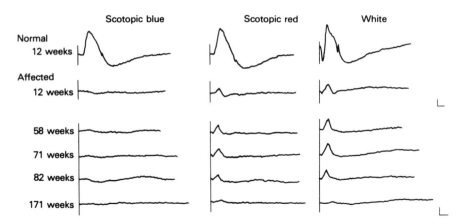

	Scotopic blue	Scotopic red	White
Normal 12 weeks			
Affected 12 weeks			
58 weeks			
71 weeks			
82 weeks			
171 weeks			

FIGURE 16–17. The ERG recorded from dark-adapted normal dogs and rod dysplasia–affected Norwegian elkhounds of different ages in response to scotopically balanced blue and red light stimuli and white light. In the affected dogs, the scotopic blue stimulus fails to elicit a recordable response. The scotopic red and white stimuli elicit low-amplitude, short-latency responses. At 171 weeks of age the peak latency of these responses has increased. Vertical black lines denote onset of 20-ms-duration light stimulus. Vertical calibration marks, 100 μV: horizontal calibration marks, 50 ms. Calibration marker at lower right applies only to the responses recorded at 171 weeks of age. (From Aguirre GD: Retinal degenerations in the dog: I. Rod dysplasia. Exp Eye Res 26:233, 1978.)

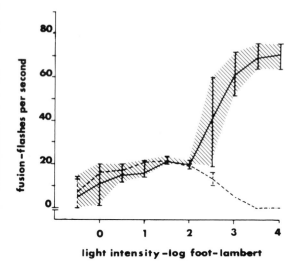

FIGURE 16–18. The flicker fusion response curve from normal control dogs and Alaskan malamutes with hemeralopia. Black line = controls; dashed line = malamutes with hemeralopia. (From Aguirre GD, Rubin LF: The electroretinogram in dogs with inherited cone degeneration. Invest Ophthalmol Vis Sci 14:840, 1975.)

FIGURE 16–19. Equipment for electroretinography Left to right: High-gain amplifier and chart recorder, oscilloscope, flash generator, and flash tube. In diagnostic electroretinography, individual responses are measured, and computer averaging techniques are unreliable.

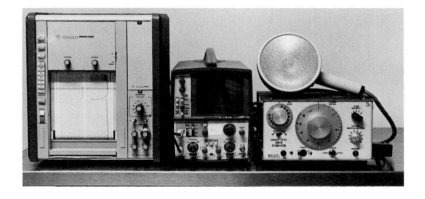

TABLE 16–5. Electroretinographic Findings in Selected Ocular Disorders

Disease	ERG Findings	Comments
Cataract	ERG slightly reduced in amplitude in animals with a normal retina	ERG very important in determining whether retina is normal or severely diseased Used before cataract extraction
Complete corneal edema	ERG normal to slightly reduced in amplitude in animals with a normal retina	ERG very important in determining whether retina is normal or severely diseased
Retinal detachment	ERG usually absent Small-amplitude a wave and no b wave seen in early cases	ERG important in cases in which retina cannot be seen
Cortical blindness	ERG normal	ERG useful in differentiating retinal from cortical blindness ERG examination must evaluate rod and cone function
Optic neuritis and optic atrophy	ERG normal	Clinical signs and ophthalmoscopy often sufficient ERG rarely necessary except in retrobulbar neuritis
Glaucoma	ERG normal in very early cases if pressure not markedly elevated ERG absent in later cases	In early cases of glaucoma causes ganglion cell loss with no change in ERG In late cases there is extensive retinal degeneration and absent ERG ERG of *no use* in prognosis for glaucoma
Hemeralopia (day blindness) in Alaskan malamutes	Rod ERG normal; cone ERG absent	ERG essential for definitive diagnosis of hemeralopia
Feline retinal degeneration due to taurine deficiency	Rod ERG normal; cone ERG depressed or absent	Diagnosed ophthalmoscopically; ERG only indicates widespread cone dysfunction that is not visible ophthalmoscopically
Congenital nyctalopia (night blindness) in appaloosas	Decreased b wave amplitude and implicit time	Clinical findings usually sufficient for diagnosis ERG confirms rod abnormality
PRD type I	ERG in early cases	ERG most useful in identifying those animals that will develop PRD months to years before the clinical disease is evident
Poodle	Rod and cone ERG present but abnormal	
Norwegian elkhound	Rod ERG absent; cone ERG normal	
Irish setter	Rod ERG absent; cone ERG present but abnormal	
PRD type II	ERG may be normal until advanced stages	Ophthalmoscopy sufficient for diagnosis; ERG of *no value*
Sudden acquired retinal degeneration	ERG amplitude reduced or absent	ERG essential for diagnosis; ophthalmoscopy nonrevealing

Modified from Aguirre GD: Electroretinography in veterinary ophthalmology. J Am Anim Hosp Assoc 9:234, 1973; and others.

Reparative Processes

As with other neural tissues, the retina has limited or no regenerative capacity. Changes in photoreceptor and neural elements are almost irreversible, limiting the scope of treatment for many disorders to prevention of further damage. Repetitive stimuli thus result in cumulative damage until vision is affected.

Retina–Optic Nerve Interaction

Diseases that result in severe and widespread retinal lesions, especially of the ganglion cell layer, eventually also cause lesions of the axons of these cells in the optic nerve—the clinical disorder of OPTIC ATROPHY. This is believed to be due to interruptions of *axoplasmic* *flow*—the flow of solutes along the axon both toward and away from the cell body. Lesions of the photoreceptors eventually result in loss of ganglion cells and intermediate layers, with optic atrophy. This transynaptic degeneration is less marked in the descending direction (toward the eye). Chronic lesions of the optic nerve cause degeneration or atrophy of the nerve fiber and ganglion cell layers.

Interactions with Choroid and Vitreous

Infectious processes in the vitreous—for example, abscess—almost always result in severe retinal damage. Inflammation of the choroid frequently extends to involve the retina and vice versa. Common examples are hematogenous bacterial and viral infections of the choroid (colibacillosis, bovine malignant catarrhal fever) that extend to the retina. Neurotrophic viral retinitis—for example, canine distemper—may proceed from retina to choroid. Neoplastic disorders—for example, lymphosarcoma—of the choroid frequently extend to the retina. The consequences of many of these disorders are often much more devastating to the retina than to the tissue from which they arose.

Gliosis

In many acute, severe insults, neural elements of the retina may be lost early, but the more resistant glial Müller cells survive and may proliferate to fill spaces left by neural cells. The end stage of many chronic retinal disorders is often a glial scar replacing the retina (Figs. 16–20 and 16–21).

Reactions of Pigment Epithelium

Reactions of pigment epithelium are frequently visible ophthalmoscopically. After a pathological insult, the two most common reactions are atrophy and proliferation, with the two sometimes occurring together. If only atrophy of the pigment epithelium occurs over the tapetum, it is not readily apparent, but if it occurs in the nontapetal area, the affected cells are visible as a depigmented or pale area (Figs. 16–22 and 16–23).

When proliferation of pigment epithelial cells occurs, with either hyperplasia or hypertrophy and increased amounts of pigment, the results are visible ophthalmoscopically as focal areas of increased pigmentation. These areas are visible in both tapetal and nontapetal areas (Figs. 16–24, 16–25, and 16–26). Hypertrophy and hyperplasia of pigment epithelial cells are usually accompanied by loss of adjacent rods and cones.

Perivascular Cuffing

In inflammatory and neoplastic diseases, inflammatory cells frequently accumulate around retinal vessels, as they do elsewhere in the nervous system (see Fig.

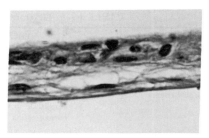

FIGURE 16–20. Glial band replacing the retina after chronic PRD in a dog.

16–26). This vasculitis or "perivascular cuffing" is visible as a white or gray sheath around vessels, which sometimes obscures their color (Fig. 16–27).

Primary Photoreceptor Disease

Many disorders in the group of "retinal atrophies" primarily affect rods and cones. These disorders frequently progress to atrophy of the entire retina, leaving a glial scar and causing similar clinical signs.

Gradual vascular attenuation in atrophic retinal disease is *secondary* to atrophy.

Increased Tapetal Reflectivity

Retinal atrophy of any cause results in increased reflection of light from the tapetum when viewed ophthalmoscopically. If the tapetum and transparent retina are compared with a mirror (tapetum) and curtain (retina), when the curtain is removed (retinal atrophy), reflectivity is increased (Fig. 16–28).

Retinal Hemorrhages[1]

Hemorrhages into and around the retina occur in many diseases and conditions, for example, anemia,

---

1. See also Chap 19.

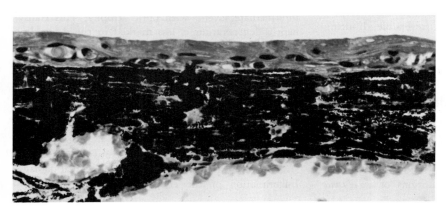

FIGURE 16–21. Glial band replacing the retina in chronic glaucoma.

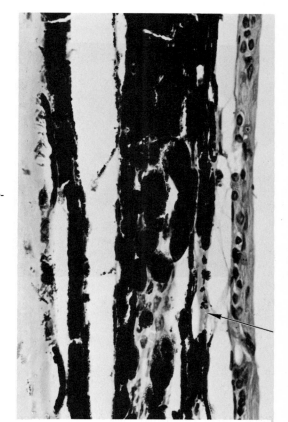

FIGURE 16–22. Focal loss of pigment (arrow) from pigment epithelial cells in the nontapetal area in a dog with PRD.

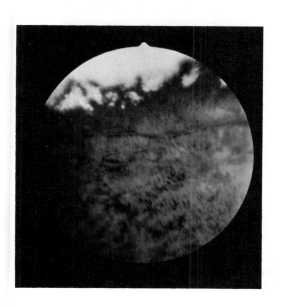

FIGURE 16–23. Ophthalmoscopic appearance of paler "punched-out" areas of depigmentation of the pigment epithelium in the nontapetal fundus in PRD.

FIGURE 16–24. Hypertrophy of pigment epithelial cells in canine pigment epithelial hypertrophy (central progressive retinal atrophy [PRA]; PRD type II).

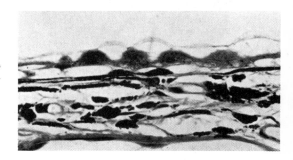

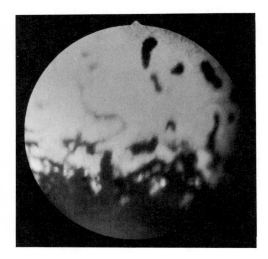

FIGURE 16–25. Focal areas of pigment epithelial hypertrophy over the tapetum in pigment epithelial dystrophy (PRD type II).

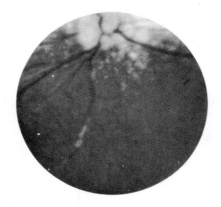

FIGURE 16–26. Perivascular cuffing of inflammatory cells around a retinal vessel. (From Rubin LF: Atlas of Veterinary Ophthalmoscopy. Lea & Febiger, Philadelphia, 1974.)

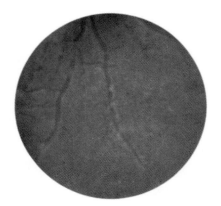

FIGURE 16–27. Grayish-white sheathing around retinal veins. (From Rubin LF: Atlas of Veterinary Ophthalmoscopy. Lea & Febiger, Philadelphia, 1974.)

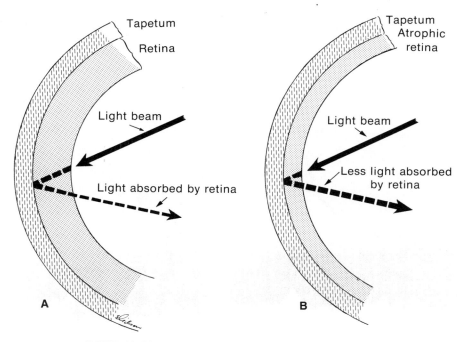

FIGURE 16–28. *Pathogenesis of increased tapetal reflectivity.*

o,p′-DDD or ethylene glycol toxicity, ehrlichiosis, monoclonal gammopathy in dogs, and thromboembolic meningoencephalitis in cattle. It is possible to localize the position of these hemorrhages ophthalmoscopically to the layer involved (Fig. 16–29).

OPHTHALMOSCOPIC VARIATIONS

Before pathological processes can be recognized, common variations in fundus appearance must be appreciated. Detailed fundus diagnosis is the province of the veterinary ophthalmologist, but familiarity with common, normal fundus variations is essential so that they can be recognized and distinguished from pathological processes by the general practitioner.

Unpigmented Nontapetal Fundus

Lack of pigment in the pigment epithelial cells of the nontapetal retina is a common variation (Plate IV*A* and *B*) and is frequently seen in subalbinotic or color-dilute animals, e.g., Siamese cat, appaloosa, merled collie. The larger choroidal vessels are visible through the retina as numerous parallel red stripes, the so-called tigroid fundus. Note that the much finer retinal vessels are visible overlying the choroidal vasculature. This type of normal fundus *must not be confused with hemorrhage.*

Tapetal Aplasia

Absence of the tapetum is common in Dalmatians and occurs sporadically in other breeds (Plate IV*C, D,* and *E*). In toy breeds, the tapetum is frequently small. There exists an inherited abnormality of the tapetum in Siamese cats, in whom the tapetum has a lower reflectivity because of disruption of the tapetal rods, and a lower zinc content has been reported. A similar recessively inherited tapetal abnormality occurs in the beagle. The normal pig has no tapetum. The nontapetal fundus is often unpigmented in association with tapetal agenesis.

Tapetal Degeneration

A recessively inherited tapetal degeneration occurs in the beagle. Degeneration begins at 21 days postpartum, is complete by 1–2 years, and can be recognized ophthalmoscopically. Retinal structure is normal. Tapetal degeneration also occurs in cats with Chediak-Higashi syndrome.

Pigment Over the Tapetum

Pigment in the normally unpigmented pigment epithelium in the tapetal area occasionally occurs and is differentiated from pathological pigmentation (Plate IV*F*). The pigmented areas are more frequent at the tapetal-nontapetal junction (Plate IV*G*).

A DEEP INTRARETINAL HEMORRHAGES

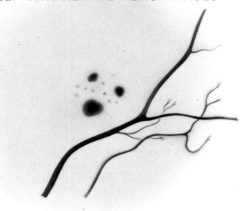

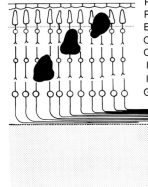

Pigment epithelium
Photoreceptors
External limiting membrane
Outer nuclear layer
Outer plexiform layer
Inner nuclear layer
Inner plexiform layer
Ganglion cell layer

Nerve fiber layer

Internal limiting membrane

Vitreous

B SUPERFICIAL INTRARETINAL HEMORRHAGES

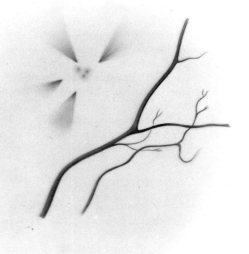

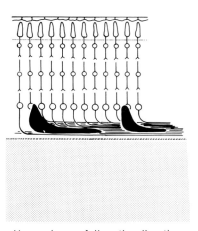

Hemorrhages follow the direction of the nerve fibers, giving a "brush- or "flame"-shaped margin

FIGURE 16–29. *Retinal hemorrhages.* A, *Deep intraretinal hemorrhage.* B, *Superficial intraretinal hemorrhage.*

C PRERETINAL (SUBHYALOID) HEMORRHAGES
(''keel-shaped'' with red cells sinking inferiorly)

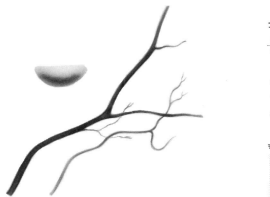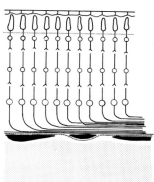

D SUBRETINAL HEMORRHAGES
(usually large and dark in color)

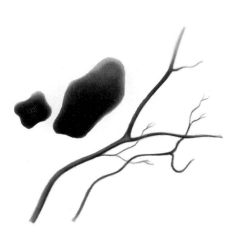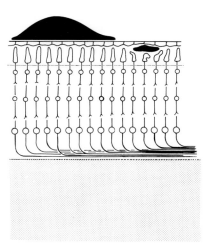

FIGURE 16–29 Continued C, *Preretinal (subhyaloid) hemorrhage.* D, *Subretinal hemorrhage.*

Variations in Color

Color variations in the tapetum are common in all species. In newborn pups, the fundus is blue (Plate IV*H*) until about 4 months of age, when the tapetum and adult colors appear.

Myelination of Nerve Fiber Layer

Myelination of optic nerve fibers usually stops at the optic disc. Occasionally, myelination spreads into the nerve fiber layer of the retina, appearing as white fan-shaped streaks radiating from the optic disc. These are differentiated clinically from papilledema and optic neuritis (see Table 17–12).

CONGENITAL RETINAL DISORDERS

Retinal Dysplasia

(For details of scleral ectasia syndrome or collie eye anomaly see Chap 11.)

Retinal dysplasia is congenital maldevelopment of the retina. It occurs in all species but is of most clinical significance in dogs and of lesser importance in cats and cattle.

In cats, retinal dysplasia occurs in kittens after infection of the queen by panleukopenia virus; cerebellar hypoplasia may also be present. In cattle, retinal dysplasia also occurs with cerebellar hypoplasia, especially in shorthorns. Retinal degeneration and atrophy and cerebellar hypoplasia are caused in newborn calves infected in utero with bovine virus diarrhea–mucosal disease virus. In dogs, spontaneous retinal dysplasia occurs most commonly in the American cocker spaniel (Plate V*A*); English springer spaniel (Plate V*B*); beagle; Labrador and golden retrievers; Bedlington, Sealyham, and Yorkshire terriers; and collie. It can occur in any breed and can be subdivided into two forms: (1) that associated with severe retinal malformation, hemorrhages, and visual deficits (Bedlington, Sealyham, and Yorkshire terriers; English springer spaniel; and Labrador retriever) when combined with skeletal chondrodysplasia and (2) that associated with combinations of retinal folds and areas of dysplasia, some of which may not be visible ophthalmoscopically at a later age (cocker spaniel, Labrador and golden retrievers).

Histologically, retinal dysplasia is characterized by retinal folds or rosettes and is nonprogressive (Fig. 16–30). The dysplastic retina may be detached. The most common reason for presentation is blindness or intraocular hemorrhage in puppies, although dysplasia or folds may be seen during routine examination programs for hereditary ocular defects in puppies and older dogs. Dysplasia is transmitted as a simple recessive trait in the Bedlington terrier and Labrador retriever and is probably recessive in the American cocker spaniel and Sealyham terrier. Cataracts may occur with retinal dysplasia in the English springer spaniel and Labrador retriever.

Animals with retinal dysplasia should not be bred.

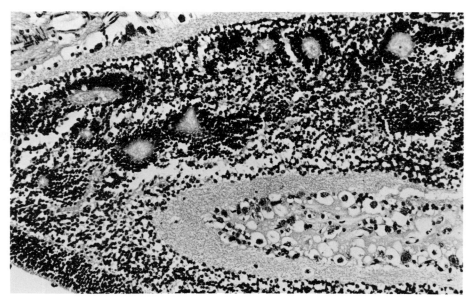

FIGURE 16–30. Retinal folds and rosettes in a kitten whose dam was affected with panleukopenia during pregnancy. Cerebellar hypoplasia was also present.

Retinal Effects of Pre- and Postpartum Irradiation in Dogs

Irradiation of the canine retina may cause retinal dysplasia and atrophy, depending on the dose and the time of irradiation. Doses between 1.0 and 3.8 Gy caused dysplasia when given at 28 and 55 days after coitus and at 2 days postpartum. Progression of the lesions occurred with time, resulting in retinal vascular attenuation. These doses considerably exceed those used in diagnostic radiology, but they may be significant in radiation therapy.

Chorioretinal Dysplasia

Chorioretinal dysplasia (abnormal development of the choroid and retina) is a major component of the scleral ectasia syndrome in collies, Shetland sheepdogs, and Australian [sic] shepherds[2] (see Chap 11).

---

2. The "Australian shepherd" does not occur in Australia.

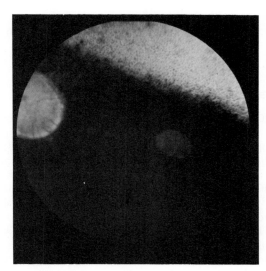

FIGURE 16–32. Small coloboma in the fundus of a 6-year-old pony, appearing as a pale area in the nontapetal fundus.

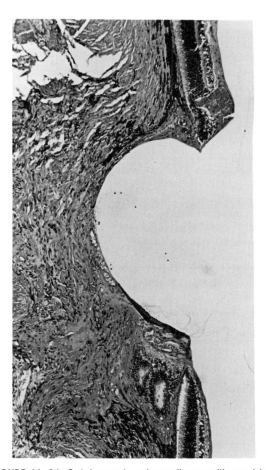

FIGURE 16–31. Coloboma in a basenji pup with persistent pupillary membrane. Note the retinal rosettes on the right side of the coloboma beneath the retina. (Tissue courtesy of Dr. J. R. Blogg.)

Colobomata

Colobomata (holes or pits) in the retina, choroid, sclera, or optic nerve are also part of the scleral ectasia syndrome in dogs. They are seen in charolais cattle and in basenjis in association with persistent pupillary membranes (Fig. 16–31). An isolated coloboma is uncommon but is seen occasionally in all species (Fig. 16–32). Colobomata are distinguished from focal areas of hypopigmentation known as "peripheral albinotic spots."

RETINOPATHY

Retinopathies fall into four major classes:
1. **DYSTROPHIES, DYSPLASIAS, AND DEGENERATIONS**
    a. PRD or PRA
    b. Rod-cone degeneration in poodles
    c. Rod dysplasia in the Norwegian elkhound
2. **ACQUIRED RETINOPATHIES**
    a. Drug toxicity (e.g., rafoxanide toxicity in sheep, o,p'-DDD toxicity in dogs)
    b. Nutritional deficiency (e.g., taurine deficiency in cats)
    c. Plant toxicity (e.g., bracken fern poisoning in sheep)
    d. Hypertensive retinopathy, (e.g., renal hypertension in cats)
    e. Atrophy secondary to glaucoma
3. **METABOLIC DISORDERS**
    a. Ceroid lipofuscinosis in dogs, cats, and sheep
    b. Mannosidosis in Aberdeen Angus cattle and cats

4. IDIOPATHIC CAUSE
   a. Sudden acquired retinal degeneration (SARD) in dogs

Retinal Degeneration

Classification of retinal disorders continues to evolve as detailed electron microscopic and electroretinographic studies are performed on specific disorders in different breeds. Initially all such disorders were termed *retinal atrophy,* a grouping that contained disorders of different clinical presentation and pathogenesis. Semantic discussions of the terms atrophy, dystrophy, abiotrophy, dysplasia, and degeneration recall the words of Duke-Elder: "Generalizations about the unknown, although satisfying to the ordered mind, are not to be interpreted as explanations or as advances in knowledge."[3]

The broad classification of the disorders in group 1 (dystrophies, dysplasias and degenerations) into PRD types I, II, and III is based on an earlier classification by Barnett (1969). It is based on similarities of clinical signs of affected animals, although diseases in each group may differ in pathogenesis and time of onset. In English and American cocker spaniels, the gene is located at the *pcrd* locus, and the condition in the two breeds is inherited with separate phenotypic characteristics, either because separate mutations have occurred at the same locus or because of the presence of undetermined modifier genes at different loci.

Elevated cyclic guanosine monophosphate and decreased levels of nucleotide phosphodiesterase have been recorded in the retinae of dogs with retinal degenerations, but their relationship to the pathogenesis is uncertain. Retinopathy caused by taurine deficiency (formerly feline central retinal degeneration) is now regarded as an acquired disorder (Figs. 16–33 and 16–34).

---

3. Duke-Elder S: System of Ophthalmology, vol 7, The Foundations of Ophthalmology, p 184. H Kimpton, London, 1962.

PRD Type I

Any breed of dog may be affected by PRD type I, even if the disease is not a severe problem in that breed.

CLINICAL SIGNS

Visual Loss. Early loss of night vision (nyctalopia), is followed by loss of day vision (hemeralopia) later in the disease. This is due to early degeneration or dysplasia of rods, and later of the cones as degeneration becomes severe (Figs. 16–35 and 16–36). In some breeds (e.g., Irish setter), rod and cone degeneration occur together. Affected animals often have difficulty seeing moving objects. From the initial diagnosis it is difficult to estimate how long it will take for the dog to become totally blind, although in general the younger the dog is when first affected, the faster the progression seems to be. Frequently, patients have severe visual defects before any change is noticed by the owner, which often happens when the dog is taken out of its familiar environment—for example, on vacation or for grooming or boarding. In appaloosas with congenital night blindness, nyctalopia is evident from birth, although ophthalmoscopically the fundus appears normal.

Dilated Pupils. In advanced disease, owners become aware that the pupils are abnormal. On examination, pupillary light reflexes are depressed or lacking.

Increased Tapetal Reflectivity and dilated pupils cause the eyes to appear greenish, silvery, or yellow to owners.

Cataracts are often noticed early by owners and are made more evident by the dilated pupil. Questioning usually reveals that there was a deficit in night vision *before* the cataracts occurred.

Early loss of night vision is due to rod degeneration.

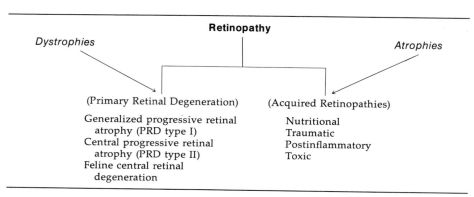

FIGURE 16–33. *Classification of retinopathies.*

Primary Retinal Degeneration (Progressive Retinal Atrophy Syndrome)

Progressive Retinal Degeneration Type I (PRD I)	Progressive Retinal Degeneration Type II (PRD II)	Progressive Retinal Degeneration Type III (PRD III)
Rod-cone dysplasia (Irish setter, miniature poodle, collie, miniature schnauzer)	Pigment epithelial dystrophy (formerly central PRA); predominantly in working breeds	Hemeralopia (Alaskan malamute, miniature poodle)
Rod dysplasia (Norwegian elkhound)		
Early retinal degeneration (Norwegian elkhound)		
Rod-cone degeneration (miniature poodle, English and American cocker spaniel, Abyssinian cat)		

Type I clinical signs:

Clinical Signs

1. Progressive loss of day then night vision
2. Increased tapetal reflectivity
3. Dilated pupils
4. Secondary cataracts in some patients
5. Retinal vascular attenuation
6. ERG affected or extinguished
7. Pupillary light reflexes absent later in the disease
8. Eventually blindness occurs

Type II clinical signs:

Clinical Signs

1. Poor near vision
2. Distance vision may be near normal
3. Pigment visible in the tapetal retina
4. Cataracts rare
5. Poor night vision not a feature
6. Pupillary light reflexes usually normal
7. ERG normal

Type III clinical signs:

Clinical Signs

1. Day blindness
2. No ophthalmoscopic signs
3. ERG used for confirmation
4. No cataracts

FIGURE 16–34. Types of primary retinal degeneration.

OPHTHALMOSCOPIC SIGNS

Attenuation of Retinal Vessels, especially arterioles, is an early and subtle sign (Plate V*C*). Variations of normal must be taken into account when interpreting this sign.

Tapetal Hyperreflectivity. As the retina atrophies, tapetal reflectivity increases and the granular appearance of the tapetum changes to a homogeneous sheen (Plate V*C;* see also Fig. 16–28). By the time reflectivity is greatly increased, vessel attenuation is severe and vision is poor (Plate V*D* and Fig. 16–37).

Pale Optic Disc. The optic disc becomes pale owing to loss of capillaries on its surface and atrophy of the nerve fibers caused by extensive degeneration of the retina (Plate V*D*).

Depigmentation of the Nontapetal Fundus. Focal depigmented areas in the nontapetal fundus are seen relatively early and may enlarge to affect the entire nontapetal fundus.

Cataract. Secondary cataracts are common in the later stages of PRD type I and appear as radial, spokelike opacities from the equator to the center of the lens (Fig. 16–38). They usually progress to maturity, but removal is contraindicated for visual purposes. Removal may be indicated if the lens luxates. Cataracts are thought to be due to substances released from the degenerating retina.

There is no treatment for PRD.

PRD type I is inherited as a simple autosomal recessive trait in those breeds in which it has been investigated. Clinical evidence suggests a similar pattern for other breeds. Although age of onset varies with breed (e.g., there is clinical evidence of PRD type I by the age of 12 months in the Irish setter and Cardigan corgi), *there is no upper age limit* after which animals will not get the disease. Electroretinography will detect the disease earlier than will ophthalmoscopy or the presence of clinical signs, but it is of little use in control of a breed problem because of expense, sophistication of the technique, and restricted availability. Breeds currently affected by PRD types I, II, III are given in Figure 16–34 and Table 16–6. Affected animals and their parents and offspring should not be used for breeding.

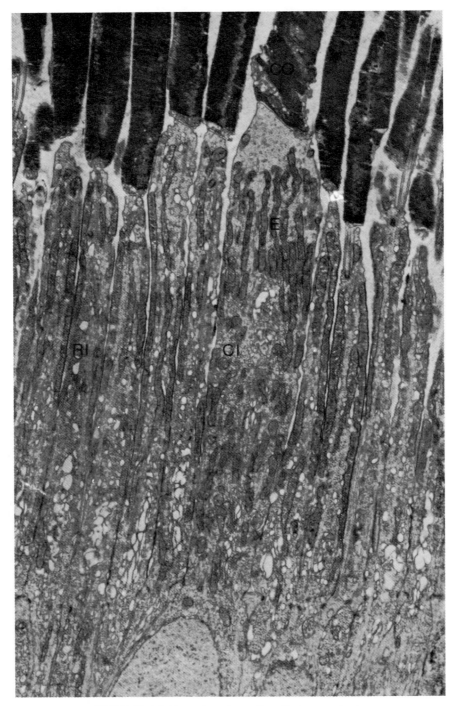

FIGURE 16–35. Normal canine retina. Photoreceptor layer of a 60-day-old normal dog. Rod and cone inner segments (RI and CI) are approximately the same length, although cones are broader and have a very distinct mitochondria-rich ellipsoid region (E) near the apex. The outer segments of rods (RO) and cones (CO) contain parallel membranous discs in a "coinstack" configuration. (From Aguirre GD: Retinal degenerations in the dog. I. Rod dysplasia. Exp Eye Res 26:233, 1978.)

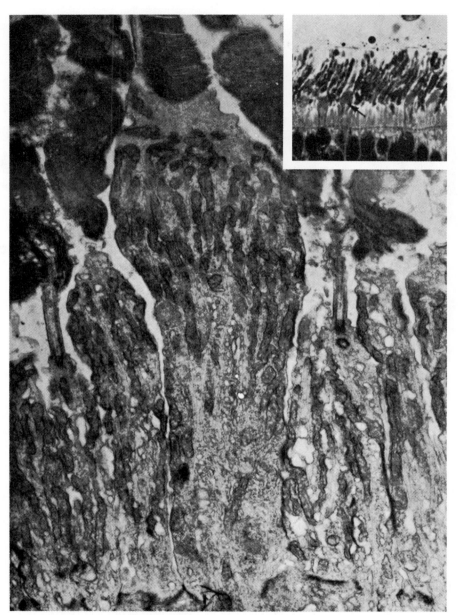

FIGURE 16–36. *Photoreceptor layer from the tapetal zone of a 12-week-old Norwegian elkhound with rod dysplasia. Cone inner and outer segments are normal, but rod inner segments are small, and outer segments are disorganized and disoriented. (From Aguirre GD: Retinal degenerations in the dog. I. Rod dysplasia. Exp Eye Res 26:233, 1978.)*

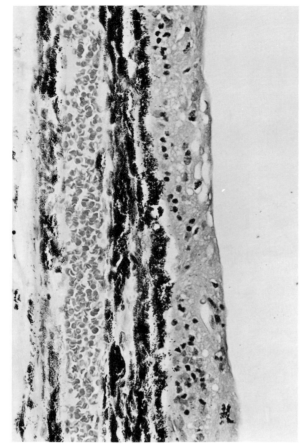

FIGURE 16–37. Advanced PRD type I. At this stage retinal degeneration from different causes appears similar histologically.

The recommended method for control of PRD type I is the certification of all breeding stock by competent observers and maintenance of an accessible central file of this information for use by veterinarians, breeders, and the animal-buying public.

PRD Type I in Cats

PRD type I occurs occasionally in cats but not frequently enough to constitute a major problem, except in the Abyssinian, in which the first signs are seen at 1 to 2 years of age. In Abyssinians in Sweden and Denmark, PRD I is a recessive trait. Ophthalmoscopic and clinical signs in cats are similar to those in dogs, although cataracts do not occur as frequently. It is believed to be a recessive trait in Persians but may not be hereditary in other breeds.

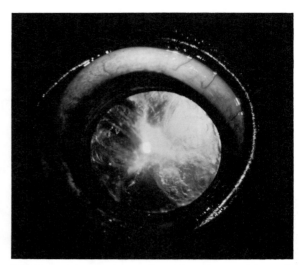

FIGURE 16–38. Immature cataract in a 6-year-old poodle with PRD type I.

Early-Onset Rod-Cone Dysplasia in Abyssinians

A separate early-onset degeneration occurs in Abyssinians, with dominant inheritance. The disease is evident ophthalmoscopically at 8–12 weeks and is preceded by mydriasis, nystagmus, and impairment of the pupillary light reflex.

PRD Type II

PRD type II affects primarily hunting and working dog breeds (see Fig. 16–34 and Table 16–6).

PRD type II is a pigment epithelial dystrophy that eventually progresses to involve the remaining retinal layers. Like PRD I, there are probably numerous conditions with differing pathogeneses in the PRD II designation.

CLINICAL SIGNS

Visual defects in PRD type II are less severe than in type I and usually do not occur until middle age. Affected animals show loss of central vision first, retaining peripheral vision until later in the disease. They are often reluctant to approach a stationary object, but see moving objects well—for example, a gun dog may see his bird fall but be unable to find it except by smell. An affected dog may see her or his owner from a distance but be unable to find her or him up close.

TABLE 16–6. Breeds Affected by Canine Progressive Retinal Degeneration

Type I		
Afghan hound	English cocker spaniel	Shetland sheepdog
Akita	English springer spaniel	Shih-Tzu
American cocker spaniel	Field spaniel	Siberian husky
Australian cattle dog	Fox terrier (wire-haired)	Soft-coated wheaten terrier
Australian [sic] shepherd	German shepherd	Spitz
Basenji	Golden retriever	Tibetan spaniel
Basset hound	Gordon setter	Tibetan terrier
Beagle	Great Dane	Toy Havanese
Bearded collie	Irish setter	Vizsla
Bedlington terrier	Italian greyhound	Welsh springer spaniel
Belgian sheepdog	Keeshond	Whippet
Bernese mountain dog	Kerry blue terrier	
Black and tan coonhound	Labrador retriever	**Type II**
Border collie	Lhasa apso	Border collie
Border terrier	Maltese terrier	Briard
Borzoi	Manchester terrier	Cardigan Welsh corgi
Boston terrier	Miniature pinscher	Chesapeake Bay retriever
Boxer	Norwegian elkhound	Collie (rough and smooth)
Briard	Nova duck tolling retriever	English setter
Brittany spaniel	Old English sheepdog	German shepherd (in Europe)
Bullmastiff	Pekingese	Golden retriever
Bull terrier	Pembroke corgi	Greyhound
Cairn terrier	Pointer	Irish setter
Cardigan Welsh corgi	Pomeranian	Jack Russell terrier
Cavalier King Charles spaniel	Poodle (miniature, toy, and standard)	Labrador retriever
Chesapeake Bay retriever	Portuguese water dog	Redbone coonhound
Chihuahua	Rottweiler	Shetland sheepdog
Collie (rough and smooth)	Saint Bernard	
Curly-coated retriever	Samoyed	**Type III**
Dachshund	Schnauzer (giant)	Alaska malamute
Doberman pinscher	Scottish terrier	Poodle (miniature)

There is little difference between day and night vision, and progression to total blindness is not common.

OPHTHALMOSCOPIC SIGNS

Focal areas of pigmentation are present in the central fundus overlying the tapetum (Plate V*E* and Fig. 16–39). The size and shape of affected areas vary. *Tapetal hyperreflectivity* occurs between the pigment spots. As the disease progresses, pigmentation and hyperreflectivity affect peripheral areas. Late in the disease, the optic disc may become pale, the vessels attenuated, and the nontapetal fundus pale and gray-brown.

ERG is often normal until late in the disease and is not used for early diagnosis. Because of the lesser visual deficits, the disease may be much more widespread than realized. The exact nature of inheritance is unknown, but it is believed to be a dominant trait with incomplete penetrance. Barnett attributes selective breeding to a decrease in incidence from 12% to 2% in large samples of dogs in Britain over an 8-year period. Affected animals and their offspring should not be used for breeding. The same certification scheme used for PRD type I is recommended.

Clinical features of PRD types I and II are compared in Table 16–7. In greyhounds descended from Irish stock in Australia that have a form of PRD II, cataracts and corneal dystrophy are occasionally seen. An ophthalmoscopically similar condition occurs in Italian greyhounds in California, but cataracts and corneal dystrophy have not been reported.

Retinal Atrophy in Sheepdogs

PRD II is distinguished from the widespread heterogeneous retinal atrophy seen in Australian and New Zealand working sheepdogs. This condition affects large areas of the retina, often leaving adjacent areas unaffected, and apparently does not impair vision. It is believed to be due to migrating parasite larvae, possibly *Toxocara canis*.

PRD Type III

PRD type III is a simple autosomal recessive disorder affecting cones in the Alaskan malamute and miniature poodle and resulting in hemeralopia. It is a rare disease and is important only because of its distinctive pathogenesis. Clinically the dogs are affected with progressive hemeralopia, but pupillary light reflexes and fundus appearance are normal. Diagnosis is confirmed by electroretinography.

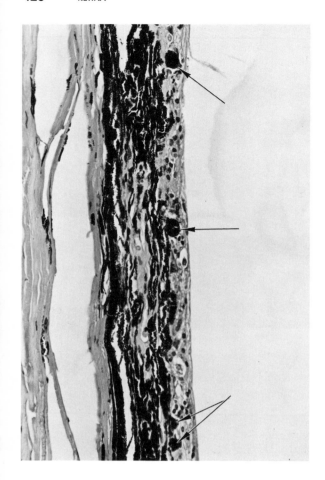

FIGURE 16–39. *Pigment epithelial dystrophy in PRD type II. Pigment epithelial cells are hyperplastic (arrows) and the overlying retina is atrophic.*

TABLE 16–7. Comparison of Clinical Features of Progressive Retinal Degeneration Types I and II

Feature	PRD Type I	PRD Type II
1. Breeds affected (see Table 16–6)	*All* breeds possible	Mostly working breeds
2. Visual defect	Poor night vision early Difficulty seeing moving objects Total blindness eventually	Early loss of central vision with temporary retention of peripheral vision Moving objects seen well; difficulty with stationary objects Vision good in dim light, but day vision gradually lost Total blindness unusual
3. Direct pupillary reflex	Eventually lost	Some activity usually retained
4. Retinal vessels	Attenuated early	Normal until late in course
5. Tapetal fundus	Hyperreflectivity	Focal hyperpigmentation with some hyperreflectivity later
6. Optic disc	Pale as disease progresses	Normal until very late in course
7. Nontapetal fundus	Focal depigmentation and mottling later	No significant changes
8. Lens	Cataracts frequent later in disease	Cataracts rare
9. ERG	Useful in diagnosis	No use in diagnosis
10. Inheritance	Recessive	Dominant with incomplete penetrance

Feline Retinal Degeneration Caused by Taurine Deficiency

Retinal degeneration resulting from dietary taurine deficiency was formerly called *feline central retinal degeneration*. The two disorders are now considered to be the same. Taurine is an essential amino acid for the cat. The lesions do not cause visual abnormalities early in the course of the disease and are usually noticed incidentally during ophthalmoscopic examination. They vary in size from a small rounded lesion that is temporal to and slightly above the disc in the area centralis to an ellipsoid lesion extending in a band from the temporal fundus across the top of the optic disc to the nasal fundus (Figs. 16–40 and 16–41). The area within the lesion is hyperreflective. Electroretinographic studies have shown widespread photoreceptor dysfunction.

Cats should not be fed taurine-deficient diets—for example, dog food. The cat is unable to synthesize taurine, unlike the dog. Taurine can be supplemented in the form of tablets or more economically with clam juice, meat, milk, or fish. The quality of commercial food does not seem to be a factor in reduction in taurine content, which is seen in foods from numerous American manufacturers. Reduced taurine also occurs in commercial cat foods. A taurine concentration of 0.1% is sufficient to prevent retinal lesions. Low plasma taurine is associated with a reversible but sometimes severe cardiomyopathy; hence, feline cardiac patients should receive an ophthalmic examination to help confirm taurine deficiency by the presence of retinal lesions.

Cats should not be fed commercial dog food.

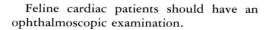

Feline cardiac patients should have an ophthalmoscopic examination.

Sudden Acquired Retinal Degeneration

Synonyms for sudden acquired retinal degneration (SARD) include silent retina syndrome and metabolic toxic retinopathy. SARD occurs in dogs and is characterized by sudden, usually total, permanent blindness of unknown cause in otherwise healthy animals. The ERG is absent, and there are no ophthalmoscopic abnormalities. Both rods and cones are affected. The ERG is necessary for diagnosis and to distinguish the condition from retrobulbar optic neuritis, as the latter disease may respond to treatment.

SARD is most common in middle-aged adult dogs, especially obese spayed females, and may be more common in winter. Within 3 to 4 months, ophthalmoscopic signs of generalized retinal atrophy are visible. A serum chemistry evaluation of affected patients is performed to eliminate other systemic diseases, but the results in SARD are usually normal. Antiretina antigens have been detected in serum from affected dogs, but they are also found in the Vogt-Koyanagi-Harada syndrome and PRD, making the significance undetermined. Affected patients often have a history of a recent, nonspecific episode of ill health. There is no known treatment.

Retinal Degeneration in Friesans

An apparently primary photoreceptor degeneration has been described in friesans in the United Kingdom (Bradley et al, 1982). The disease results in blindness,

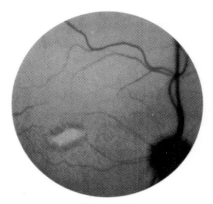

Fig. 16–40

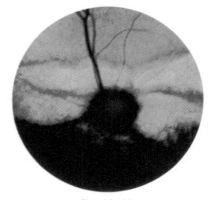

Fig. 16–41

FIGURE 16–40. *A small lesion temporal to the optic disc in a 7-year-old domestic shorthair cat. (From Rubin LF: Atlas of Veterinary Ophthalmoscopy. Lea & Febiger, Philadelphia, 1974.)*

FIGURE 16–41. *A band-shaped area of feline retinal degeneration due to taurine deficiency extending across the top of the optic disc in a 6-year-old male cat. (From Rubin LF: Atlas of Veterinary Ophthalmoscopy. Lea & Febiger, Philadelphia, 1974.)*

increased tapetal reflectivity, sluggish pupillary reflexes, attenuation of retinal vessels, and behavioral abnormalities. Although it is probably hereditary, the pattern is not simple.

Acquired Noninflammatory Retinopathies

HYPERTENSIVE RETINOPATHY

Hypertensive retinopathy is important in dogs and cats (see Chap 19).

NEURONAL CEROID LIPOFUSCINOSIS

Ceroid lipofuscinosis occurs in colonies of sheep (Hampshire), cattle (Devon), and dogs (border collie, Irish setter, and Dalmatian). Although retinal and central nervous system (CNS) lesions occur, the significance and frequency are undetermined. Affected animals show visual disturbances, gait abnormalities, and ophthalmoscopic signs. Definitive diagnosis is by histopathological examination.

DRUG AND PLANT TOXICITIES

Numerous chemical agents induce retinopathy in different animals, but only those of immediate clinical interest are discussed here.

"Bright Blindness" in Sheep. Bright blindness caused by chronic ingestion of bracken fern (*Pteris aquilina*) occurs widely in the United Kingdom. It affects only ewes, presumably because of different husbandry methods and plant exposure, and causes dilated pupils, depressed pupillary light reflexes, tapetal hyperreflectivity (Plate VF), pale optic discs, and narrowing of retinal blood vessels. Outer retinal layers are destroyed, and inner layers are spared. All confirmed cases have been in animals older than 1 year of age, and up to 5% of flocks are affected.

Bright blindness is distinguished from other causes of blindness in sheep that lack retinal lesions, such as:[4]

1. Infectious Ovine Keratoconjunctivitis
   a. Seen in all ages of sheep
   b. Obvious keratitis and conjunctivitis
   c. Corneal scars remain but no permanent blindness
2. Coenurosis (Gid)
   a. Usually younger sheep affected
   b. In the acute form there may be blindness or CNS signs without circling, but some months later sheep begin circling and die
3. Pregnancy Toxemia
   a. Affects pregnant ewes
   b. Usually other symptoms in addition to blindness

4. Cerebrocortical Necrosis
   a. Usually younger sheep affected
   b. Rapidly progressive, with CNS signs (e.g., head pressing, dummy syndrome)
   c. Trochlear nerve paralysis, causing dorsal oblique palsy and extorsion (lateral rotation of the globe) (see Fig. 17–5)
5. Cataract
   a. Obvious lens opacity

"Blindgrass" *(Stypandra imbricata)* **in Sheep and Goats.** "Blindgrass" toxicity occurs in western Australia and affects sheep and goats. The toxic principle is unknown. Most animals are affected with posterior paresis and some die, but survivors become blinded by lesions in the photoreceptor layer, optic nerve, and optic tracts. Animals graze on the plant only when it is freely available and other feed is restricted.

Rafoxanide Toxicity in Sheep. Rafoxanide is used to treat *Oestrus ovis* infections in sheep in South Africa. Overdosage causes blindness. Experimentally, rafoxanide is neurotoxic and causes blindness in dogs.

Hexachlorophene Toxicity in Sheep and Cattle. Hexachlorophene is used to kill liver flukes in sheep and cattle. Acute signs of toxicity are seen within 12 to 30 hours of treatment and include dullness, incoordination, diarrhea, and muscular weakness. Survivors are blind and lack pupillary reflexes as a result of retinal, optic nerve, and CNS lesions.

Oxygen Toxicity in Cats and Dogs. Young kittens (less than 3 weeks) exposed to high oxygen concentrations develop an abnormality of retinal vasculature and consequent retinopathy termed **RETROLENTAL FIBROPLASIA**. Several days of oxygen therapy at concentrations approaching 100% are required. In adult dogs, exudative retinal detachments occur after 3 or 4 days in a high-oxygen environment. Chlorpromazine greatly increases the incidence of retinal detachments caused by oxygen toxicity in dogs.

POST-TRAUMATIC CHORIORETINOPATHY IN HORSES

A syndrome of **CHORIORETINAL ATROPHY** occurs in young horses after severe blood loss and trauma. Ophthalmoscopic signs include (1) focal pigment proliferations in the tapetal retina, (2) pigment proliferations and areas of extensive atrophy and depigmentation in the nontapetal fundus (Fig. 16–42), (3) increased tapetal reflectivity in advanced stages, and (4) optic atrophy and disappearance of retinal vessels (variable).

Most affected animals are 2 years of age or younger. Vision is often severely affected, although traumatic lesions in the central visual pathways can coexist. The condition is nonprogressive, but some animals become completely blind. The history of hemorrhage from the nasal cavity after trauma to the top of the head—for example, from rearing up and falling over backward onto a hard surface—is common.

---

4. Modified from Watson WA, et al: Progressive retinal degeneration (bright blindness) in sheep: A review. Vet Rec 91:665, 1972.

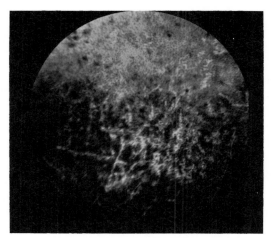

FIGURE 16–42. *Pigment proliferation and atrophy in the nontapetal fundus of a horse after head trauma and hemorrhage.*

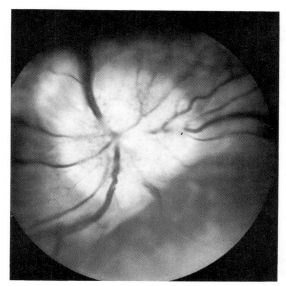

FIGURE 16–43. *Papilledema and pigment disruption in the nontapetal region of a blind steer with vitamin A deficiency. (From Divers TJ, et al: Blindness and convulsions associated with vitamin A deficiency in feedlot steers. J Am Vet Med Assoc 189:1579, 1986.)*

The exact pathogenesis of the syndrome is unknown, but it probably results from hypotension after hemorrhage (which causes retinal hypoxia because of the poorly developed equine retinal vasculature) combined with trauma to the ciliary vessels and parent vessels in the orbit.

VITAMIN A DEFICIENCY IN CATTLE AND PIGS

In clinical practice, vitamin A deficiency is of ocular significance in cattle and pigs only. In pigs, deficiency in pregnant sows causes microphthalmia and blindness in piglets. Deficiency in adults can also cause nyctalopia late in the disease.

In cattle, nyctalopia (especially at twilight) is an important sign of hypovitaminosis A (Table 16–8). In addition, poor reproductive efficiency, skin and CNS lesions, and conjunctivitis are encountered. Plasma levels of vitamin A fall only after depletion of hepatic reserves. Diagnosis can be made if liver levels are less than 2.0 µg/g of liver, or if plasma levels fall to less than 5 µg/dl.

TABLE 16–8. Ocular Signs of Hypovitaminosis A in Cattle

Young Calves	Adult Cattle
Papilledema (Fig. 16–43) (both congenital and in growing calves)	Papilledema
	Tapetal pallor
	Mottling of nontapetal fundus
Retinal venous congestion	Nyctalopia
Focal superficial retinal hemorrhages	Complete blindness rare; changes usually reversible
Optic atrophy in advanced cases (Fig. 16–44)	
Fixed, dilated pupils	
Apparent exophthalmia	
Lid retraction	
Nyctalopia	

Miscellaneous Retinopathies

In cats, numerous small retinal hemorrhages occur with anemia of various kinds. The hemorrhages are small and often multiple and may be superficial or deep. The cause is unknown.

In many of the storage diseases described in Table 17–14 (e.g., GM_1 gangliosidosis, mannosidosis, ceroid lipofuscinosis, glycogen storage disease type II), retinal lesions are present and of diagnostic value.

After focal inflammation or hemorrhage, atrophy of the surrounding retina frequently occurs, appearing as an area of hyperreflectivity, with or without pigmen-

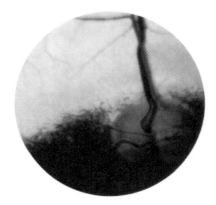

FIGURE 16–44. *Optic atrophy with a pale gray optic disc after long-standing vitamin A deficiency in a calf. (From Rubin LF: Atlas of Veterinary Ophthalmoscopy. Lea & Febiger, Philadelphia, 1974.)*

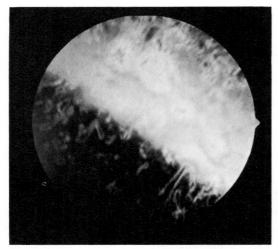

FIGURE 16–45. Inactive areas of focal pigmentation and surrounding atrophy in the tapetal and nontapetal areas of a foal.

tation in the tapetal fundus (Fig. 16–45) or as areas of depigmentation in the nontapetal fundus, or both. Such areas are seen relatively frequently in older animals, especially in dogs, in the course of routine ophthalmoscopic examination. The cause is usually unknown.

RETINITIS

The retina rarely shows isolated inflammation. The choroid is nearly always involved as well, resulting in either **RETINOCHOROIDITIS** or **CHORIORETINITIS**. Retinochoroiditis is inflammation of the choroid that has spread to adjacent areas of the retina, for example, as in canine distemper. Chorioretinitis is inflammation of the choroid that has spread to adjacent areas of the retina, for example, as in pyosepticemic chorioretinitis in cattle.

Retinitis may be either *active* or *inactive*. Distinguishing clinical signs of each will be discussed.

Ophthalmoscopic and Clinical Signs

ACTIVE RETINITIS[5]

1. Cellular Infiltration
   a. Tapetum:
      Dark colored; shows dull gray areas with indistinct borders (see Plate IVF).

   b. Nontapetal fundus:
      Gray or white areas with indistinct borders. Nontapetal retina appears dull. Perivascular sheathing of vessels has a white appearance.
2. Edema
   a. Tapetum:
      Focal gray areas, often well demarcated.
   b. Nontapetal fundus:
      Gray areas.
3. Retinal Exudates or Focal Granulomata
   a. Tapetum:
      Focal gray areas.
   b. Nontapetal fundus:
      Focal white areas. "Cotton wool spots" (infrequently seen in animals) are areas of ischemic necrosis in the inner retinal layers.
4. Retinal Hemorrhages
   a. Appearance depends on depth within the retina (see Fig. 16–29).
5. Retinal Detachment
   a. Cystic spaces between retina and pigment epithelium or large, pale, curtainlike folds of retina.
6. Progressive Enlargement of a Lesion or Satellite Lesion
7. Haziness of Adjacent Vitreous
8. Defective Vision
9. Uveitis
   a. Frequently concurrent.

INACTIVE RETINITIS[6]

1. Retinal Atrophy
   Tapetum:
      Tapetal hyperreflectivity.
   Nontapetal fundus:
      Pale, light-brown areas of depigmentation.
2. Pigment Epithelial Hypertrophy, Hyperplasia, and Migration
   Tapetum:
      Focal, multifocal, or diffuse pigmentation, usually within hyperreflective areas.
   Nontapetal fundus:
      Focal, multifocal, or diffuse pigmentation within pale or pigmented areas.
3. Vascular Thinning: Sclerosis
   Tapetum:
      Decrease in size of blood vessels.
   Nontapetal fundus:
      Decrease in size of blood vessels. Sclerotic choroidal vessels appear as radiating thin white lines through a depigmented retina and choroid.

5. Modified from Aguirre GD: The retina: Practical ophthalmology. Proc Am Anim Hosp Assoc, Elkhart, IN, 1974; and Blogg JR: The Eye in Veterinary Practice. VS Supplies, North Melbourne, Victoria, Australia, 1975.

6. Modified from Aguirre GD: The retina: Practical ophthalmology. Proc Am Anim Hosp Assoc, Elkhart, IN, 1974; and Blogg JR: The Eye in Veterinary Practice. VS Supplies, North Melbourne, Victoria, Australia, 1975.

TABLE 16–9. Systemic Disorders of the Retina

Dog	Sheep
Blastomycosis	Scrapie
Coccidioidomycosis	**Cow**
Cryptococcosis	Malignant catarrhal fever
Distemper	Rift Valley fever
Ehrlichiosis	Rinderpest
Histoplasmosis	Thromboembolic
Hypertension	meningoencephalitis
Larva migrans (*Toxocara*	**Pig**
spp)	African swine fever
Leishmaniasis	Hog cholera
Lymphosarcoma	**Horse**
Multiple myeloma	Recurrent equine uveitis
Toxoplasmosis*	Guttural pouch mycosis
Cat	Leptospirosis
Blastomycosis	Lymphosarcoma
Cryptococcosis	Strangles
Feline infectious peritonitis	Toxoplasmosis
Histoplasmosis	
Hypertension	
Lymphosarcoma—both	
FELV (feline leukemia	
virus) positive *and*	
negative	
Toxoplasmosis	
Tuberculosis	

*A newly recognized fatal protozoan disease caused by *Neosporum caninum* has been found to be the cause in some infections previously diagnosed as toxoplasmosis in dogs. The clinical sigificance is undetermined.

SYSTEMIC DISORDERS

Common systemic disorders affecting the retina are discussed in Chapter 19 and are listed in Table 16–9.

RETINAL DETACHMENT

Retinal detachment is separation of the retina from the underlying choroid, which usually occurs between the photoreceptor layer and the pigment epithelium. The outer layers of the retina are separated from their source of nutrition in the choroid, and the photoreceptors are separated from the pigment epithelium. The intimate contact between the rods and cones and pigment epithelial cells is disrupted, and metabolites are no longer available from the choroid, nor can end products of metabolism be removed. Severe irreversible changes in the retina begin early because of its high metabolic rate.

Causes

1. Congenital: Retinal dysplasia, scleral ectasia syndrome (in collies), and multiple congenital anomalies are examples of congenital disorders that cause retinal detachment (Fig. 16–46).

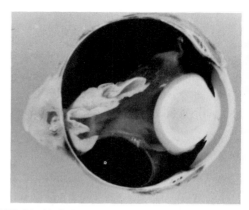

FIGURE 16–46. *Retinal detachment in a collie with scleral ectasia syndrome. The retina has remained attached at the optic disc and ora ciliaris retina. (Courtesy of Dr. G. A. Severin.)*

2. Serous detachments: Accumulations of fluid beneath the retina push it away from underlying tissues (e.g., the Vogt-Koyanagi-Harada syndrome in dogs, hypertension in dogs and cats, and inflammatory exudates of various causes).

3. Traction detachments: Contraction of scar tissue within the vitreous pulls the retina off. Inflammatory exudates frequently leave such scar tissue (e.g., in equine recurrent uveitis).

4. Solid detachments: Accumulations of inflammatory or tumor cells or microorganisms in the retina or choroid force the retina to detach (e.g., in lymphosarcoma).

5. Extraocular pressure: Focal pressure on the globe from tumors or space-occupying lesions in the orbit may cause detachment. Early signs of this pressure are wrinkles or folds in the retina over the site of the pressure.

6. Severe trauma is another cause.

7. Severe intraocular inflammation (Plate V*E*) can also cause retinal detachment.

8. Vitreous degeneration: Liquefaction of the vitreous is important in the pathogenesis of human retinal detachment. The exact role of syneresis in spontaneous retinal detachment in aged animals is poorly understood.

9. Holes in the retina are believed to be important in the pathogenesis of detachment, as in humans. Detachments associated with holes are termed *rhegmatogenous;* those in which no hole is present are called *nonrhegmatogenous.* Fluid is thought to leak from the vitreous through the hole and thereby elevate the retina.

Rhegmatogenous tears with proliferative vitreoretinopathy, cataract, axial myopia, vitreous liquefaction, and detachment have been described as an entity in Labrador retrievers with skeletal abnormalities. The cause of the tears was believed to be vitreoretinal detachment. The end result was fibrocellular membranes on the surface of the vitreous with a totally detached retina. The frequency and importance of this occurrence in Labrador retrievers are undetermined.

Signs

1. Loss of vision occurs (if the detachment is large or total).
2. There may be appearance of a white mobile structure behind the lens (Plate V*E*).
3. Retinal vessels are clearly visible through the pupil.
4. Increased systolic blood pressure is frequent.

Treatment

Spontaneous unilateral retinal detachment in animals is usually found incidentally during examination, is of long standing, and is therefore rarely amenable to surgical correction. Patients may be presented for sudden loss of vision due to retinal detachments, and the vision of these animals can often be saved through medical therapy.

Initial diagnostic attempts are directed at determining the cause. Patients with bilateral detachments should receive a hematological and serum chemistry profile to evaluate renal function, as well as complete eye and physical examinations systolic blood pressure measurements, and serological evaluation for possible responsible microorganisms (see previous discussion).

Initial therapy consists of an oral diuretic—for example, furosemide, 2.5 mg/kg by mouth 3 times daily—broad-spectrum antibiotic therapy, and corticosteroids if an infectious cause is unlikely[7] (e.g., dexamethasone, 0.25 mg/kg twice daily). A steroid with anti-inflammatory glucocorticoid and *low* mineralocorticoid activity should be used until hypertension is ruled out.[8] If the Vogt-Koyanagi-Harada syndrome is diagnosed, initial therapy with oral azathioprine, 0.5 mg/kg daily, is also indicated in severe cases, with regular monitoring of total white cell count and serum indices of hepatic function.

If hypertension is confirmed at the initial examination, antihypertensive therapy is indicated, with the owner being warned of possible side effects of medication, especially if cardiac or respiratory disease is present (e.g., in cats, propranolol, 5 to 10 mg orally 3 times daily, and captopril, up to 12.5 mg 3 times daily, either separately or together).

Once initial therapy is instituted, the response is observed, and suitable diagnostic attempts are continued to determine the cause.

---

7. Because delay in therapy may prejudice results, it is often necessary to decide whether steroids can be used prior to receiving laboratory data.
8. Avoid prednisolone and prednisone.

REFERENCES

Acland GM (1988): Diagnosis and differentiation of retinal diseases in small animals by electroretinography. Semin Vet Med Surg 3:15.

Acland GM, Aguirre GD (1987): Retinal degeneration in the dog IV. Early retinal degeneration (erd) in Norwegian elkhounds. Exp Eye Res 44:491.

Aguirre GD (1978): Retinal degenerations in the dog. I. Rod dysplasia. Exp Eye Res 26:233.

Aguirre GD, Acland GM (1988): Variation in retinal degeneration phenotype inherited at the prcd locus. Exp Eye Res 46:663.

Aguirre GD, Laties A (1976): Pigment epithelial dystrophy in dogs. Exp Eye Res 23:247.

Aguirre GD, Rubin LF (1971): The early diagnosis of rod dysplasia in the Norwegian elkhound. J Am Vet Med Assoc 159:429.

Aguirre GD, Rubin LF (1971): Progressive retinal atrophy (rod dysplasia) in the Norwegian elkhound. J Am Vet Med Assoc 158:208.

Aguirre GD, Rubin LF (1972): Progressive retinal atrophy in the miniature poodle: an electrophysiologic study. J Am Vet Med Assoc 160:191.

Aguirre GD, Rubin LF (1974): Pathology of hemeralopia in the Alaskan malamute dog. Invest Ophthalmol Vis Sci 13:231.

Aguirre GD, Rubin LF (1975): The electroretinogram in dogs with inherited cone degeneration. Invest Ophthalmol Vis Sci 14:840.

Aguirre GD, Schmidt SY (1978): Retinal degeneration associated with the feeding of dog food to cats. J Am Vet Med Assoc 172:791.

Aguirre GD, et al (1978): Rod-cone dysplasia in Irish setters: A cyclic GMP metabolic defect of visual cells. Science 201:1133.

Aguirre GD, et al (1982): Hereditary retinal degenerations in the dog: Specificity of abnormal cyclic nucleotide metabolism to diseases of arrested photoreceptor development. Birth Defects 18:119.

Aguirre GD, et al (1982): Pathogenesis of rod-cone degeneration in miniature poodles. Invest Ophthalmol Vis Sci 23:610.

Aguirre GD, et al (1982): Retinal degeneration in the dog. III. Abnormal cyclic nucleotide metabolism in rod-cone dysplasia. Exp Eye Res 35:625.

Anderson PA, et al (1979): Biochemical lesions associated with taurine deficiency in the cat. J Anim Sci 49:1227.

Armstrong D, et al (1978): Studies on the retina and pigment epithelium in hereditary canine ceroid lipofuscinosis. Invest Ophthalmol Vis Sci 17:608.

Ashton N, et al (1968): Retinal dysplasia in the Sealyham terrier. J Path Bact 96:269.

Barlow RM, et al (1981): Mannosidosis in Aberdeen Angus cattle in Britain. Vet Rec 109:441.

Barnett KC (1965): Canine retinopathies. I. History and review of the literature. J Sm Anim Pract 6:41.

Barnett KC (1965): Canine retinopathies. II. The miniature and toy poodle. J Sm Anim Pract 6:93.

Barnett KC (1965): Canine retinopathies. III. The other breeds. J Sm Anim Pract 6:185.

Barnett KC (1965): Canine retinopathies. IV. Causes of retinal atrophy. J Sm Anim Pract 6:229.

Barnett KC (1969): Primary retinal dystrophies in the dog. J Am Vet Med Assoc 154:804.

Barnett KC, Watson WA (1970): Bright blindness in sheep. A primary retinopathy due to feeding bracken (*Pteris aquilina*). Res Vet Sci 11:289.

Barnett KC, et al (1970): Hereditary retinal dysplasia in the Labrador retriever in England and Sweden. J Sm Anim Pract 10:755.

Barnett KC, et al (1970): Ocular changes associated with hypovitaminosis A in cattle. Br Vet J 126:561.

Bedford PGC (1982): Multifocal retinal dysplasia in the Rottweiler. Vet Rec 113:304.

Bedford PGC (1983): Feline central degeneration in the United Kingdom. Vet Rec 112:456.

Beehler CC, Roberts W (1968): Experimental retinal detachments induced by oxygen and phenothiazines. Arch Ophthalmol 79:759.

Bellhorn RW, Fischer CA (1970): Feline central retinal degeneration. J Am Vet Med Assoc 157:842.

Bellhorn RW, et al (1974): Feline central retinal degeneration. Invest Ophthalmol Vis Sci 13:608.

Bellhorn RW, et al (1975): Hereditary tapetal abnormality in the beagle. Ophthalmic Res 7:250.

Bellhorn RW, et al (1988): Anti-retinal immunoglobulins in canine ocular diseases. Semin Vet Med Surg 3:28.

Berson EL, et al (1976): Retinal degeneration in cats fed casein. II. Supplementation with methionine, cysteine, or taurine. Invest Ophthalmol Vis Sci 15:52.

Blair NP, et al (1985): Rhegmatogenous retinal detachment in Labrador retrievers. I. Development of retinal tears and detachment. Arch Ophthalmol 103:842.

Blair NP, et al (1985): Rhegmatogenous retinal detachment in Labrador retrievers. II. Proliferative retinopathy. Arch Ophthalmol 103:848.

Blood DC, et al (1983): Veterinary Medicine, 5th ed. WB Saunders Co, Philadelphia.

Brach V (1975): The effect of intraocular ablation of the pecten oculi of the chicken. Invest Ophthalmol Vis Sci 14:166.

Bradley R, et al (1982): The pathology of a retinal degeneration in Friesan cows. J Comp Pathol 92:69.

Burns MS, et al (1988): Development of hereditary tapetal degeneration in the beagle dog. Curr Eye Res 7:103.

Buyukmihci N, et al (1982): Retinal degenerations in the dog. II. Development of the retina in rod-cone dysplasia. Exp Eye Res 30:575.

Carrig CB, et al (1977): Retinal dysplasia associated with skeletal abnormalities in Labrador retrievers. J Am Vet Med Assoc 170:49.

Clegg FG, et al (1981): Blindness in dairy cows. Vet Rec 109:101.

Collier LC, et al (1985): Tapetal degeneration in cats with Chediak-Higashi syndrome. Curr Eye Res 4:767.

Curtis R, et al (1987): An early onset retinal dystrophy with dominant inheritance in the Abyssinian cat. Clinical and pathological findings. Invest Ophthalmol Vis Sci 28:62.

Dice PF (1980): Progressive retinal atrophy in the Samoyed. Mod Vet Pract 61:59.

Divers TJ, et al (1986): Blindness and convulsions associated with vitamin A deficiency in feedlot steers. J Am Vet Med Assoc 189:1579.

Duddy JA, et al (1983): Hyaloid patency in neonatal beagles. Am J Vet Res 44:2344.

Duke-Elder S (1958): System of Ophthalmology, vol 1, The Eye in Evolution. H Kimpton, London.

Duke-Elder S (1968): System of Ophthalmology, vol 6, The Physiology of the Eye and of Vision. H Kimpton, London.

Fischer CA (1970): Retinopathy in anemic cats. J Am Vet Med Assoc 156:1415.

Flower RW, Patz A (1971): Oxygen studies in retrolental fibroplasia. IX. The effects of elevated arterial oxygen tension on retinal vascular dynamics in the kitten. Arch Ophthalmol 85:197.

Fox LE, et al (1987): Reversal of ethylene glycol—induced nephrotoxicosis in a dog. J Am Vet Med Assoc 191:1433.

Goebel HH, Dahme E (1986): Ultrastructure of retinal pigment epithelial and neural cells in the neuronal ceroid-lipofuscinosis affected Dalmatian dog. Retina 6:179.

Graydon RJ, Jolly RD (1984): Ceroid-lipofuscinosis (Batten's disease). Sequential electrophysiologic and pathologic changes in the retina of the ovine model. Invest Ophthalmol Vis Sci 25:294.

Harper PA, et al (1988): Neurovisceral ceroid-lipofuscinosis in blind Devon cattle. Acta Neuropathol 75:632.

Heywood R, Wells GAH (1970): A retinal dysplasia in the beagle dog. Vet Rec 87:178.

Hughes PL, et al (1987): Multifocal retinitis in New Zealand sheep dogs. Vet Pathol 24:22.

Jolly R, et al (1987): Mannosidosis: Ocular lesions in the bovine model. Curr Eye Res 6:1073.

Keep JM (1972): Clinical aspects of progressive retinal atrophy in the Cardigan Welsh corgi. Aust Vet J 48:197.

Kirk GR, Jensen HE (1975): Toxic effects of o,p'-DDD in the normal dog. J Am Anim Hosp Assoc 11:765.

Koch E (1974): Retinal Dysplasia—A Comparative Study in Human Beings and Dogs. Karolinska Institute, Stockholm.

Koch SA, Rubin LF (1972): Distribution of cones in retina of the normal dog. Am J Vet Res 33:361.

Lahav M (1973): Clinical and histopathologic classification of retinal dysplasia. Am J Ophthalmol 75:648.

Lavach JD, et al (1978): Retinal dysplasia in the English springer spaniel. J Am Anim Hosp Assoc 14:192.

Leber T (1903): Die Circulations und Ernahrungsverhaltnisse des Auges. In von Graefes A, Saemisch T (eds): Handbuch der gesamten Augenheilkunde, vol 2, 2nd ed. Englemann, Leipzig.

MacMillan AD (1976): Acquired retinal folds in the cat. J Am Vet Med Assoc 168:1015.

MacMillan AD, Lipton DE (1978): Heritability of multifocal retinal dysplasia in American cocker spaniels. J Am Vet Med Assoc 172:568.

Millichamp NJ (1988): Progressive retinal atrophy in Tibetan terriers. J Am Vet Med Assoc 192:769.

Narfstrom K (1983): Hereditary progressive retinal atrophy in the Abyssinian cat. J Hered 74:273.

Narfstrom K, Nilsson SE (1987): Hereditary rod-cone degeneration in a strain of Abyssinian cats. Prog Clin Biol Res 247:349.

Narfstrom K, et al (1985): Progressive retinal atrophy in the Abyssinian cat: Studies of the DC-recorded electroretinogram and the standing potential of the eye. Br J Ophthalmol 69:618.

Nelson DL, Macmillan AD (1983): Multifocal retinal dysplasia in field trial Labrador retrievers. J Am Anim Hosp Assoc 19:388.

O'Toole D, Roberts SM (1984): Generalized progressive retinal atrophy in two Akita dogs. Vet Pathol 21:457.

O'Toole DO, et al (1983): Retinal dysplasia of English springer spaniel dogs: Light microscopy of the postnatal lesions. Vet Pathol 20:298.

Moses RA (1970): Adler's Physiology of the Eye, 5th ed. WB Saunders Co, Philadelphia.

Pion PD, et al (1987): Myocardial failure in cats associated with low plasma taurine: A reversible cardiomyopathy. Science 237:764.

Prozesky L, Pienaar JG (1977): Amaurosis in sheep resulting from treatment with rafoxanide. Onderstepoort J Vet Res 44:257.

Rabin AR, et al (1973): Cone and rod responses in nutritionally induced retinal degeneration in the cat. Invest Ophthalmol Vis Sci 12:694.

Roberts SR (1971): Chorioretinitis in a band of horses. J Am Vet Med Assoc 158:2043.

Roeder PL, et al (1986): Pestivirus fetopathogenicity in cattle: Changing sequelae with fetal maturation. Vet Rec 118:44.

Rubin LF (1963): Atrophy of rods and cones in the cat retina. J Am Vet Med Assoc 142:1415.

Rubin LF (1968): Heredity of retinal dysplasia in Bedlington terriers. J Am Vet Med Assoc 152:260.

Rubin LF (1971): Clinical features of hemeralopia in the adult Alaska malamute. J Am Vet Med Assoc 158:1696.

Rubin LF (1971): Hemeralopia in Alaskan malamute pupa. J Am Vet Med Assoc 158:1699.

Rubin LF, Lipton DE (1973): Retinal degeneration in kittens. J Am Vet Med Assoc 162:467.

Santo-Anderson R, et al (1980): An inherited retinopathy in collies: A light microscopic study. Invest Ophthalmol Vis Sci 19:1281.

Sarv AR (1986): Progressive retinal atrophy in the Abyssinian cat. Nord Vet Med 38:388.

Schaffer EH, Wallow IHL (1975): Rhegmatogenous bilateral retinal detachment in a poodle dog. J Comp Pathol 85:195.

Scheie HG, Albert DM (1977): Textbook of Ophthalmology, 9th ed. WB Saunders Co, Philadelphia.

Schmidt GM, et al (1979): Inheritance of retinal dysplasia in the English springer spaniel. J Am Vet Med Assoc 174:1089.

Schmidt SY, et al (1976): Retinal degeneration in cats fed casein. I. Taurine deficiency. Invest Ophthalmol Vis Sci 15:47.

Schweitzer DJ, et al (1987): Retinal dysplasia and progressive atrophy in dogs irradiated during ocular development. Radiat Res 111:340.

Slatter DH et al (1980): Progressive retinal degeneration in the greyhound. Aust Vet J 56:106.

Slatter DH, et al (1980): *Stypandra* spp ("blindgrass") poisoning in ruminants—Ocular and neurological findings in spontaneous cases. Aust Vet J 57:132.

Stades FC (1978): Hereditary retinal dysplasia in a family of Yorkshire terriers. Tijdschr Diergeneeskd 103:1087.

Taylor RM, Farrow BR (1988): Ceroid-lipofuscinosis in border collie dogs. Acta Neuropathol 75:627.

Vainisi SJ, Campbell LH (1969): Ocular toxoplasmosis in cats. J Am Vet Med Assoc 154:141.

Watson WA, et al (1972): Progressive retinal degeneration (bright blindness) in sheep: A review. Vet Rec 91:665.

Wen GY, et al (1982): Hereditary abnormality of the tapetum lucidum of the Siamese cats. Histochemistry 75:1.

West-Hyde L, Buyukmihci N (1982): Photoreceptor degeneration in a family of cats. J Am Vet Med Assoc 181:243.

Witzel DA, et al (1977): Night blindness in the Appaloosa: Sibling occurrence. J Eq Med Surg 1:383.

Witzel ED, et al (1977): Electroretinography of congenital night blindness in an Appaloosa filly. J Eq Med Surg 1:266.

Wolf ED, et al (1978): Rod-cone dysplasia in the collie. J Am Vet Med Assoc 173:1331.

Woodford BJ, et al (1982): Cyclic nucleotide metabolism in inherited retinopathy in collies. Exp Eye Res 34:703.

Yanoff M, et al (1970): Oxygen poisoning of the eyes. Comparison in cyanotic and acyanotic dogs. Arch Ophthalmol 84:627.

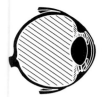

17

Neuro–Ophthalmology

In collaboration with Alexander deLahunta

REACTIONS OF NERVOUS
    TISSUE TO DISEASE
CRANIAL NERVES OF
    OPHTHALMIC SIGNIFICANCE
EXAMINATION OF THE NEURO-
    OPHTHALMIC PATIENT

CLINICAL SIGNS OF
    DYSFUNCTION OF CRANIAL
    NERVES III, IV, AND VI
AUTONOMIC INNERVATION
    AND ABNORMALITIES

THE VESTIBULAR SYSTEM
THE CEREBELLUM
CENTRAL VISUAL PATHWAYS
DISEASES OF THE VISUAL
    SYSTEM

Neuro-ophthalmology can be confusing and complicated for the clinician. Simple recognition is rarely sufficient to arrive at a diagnosis. If anatomy, physiology, and pathology are understood, a diagnosis can be reached by deduction and elimination rather than from memory. The reader should refer to a basic pathology text to review the reactions of nervous tissues to disease processes, which is beyond the basic summary given here.[1]

REACTIONS OF NERVOUS TISSUES TO DISEASE[2]

Elements of Nervous Tissue

Nervous tissue is composed of three elements: neurons, neuroglia (astrocytes, oligodendrocytes, microglia), and vascular connective tissue (Fig. 17–1).

NEURONS

Neurons—for example, retinal ganglion cells—have large cell bodies with huge nuclei and prominent nucleoli. Dendrites conduct impulses toward the cell body—for example, the inner plexiform layer of the retina—and axons transmit impulses away from it—for example, fibers of the optic nerve. Axons in the nerve fiber layer of the retina have no myelin sheath but are myelinated in the optic nerve by oligodendrocytes. Myelin in the optic nerve differs from that in peripheral nerves, in which lemmocytes (Schwann cells) form the myelin. Diseases affecting Schwann cells do not influence the optic nerve, and diseases that affect oligodendrocytes of the optic nerve do not affect peripheral nerve myelin.

Axoplasmic flow of metabolites and cell organelles occurs in both directions in the axon—to and from the cell body. Interruption of this flow is significant in the pathogenesis of *papilledema.*

Acute Neuronal Degeneration. Because neurons are specialized and have little ability to regenerate or proliferate, the alterations seen are the result of degeneration or necrosis. Severe, acute insults cause immediate damage and destroy the cell. Duration of the insult is more important than the cause. The sequence is

$$\text{Acute insult} \rightarrow \left.\begin{array}{l}\text{Swelling}\\\text{fragmentation}\\\text{dissolution}\end{array}\right\} \text{of cell bodies} \rightarrow \text{necrosis}$$

Tissues become edematous or cystic and later collapse and shrink. There is minimal reactive proliferation, and remnants of disintegrating ganglion cells are phagocytized by microglia. Neuroglial cells may fill in the defect ("gliosis").

Chronic Neuronal Degeneration. There are more identifiable stages in this process than in acute degeneration. Neurons may swell and accumulate cytoplasmic lipoidal vacuoles. Others may shrink, losing cell bodies and processes, and leave only a pyknotic nucleus.

---

1. Spencer WH (ed): Ophthalmic Pathology, vols 1–3. WB Saunders Co, Philadelphia, 1985.
2. Modified from Hogan MJ, Zimmerman LE: Ophthalmic Pathology, 2nd ed. WB Saunders, Philadelphia, 1962.

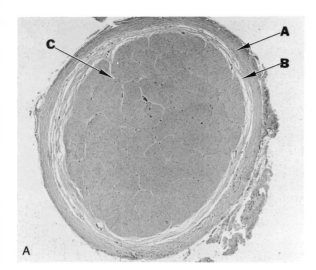

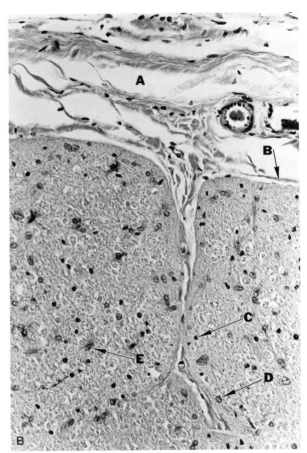

FIGURE 17–1. Normal canine optic nerve. A, Transverse section, showing dura mater (A), arachnoid (B), and pial septum (C). B, Transverse section (higher power), showing subarachnoid space (A), pial sheath (B), microglia (C), oligodendrocyte (D), and astrocyte (E). C, Longitudinal section. D, Longitudinal section (higher power), showing astrocyte (A), oligodendrocyte (B), and microglia (C).

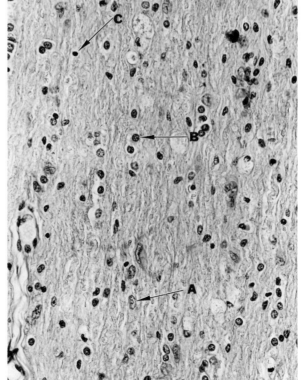

Axonal Degeneration. Lesions and degenerative processes may occur in axons distant from the cell body. Numerous degenerative conditions affect the optic nerve, which is a collection of axons, before the retinal ganglion cell is affected. Segments distal to the injury shrink rapidly, but proximal segments attached to the cell body survive longer and develop bulblike swellings at the site of injury. These bulblike swellings ("cytoid bodies") are visible ophthalmoscopically in the retina and are termed *cotton wool spots*. They do not persist, and eventually both proximal and distal portions of the neuron, including the cell body, disappear. Chronic atrophy of the optic nerve eventually leads to disappearance of the nerve fiber and ganglion cell layers of the retina. Similarly, loss of the retinal ganglion cells causes atrophy and disappearance of the corresponding axons in the optic nerve.

Wallerian Degeneration and Regeneration. Wallerian degeneration is the early disappearance of the distal segment of an injured axon and the more gradual loss of the proximal segment and cell body. Because transynaptic degeneration rarely occurs, the inner layers of the retina or those beyond the lateral geniculate body are not affected by optic neuropathy. Regeneration is limited in the optic nerve, but it may take place in the peripheral nerves of ophthalmic importance, for example, in branches of the facial nerve (cranial nerve VII).

Myelin Degeneration. Destruction of the optic nerve causes alterations in the myelin sheath. The complex lipids in myelin turn into simple lipids. These simple lipids are lost during routine histological processing, leaving spaces (Fig. 17–2). Macrophages phagocytize the lipid (Fig. 17–3).

NEUROGLIA

Pathological Reactions. Neuroglia are the supporting cells of the central nervous system (CNS) and are classified by characteristics of their cytoplasmic processes. *Astrocytes* proliferate when stimulated, although severe, acute degeneration of the retina may destory both neurons and neuroglia. In the retina, the astrocytes become larger, proliferate, and fill in defects caused by the disappearance of other neuronal tissues, forming "glial scars" or areas of "gliosis." Histiocytes or fixed macrophages of the CNS are termed *microglia*. They phagocytize fatty materials released during degeneration of nervous tissue and become large and rounded with vacuolated cytoplasm (gitter cells).

CRANIAL NERVES OF OPHTHALMIC SIGNIFICANCE

The following cranial nerves are significant in relation to ocular functions:

Optic nerve	Cranial nerve II
Oculomotor nerve	Cranial nerve III

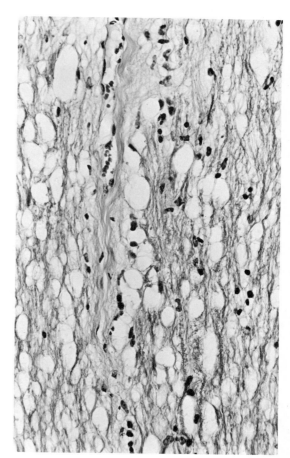

FIGURE 17–2. Myelin degeneration in the optic nerve of a horse with recurrent equine uveitis.

Trochlear nerve	Cranial nerve IV
Trigeminal nerve	Cranial nerve V
Abducens nerve	Cranial nerve VI
Facial nerve	Cranial nerve VII

Function of the Extraocular Muscles

To understand signs that result from lesions of the three cranial nerves that innervate the extraocular muscles, normal innervation of the muscles must be understood (Table 17–1).

The globe has three axes of rotation, and the muscles are grouped into three opposing pairs. Each muscle in the pair acts in a reciprocal manner with its partner, similar to flexor and extensor muscles in the limbs. Such a pair of extraocular muscles are termed YOKE MUSCLES. When both eyes move in the same direction, the movement is called CONJUGATE. Around a horizontal axis, passing transversely through the center of the globe, the medial rectus muscle *adducts* and the lateral rectus muscle *abducts* the globe. Around the anterior-posterior axis, through the center of the globe, the dorsal oblique muscle *intorts* the globe (rotates the

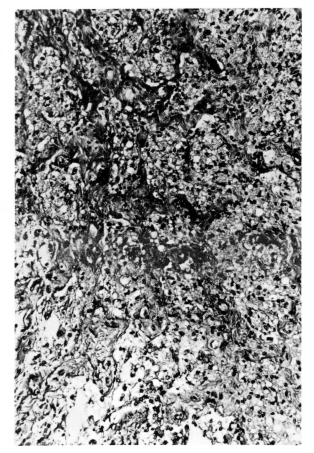

FIGURE 17–3. Severe acute toxic optic neuropathy in a sheep poisoned with Stypandra imbricata ("blindgrass"). Note the loss of normal architecture, loss and disorganization of axons, and presence of gitter cells (fat-laden macrophages).

lateral recti in horizontal conjugate movement (Fig. 17–4).

When the eyes move conjugately to the right, facilitation of abducent neurons to the lateral rectus of the right eye, and inhibition to those of the left eye, is required in conjunction with inhibition of the oculomotor neurons to the medial rectus of the right eye and facilitation to those of the left eye. The MEDIAL LONGITUDINAL FASCICULUS functions in coordinating this activity.

The function of any muscle at a specific time depends on the position of the eye. Functions of the extraocular muscles in domestic animals do not compare exactly with those in humans because of anatomical differences in the position of the eye with respect to the muscle insertion.

EXAMINATION OF THE NEURO-OPHTHALMIC PATIENT

Examination of the eye and its adnexa is a major component of the neurological examination of a patient. Many cranial nerves are involved in the innervation of these structures, and the central visual pathway comprises a significant portion of the prosencephalon. One of the most reliable indicators of a cerebral lesion is loss of vision with preservation of pupillary light responses. This discussion of neuro-ophthalmology follows the method of examination of the eye in the neurological examination of a patient.

The order in which one performs the neurological examination depends on the nature of the patient's disability. If the patient is ambulatory, the gait and postural reactions are usually examined first. While watching a small animal walk through the corridors of the hospital and around objects, a visual deficit may be apparent only if it is severe. Even almost completely blind animals often avoid objects well in a familiar environment. Owners rarely recognize a visual deficit until it is totally bilateral. This often results in a complaint of a sudden onset of blindness. A maze can be set up for any of the domestic animals, but evaluation is most difficult in cats. In routine evaluation, the menace response is the most reliable test for vision.

dorsal portion medially toward the midline), and the ventral oblique muscle *extorts* the globe (moves the same point laterally away from the midline). These muscles do not function alone but act together in a synergistic or antagonistic manner to provide conjugate movements of both eyes in the same direction at the same time. This is demonstrated by the action of the medial and

TABLE 17–1. Extraocular Muscles—Actions and Innervations

Muscle	Innervation	Action
Superior (dorsal) rectus m	Oculomotor III	Elevates globe
Inferior (ventral) rectus m	Oculomotor III	Depresses globe
Medial rectus m	Oculomotor III	Turns globe nasally
Lateral rectus m	Abducens VI	Turns globe temporally
Superior (dorsal) oblique m	Trochlear VI	Intorts globe (rotates 12 o'clock position nasally)
Inferior (ventral) oblique m	Oculomotor III	Extorts globe (rotates 12 o'clock position temporally)
M retractor bulbi	Abducens VI	Retracts globe
M levator superioris	Oculomotor III	Elevates upper lid

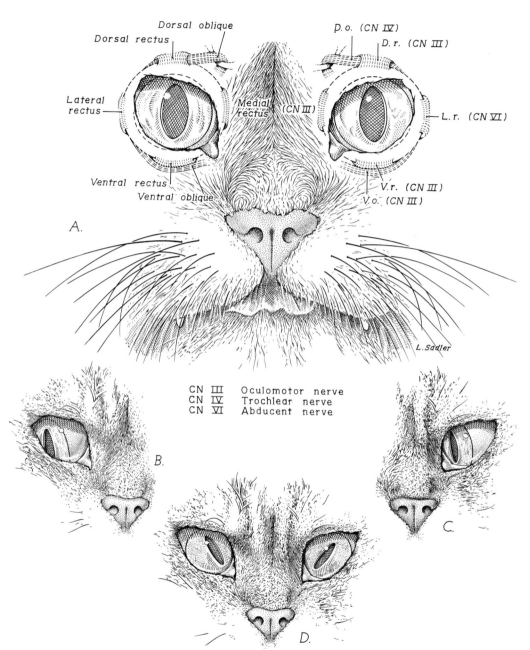

Dorsal oblique
Dorsal rectus
D.o. (CN IV)
D.r. (CN III)

Lateral rectus
Medial rectus (CN III)
L.r. (CN VI)

Ventral rectus
Ventral oblique
V.r. (CN III)
V.o. (CN III)

A.

CN III   Oculomotor nerve
CN IV   Trochlear nerve
CN VI   Abducent nerve

L.Sadler

B.

C.

D.

FIGURE 17–4. A, Functional anatomy of the extraocular muscles. Directions of strabismus are shown following paralysis of the oculomotor (B), abducent (C), and trochlear (D) neurons. (From deLahunta A: Veterinary Neuroanatomy and Clinical Neurology, 2nd ed. WB Saunders Co, Philadelphia, 1983.)

A diagnostic approach is outlined in Figure 17–5 based on the signs observed in the order in which the eye is examined. Further details of some of the conditions mentioned are given later in this chapter, discussed by the condition rather than by the clinical signs.

Menace Response
(See Fig. 17–18)

The cranial nerve examination begins with the eye and the animal's response to a menacing gesture. Most small animals are examined as you face them from the front or by standing over them and gently extending the head and neck so that both eyes can be seen. In recumbent large animals, the eye on the recumbent side may be severely traumatized, limiting some aspect of this examination. The menace response is performed by making a threatening gesture with the hand at each eye while the other hand covers the opposite eye. If you do not cover the other eye, an alert animal who is blind in the eye being tested may observe the threat with its normal eye and respond by blinking bilaterally. This is not necessary in cattle and horses. It is crucial to the validity of this test that the threatening hand does not touch the patient or create enough air current to be felt by the patient. Avoid the long cilia (eyelashes) in some horses and dogs.

The normal response to this threat is a rapid blink and closure of the palpebral fissure. The motor component is mediated through the facial nerve and its nucleus in the medulla. The afferent side of this response is extensive and involves a cerebral pathway, which implicates this as a learned response. Therefore, this response may not become fully developed until 10 to 12 weeks in some small animals. It is usually present by 5 to 7 days in foals and calves. The following structures must be normal for the impulses to be generated by the threat and ultimately reach the facial motor neurons in the medulla: the cornea, aqueous, lens, vitreous, retina, optic nerve, optic chiasm (65% of optic nerve axons cross in the cat, 75% in the dog,

80–90% in large animals), optic tract, and the lateral geniculate nucleus, optic radiation, and visual cortex of the occipital lobe. It is assumed that the visual cortex projects to the motor cortex, which, in turn, projects via the internal capsule and crus cerebri to the facial nuclei in the medulla.

Because the majority of optic nerve axons cross in the optic chiasm, the impulses generated in the retina of the threatened eye primarily project to the opposite optic tract, lateral geniculate nucleus, optic radiation, and visual cortex. Therefore, a loss of menace response on one side is a reliable indicator of a lesion in the opposite central visual pathway, even though there are still intact optic nerve axons projecting ipsilaterally. Most of the optic nerve axons that cross in the chiasm arise from the ganglion cell layer of the medial two thirds of the retina, and those that project ipsilaterally come from the lateral retina. Ideally, they could be tested separately by a threat from the lateral and medial visual fields, respectively. However, this is unreliable, and a close relationship exists between a unilateral menace deficit and a contralateral central lesion.

Because of the close interaction between the cerebrum and the cerebellum, serious cerebellar lesions prevent the menace response but do not interfere with visual perception. Animals with this condition have significant signs of cerebellar ataxia. A unilateral cerebellar lesion causes an ipsilateral menace deficit with normal vision. This occurs because of the crossing of the visual pathway in the optic chiasm and the reciprocal interaction between the cerebrum on one side and the opposite cerebellar hemisphere.

If the menace response does not occur, check the facial nerve innervation of the orbicularis oculi by touching the eyelids to see that they close the fissure normally. If facial paralysis exists, observe forehead or eye retraction when that eye is threatened. With slight retraction of the eye, the third eyelid passively protrudes. A patient with "flashing third eyelids" may have facial paralysis, and this is an indication that vision is intact. If there is no facial paralysis and no menace response occurs, lightly strike the animal two to three times with the threatening hand and repeat the threat without touching the patient. This often arouses and directs the attention of the patient and is then followed by a normal response.

Moving Objects

With all young, small animals who may not yet have learned the menace response, and occasionally with stoic older animals, vision can be assessed by rolling a cylinder of tape past them on the floor from different directions. A normal, alert young animal that may not respond to a menace readily follows the tape. The same can be accomplished by dropping cotton balls. Young hungry calves and foals often follow your hand or a nursing bottle.

EXAMINATION	1. Menace response
	2. Moving objects
	3. Visual placing postural reaction
	4. Pupillary light reflex
FINDINGS	5. Lesions with normal pupils
	6. Lesions with abnormal pupils
	7. Pupil size
	8. Intracranial injury
	9. Palpebral fissure
	10. Third eyelid
	11. Strabismus
	12. Nystagmus
	13. Palpebral reflex

FIGURE 17–5. Fundamentals of neuro-ophthalmic diagnosis.

Visual Placing Postural Reaction

The animal is held off the ground and brought to a table edge. If it sees the table, it elevates its limbs to place them on the table's surface before the limbs touch the table. A blind animal will not elevate the limbs until they touch the table's edge. As a rule, suspect total blindness when the patient does not direct its eyes at you during the examination.

Pupillary Light Reflex
(See Figs. 17–11 to 17–15)

The size and response of pupils to light is assessed after the menace test. If there is a visual deficit, further location of the lesion depends on a careful examination of the eyes and the pupils. It is important to evaluate the size of the pupils in normal room light before stimulating the retina with a strong light source. If the pupils cannot be seen without extra light, hold a penlight rostral to the nose of the patient and at a distance that will just allow you to see the pupillary margins. Assess the size of the pupils and compare them with each other. The pupillary light reflex is remarkably resistant to serious ocular diseases. Animals with extensive retinal or optic nerve disease (optic neuritis, progressive retinal degeneration) can be functionally blind, and yet the pupils may still respond to bright light. If you are not aware of this point, you may direct a strong light source into the fundus of a blind dog, observe a pupillary response, and erroneously diagnose a lesion in the central visual pathways. Although animals with retinal or optic nerve disease are blind and have pupils that respond to a bright light source, their pupils are dilated more than normal in room light. This can be verified by comparison with other animals with normal vision in the same room light.

Lesions in Animals With Normal Pupils

Based on this concept of the pupillary light reflex pathway, the size of the pupils and their response to light will be normal in animals with cerebral disease or disease limited to the lateral geniculate nuclei.

Bilateral cerebral lesions that cause blindness include prosencephalic hypoplasia with no cerebral hemispheres (calves), hydranencephaly (calves, lambs), anoxia, acute lead or chronic mercury poisoning, polioencephalomalacia–thiamine deficiency (ruminants), salt intoxication–water deprivation (pigs, ruminants), cerebral contusion, cerebral edema (injury, space-occupying lesions), leukoencephalomalacia (mycotoxicosis in horses), viral encephalitis, thrombotic meningoencephalitis (*Haemophilus somnus*) in cattle, and storage diseases.

The most common causes of a unilateral cerebral lesion with contralateral visual deficit are neoplasms in small animals and abscesses in large animals. Other causes include ischemic encephalopathy–cerebral infarction (most common in cats), protozoal encephalitis in horses, chronic canine distemper encephalitis, *Toxoplasma* granulomata, granulomatous meningoencephalitis in dogs, thrombotic meningoencephalitis in cattle, and parasitic cysts (coenurosis in sheep) or migrations.

Lesions in Animals With Abnormal Pupils

It takes a serious lesion of the afferent side of this reflex to cause an abnormality. It is rare for this reflex to be abnormal in an animal with an afferent lesion that was not blind in that eye. As a rule, afferent lesions that interrupt this reflex occur in the eye, optic nerve, or optic chiasm. Rarely, both optic tracts are affected sufficiently to cause pupillary abnormalities. A single optic tract lesion is rare and may cause no pupillary light reflex abnormality or may cause a depressed response when the eye opposite the lesion is stimulated.

A patient with a unilateral lesion in the retina or optic nerve has no menace response in that eye. Frequently there is no asymmetry of pupil size, or the pupil in that eye is slightly larger. Light directed into the affected eye causes no response in either eye. Light directed into the unaffected eye elicits a bilateral response. To assess direct and indirect responses, direct the light back and forth between the eyes. As the light is directed from the unaffected to the affected eye in the animal with a unilateral lesion, the pupil in the affected eye will be dilating back to the resting state created by the room light. This is because the strong light source was taken away from the unaffected eye and the lesion in the affected eye has interrupted the afferent pathway for this reflex. This phenomenon is readily apparent as the light is repeatedly moved between the eyes. Further confirmation of a unilateral lesion is made by covering the normal eye and observing further dilation of the pupil in the affected eye.

Unilateral lesions include congenital optic nerve hypoplasia or atrophy, optic nerve coloboma (part of the scleral ectasia syndrome of collies and Shetland sheepdogs and charolais cattle), ocular or optic nerve injury, and ocular or retrobulbar neoplasia.

Severe bilateral ocular, optic nerve, or optic chiasm lesions cause blindness with dilated pupils that are unresponsive to light. This occurs with bilateral congenital lesions (hypoplasia or atrophy, colobomata) and extensive retinal degeneration. Both optic nerves are subject to traumatic injury, causing direct avulsion of the axons at the level of the optic canals or optic chiasm or interference with the vascular supply of the intracanalicular part of the optic nerve. This may be more common in horses. In the chronic stage in the horse, fundic examination often shows optic disc atrophy, hypovascularity, and a linear hypopigmentation just ventral to the disc in the nontapetal area. Vitamin A deficiency in young cattle causes optic nerve compression from stenosis of the optic canals. Rarely in cats, the ischemic encephalopathy syndrome results in infarction of the optic chiasm.

Optic neuritis from canine distemper infection or idiopathic granulomatous meningoencephalitis can affect both optic nerves and the optic chiasm. If the lesion is severe enough, a visual deficit results. This is more common with granulomatous inflammation. Hypophyseal fossa neoplasms occasionally compress the optic chiasm sufficiently to cause a visual deficit.

A lesion of the efferent pathway in the parasympathetic component of the oculomotor nerve causes a widely dilated pupil in the ipsilateral eye at rest. The menace response is normal in each eye. Light directed into either eye causes constriction of the pupil in the eye on the side opposite the lesion only.

The optic chiasm and the oculomotor nerves may be compressed by extramedullary space-occupying lesions near the hypophyseal fossa. These lesions include pituitary neoplasms and germ cell neoplasms (teratomata). The latter are more common in dogs less than 5 years of age. A retrobulbar or intracranial lesion that affects both the optic nerve and the parasympathetic part of the oculomotor nerve causes a widely dilated pupil in the ipsilateral eye at rest. There is no menace response from this affected eye. Light directed into the affected eye elicits no response in either eye. Light directed into the unaffected eye causes pupillary constriction in that eye only. A complete oculomotor nerve deficit includes ventrolateral strabismus and ptosis.

Pupil Size

It is apparent that it is important to evaluate and compare the size of the pupils in room light or under an equal amount of light from an accessory source. The influence of lesions in the eye, optic nerve, and oculomotor nerve has been considered. The remaining neurological component that can influence the size of the pupil is the sympathetic innervation of the iris smooth muscle that dilates the pupil. The size of the pupil at rest represents a balance between the amount of light stimulating the retina and influencing the oculomotor neurons to constrict the pupil and the emotional status of the patient, which influences the sympathetic system and causes pupillary dilation.

A defect in the sympathetic innervation of the structures of the head is referred to as Horner's syndrome (discussed later in this chapter).

Intracranial Injury

Evaluation of the size of the pupils is important in assessing the location and extent of brain damage from intracranial injury and also in following the response to therapy. Brain stem contusion with hemorrhage and laceration of the midbrain and pons is a common result of serious injury. This interrupts the parenchymal components of the oculomotor neurons, causing bilateral widely dilated, unresponsive pupils, which are a grave sign. These animals are also recumbent and semicomatose or comatose. Injuries that predominately involve the prosencephalon often result in very miotic pupils, which is assumed to represent a release of the parasympathetic oculomotor neurons from upper motor neuron inhibition. These miotic pupils can change rapidly to dilated, unresponsive pupils if there is progressive brain stem edema or hemorrhage. They can just as readily return to normal size if the cerebral edema resolves. Frequently, there is remarkable anisocoria with one mydriatic and one miotic pupil. Usually each shows a slight response to light. Pupils in this state should be watched carefully as an indication of whether to treat the patient more vigorously or not. Severe caudal brain stem lesions that are life-threatening often result in partly dilated, fixed, and unresponsive pupils.

Palpebral Fissure

Lesions that decrease the size of the palpebral fissure include:
1. Facial paralysis or paresis
2. Atrophy of the muscles of mastication
3. Horner's syndrome
4. Hemifacial spasm
5. Tetanus

In small animals, the size of the palpebral fissure primarily depends on normal tone in the levator palpebrae superioris muscle innervated by the oculomotor nerve and in the smooth muscle innervated by the sympathetic neurons. In large animals, superficial facial muscles innervated by the facial nerve (cranial nerve VII) insert in the upper eyelid and help keep the fissure open. The orbicularis oculi, innervated by the facial nerve, is responsible for closure of the fissure. Its function was observed when the menace response was tested. In facial paralysis in small animals, the size of the palpebral fissure is usually unchanged or slightly larger because of loss of tone in the orbicularis oculi. Facial paralysis is further discussed on page 447.

In small animals, a small palpebral fissure or ptosis results from a lesion in the oculomotor or sympathetic neurons that supply the eye. With complete oculomotor paralysis, the ipsilateral pupil is dilated and unresponsive to light directed into either eye. There is also a lateral and slightly ventral strabismus with decreased ability to adduct the eye normally. A lesion in the sympathetic innervation also produces an elevated third eyelid and miosis. Ptosis in large animals can have the same causes but also will occur with facial paralysis. The latter is easily determined by recognizing the accompanying inability to close the fissure. Otitis media can affect facial neurons in all large animals, and rarely guttural pouch mycosis can involve these neurons in horses.

A small palpebral fissure occurs indirectly when extensive atrophy of the muscles of mastication occurs and the eye retracts into the orbit. This atrophy can result from an extensive myositis of these muscles or from their denervation when lesions affect the mandibular nerve component of the trigeminal nerve.

A narrowed palpebral fissure occurs with spasm of the facial muscles on one side (see p 448).

Occasionally, animals with serious cerebellar disease that involves the cerebellar nuclei will have one palpebral fissure that is slightly wider or a mildly elevated third eyelid. This has also been produced experimentally with lesions in the nuclei of the cerebellum.

Third Eyelid

Normally, the third eyelid is maintained in its position ventromedial to the eye by the tone in its smooth muscle, which keeps it retracted. This is a function of its sympathetic innervation. The normally protruded position of the eye in the orbit also contributes to the normal position of the third eyelid. Lesions of the sympathetic neurons cause a constant protrusion of the third eyelid, which is a feature of Horner's syndrome. The third eyelid also passively protrudes if the eye is actively retracted, as in tetanus, or if the eye sinks in the orbit from atrophy of the muscles of mastication (chronic myositis or trigeminal nerve paralysis).

Strabismus

Strabismus is an abnormal position of the eye and results from lesions of the cranial nerves that innervate the striated extraocular muscles (cranial nerves III, IV, and VI) or occurs in some head positions with lesions in the vestibular system. Oculomotor nerve lesions cause a lateral and slightly ventral strabismus—EXOTROPIA—primarily from loss of innervation of the medial rectus and secondarily from the denervation of the dorsal and ventral rectus muscles and the ventral oblique muscle. Eye adduction is deficient and will be observed on testing normal vestibular nystagmus. As the head is moved in a dorsal plane, side to side, the eyes normally develop a jerk nystagmus with the quick phase in the direction of the head movement. The jerklike movement toward the nose is adduction from the action of the medial rectus innervated by the oculomotor nerve (cranial nerve III).

The same abrupt movement away from the nose, adduction, is a function of the lateral rectus innervated by the abducent nerve (cranial nerve VI). The latter is deficient in lesions of the abducent neurons and ESO-TROPIA is observed.

Ptosis and a dilated unresponsive pupil accompany a complete loss of oculomotor nerve function.

Trochlear nerve (cranial nerve IV) lesions are rare. Denervation of the dorsal oblique muscle results in a strabismus that is difficult to recognize in the dog because of the animal's round pupil, and it may recover rapidly because of the compensatory activity of the other extraocular muscles. In ruminants and horses, the medial end of the normally horizontal pupil will be directed dorsally—dorsomedial strabismus. This is seen in polioencephalomalacia in ruminants and is thought to represent a unique susceptibility of the trochlear neurons to this metabolic encephalopathy. In cats, with vertical pupils, the dorsal aspect of the pupil deviates laterally with a lesion of the trochlear neurons. In the dog, a fundic examination may reveal a similar lateral displacement of the superior retinal vein.

Exotropia is often seen in hydrocephalic animals that have an enlarged cranial cavity. Both eyes often deviate ventrolaterally. This is thought to result from a malformation of the orbit that occurs when the cranial cavity is distorted by the early development of the brain abnormality. These eyes will adduct and abduct normally on testing normal vestibular nystagmus, and no ptosis or pupillary abnormality is present.

Strabismus can also occur in some positions of the head with lesions in the vestibular system. It can occur peripherally with lesions in the inner ear and vestibulocochlear nerve (cranial nerve VIII) or centrally with lesions in the vestibular nuclei of the medulla or vestibular pathways in the cerebellum. This involves the eye on the same side as the vestibular abnormality, is usually a ventrolateral strabismus, and is only present when the head is in certain positions. It is most evident when the head and neck are extended and the eye on the affected side fails to elevate normally in the palpebral fissure. Sclera is evident dorsally in the "dropped" eye. Normally in small animals, both eyes elevate and remain in the center of the fissure so that no sclera is visible. This normal ocular elevation is less in horses and even less in cattle. The ventrolateral exotropia associated with vestibular disease can be differentiated from the strabismus of an oculomotor nerve lesion by the presence of signs of vestibular system disturbance and the maintenance of the ability to adduct the eye normally on testing normal nystagmus.

Nystagmus

See page 461.

Palpebral Reflex

The palpebral reflex is used to test the ability of the animal to close its eyelids. It tests both sensory (cranial

TABLE 17–2. Summary of Neuro-Ophthalmic Examination

Test or Observation	Neurological Components
Menace response	Cranial nerve II—central visual pathway—cranial nerve VII (cerebellum)
Size of pupils	Cranial nerves II, III, sympathetics, diencephalon-mesencephalon (cerebellum)
Pupillary light reflex	Cranial nerve II—pretectal nuclei—cranial nerve III
Eyelids (size of fissure)	Cranial nerve III, sympathetics, cranial nerve VII Masticatory muscle atrophy (cerebellum)
Third eyelid	Sympathetics Masticatory muscle atrophy (cerebellum)
Position of eyes	Cranial nerves III, IV, VI, vestibular system orbit
Normal nystagmus	Cranial nerve VIII—brain stem—cranial nerves III, VI
Abnormal nystagmus	Vestibular system Congenital—Visual system
Palpebral reflex	Cranial nerve V—cranial nerve VII

nerve V) and motor (cranial nerve VII) innervation of the eyelids. Sensory innervation is via branches of the ophthalmic and maxillary nerves from the trigeminal nerve (cranial nerve V). Although the ophthalmic nerve branches are predominantly medial and the maxillary nerve branches are lateral, there is extensive overlap so that the only autonomous zone of the ophthalmic nerve is a small area of skin dorsomedial to the medial angle of the eyelids. For the maxillary nerve branches, this zone is ventrolateral to the lateral angle of the eyelids. Sensory deficits are uncommon when compared with facial paralysis and can be mistaken for the latter. Animals with only a trigeminal nerve lesion blink spontaneously when the eye is menaced provided that they can see. Loss of ophthalmic nerve innervation to the cornea via ciliary nerves may result in a neurotrophic keratitis.

Diseases that predominate in the brain stem may cause various combinations of cranial nerve deficits that are observed in the ocular examination. The most common of these is listeriosis in cattle. Others include protozoal encephalitis in horses, thrombotic meningoencephalitis in cattle, granulomatous meningoencephalitis in dogs, and intramedullary or extramedullary neoplasia in all animals.

Table 17–2 summarizes the neuro-ophthalmic examination.

CLINICAL SIGNS OF DYSFUNCTION OF CRANIAL NERVES III, IV, AND VI

Strabismus

Abducent Paralysis. Lesions of the abducent nucleus or nerve cause paralysis (palsy) of the lateral rectus and retractor bulbi muscles. Paralysis of the lateral rectus muscle causes unilateral esotropia (medial strabismus), which is an abnormal position of the affected eye that results in asymmetry. Compared with the normal eye, the affected eye cannot be abducted fully.

This is detected by moving the patient's head from side to side in a horizontal plane and observing the degree of abduction and adduction of each eye. Strabismus may be caused by neural dysfunction or mechanical and muscular disorders within the orbit.

Trochlear Paralysis. Lesions of the trochlear nucleus or nerve paralyze the dorsal oblique muscle. In species with round pupils, no strabismus is observed; however, ophthalmoscopic examination may show the superior retinal vein to be deviated laterally from its normal vertical position because of the abnormal rotation caused by the tone in the unopposed ventral oblique muscle. In cattle and sheep, which have horizontal pupils, the medial portion of the pupil is deviated dorsally (Fig. 17–6). This is called EXTORSION and is seen in ruminants with polioencephalomalacia.

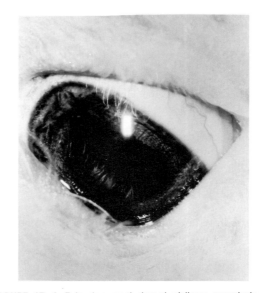

FIGURE 17–6. Extorsion and dorsal oblique paralysis in a sheep with polioencephalomalacia. Note elevation and lateral rotation of the medial part of the elliptical pupil (left eye). (Courtesy of Dr. E. Thornber.)

Oculomotor Paralysis. Paralysis of the intraocular muscles is called INTERNAL OPHTHALMOPLEGIA, and paralysis of the extraocular muscles is called EXTERNAL OPHTHALMOPLEGIA. Each type may occur alone. Lesions of the oculomotor nucleus or nerve produce a lateral and ventral strabismus resulting from the paralysis of the extraocular muscles and ptosis resulting from paralysis of the levator palpebrae muscle. In addition, loss of function of the general visceral efferent neurons controlling the intraocular muscles, which are also a component of this nerve, causes a dilated, unresponsive pupil. There is experimental evidence to support the direction of this strabismus, although it is difficult to explain the ventral deviation on the basis of the anatomy of the oblique muscle.

When strabismus is suspected, the eye movements are tested to verify the paralysis of the extraocular muscles. This is done by moving the head of the patient vertically or horizontally and watching for symmetry of ocular movements. The vestibular and cervical proprioceptive systems exert considerable influence on the nuclei of the cranial nerves that innervate the extraocular muscles. Movements of the head require a simultaneous conjugate response by the eyes to maintain fixation on objects in the visual field. One of the major pathways involved in connecting the vestibular system to these nuclei is the MEDIAL LONGITUDINAL FASCICULUS.

Lesions of the vestibular system or of the medial longitudinal fasciculus may cause an abnormal ocular position when the head is in certain positions. This appears as strabismus but can usually be corrected by repositioning the head. Strabismus resulting from faulty extraocular muscle innervation persists in *all* positions of the head.

Trigeminal Dysfunction. Bilateral disease of these motor neurons (NEURAPRAXIA) causes a dropped jaw that cannot be closed. The patient has difficulty grasping food or retaining it in the oral cavity. Manipulation of the jaw reveals muscle atonia, and neurogenic atrophy of the temporal muscles follows if paralysis persists. Unilateral disease may be difficult to discover until muscle atrophy appears. The lower jaw may be directed toward the side of the lesion by the unopposed tone in the normal pterygoid muscles, and chewing may be asymmetrical, but this is difficult to detect. Bilateral neurapraxia of the mandibular branch has been seen in dogs after prehension of large objects. The condition resolves spontaneously in 4–5 weeks if the dog is fed soft foods and the mandible is fastened to the maxilla. Involvement of the ophthalmic branch of the trigeminal nerve has been observed concurrently, causing bilateral loss of corneal sensitivity and the corneal reflex. Recovery of the corneal reflex is slower than return of mandibular control.

Damage to the sensory portions of the trigeminal nerve, usually resulting from trauma, may cause corneal insensitivity with resulting ulceration from local persistent minor trauma or neurotrophic keratitis. (See Chap 11.)

Facial Nerve Dysfunction

Facial Paralysis. Lesions of the nucleus or of the nerve up to the level of its termination into branches that supply the different muscle groups result in complete facial palsy or paralysis, with inability to move these muscles normally.

Clinical Signs

1. FACIAL ASYMMETRY. Paralysis is evident in the asymmetrical position of the ears, eyelids, lips, and nose, the ear drooping in those animals with normally erect ears. If the ear cartilage is stiff, as in most cats and some dogs, it may keep the ear erect despite paralysis.

2. DROOLING OF SALIVA. The lip may droop on the affected side, allowing saliva to drip from the corner of the mouth. It is helpful to extend the head with a finger between the mandibles and examine the corner of the lips for asymmetry. On the paralyzed side, more mucosa is exposed, and drooling may be apparent.

3. DISPLACEMENT OF THE NASAL PHILTRUM. The nose may be *pulled toward the normal side,* owing to the unopposed nasal muscles, especially in horses. In dogs, there is slight deviation of the philtrum from its normal vertical position. During inspiration, the nostril may not be opened as wide as usually on the affected side.

4. LOSS OF CORNEAL AND PALPEBRAL REFLEXES. The palpebral fissure in small animals is usually slightly wider than normal and fails to close on stimulation of the cornea or eyelids (corneal and palpebral reflexes), owing to paralysis of the orbicularis oculi. In facial paralysis, this closure is weak. In large animals, the loss of tone in the frontalis muscle, which contributes fibers that elevate the upper eyelid, causes slight ptosis. The eyelids of both sides are palpated simultaneously for strength of closure when examining for asymmetry in facial paresis.

5. CORNEAL DESSICATION AND ULCERATION. This condition occurs in chronically affected animals and may be the major clinical difficulty in management.

Lesions of individual branches of the facial nerve along their course produces paralysis restricted to those muscle groups. Injury to the buccal branches of the facial nerve on the side of the masseter muscle causes the lips to droop and the nose to be pulled toward the normal side. This occurs when horses undergo surgery for prolonged periods in a recumbent position without padding for the head. Eyelid and ear function are normal. Injury to the auriculopalpebral nerve at the zygomatic arch causes paresis of the ear and eyelid muscles.

The *facial and vestibulocochlear nerves* are closely associated and may be affected by the same lesion in or on the medulla or in the petrosal bone. It is important to distinguish between the two locations because of the poor prognosis of medullary lesions. Both a medullary neoplasm and otitis media and otitis interna can affect the function of these two cranial nerves. Medullary lesions usually affect other brain stem structures, which aids in locating the lesion. Structures that may be affected by medullary neoplasms include the upper motor neuron, causing tetra- or hemiparesis; the ascending reticular activating system, resulting in signs ranging from depression to coma; and the abducent nucleus, causing esotropia. General proprioception may also be affected, resulting in ataxia. Facial paralysis on one side of the face must be distinguished from the syndrome of hemifacial spasm on the other side.

In dogs (and less commonly in cats), *permanent or temporary spontaneous facial paralysis* of unknown cause occurs. Cocker spaniels, Pembroke corgis, boxers, and English setters are at greater risk, with dogs greater than 5 years of age being predisposed. Temporary cases resolve within 4–6 weeks, during which time systemic corticosteroids should be administered. Tarsorrhaphy, third eyelid flap, and topical therapy may be necessary to treat corneal ulceration. An association with hypothyroidism *in some cases* has been confirmed in dogs.

Table 17–3 lists signs and causes that were recorded by Kern and Erb.

Enucleation may be necessary in permanent paralysis. In cats and horses, facial paralysis is more commonly traumatic. In all species, otitis media may involve the facial nerve as it passes through the facial canal in the petrosal bone close to the tympanic bulla. The entire area of distribution of the facial nerve is usually affected with paresis or paralysis. Signs of vestibular ataxia are usually present, as the vestibulocochlear nerve in the inner ear is also involved. Table 17–4 summarizes the common clinical signs of facial paralysis in the dog, cat, and horse.

TABLE 17–4. Summary of Clinical Signs of Facial Paralysis

Dog and Cat	Horse
Paralyzed side of face is pulled toward normal side.	Paralyzed side of face is pulled toward normal side.
Deviation of philtrum is slight.	Drooping of ear on affected side.
Drooping of ear on affected side (Fig. 17–7).	Ptosis (paralysis of frontalis muscle).
Drooling of saliva and visible mucosa on affected side. Self-mutilation during chewing in some dogs.	
Palpebral fissure is wider, and lower lid droops (Fig. 17–19).	
Loss of corneal and palpebral reflexes.	
Desiccation of cornea and ulceration in chronic cases (Fig. 17–7).	

Injury to the petrosal bone may cause hemorrhage in the middle and inner ears and bleeding from the external ear canal through a ruptured tympanum, usually associated with fracture of the basioccipital or petrosal bone. Facial and vestibulocochlear nerve function may be affected. In guttural pouch mycosis in horses, extensive inflammation may cause paralysis of the adjacent facial nerve, in addition to Horner's syndrome.

Hemifacial Spasm. In chronic otitis media and otitis interna in dogs, hypersensitivity of the facial

TABLE 17–3. Signs and Causes of Facial Paralysis

Feature	Dog (79 cases) %	Cat (16 cases) %
Cause		
Idiopathic	25.0	25.0
Surgery	8.9	12.5
Trauma	5.1	31.3
Neoplasia	2.5	25.0
Otitis media	—	6.3
Neuropathy as the Only Sign	39.2	50.0
Associated Signs		
Hypothyroidism	25.0	0.0
Keratoconjunctivitis sicca	18.8	12.5
Otitis media	14.6	37.5
Horner's syndrome	14.6	25.0
Other cranial nerve neuropathies	8.3	—
Vestibular signs	6.7	87.5

From Kern TJ, Erb N: Facial neuropathy in dogs and cats: 95 cases (1975–1985). J Am Vet Med Assoc 191:1604, 1987.

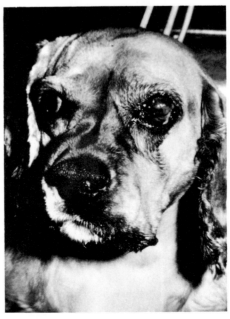

FIGURE 17–7. Unilateral facial paralysis (idiopathic) in a dog. Note the widened palpebral fissure. (Courtesy of Dr. G.A. Severin.)

nerve may occur, causing spasm of facial muscles on the affected side.

Clinical Signs

1. Blepharospasm, possibly resulting in spastic entropion.

2. Elevated, wrinkled upper lip with caudal displacement of the commissure, which gives the animal a "grinning" appearance.

3. Elevation of the ear.

4. Deviation of the nose toward the affected side.

5. Often ipsilateral Horner's syndrome, but without signs of vestibular dysfunction.

Treatment

1. Routine medical and surgical treatment of otitis.

2. Surgical correction of spastic entropion, if necessary.

3. Blocking of the palpebral branch of the facial nerve with ethyl alcohol. This should not be performed in exophthalmic breeds, as lagophthalmos and exposure keratitis may result.

4. Supportive therapy for the cornea, including regular cleansing and topical antibiotics.

Multiple Cranial Nerve Disorders

Numerous conditions result in disorders of one or more of the nerves associated with the eye and the adnexa. For relevant details of myasthenia gravis, listeriosis, equine focal protozoal encephalitis, and polioencephalomalacia in ruminants see Chapter 19.

AUTONOMIC INNERVATION AND ABNORMALITIES

The autonomic nervous system is a physiological and anatomical system with central and peripheral components. It includes higher centers situated in the hypothalamus, midbrain, pons, and medulla. The hypothalamus is the primary integrating center for the autonomic nervous system. Nuclei in its rostral portion subserve the parasympathetic division of the autonomic system. These hypothalamic nuclei receive afferents from the cerebrum (by numerous pathways), thalamic nuclei, and ascending general visceral afferent pathways. The hypothalamus influences the activity of the metabolic centers in the reticular formation of the midbrain, pons, and medulla.

Autonomic innervation is composed of two neurons interposed between the CNS and the organ innervated. The cell body of the first neuron is located in the gray matter of the CNS, and its axon passes through a cranial or spinal nerve to the peripheral ganglion, at which point it connects with the cell body of the second neuron. The first neuron is called the PREGANGLIONIC NEURON. The second neuron has its cell body and dendritic zone in a peripheral ganglion, and its axon, the POSTGANGLIONIC AXON, terminates in the innervated structure.

The autonomic system is grouped into two divisions physiologically and anatomically. The SYMPATHETIC SYSTEM (thoracolumbar) has cell bodies of preganglionic neurons in the intermediate gray column of the spinal cord from approximately the first thoracic to the fifth lumbar spinal cord segment. With few exceptions, the neurotransmitter elaborated at the postganglionic axon in the sympathetic system is NOREPINEPHRINE. The PARASYMPATHETIC SYSTEM (craniosacral) has cell bodies of preganglionic neurons in sacral segments of the spinal cord and in the nuclei of the brain stem associated with cranial nerves III, VII, IX, and XI. The neurotransmitter released at the postganglionic axon in the parasympathetic system is ACETYLCHOLINE (see Figs. 3–11 and 3–12).

Control of Pupils

In clinical neuro-ophthalmology, knowledge of pupil innervation is important in understanding pupillary size and responsiveness to light, excitement, and disease processes. The parasympathetic innervation of the pupil responds to incident light, whereas sympathetic innervation is stimulated by factors that elicit excitement, fear, or anger. In the resting pupil, both pupillary dilator (sympathetic) and the antagonistic pupillary sphincter (parasympathetic) muscles are active. The relative resting parasympathetic and sympathetic innervation and resulting muscle tone determine the size of the pupil (Fig. 17–8). The pupillary sphincter (or constrictor) is the *more powerful* of the two muscles.

Disorders of the autonomic nervous system are now considered under sympathetic and parasympathetic innervation.

Sympathetic Lower Motor Neuron Innervation[3]

Preganglionic cell bodies are located in the first three or four segments of the thoracic spinal cord. Axons join the ventral roots of these segments and the proximal portion of the segmental spinal nerve. These preganglionic axons leave the spinal nerve in the segmental rami communicantes, join the thoracic sympathetic trunk inside the thorax (ventrolateral to the vertebral column), and pass cranially without forming a synapse. They pass *through* the cervicothoracic and middle cervical ganglia and forward in the cervical sympathetic trunk, as part of the vagosympathetic trunk. Medial to the origin of the digastric muscle and ventromedial to the tympanic bulla, the cervical sympathetic trunk separates from the vagus and terminates in the CRANIAL CERVICAL GANGLION *at which point the preganglionic axons connect.* The cell body of the postganglionic axon is in the cranial cervical ganglion.

---

3. See Figs. 1–18 and 1–19.

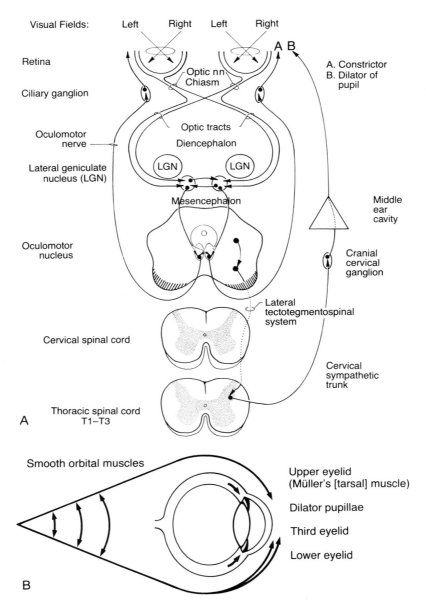

FIGURE 17–8. Neuroanatomical pathway for pupillary control. A, *Parasympathetic and sympathetic pathways.* B, *Structures in the eye and orbit with sympathetic innervation.*

The axons for ocular innervation in dogs and cats pass rostrally through the tympano-occipital fissure with the internal carotid artery and pass between the tympanic bulla and the petrosal bone into the middle ear cavity, closely associated with the ventral surface of the petrosal bone. The axons continue rostrally between the petrosal bone and basisphenoid to join the trigeminal ganglion and ophthalmic nerve. The ophthalmic nerve enters the periorbita through the orbital fissure.

Postganglionic sympathetic axons are distributed by ophthalmic nerve branches to smooth muscles of the orbit, Müller's muscle of the upper lid (and analogous sympathetically innervated tissue in the lower lid), third eyelid, ciliary muscle, pupillary dilator, and receptors in the iridocorneal (drainage) angle. The exact function of autonomic innervation in control of aqueous outflow facility in the drainage angle is unknown. Normal tone of sympathetically innervated ocular structures keeps the eye protruded, the palpebral fissure widened, the third eyelid retracted, and the pupil partially dilated.

FELINE DYSAUTONOMIA (Key-Gaskell Syndrome)

Synonyms: Dilated pupil syndrome, feline autonomic polyganglionopathy

Feline dysautonomia is a disturbance of systemic autonomic innervation with a marked reduction in the number of neurons in autonomic ganglia, resulting in complete autonomic denervation of the eye (and other organs). The majority of affected cats are less than 3 years of age. The condition is more common in domestic shorthaired cats and in males. The onset is usually acute and sporadic.

Diagnosis. Feline dysautonomia is diagnosed by its clinical signs, especially *protrusion of the third eyelids with dilated pupils.* Together with the other signs, this differentiates it from Horner's syndrome, in which the denervation is limited to the sympathetic system and is usually unilateral. To date, the condition has been reported in the United Kingdom and in cats imported to the United States from the British Isles.

Pharmacological testing can be used to demonstrate *denervation hypersensitivity* of both sympathetic and parasympathetic systems. The procedure is as follows:

Parasympathetic Denervation

Synonyms: Adie's pupil, pupillatonia

1. Instill a drop of 0.1% pilocarpine and measure pupillary diameter every 5 minutes. If denervation is present, immediate miosis can be expected when compared with a normal control animal.

2. Instill a drop of 0.06% echothiophate iodide (Phospholine Iodide). The denervated eye will show no change in pupillary diameter, but miosis will occur in the control cat.

Sympathetic Denervation

1. Instill one drop of 1:10000 epinephrine. The third eyelid will retract in the denervated eye because of hypersensitivity of the orbital smooth muscle to the epinephrine.

Clinical Signs.
1. Dilated unresponsive pupils
2. Protrusion of the third eyelids
3. Blepharospasm
4. Keratoconjunctivitis sicca
5. Dry crusted nose
6. Dry oral mucous membranes and oral cavity
7. Anorexia and lethargy
8. Megaesophagus and difficulty in swallowing
9. Vomiting-regurgitation
10. Slow gastric emptying
11. Fecal and urinary incontinence
12. Bradycardia
13. Distended bladder

Treatment. The prognosis is poor.
1. General supportive therapy, including subcutaneous and oral fluids.
2. Routine topical agents for keratoconjunctivitis sicca, including compound KCS drops and artificial tears.
3. Laxatives

HORNER'S SYNDROME

Clinical Signs. Loss of sympathetic innervation causes a lack of tone in the orbital smooth muscle and the eye retracts slightly, producing ENOPHTHALMOS. Loss of tone in Müller's muscle causes slight narrowing of the palpebral fissure resulting from incomplete elevation of the upper lid (PTOSIS). Lack of retraction causes PROTRUSION OF THE THIRD EYELID and lack of normal sympathetic tone in the pupillary dilator with MIOSIS and anisocoria (Fig. 17–9). These four signs collectively are called HORNER'S SYNDROME and are associated with lesions in any portion of this pathway from the hypothalamus to the cranial thoracic spinal cord segments to the effector muscle in the eye or orbit.

In addition to signs of denervation of orbital smooth

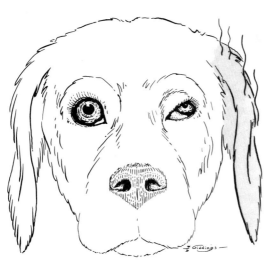

Miosis

Protrusion of the third eyelid

Ptosis

Enophthalmos

Dermal vasodilatation and hyperthermia

Ipsilateral sweating in horses

FIGURE 17–9. Signs of Horner's syndrome.

muscle, *peripheral vasodilation* occurs and may cause increased warmth, a pink skin color best observed in the ear, and congestion of ipsilateral nasal mucosa. These signs may be difficult to detect.

Pre- or postganglionic destruction of sympathetic innervation of the head in horses causes profuse sweating of the ipsilateral half of the face and cranial neck. The same area is hyperthermic, and the nasal and conjunctival mucosae are congested. Hyperthermia is determined by palpation of the ears. There is a prominent ptosis of the upper eyelid but only slight protrusion of the third eyelid and slight miosis. In cattle, sheep, and goats, the most constant signs are hyperthermia detected on ear palpation, and ptosis. Miosis and third eyelid protrusion are subtle. In cattle *less sweating* is visible on the surface of the nose on the denervated side.

Etiology (Table 17–5).

1. Injury, infarction, or neoplastic involvement of the cranial thoracic spinal cord causes signs of paresis or paralysis of the pelvic limbs and mild deficits in the thoracic limbs in addition to ipsilateral Horner's syndrome. Unilateral infarction of the lateral funiculus of the cervical spinal cord from fibrocartilaginous emboli may cause a persistent Horner's syndrome, along with hemiplegia, in dogs.

2. Avulsion of the brachial plexus roots in dogs and cats, with resultant thoracic limb paralysis, occurs after car accidents. Ipsilateral Horner's syndrome indicates that the injury to the nerves innervating the thoracic limb is in the cranial thoracic spinal cord.

3. Thoracic inlet or cranial mediastinal lesions (such as lymphosarcoma) involving the cranial thoracic sympathetic trunk or caudal cervical sympathetic trunk, or both, may cause Horner's syndrome.

4. Injury to the cervical sympathetic trunk from a dog bite or from surgical exposure of cervical intervertebral discs causes an ipsilateral Horner's syndrome that is usually transient (Fig. 17–10). Neoplasms involving the cervical sympathetic trunk, such as thyroid adenocarcinoma, are another cause.

5. Mycosis of the guttural pouch in horses may involve the cranial cervical ganglion or internal carotid nerve and produce ipsilateral Horner's syndrome.

6. Otitis media may produce Horner's syndrome,

often accompanied by signs of peripheral vestibular disturbance or facial paresis, or both.

7. Retrobulbar injury, neoplasia, and abscess are common causes of this syndrome.

8. Peripheral neuropathy caused by diabetes mellitus has been associated with Horner's syndrome in a bitch.

9. Routine venipuncture without administration of drugs has caused transient ipsilateral Horner's syndrome in horses.

The majority of cases of Horner's syndrome in dogs are idiopathic and postganglionic and resolve spontaneously within 6–8 weeks. Other causes should not be dismissed, however.

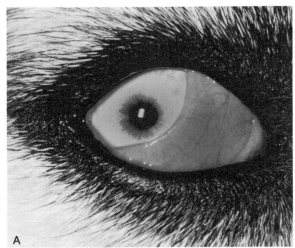
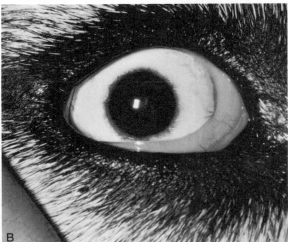

FIGURE 17–10. *Preganglionic Horner's syndrome in the left eye of an Alaskan malamute. A, Before instillation of epinephrine. B, Mydriasis 35 minutes after application of 0.1 ml of 0.0001% epinephrine solution. The lesion was preganglionic and associated with trauma resulting from vigorous lunging on a chain. It resolved spontaneously in 5–6 weeks.*

TABLE 17–5. Causes of Horner's Syndrome

Cause	Dog (18 cases) %	Cat (8 cases) %
Idiopathic	44.4	25.0
Car accidents	22.2	25.0
Bites	11.1	12.5
Cervical disc protrusion	11.1	—
Otitis media	5.6	—
Foreign body	—	12.5
Spinal neoplasia	—	12.5
Iatrogenic	—	12.5

Modified from van den Brock AHM: Horner's syndrome in cats and dogs: A review. J Sm Anim Pract 28:929, 1987.

Lesions causing Horner's syndrome, their location, and associated neurological deficits are summarized in Table 17–6.

DENERVATION HYPERSENSITIVITY is a phenomenon peculiar to smooth muscle innervated by the general visceral efferent system. Increased sensitivity of the muscle to neurotransmitters occurs and is evident in smooth muscle innervated by sympathetic neurons when the postganglionic axon is affected. Such denervated muscle shows hypersensitivity to the application of epinephrine or to circulating epinephrine released during excitement. This phenomenon has been studied in the dog with lesions of sympathetic innervation of the ocular smooth muscles. *Greater hypersensitivity* is present with lesions of postganglionic axons or their cell bodies than with lesions of preganglionic neurons, and this effect is used in differential diagnosis.

Topical application of 0.1 ml of 0.001% epinephrine causes pupillary dilation in 20 minutes with lesions of postganglionic axons or their cell bodies, and in 30 to 40 minutes with lesions of preganglionic neurons.[4] This test is useful to determine the location of the lesion in Horner's syndrome (see Fig. 17–10). Pharmacological testing can also be used to confirm complete autonomic denervation in feline dysautonomia.

---

4. Use of topical hydroxyamphetamine (Paredrine) for differential diagnosis of Horner's syndrome in dogs is based on human observations, is not substantiated by experimental findings in dogs, gives conflicting results, and is *not recommended.*

Treatment. The most important task is to determine the site of the Horner's syndrome. In general, preganglionic lesions have a less favorable prognosis than do postganglionic lesions. With postganglionic Horner's syndrome, in which an exact cause cannot be determined, symptomatic treatment may be instituted with phenylephrine drops (0.125% or 10%) as necessary to relieve the clinical signs. Most cases of postganglionic Horner's syndrome resolve spontaneously within 6 weeks. If the lesion is preganglionic, additional diagnostic procedures are undertaken to determine the site and cause, for example, cervical and thoracic radiographs, serum chemistry profile, neurological examination, and computerized axial tomography (CAT) scans of the neck if available. Because of the frequency of lymphosarcoma with cranial mediastinal lesions, thoracic radiographs are routinely taken in cats affected with Horner's syndrome.

Horner's syndrome must be distinguished from other common disorders of the third eyelid (see Chap 9).

Parasympathetic Lower Motor Neuron Innervation

OCULOMOTOR NERVE (CRANIAL NERVE III)

The cell bodies are located in the parasympathetic oculomotor nucleus adjacent to the motor component of this nucleus in the rostral colliculus and pretectal

TABLE 17–6. Horner's Syndrome—Summary of Lesions

Location	Lesion	Associated Neurological Deficit
Cervical spinal cord	External injury Focal leukomyelomalacia (ischemic)	Tetraplegia—spastic Hemiplegia—ipsilateral, spastic
T1–T3 spinal cord	External injury Neoplasm Focal poliomyelomalacia (ischemic)	Pelvic and thoracic limb paresis or paralysis with lower motor neuron deficit in thoracic limbs and upper motor neuron deficit in pelvic limbs
	Diffuse myelomalacia (ascending and descending)	Lower motor neuron deficit and analgesia of tail, anus, pelvic limbs, abdomen, and thorax with paretic thoracic limbs
T1–T3 ventral roots Proximal spinal nerves	Avulsion of roots of brachial plexus	Brachial plexus paresis or paralysis of the thoracic limb on the same side
Cranial thoracic sympathetic trunk	Lymphosarcoma Neurofibroma	None if confined to the trunk
Cervical sympathetic trunk	Injury from surgical intervention in the area or from dog bites	None if unilateral; bilateral lesions interfere with laryngeal and esophageal function because of vagal involvement
	Neoplasm (thyroid adenocarcinoma)	
Middle ear cavity	Otitis media	Signs of peripheral vestibular disturbance: Ipsilateral ataxia, head tilt, nystagmus, and sometimes facial palsy, or hemifacial spasm
Retrobulbar	Contusion Neoplasia	Varies with degree of contusion to the optic and oculomotor nerves, which also influences pupillary size

From deLahunta A: Veterinary Neuroanatomy and Clinical Neurology, 2nd ed. WB Saunders Co, Philadelphia, 1983.

area. This portion of the oculomotor nucleus is called the EDINGER-WESTPHAL NUCLEUS. The parasympathetic axons leave the mesencephalon with the motor axons. In the canine oculomotor nerve, these parasympathetic axons are superficial on the medial side of the nerve and are especially susceptible to compression of the nerve from midbrain swelling or displacement. The nerve passes through the orbital fissure into the periorbita. The CILIARY GANGLION is located at the rostral end of the oculomotor nerve, ventral to the optic nerve (see Figs. 1–18 and 1–19).

Preganglionic parasympathetic axons of the oculomotor nerve connect here with the cell bodies of the postganglionic axons. The postganglionic axons pass via short ciliary nerves adjacent to the optic nerve to the globe to innervate the ciliary body and pupillary constrictor muscles.

Parasympathetic axons in the canine oculomotor nerve are superficial and medial in the nerve. They are susceptible to compression during midbrain swelling or displacement.

ABNORMALITIES OF THE PUPILLARY LIGHT REFLEX

The Normal Reflex. Stimulation of the retina of one eye with a bright source of light causes constriction of both pupils. Constriction in the eye being stimulated is the DIRECT PUPILLARY REFLEX. Constriction of the opposite pupil is the CONSENSUAL REFLEX. The afferent pathway to the parasympathetic oculomotor nucleus is via the optic nerve to the optic chiasm, at which point some crossing occurs, through both optic tracts, over the lateral geniculate nuclei without forming a synapse, and ventrally into the region between the thalamus and the rostral colliculus, called the pretectal area. A synapse is formed in the pretectal nuclei. Crossing *between sides* occurs between the pretectal nuclei via the caudal commissure. Axons of the pretectal cell bodies pass to the Edinger-Westphal (parasympathetic oculomotor) nucleus of both sides, activating these preganglionic neurons, which causes bilateral pupillary constriction. To evaluate the pupillary light reflex, a strong light source is used, and the patient should be relaxed. Circulating epinephrine may interfere with the speed and degree of response. For a discussion of the normal reflex, see also Chapter 1.

Pupillary Light Reflexes in Disorders of the Visual System (Figs. 17–11 to 17–15). Lesions restricted to visual pathways in the cerebral hemispheres cause blindness, with pupillary responses remaining normal.

Diseases Associated With Anisocoria. Anisocoria means inequality of pupil size. It is first necessary to determine which pupil is dilated and which is constricted.

Some of the causes include:

1. A unilateral oculomotor nerve lesion producing ipsilateral severe mydriasis that is unresponsive to light directed into either eye.

2. Unilateral severe retinal or optic nerve lesions, resulting in partial ipsilateral mydriasis that responds to light directed into the opposite eye. No miosis occurs in either eye from light directed into the affected eye.

3. Iris degeneration with atrophy causing ipsilateral mydriasis with a variable response to light (sometimes none). (This is more common in older animals and in certain breeds, e.g., miniature schnauzers and miniature poodles, and Siamese cats.)

4. Glaucoma with ipsilateral mydriasis as increased intraocular pressure paralyzes the pupillary sphincter. The eye is unresponsive to light. The consensual reflex is often lacking, as sustained elevation of intraocular pressure damages retinal function.

5. Anterior uveitis causing stimulation of pupillary constrictor and ciliary muscles, resulting in miosis.

6. A unilateral lesion of sympathetic innervation of the pupil, causing ipsilateral miosis that dilates slightly in reduced light (part of Horner's syndrome).

7. Unilateral ocular disorders causing pain (e.g., keratitis), which induces activation of the oculopupillary reflex and ipsilateral miosis.

Pupils in Acute Brain Disease. Pupillary abnormalities are common following intracranial trauma and often accompany severe, acute brain lesions such as those found in polioencephalomalacia and lead poisoning in ruminants. They do not necessarily reflect destruction of the parasympathetic oculomotor neurons or of the origin of the lateral tectotegmentospinal (sympathetic) system. Severe bilateral miosis is a sign of acute, extensive brain disturbance, which by itself is not necessarily of any localizing value. The return of the pupils to normal size and response to light is a favorable prognostic sign and indicates recovery from the brain disturbance, especially if caused by trauma. With trauma, progression from bilateral miosis to bilateral mydriasis with fixed pupils that are unresponsive to light indicates that the brain disturbance is advancing and the oculomotor neurons in the midbrain are nonfunctional. This often accompanies *severe contusion of the midbrain* with hemorrhage, usually along the midline. This may follow *brain swelling and herniation of the occipital lobes ventral to the tentorium cerebelli,* accompanied by compression and displacement of the midbrain or oculomotor nerve (or both).

The cause of unilateral or bilateral miotic pupils in acute brain disease is not known. It probably represents facilitation of the oculomotor parasympathetic neurons released from higher center inhibition owing to its functional disturbance. Pupillary changes may take place hourly following head trauma. Unilateral my-

Text continued on page 460

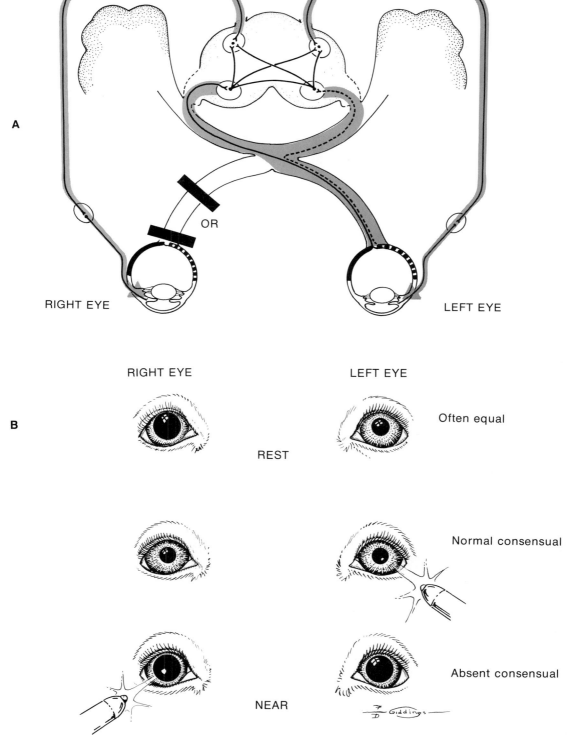

FIGURE 17–11. *Lesion of retina or optic nerve. A lesion in the right retina or optic nerve causes the pupil of the right eye to be partially dilated, and light stimulation of the left eye induces constriction of both pupils. Light stimulation of the right eye produces no change in either pupil because of the interference with the sensory limb of the reflex in the optic nerve.*

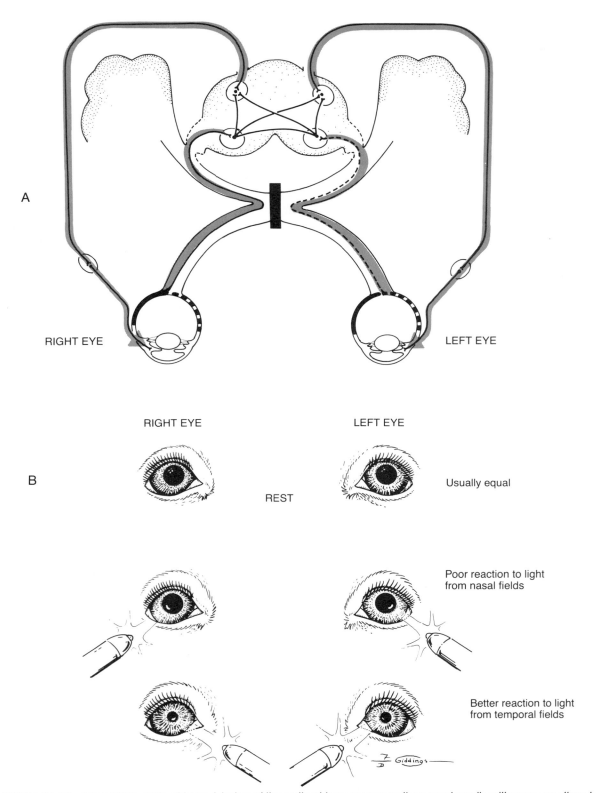

A

B

RIGHT EYE

LEFT EYE

RIGHT EYE

LEFT EYE

REST

Usually equal

Poor reaction to light
from nasal fields

Better reaction to light
from temporal fields

FIGURE 17–12. *Lesion of the optic chiasm. A lesion of the optic chiasm causes resting equal pupils, with poor reactions to light when directed into the nasal visual fields and a better reaction from the temporal fields.*

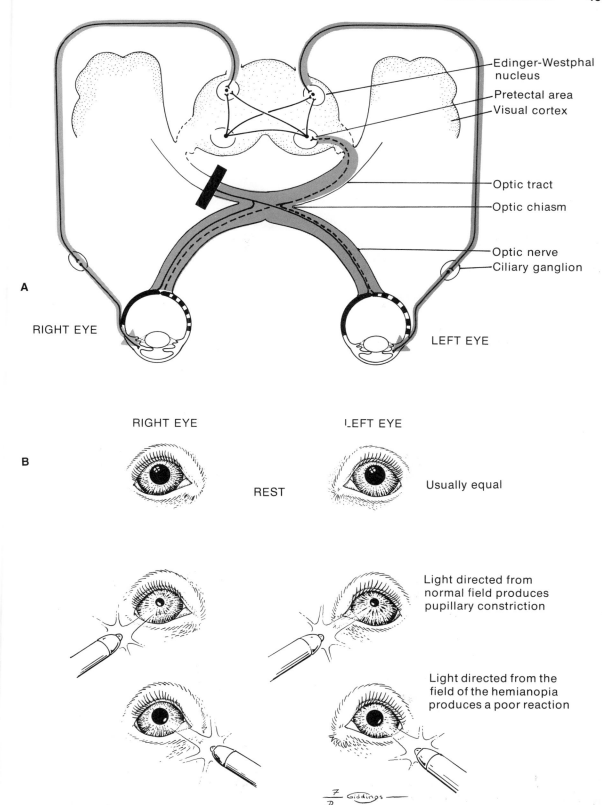

FIGURE 17–13. Lesion of the optic tract. A lesion of the right optic tract causes equal resting pupils; light directed from the normal visual field gives bilateral constriction, from the field of hemianopia (no vision) a lesser or no reaction.

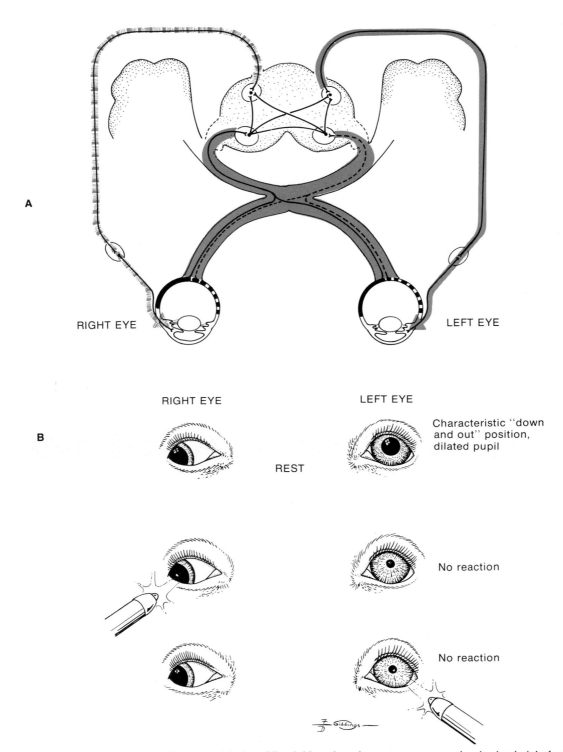

RIGHT EYE

LEFT EYE

RIGHT EYE

LEFT EYE

Characteristic "down and out" position, dilated pupil

REST

No reaction

No reaction

FIGURE 17–14. Lesion of the oculomotor nerve. A lesion of the right oculomotor nerve causes exotropia due to interference with innervation of the rectus muscles and an ipsilateral dilated pupil. There is no direct pupillary reflex, but the consensual reflex is normal. When the light is directed into the contralateral eye, the direct reflex is normal, but the contralateral reflex is absent.

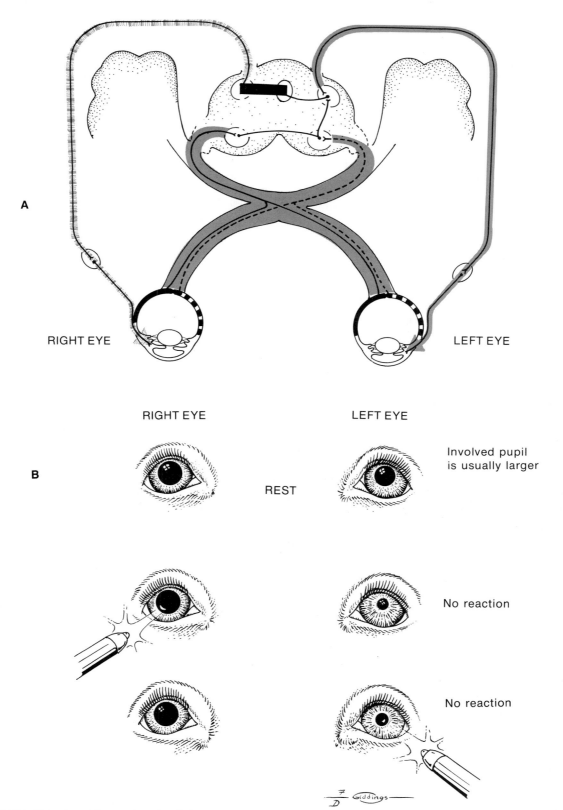

FIGURE 17–15. *Lesion of the oculomotor (Edinger-Westphal) nucleus. A lesion in the right Edinger-Westphal nucleus causes a widely dilated, resting right pupil. There is no direct reflex in the ipsilateral eye, but the consensual reflex is normal. In the contralateral eye, the direct reflex is normal, but the consensual reflex is absent.*

driasis, which in some cases may be accompanied by miosis of the opposite pupil, is probably brought about by compression of the ipsilateral oculomotor nerve. Experiments in dogs have shown that compression of the brain stem tectum at the level of the rostral colliculus causes miosis. Compression of cranial nerve III produces mydriasis. Pupil size and prognosis in intracranial injury are shown in Table 17–7.

> Return to normal pupillary size and light response is a favorable prognostic sign indicating recovery from the brain disturbance, especially after trauma. Progression from bilateral miosis to bilateral fixed mydriasis indicates damage to the parasympathetic oculomotor nuclei and progression of the pathological process.

Protrusion of the Third Eyelid. The third eyelid may protrude for a number of reasons. This protrusion is a passive event, except possibly in the cat. The third eyelid protrudes passively when the globe is retracted actively by the retractor bulbi (cranial nerve VI) and other extraocular muscles (cranial nerves III, IV, and VI). In the cat, slips of striated muscle from the lateral rectus and levator palpebrae superiorus attach to the two extremities of the membrane and may contract and contribute actively to this protrusion.

Protrusion of the third eyelid is a typical feature in

1. *Horner's syndrome.* A constant partial protrusion of the third eyelid occurs in Horner's syndrome because of loss of the sympathetic innervation of the smooth muscle that normally keeps it retracted.

2. *Tetanus.* Brief, rapid, passive protrusions ("flashing") of the third eyelid occur in tetanus owing to the effect of tetanus toxin on neurons that innervate the extraocular muscles. This causes brief contractions of the muscles, especially if the animal is startled. The reaction is most noticeable in horses but also occurs in other species.

3. *Facial paralysis.* When the animal with facial paralysis is threatened, the orbicularis oculi is paralyzed and the efferent branch of the reflex arc is interrupted, preventing the blink reflex. However, the globe is retracted, causing a brief rapid protrusion of the third eyelid. Paralysis of the orbicularis oculi, with ventral relaxation of the lower lid, may give the appearance of a protruded third eyelid when it is actually in its normal position.

4. *Haws syndrome.* Cats with severe systemic disease and depression often have persistent bilateral protrusion of the third eyelid. the cause is unknown, but may be due to dehydration. The so-called haws syndrome in cats consists of bilateral protrusion of the third eyelid. The condition is often associated with diarrhea and loose stools and may persist for 4–6 weeks but is usually self-limiting. Protrusion of the third eyelid may be treated symptomatically with topical sympathomimet-

TABLE 17–7. Pupillary Reactions in Intracerebral Injury

Condition	Pupil Size		Prognosis
Normal	⊙	⊙	Good
Unilateral oculomotor nuclear or nerve contusion or compression*	⦾	⊙	Guarded
Compression of midbrain tectum†	⊙	⊙	Guarded
Bilateral oculomotor nuclear or nerve contusion or compression	⦾	⦾	Grave

*Asymmetrical interference with cerebral control of oculomotor neurons or the sympathetic upper motor neuron system, or both.
†Bilateral sympathetic upper motor neuron deficiency or loss of facilitation, bilateral release, of oculomotor general visceral efferent neurons from cerebral inhibition.

ics (1% phenylephrine solution as necessary). If diarrhea is present, it is treated symptomatically.

The cause of this syndrome is unknown, but it can be distinguished from bilateral protrusion of the third eyelid in cats with severe systemic disease or dehydration, or both. It has been proposed that the condition is caused by an imbalance in sympathetic and parasympathetic tone, that is, a decrease in sympathetic tone, causing the protrusion of the third eyelids, and an increase in parasympathetic tone, causing increasing intestinal motility, decreased fecal passage time, and diarrhea.

5. *Atrophy of the muscles of mastication.* Atrophy of the temporal and pterygoid muscles after eosinophilic myositis and in senility can cause secondary protrusion of the third eyelid together with enophthalmos.

6. *Shrinkage of orbital contents.* After trauma, inflammation and senile atrophy of orbital fat enophthalmos and protrusion of the third eyelid may occur. Severe dehydration has a similar effect.

7. *Feline dysautonomia.* In this condition, bilateral protrusion of the third eyelids occurs because of sympathetic denervation, but *dilated pupils* occur, in contrast to Horner's syndrome. For further details see page 451.

THE VESTIBULAR SYSTEM

The vestibular system maintains the position of the eyes, trunk, and limbs in reference to head position or movement. It consists of receptors and cell bodies in the vestibular ganglion in the petrosal bone (inner ear), axons in cranial nerve VIII, neurons in the vestibular nuclei of the cerebellum, and axons in the medial longitudinal fasciculus. The medial longitudinal fasciculus connects vestibular neurons with neurons in the brain stem nuclei that innervate extraocular muscles (cranial nerves III, IV, and VI). Normal vestibular nystagmus depends on this pathway. Figure 17–16 illustrates prominent features of the system.

Nystagmus (Table 17–8)

NORMAL VESTIBULAR NYSTAGMUS

Nystagmus is involuntary, rhythmic ocular movement. It can be induced by slowly moving the head from side to side or up and down. Such head movement induces impulses in the vestibular component of cranial nerve VIII from the stimulus to the receptors in the

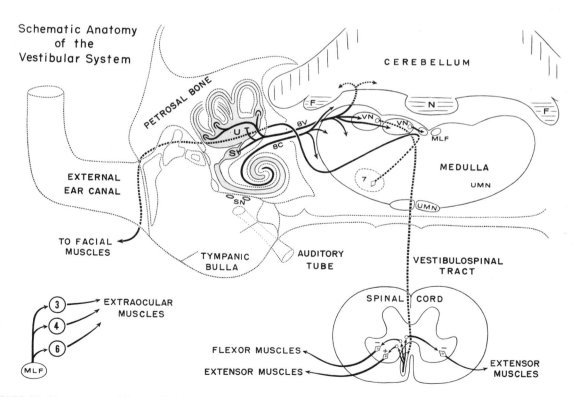

FIGURE 17–16. Anatomy of the vestibular system. N = nodulus; F = flocculus; UMN = upper motor neuron; MLF = medial longitudinal fasciculus; VN = vestibular nucleus; 8V = cranial nerve VIII, vestibular portion; 8C = cranial nerve VIII, cochlear portion; U = utricle; S = saccule; SN = sympathetic neurons; 3 = oculomotor nucleus; 4 = trochlear nucleus; 6 = abducens nucleus; 7 = facial nucleus. (From deLahunta A: Veterinary Neuroanatomy and Clinical Neurology, 2nd ed. WB Saunders Co, Philadelphia, 1983.)

TABLE 17–8. Characteristics of Nystagmus

Normal
    Occurs with head movement
    Quick phase in same direction as head movement
    Horizontal plane → horizontal nystagmus
    Vertical plane → vertical nystagmus

Abnormal
    Occurs *spontaneously* or with head held flexed laterally or extended
        (*positional nystagmus*)
    Peripheral receptor disease: Quick phase constantly to side opposite
        from lesion, either horizontal or rotatory (direction from 12
        o'clock point on globe)
    Central vestibular disease (pons, medulla, cerebellum): Quick phase
        constantly in any one direction, opposite from or toward side
        of lesion, or vertical
    Quick phase varying in direction with different positions of the
        head
    Lack of any response to head movements or rapid rotation
        indicates severe bilateral receptor or severe brain stem disease
    Lack of any response to cold water irrigation of *one* of the external
        auditory canals (caloric test) indicates a severe lesion in the
        receptor of that side

semicircular ducts. The afferent neuronal pathway that results in nystagmus continues through the vestibular nuclei in the medulla and via the medial longitudinal fasciculus to the brain stem nuclei, whose axons innervate the extraocular muscles. Normal vestibular nystagmus is tested by slowly moving the head from side to side and observing the limbus to note nystagmus. This form of nystagmus has a *rapid phase in one direction and a slow phase in the opposite direction.*

The direction of nystagmus is defined by the direction of the rapid phase.

The *rapid phase of nystagmus is in the same direction as the movement of the head—left movement causes left nystagmus, and ventral movement causes ventral nystagmus.* Normal vestibular nystagmus occurs only as the head is being moved. Both eyes are affected and move simultaneously in conjugate fashion. Testing normal vestibular nystagmus evaluates the animal's ability to abduct and adduct each eye. It is abnormal if nystagmus persists after the head movement is stopped or if the head is extended or flexed laterally and nystagmus develops in that position.

Lesions that destroy the vestibular system, the medial longitudinal fasciculus, or neurons of cranial nerves III, IV, and VI cause loss of normal vestibular nystagmus.

In the neurological evaluation after intracranial injury, it is important to distinguish between signs of diffuse cerebral edema and brain stem contusion. Loss of vestibular nystagmus indicates a severe lesion in the

brain stem affecting the vestibular nuclei, medial longitudinal fasciculus, or the nuclei of cranial nerves III, IV, and VI.

Observation of ocular movements in normal nystagmus also allows evaluation of specific extraocular muscles. With a right abducent nerve paralysis, there is esotropia of the right eye and failure of the eye to abduct fully on moving the head to the right.

ABNORMAL NYSTAGMUS

When the head is held extended, flexed laterally to either side, or extended fully, no nystagmus is found. In *vestibular disease,* nystagmus may be observed.

Spontaneous nystagamus   induced when the head
                                        is extended

Positional nystagmus   induced in lateral flex-
                                   ion or full extension

In *peripheral receptor disease,* the nystagmus is either horizontal or rotatory, and it is always in a direction (quick phase) away from the side of the lesion. The direction of rotatory nystagmus is defined by the change in the dorsal limbus during the quick phase. This direction does not change when the position of the head is changed.

With *disease of the vestibular nuclei or vestibular pathways* in the cerebellum, the nystagmus may be *horizontal, rotatory, or vertical* and may change in direction with position of the head; any of these types of nystagmus suggests central involvement of the vestibular system.

Peripheral receptor disease is suggested if the direction of nystagmus does not change when the position of the head is changed. Vertical nystagmus or nystagmus that changes direction if the position of the head is changed suggests a central disorder of the vestibular system.

Postural Reactions in Vestibular Disease

Most postural reactions remain intact, except for the righting response. Usually the patient experiences difficulty righting itself, with an exaggerated response toward the side of the lesion. When the head is extended in the tonic neck reaction, the eyes should remain in the center of the palpebral fissure in the dog and cat. This often fails to occur on the side of the vestibular disturbance and results in a drooling or ventrally deviated eye.

In ruminants, it is normal for the eyes to deviate ventrally on neck extension. In horses, there is normally a slight ventral deviation, which is more pronounced in the eye ipsilateral to a vestibular system lesion. Occasionally in vestibular disease, an eye is deviated ventrally (hypotropia) or ventrolaterally without extension of the head and neck. This appears as a lower motor neuron strabismus, but it can be corrected by moving the head into a different position or by inducing the patient to move its eyes to gaze in different directions. This is referred to as a vestibular strabismus. There is no paralysis of the cranial nerves that innervate the extraocular muscles. The ventrally deviated eye is on the side of the lesion in the vestibular system. Sometimes the opposite eye may appear to be deviated dorsally (hypertropia).

Disorders of the Vestibular System

FELINE VESTIBULAR DISEASE

For the first 72 hours, spontaneous nystagmus occurs opposite the head tilt. This is usually horizontal, occasionally rotatory. At the onset, a head oscillation may occur simultaneously with nystagmus. After 3 or 4 days, spontaneous nystagmus disappears, but abnormal positional nystagmus may be elicited on altering the position of the head. The direction remains opposite the head tilt.

OTITIS MEDIA AND OTITIS INTERNA

Vestibular signs occur in animals when middle ear inflammation indirectly or directly affects the function of the membranous labyrinth. Varying degrees of unilateral vestibular disturbance appear, which consist of asymmetrical ataxia with strength preservation. Sometimes only a head tilt and positional nystagmus are evident. Occasionally, these signs are accompanied by an ipsilateral facial paresis or palsy or by Horner's syndrome, or by both. They occur if the otitis media disturbs the function of the facial and sympathetic nerves, respectively, which pass adjacent to or through the middle ear in the dog and cat. Unilateral deafness may occur but is difficult to determine clinically.

CENTRAL DISORDERS

Signs of vestibular system disturbance referable to disease of the vestibular nuclei or their pathways are similar to those seen in diseases of the peripheral vestibular system.

Vestibular signs usually seen only with diseases of the central pathways include:

1. Consistent vertical nystagmus
2. Nystagmus that changes direction with different positions of the head
3. Tendency to roll in one direction (may also occur to a limited degree with peripheral disease)

The lesion is localized to the central pathways mostly by the presence of signs that accompany the brain stem involvement of other functional systems. In ruminants, *Listeria monocytogenes* causes inflammation of the brain stem with signs referable to this location, including vestibular disturbance. Varying degrees of upper motor neuron paresis, head tilt, abnormal nystagmus, and facial paresis are typical.

TRAUMA

Intracranial injury may affect the central vestibular pathways in addition to other systems in the brain stem. The degree of vestibular disturbance manifested depends on the degree of disturbance of other systems, which may mask the vestibular disturbance. Abnormal nystagmus may be the only sign of vestibular disturbance evident in the tetraplegic semicomatose patient.

CONGENITAL NYSTAGMUS

Congenital nystagmus occurs in humans as an inherited functional abnormality or secondary to congenital lesions in the visual system of the infant. The nystagmus is usually pendular. Similar nystagmus has been described in dogs. In cattle, PENDULAR NYSTAGMUS occurs in the Holstein-Friesan, Jersey, Guernsey, and Ayrshire. It is significant for diagnostic purposes only and does not affect vision.

Congenital nystagmus occurs in young animals with severe visual deficit during the early postnatal period, for example, in pups with scleral ectasia syndrome (collie eye anomaly) and retinal detachment or intraocular hemorrhage.

THE CEREBELLUM

Neuro-Ophthalmic Signs of Cerebellar Disease

1. Involvement of the cerebellum may cause vestibular disturbance with loss of equilibrium, nystagmus, bizarre postures, and a broad-based staggering gait with jerky movements and a tendency to fall to the side or back, especially if the thoracic limbs are elevated. Abnormal nystagmus is observed only occasionally.

2. Animals with significant cerebellar cortical disease have no menace response, which is often used to test the visual system. The central visual pathway to the visual cortex as well as the facial neurons of cranial nerve VII, must be intact for this response to occur. It is assumed that the pathway between the visual cortex and the facial nucleus must pass through the cerebellum.

Disorders With Neuro-Ophthalmic and Cerebellar Signs

Interested readers are referred to standard texts on veterinary neurology for discussion of bovine cortical abiotrophy and progressive equine cerebellar ataxia.

CENTRAL VISUAL PATHWAYS

Anatomy of the central visual pathways is discussed in Chapter 1 and is summarized in Figure 1–7 and Figure 17–17.

Clinical Signs of Central Visual Pathway Disease Disorders
(Table 17–9; see also Figs. 17–11 to 17–15)

Complete bilateral lesions in the optic tracts or lateral geniculate nucleus produce total blindness with dilated, unresponsive pupils. More often the lesions are partial, and clinical signs are difficult to determine. Canine distemper encephalitis often produces extensive lesions in the optic tracts without obvious clinical deficit of vision or pupillary functions. Chromophobe adenomata in budgerigars and granulomata in parrots have been reported as causes of central blindness when eye lesions are lacking.

The degree of visual deficit depends on location and extent of the lesion in the visual pathway.

Lesions that destroy the retina or optic nerve in one eye cause blindness and a partially dilated pupil in that eye (see Fig. 17–11). This does not cause disorientation of gait nor any head tilt or neck curvature. the menace, direct, and consensual light reflexes are lost in the affected eye but are retained in the contralateral eye. In the pupillary reflex pathway, the afferents cross in the optic chiasm and in the pretectum to influence both oculomotor nuclei. It is through this pathway that ambient light causes partial constriction of the pupil of the blind eye.

Total bilateral retinal or optic nerve destruction causes complete blindness, with both pupils widely dilated and unresponsive to light directed into either eye, caused, for example, by brain abscesses due to *Corynebacterium pyogenes* in cattle. Retinal degenerations are the most common cause of this deficit. Unilateral lesions in the optic tract, lateral geniculate nucleus, optic radiation, or visual cortex cause a visual deficit in the contralateral visual field. This is referred to as a HEMIANOPIA, because the visual deficit affects 50% of the visual field. In the dog, this represents about a 25% dysfunction in the contralateral eye because of decussation at the chiasm.

In dogs and cats, the visual deficit is difficult to detect as the animal moves in its surroundings. Occasionally, an object may be bumped on the side opposite the lesion, but often there is *no evidence* of visual deficit.

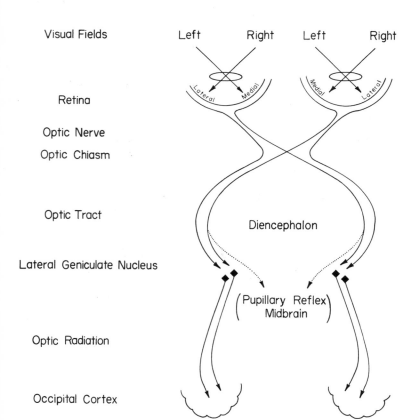

FIGURE 17–17. Central visual pathway for conscious perception. (From deLahunta A: Small animal neuro-ophthalmology. Vet Clin North Am 3:491, 1973.)

TABLE 17–9. Clinical Signs of Visual Deficit

	Lesions				
Test	*Right Optic Nerve*	*Right Cranial Nerve III*	*Right Postorbital*	*Right Optic Tract*	*Right Visual Cortex*
Left Eye (OS)					
Pupil	Normal size	Normal size	Normal size	Normal size	Normal size
	Light in OS	Light in OS	Light in OS	Light in OS	Light in OS
	Both constrict	Only OS constricts	Only OS constricts	Both constrict	Both constrict
Menace	Present	Present	Present	Mostly absent	Mostly absent
Right Eye (OD)					
Pupil	Partial dilation	Complete dilation	Complete dilation	Normal size	Normal size
	Light in OD	Light in OD	Light in OD	Light in OD	Light in OD
	Neither constricts	Only OS constricts	Neither constricts	Both constrict	Both constrict
Menace	Absent	Present	Absent	Mostly present	Mostly present

From deLahunta A: Veterinary Neuroanatomy and Clinical Neurology, 2nd ed. WB Saunders Co, Philadelphia, 1983.

Unilateral blindfolding and maze testing of the animal may help demonstrate the deficit. In horses, sheep, and cattle with 80–90% decussation of optic nerve axons, there is a greater tendency to walk into objects on the side of the visual deficit, contralateral to the lesion. In all domestic animals there is a poor or lacking menace reflex contralateral to the lesion (Fig. 17–18). It is important to cover the eye not being tested and to menace the other eye from both nasal and temporal sides. The deficit is pronounced from the temporal side (visual field) when there are contralateral lesions in the central visual pathway.

In all unilateral lesions caudal to the optic chiasm, the pupillary light reflex responses are usually normal because of decussation at the chiasm, pretectal area, and Edinger-Westphal nuclei. Bilateral lesions in the optic radiation or the visual cortex, or both, cause complete blindness with normal pupillary light reflexes.

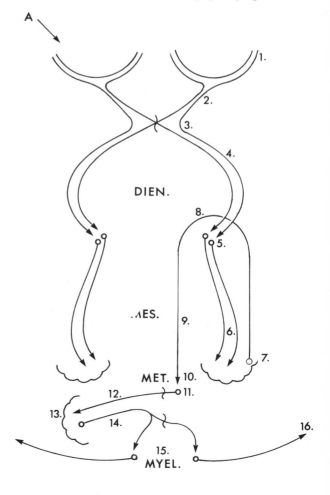

FIGURE 17–18. *Anatomical pathway of the menace response: 1 = retina; 2 = optic nerve; 3 = optic chiasm; 4 = optic tract; 5 = lateral geniculate nucleus; 6 = optic radiation; 7 = visual cortex; 8 = internal capsule; 9 = crus cerebri; 10 = longitudinal fibers of pons; 11 = pontine nucleus; 12 = transverse fibers of pons and middle cerebellar peduncle; 13 = cerebellar cortex; 14 = efferent cerebellar pathway; 15 = facial nuclei; 16 = facial muscles—orbicularis oculi. ⌒ indicates axons crossing the midline of the brain. A lesion in the left cerebellar hemisphere prevents a menace response directed at the left eye from its lateral field (A), because 65–90% of the optic nerve axons cross in the chiasm. (From deLahunta A: Veterinary Neuroanatomy and Clinical Neurology, 2nd ed. WB Saunders Co, Philadelphia, 1983.)*

TABLE 17–10. Clinical Signs of Meningitis

Disorder	Neuro-Ophthalmic Signs	Other Signs
Steroid-responsive suppurative meningitis (large breeds less than 2 years old)	—	Cervical rigidity, cervical pain, fever, neutrophilia
Necrotizing vasculitis (German short-haired pointers, Bernese mountain dogs)	Blindness	Cervical rigidity and pain, paralysis, seizures, neutrophilia
Pyogranulomatous meningoencephalitis (adult pointers)	Cranial nerve deficits	Ataxia, stiff gait, cervical rigidity, hyperesthesia
Granulomatous meningoencephalitis (poodles and terriers)	Blindness, facial paresis, trigeminal paralysis, nystagmus	Cervical pain, fever, ataxia, seizures, circling, head tilt
Bacterial meningitis	Nystagmus, blindness	Cervical rigidity, hyperesthesia, fever, vomiting, bradycardia, seizures, hyperreflexia, paralysis, paresis, head tilt

Modified from Meric SM: Canine meningitis: A review. J Vet Int Med 2:26, 1988.

Meningitis

Canine meningitis may cause neuro-ophthalmic signs in several ways, which are described in Table 17–10.

DISEASES OF THE VISUAL SYSTEM

Optic Nerve

PAPILLEDEMA

Papilledema ("choked disc") is not a disease but edema of the optic nerve head. It occurs in various conditions and is not accompanied by inflammation. The exact pathogenesis of papilledema is undetermined, but several theories have been advanced, including:

1. Obstruction of vascular drainage from the disc
2. Obstruction of lymphatic drainage from the disc
3. Blockage of axoplasmic transport in nerve fibers at the lamina cribrosa
4. Edema of the cerebral white matter extending along the myelin sheaths of the optic nerve

Explanations determined for the primate eye cannot be transposed because of extensive differences in the vascular anatomy of the optic disc and the lamina cribrosa.

Clinical Signs

1. Enlargement of the disc.
2. Elevation of the surface of the disc above the surrounding retina.
3. Indistinct and fluffy disc margins.
4. Retinal arterioles and veins show a distinct kink as they pass down over the edge of the disc into the retina.
5. Disc has a "watery-pink" appearance.
6. Retinal veins are congested, dilated, and tortuous, and many more fine veins are visible.
7. Small flame-shaped hemorrhages may be present on or near the disc margin. In animals, papilledema is less common than optic neuritis, from which it must be distinguished clinically.

Papilledema itself does not cause visual deficit.

In the past it has been incorrectly stated that papilledema is not associated with increased intracranial pressure (and neoplasia) in animals, as it is in humans.

Palmer and coworkers (1974) showed a 47.6% incidence of papilledema in 21 dogs with brain tumor. Visual defects occurred in 71.4%, and 33.3% showed hemianopia (Table 17–11). (Of the 21 dogs, 11 were boxers.)

Locomotor deficiency and change in temperament in a dog with visual dysfunction and papilledema is highly suggestive of an intracranial space-occupying lesion.

In addition to intracranial neoplasia, papilledema occurs in lead poisoning and vitamin A deficiency

TABLE 17–11. Clinical Signs in 21 Cases of Canine Brain Tumor

Clinical Sign	Affected %
Papilledema	47.6
Visual defect (including pupils)	71.4
Hemianopia	33.3
Nystagmus	28.5
Ocular deviation and cranial nerve paralysis	33.3
Change of temperament	80.9
Locomotor deficiency	80.9
Circling	42.6
Hemiplegia	38.1
Convulsions	38.1
Head turn or tilt	33.3
Sensory deficit	19.0
Pituitary signs	14.3

From Palmer AC, et al: Clinical signs including papilledema associated with brain tumors in twenty-one dogs. J Sm Anim Pract 15:359, 1974.

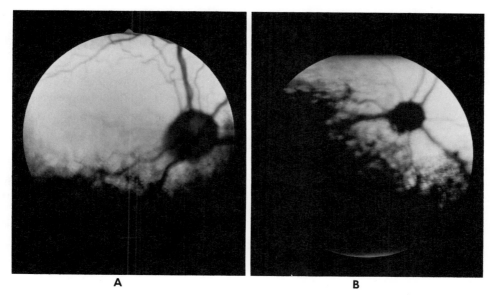

FIGURE 17–19. A, *Normal right optic disc in a 12-month-old collie with anisocoria since birth.* B, *Optic nerve hypoplasia with micropapilla in the left eye (with mydriatic pupil) of the same dog.*

in cattle, in orbital inflammations and neoplasms (including optic nerve neoplasms), and in some forms of toxic optic neuropathy (e.g., male fern poisoning in cattle).

CONGENITAL ANOMALIES

Aplasia and Hypoplasia

Aplasia and hypoplasia of the optic nerve occur infrequently in dogs, cats, horses, and cattle, and may be uni- or bilateral. The condition is more common in collies but is not usually associated with the scleral ectasia syndrome. Associated ocular defects are not uncommon (see hypovitaminosis A in cattle and pigs. Prenatal infection with bovine viral diarrhea-mucosal disease may cause congenital optic nerve atrophy. The number of retinal ganglion cells is usually also decreased and the nerve fiber layer is thin.

Diagnosis

1. Animals usually present with a history of visual deficit since birth if the condition is bilateral. In unilateral cases, an intermittent visual deficit that is more pronounced on one side (hemianopia) or anisocoria is often noticed by the owner.

2. In aplasia, the optic disc is entirely lacking. If retinal vessels are present, hypoplasia is more likely, with a small remnant of the optic disc present. In horses, few, if any, retinal vessels are present in either hypoplasia or aplasia. In hypoplasia, the size of the disc is normal but it is gray and lacks vessels. The hypoplastic disc may be heavily pigmented (Fig. 17–19).

3. Aplasia-hypoplasia should be differentiated from atrophy, which usually is not present in young animals.

Histologically, the presence of retinal gliosis, inflammatory cells, or degenerative changes in retinal ganglion cells indicates atrophy rather than aplasia-hypoplasia.

4. In the affected eye, the pupil is partially dilated. Light directed into the affected eye will not elicit a direct or consensual response. Light in the normal eye causes both pupils to constrict. In bilateral aplasia-hypoplasia, direct and consensual reflexes are lacking in both eyes, and both pupils are enlarged (Fig. 17–20).

5. In cats, the number of caudal vertebrae may be grossly reduced in association with bilateral aplasia.

6. The condition may be hereditary, for example, in the miniature schnauzer, or may occur in certain breeds, for example, the American cocker spaniel, beagle, collie, dachshund, German shepherd, Irish setter, and miniature, toy, and standard poodles.

7. Radiographic examination of the optic canal demonstrates a reduction in size with optic nerve hypoplasia (Ernest, 1976).

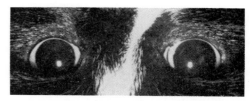

FIGURE 17–20. *Mydriasis in a cat with bilateral aplasia of the optic nerves. The two eyes are similar, normal in size, and have dilated pupils. (From Barnett KC, Grimes TD: Bilateral aplasia of the optic nerve in a cat. Br J Ophthalmol 57:663, 1974.)*

Coloboma

Colobomata are pits or excavations in the optic disc and peripapillary area caused by incomplete closure of the embryonic fissure (see Chap 2). They are *typical* if seen in the inferior medial portion of the disc and *atypical* if located elsewhere. Colobomata occur most commonly in the scleral ectasia syndrome in collies and Shetland sheepdogs and in charolais cattle, but they do occur sporadically, for example, in horses, and are inherited as separate distinct entities, for example, in basenjis. The lesions are congenital and nonprogressive and vary in size from small pits to excavations several times the size of the normal optic disc. If they are large enough, vision is affected because the nerve fiber layer is disrupted as it enters the optic nerve head. Small colobomata have minimal effect on vision. Colobomata must be distinguished from glaucomatous cupping.

INFLAMMATORY DISORDERS (Fig. 17–21)

Optic Neuritis (Neuropathy)

The term OPTIC NEURITIS may be applied to degenerative conditions more correctly termed OPTIC NEUROPATHY. Optic neuritis may occur in any species. Proliferative optic neuropathy and exudative optic neuritis in horses are classified separately. Optic neuritis may be subclassified into optic papillitis, in which the optic disc is affected, and retrobulbar neuritis, in which ophthalmoscopically visible lesions are lacking.

Etiology

1. Diseases affecting other nervous tissues, for example, canine distemper, cryptococcosis, hog cholera, toxoplasmosis, feline infectious peritonitis.

2. Neoplastic disorders, for example, primary reticulosis in dogs, feline lymphosarcoma, orbital neoplasms.

3. Exogenous toxins, for example, optic neuropathy in cattle from the ingestion of male fern and in sheep from the ingestion of *Stypandra imbricata* ("blindgrass").

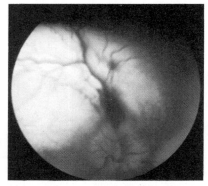

FIGURE 17–21. Optic neuritis with papilledema and hemorrhages in a Weimaraner with acute onset of visual loss and mydriasis.

In humans, numerous drugs, for example, chloramphenicol, alcohol, and nicotine, cause optic neuropathy and drugs are often suspected but unproven causes in sporadic cases in animals.

4. Vitamin A deficiency (cattle, pigs, dogs).

5. Trauma—especially after proptosis of the globe.

6. Orbital diseases, for example, orbital cellulitis and orbital abscess.

7. Hypotony after penetrating wounds.

8. Unknown. Many cases, especially in dogs, are of unknown cause.

Clinical Signs

1. Acute bilateral loss of vision. This is distinguished from bilateral retinal detachment and central cortical blindness, which may cause similar acute visual loss. In dogs, sudden acquired retinal degeneration (SARD) gives similar clinical signs.

2. Mydriasis, depending on the degree of damage to pupillary fibers in the optic nerve.

3. Papilledema and peripapillary retinal edema.

4. Hemorrhages on or around the optic disc.

5. Sluggishness or lack of direct and consensual pupillary light reflexes.

6. Retinochoroidal degeneration, especially in peripapillary areas.

7. Peripapillary retinal folds appearing as concentric rings or lines near the disc.

8. Optic atrophy in advanced cases.

9. Concurrent signs of CNS disease.

10. Exudation and haze in the adjacent vitreous.

Note: In retrobulbar neuritis, ophthalmoscopic signs may be lacking.

Optic neuritis, if untreated or uncontrolled, frequently leads to optic atrophy with a pale, grayish, shrunken optic disc and attenuation of blood vessels. Optic neuritis in dogs frequently recurs, with cumulative visual loss and damage to the nerve with each relapse.

Differential Diagnosis

Optic neuritis is distinguished from papilledema and from myelination of the nerve fiber layer of the retina surrounding the optic disc (Fig. 17–22, Table 17–12).

Treatment

The most significant therapeutic feature is the importance of early diagnosis and intensive anti-inflammatory therapy with corticosteroids to limit permanent optic nerve damage. Clients should be advised that recurrence is frequent, and early vigorous treatment of recurrences is necessary.

1. Attempt to determine the cause and institute specific therapy.

2. Symptomatic therapy—oral dexamethasone (0.2 mg/kg) or prednisolone (2 mg/kg) daily, decreasing over 4–5 weeks. If neuritis occurs because of traumatic proptosis, retrobulbar injection of 10–20 mg of triamcinolone is indicated when the globe is replaced.

3. Systemic broad spectrum antibiotics—oral chloramphenicol, 20–30 mg/kg.

TABLE 17–12. Differentiation of Common Optic Nerve Conditions

Feature	Optic Neuritis	Papilledema	Myelination of the Nerve Fiber Layer
Age	Middle-aged dogs	No specific age group unless associated with cerebral neoplasia, which is more common in older dogs	Present from birth, nonprogressive, and not pathological
Vision	Severely affected or absent	No effect	No effect
Direct pupillary light reflex	Depressed or absent	Present	Present
Disc hemorrhages	Usually present	Rarely present	Absent
Peripapillary chorioretinitis	Often present	Absent (edema may be present)	Absent
"Kink" in vessels at disc margin	Often present	Often present	Absent
Vitreous haze	Often present	Absent	Absent

4. Withdrawal of suspected toxic agents, for example, lead.

The prognosis for optic neuritis is guarded. If no response or return of vision occurs by 4 weeks, prospects of further improvement are limited.

Equine Exudative Optic Neuritis (Fig. 17–23)

Exudative optic neuritis is usually seen in horses older than 15 years of age and is characterized by:

1. Sudden, bilateral onset of blindness.

2. Multiple round or oval yellowish bodies protruding from the borders of the optic disc. The bodies are mobile, extend into the vitreous, and remain attached to the optic disc.

3. Pupillary dilation and loss or depression of pupillary light reflexes.

4. Hemorrhage on or around the optic disc that may precede or accompany appearance of the yellow bodies.

Because the condition is uncommon, cumulative experience in its treatment is lacking, although optic atrophy is the usual sequel. Affected horses should receive systemic and possibly retrobulbar steroids and should be kept out of bright light. A unilateral condition with similar signs is seen after orbital trauma in horses.

Equine Proliferative Optic Neuropathy (Fig. 17–24)

This condition is differentiated from exudative optic neuritis (Table 17–13). Affected animals are also older than 15 years of age. It is characterized by

1. Lack of visual disturbance. The condition is usually found incidentally during fundus examination.

2. Unilateral lesions only.

3. Nonprogressive course.

4. Single grayish-white, raised lesions on or near the optic disc.

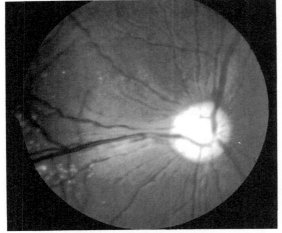

FIGURE 17–22. Myelination of the nerve fiber layer of the retina in a dog. This must be distinguished from papilledema and optic neuritis. Clinical signs are lacking, and vision is normal. (Courtesy of Dr. G. A. Severin.)

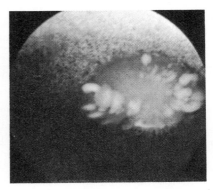

FIGURE 17–23. Exudative optic neuritis. (Courtesy of Dr. G.A. Severin.)

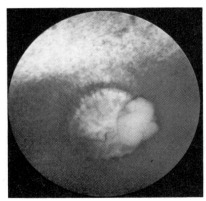

FIGURE 17–24. Proliferative optic neuropathy. (From Rubin LF: Atlas of Veterinary Ophthalmoscopy. Lea & Febiger, Philadelphia, 1974.)

5. Not preceded or accompanied by hemorrhages around the disc.

Proliferative optic neuropathy was formerly reported as astrocytoma, but histological studies indicate it is a lipid storage disorder.

OPTIC ATROPHY

Etiology

Optic atrophy has numerous causes and is the end stage of numerous pathological processes. Some of the more common follow:

1. Intraorbital nerve damage secondary to traumatic proptosis in dogs and cats. In severe proptosis or traction during enucleation of the contralateral eye, the optic chiasm may be traumatized.

2. Advanced retinal degeneration of any type.

3. Prolonged papilledema.

4. Sequel to optic neuritis and optic neuropathy.

5. Intraorbital and intracranial neoplasia.

6. Orbital disorders, for example, retrobulbar abscess, orbital cellulitis, canine eosinophilic myositis.

Clinical Signs

1. Pale, grayish white, shrunken disc.

2. Slight depression of the disc surface.

3. Exposure and increased visibility of the lamina cribrosa.

4. Attenuation of retinal vessels.

5. Pigmentation of the optic disc or surrounding it.

Treatment has no effect except to prevent further damage to the nerve by the original cause.

NEOPLASMS

Neoplasms affecting the optic nerve include meningioma, glioma, and astrocytoma. They are uncommon in all species.

Clinical Signs

1. Mydriasis and abolition of the direct pupillary light reflex in the affected eye. With a large infiltrating orbital mass, the consensual reflex from the contralateral eye to the affected eye may be abnormal because of destruction of afferent nerves.

2. Optic atrophy. Orbital neoplasms may cause papilledema, optic neuropathy, or optic neuritis.

3. Proptosis of the globe. Position of the globe and direction of the visual axis may assist in determining the position of the mass.

4. Retinal edema and folds resulting from pressure exerted by orbital masses on the posterior portion of the globe.

Treatment

Treatment is by anterior or lateral orbitotomy if the globe is to be saved or by orbital exenteration if the neoplasm is too extensive or infiltrates the globe or if secondary lesions are present in the globe.

Optic Chiasm

In domestic animals, unlike humans, most pituitary neoplasms grow into the hypothalamus. The normal canine pituitary gland projects caudally from the optic chiasm, and enlargement usually does not affect the chiasm. Occasionally, the cerebral infarction syndrome

TABLE 17–13. Differential Diagnosis of Equine Exudative Optic Neuritis and Proliferative Optic Neuropathy

Feature	Exudative Optic Neuritis	Proliferative Optic Neuropathy
Vision	Severe disturbance	No disturbance
Age	15 years or over	15 years or over
Symmetry	Bilateral (unless traumatic)	Unilateral
Course	Progressive, often leading to optic atrophy	Stationary
Appearance	1. Multiple movable bodies 2. Hemorrhages often present 3. Vitreous haze may be present	1. Single stationary body 2. No hemorrhages 3. No vitreous haze
Pupil and direct light reflex	Mydriasis and depressed direct pupillary light reflex	No pupillary or reflex abnormalities

in cats causes ischemic necrosis of the optic chiasm, with blindness and dilated unresponsive pupils.

TRAUMATIC OPTIC NERVE BLINDNESS

Excessive tension on the optic nerve caused by traumatic proptosis or during enucleation, especially in cats, may tear fibers in the chiasm, and cause either partial or complete blindness.

In horses, rupture of optic nerve axons may occur after traumatic posterior movement of the brain, stretching the nerve between the fixed canalicular portion and the optic chiasm. Clinical signs include:

1. Sudden onset of blindness, either unilateral or bilateral.

2. Dilated fixed pupils.

3. Lack of menace reflex.

4. After 3–4 weeks, the optic disc becomes paler, and retinal vasculature attenuates. Treatment is unsuccessful.

Optic Tracts

BILATERAL DISEASE

1. Incomplete bilateral lesions may produce partial bilateral visual deficit with variable pupillary responses. This is typical of the inflammation and necrosis caused by canine distemper, which has a predilection for the optic tracts. Often, no clinical visual deficit is observed. Such distemper lesions may occur in adult dogs with no overt signs of distemper. The diagnosis is confirmed either by serological evaluation of serum or cerebrospinal fluid or histologically.

2. In humans, pituitary neoplasms commonly cause compression of the optic chiasm and tracts because of the rostral location of the pituitary directly ventral to the chiasm and the lack of a meningeal barrier. In domestic animals, involvement of the optic chiasm is uncommon because of the caudal position of the pituitary gland and the restrictive dural diaphragm sellae in ruminants. Occasionally, canine pituitary neoplasms affect the optic tracts when the hypothalamus is invaded or compressed by the neoplasm.

UNILATERAL DISEASE

1. Unilateral neoplasms in the hypothalamus and thalamus may encroach on one optic tract, causing a visual deficit in the contralateral eye, but pupillary light reflexes are unaffected. Because of close approximation of the internal capsule and rostral crus cerebri to the optic tract, space-occupying lesions in the lateral hypothalamus or thalamus, or both, that affect the optic tract usually also affect the internal capsule and rostral crus cerebri. This causes mild contralateral hemiparesis, which is often not evident in the gait but demonstrable by asymmetry in postural testing.

2. Traumatic lesions that cause necrosis of these tissues on one side can result in the same residual neurological signs—that is, contralateral visual deficit and postural reaction deficit ("hemiparesis").

Lateral Geniculate Nucleus

Destruction of the lateral geniculate nucleus produces signs similar to those observed with optic tract lesions. An abnormality in the retinogeniculate projections and neuronal organization in this nucleus occurs in albinotic cats of all sizes, from Siamese cats to tigers, and in mink. In some animals it is associated with congenital esotropia.

Optic Radiation and Visual Cortex

UNILATERAL DISEASE

Unilateral lesions produce hemianopia in the contralateral visual field. Pupillary size and response to light are normal.

1. *Neoplastic lesions.* Neoplasms produce progressive signs of neurological deficit. Convulsions or changes in behavior may accompany the visual deficit.

2. *Trauma.* Traumatic lesions causing necrosis may leave a residual neurological defect limited to a contralateral visual deficit. If the entire hemisphere is involved, a contralateral postural reaction deficiency may be seen on neurological examination. Immediately following an injury, the neurological signs may be more extensive, suggesting diffuse cerebral disturbance. As hemorrhage and edema subside, residual neurological deficits relate to areas of necrotic tissue.

3. *Feline cerebral vascular disease.* This is a syndrome of peracute signs of unilateral cerebral disturbance in adult cats of all ages and both sexes caused by extensive cerebral necrosis. The onset is variable, but some animals show only severe depression with mild ataxia or circling, or both, while others circle continuously. Others begin with seizures, which consist of tonic or clonic activity of the muscles on one side of the head, trunk, and limbs. Changes in attitude and behavior are common and may involve severe aggression. Pupils are often dilated, and blindness may be apparent. For the first 1–2 days, observable hemiparesis may be present. Acute signs usually resolve in a few days, leaving signs of a nonprogressive unilateral cerebral lesion. The loss of visual cerebral cortex or optic radiation causes contralateral loss of the menace reflex, with normal pupillary reflexes. Unilateral cerebral lesions are usually in the frontal lobe. Occasionally, bilateral blindness persists with dilated unresponsive pupils because of ischemic necrosis of the optic chiasm. Examination may reveal a unilateral facial hypalgesia contralateral to the cerebral lesion. No other cranial nerve deficits have been observed. Ischemic necrosis of the cerebral hemi-

sphere is variable and usually unilateral, but occasionally it is bilateral. The necrosis may be multifocal, or the infarction may involve up to two thirds of one entire cerebrum. Vascular occlusion occurs most frequently in the middle cerebral artery. Most cats with cerebral vascular disease survive, but behavioral changes and uncontrollable seizures may persist.

4. *Unilateral cerebral abscess.* In horses, abscesses caused by *Streptococcus equi* may affect the optic radiation and cause a contralateral visual deficit with normal pupillary reflexes. Expansion of the lesion with accompanying cerebral edema increases intracranial pressure and causes the occipital lobes to herniate ventral to the tentorium cerebelli. This further compromises function of the visual cortex bilaterally, and total blindness results if both sides are affected. Similar signs occur in ruminants with *Corynebacterium pyogenes* abscess.

5. *Encephalitis.* In encephalitis caused by *Toxoplasma gondii,* a space-occupying granuloma may be produced in the optic radiation and cause a contralateral visual deficit. Cerebrospinal fluid (CSF) should contain inflammatory cells, often with neutrophils and increased amounts of protein. Occasionally, focal encephalitis produced in horses by an unidentified protozoan is severe enough in one hemisphere to cause swelling and necrosis and a contralateral visual deficit.

BILATERAL DISEASE

Total blindness with normal pupillary light reflexes is characteristic of bilateral visual cortex lesions.

1. *Tentorial herniation.* The same explanation for bilateral signs of visual deficit from tentorial herniation can be offered for any space-occupying cerebral lesion or cerebral swelling following injury. Head injury that causes progressive cerebral edema causes blindness. The pupillary activity varies with the degree of brain stem involvement.

2. *Hypoplasia of the prosencephalon* in calves. The rostral portion of the malformed diencephalon protrudes through a defect in the calvaria and is attached to the adjacent skin. The skull is flatter than normal to conform to the malformed brain, which consists of a brain stem with a small cerebellum and no cerebral hemispheres. The lack of cerebral tissue causes visual deficit, despite a functional brain stem. These animals may be able to stand and usually live for a few days.

3. *Hydranencephaly.* In this condition, the cerebral hemispheres are reduced to a membranous sac filled with CSF, which may cause a "dummy" syndrome in calves and lambs with ataxia and visual deficit. It has been caused by Akabane virus in cattle and bluetongue virus in sheep.

4. *Obstructive hydrocephalus* compromises the optic radiation in the internal capsule, in which it forms the lateral wall of the dilated lateral ventricle. Bilateral visual deficit and ataxia are common signs, reflecting attenuation of the cerebral white matter, optic radiation, and visual cortex.

5. *Ischemic necrosis of cerebrum.* During recovery from diffuse ischemic necrosis of the cerebrum caused by anesthetic overdose and prolonged apnea and cardiac arrest, the only residual deficit may be blindness with intact pupillary reflexes.

6. *Polioencephalomalacia in cattle and sheep.* This condition causes severe cerebral disturbance, including frequent blindness. The visual deficit is due to necrosis of the visual cortex caused by an abnormality in thiamine (vitamin B_1) metabolism. *Lead poisoning* causes similar acute necrosis of the cerebral cortex and an associated blindness. Similarly, severe *water intoxication* with cerebral disturbance may cause blindness.

7. *Fungicide toxicity.* Intoxication by wheat seed fungicide containing mercury causes chronic degeneration of neurons in the cerebral cortex and replacement of astrocytes. Convulsions and blindness may appear in the chronic stages.

8. *Canine distemper.* When this condition causes chronic encephalitis, demyelination and astrocytosis of the optic radiation may result. This is a sclerosing encephalitis that may produce a unilateral or bilateral visual deficit with normal pupillary function. Chorioretinitis may be visible ophthalmoscopically.

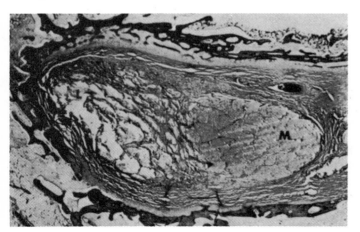

FIGURE 17–25. *Transverse section of left optic nerve and bony canal, showing progression of malacia from acute lateral angle of canal (L) where vascular supply is most prone to compression. Viable nerve is present in medial aspect (M). (From Hayes KC, et al: Pathogenesis of the optic nerve lesion in vitamin A–deficient calves. Arch Ophthalmol 80:777, 1968. Copyright 1968, American Medical Association.)*

TABLE 17–14. Storage Diseases of Ophthalmic Significance

Species	Breed	Syndrome	Synonyms	Clinical Signs	Substance Accumulated	Biochemical Defect	Genetic Classification	References
Dog	Australian silky terrier	Neurovisceral glucocerebroside storage disease	Gaucher's disease	Incoordination, hyperkinesis, exaggeration of spinal reflexes at 8 months	Glucocerebroside	Glucocerebrosidase	—	Hartley and Blakemore (1973)
	Beagle	Globoid cell leukodystrophy	Krabbe's disease	Paraparesis and dysmetria at 4 months	—	—	—	Johnson et al (1975)
	Bluetick hound	Globoid cell leukodystrophy	Krabbe's disease	Ascending paresis, tremors; proprioceptive deficit and death by 8 months of age	—	β-galactocere-brocidase	Familial	Boysen et al (1974)
	Border collie	Ceroid lipofuscinosis disease	Batten's disease	Visual abnormalities, gait abnormalities	Unknown	—	Recessive	Taylor and Farrow (1988) Harper et al (1988)
	Cairn and West Highland white terrier	Globoid cell leukodystrophy	Krabbe's disease	Ascending paresis and ataxia at 3–6 months of age; cerebellar ataxia and visual deficit Death before 12 months	Galactosyl ceramide	β-galactosidase	Recessive	Fletcher et al (1966)
	Chihuahua	Neuronal ceroid lipofuscinosis	Kuf's disease	Incoordination, restlessness, progressing blindness to 24 months	—	—	—	Rae and Giesicke (1975)
	Dachshund	Neuronal ceroid lipofuchsinosis	Kuf's disease	Cerebellar ataxia, onset at 3 years, still progressing at 4–5 years	—	—	—	Cummings and deLahunta (1977)
	English setter	Lipodystrophy (neuronal ceroid lipofuchsinosis)	Juvenile amaurotic familial idiocy	Ataxia and visual deficit at 6–12 months; "dummy" attitude, convulsions, and death by 2 years	—	Phenylene-diamine-mediated peroxidase	Hereditary	Koppang (1970, 1973)
	English spaniel	Fucosidosis	—	Visual disorders, ataxia, hearing loss, behavioral changes, dysphagia, weight loss; gait abnormalities	—	α-1-fucosidase	Hereditary	Taylor et al (1987)
	German short-haired pointer	(Lipodystrophy) GM₂ gangliosidosis	Juvenile amaurotic familial idiocy	As for English setter	GM₂ gangliosides	Hexosaminidase A (?)	Hereditary	Karbe and Schiefer (1967)
	Lapland	Glycogen storage disease type II	Pompe's disease	Dysphagia and vomiting at 1½ years	Glycogen	α-1:4-glucosidase	Familial	Mostafa (1970)
	Plott hound	Mucopoly-saccharidosis I	—	Severe joint disease, stunted growth, bilateral corneal opacity	Mucopolysac-charide	α-L-iduronidase	—	Shull et al (1982)
Cat	Domestic short hair	GM₁ gangliosidosis (similar to lipidoses and mucopoly-saccharidosis)	—	Ataxia and tremor at weaning; lethargy, gross ataxia and hypermetria, intention tremor, and visual deficit at 2–3 months; corneal opacity and retinal spots	GM₁ ganglioside	—	—	Murray et al (1983)

Table continued on following page

TABLE 17–14. Storage Diseases of Ophthalmic Significance *(Continued)*

Species	Breed	Syndrome	Synonyms	Clinical Signs	Substance Accumulated	Biochemical Defect	Genetic Classification	References
	—	Mucopolysac-charidosis I (MPS I)	Hunter's syndrome	Facial dysmorphia, bilateral corneal opacity, bilateral hip luxation, pectus excavatum, gait abnormalities	Mucopolysac-charides	α-1-iduronidase	Hereditary	Haskins et al (1983)
	Siamese	Mucopolysac-charidosis VI	—	Facial joint and skeletal deformities, multifocal spinal cord disease, cloudy cornea, and retinal atrophy Positive toluidine blue spot test	Acid mucopoly-saccharides	Arylsulfatase B	Hereditary	Cowell et al (1976) Haskins et al (1979) Aguire et al (1983)
	—	Spingomyelin lipidosis	Niemann-Pick disease	Cerebellar disturbance at 4 months progressing to death at 9 months	Spingomyelin	Sphingomyelinase	—	Chrisp et al (1970)
	—	GM$_1$ gangliosidosis	—	Tremors, progressive paresis, and ataxia at 4 months; tetraplegia at 6 months	GM$_1$ ganglioside	β-galactosidase	—	Baker et al (1971) Jortner (1971) Sandstrom (1969)
	—	Globoid cell leukodystrophy	Krabbe's disease	—	—	β-galactosidase	—	Johnson (1970)
		Glycogen storage disease type II	Pompe's disease	—	Glycogen	α-1:4-glucosidase	—	Sandstrom (1969)
Sheep	Corriedale	Glycogen storage disease type II	Pompe's disease	Incoordination, lethargy, emaciation, drooping ears by 6–10 months of age	Glycogen	α-1:4-glucosidase	—	Mankletow and Hartley (1975)
		Glucocerebroside storage disease	Gaucher's disease	—	Glucocerebrosides	Glucocerebrosidase	—	Laws and Saal (1968)
	South Hampshire	Neuronal ceroid lipofuscinosis	—	Amaurosis, mild ataxia, and generalized tremor	Unknown	Unknown	Unknown	Jolly and West (1976) Mayhew et al (1986)
Cattle	Aberdeen Angus	Mannosidosis	Pseudolipidosis	Ataxia, incoordination, intention tremor, and death before 12 months	Oligosaccharides containing mannose	α-mannosi-dase	Hereditary	Hocking et al (1972) Whitlem and Walker (1975)
	Beef master	Neuronal lipodystrophy	Juvenile or infantile amaurotic familial idiocy	Blindness and circling at 12 months	—	—	—	Read and Bridges (1969)
	Charolais	—		Stiff gait, progressive incoordination	Myelinlike lipid	—	—	Palmer et al (1972)
	Devon	Ceroid lipo-fuscinosis disease	Batten's disease	Gait abnorma-lities, blindness	Unknown	—	Recessive	Jolly et al (1987) Harper et al (1988)
	Fresian	GM$_1$ gangliosidosis	—	Incoordination and progressive loss of motor function, 3–9 months of age	—	α-galactosidase	—	Donnelly et al (1973)
	Shorthorn	Glycogen storage disease Type II	Pompe's disease	Muscle weakness, incoordination	Glycogen	α-1:4-glucosidase	Hereditary	Richards et al (1977)
Pig	Yorkshire	Cerebrospinal lipodystrophy	Similar to Tay Sach's disease	—	—	—	—	Read and Bridges (1968)
	—	Glucocerebroside storage disease	Gaucher's disease	—	Glucocerebrosides	Glucocerebrosidase	—	Sandison and Anderson (1970)

9. *Thromboembolic meningoencephalitis.* Infarction of the cerebral white matter by septic emboli occurs in cattle afflicted with thromboembolic meningoencephalitis caused by *Hemophilus somnus.* Visual deficits may result. Severe *ophthalmoscopically visible retinal lesions* are the probable cause of visual deficits and are of considerable use in diagnosis.

Vitamin A Deficiency

Vitamin A deficiency is of clinical ophthalmic and economic significance in cattle, pigs, and sheep only.

Clinical Signs

In cattle, signs depend on age.

Young Growing Calves

1. Night blindness (nyctalopia), which is reversible until severe lesions have occurred in advanced disease.

2. Loss of rod and cone layers of the retina.

3. Papilledema with occasional hemorrhages. Papilledema develops over many months and is caused by constriction of the optic nerve as it passes through the optic canal in the sphenoid bone. CSF pressure is increased, presphenoid bone growth is altered, and the dura mater surrounding the nerve thickens, causing ischemic necrosis of the nerve as it passes through the canal (Fig. 17–25). Papilledema may be seen in calves born to vitamin A–deficient dams. As the deficiency progresses, papilledema becomes worse. The disc enlarges and becomes pink and pale, and details of the central disc are obscured. In the later stages, or if treatment is not given, irreversible optic atrophy occurs, and the disc becomes gray, flat, and shrunken, with attenuated retinal vessels. Focal streaks or dots of retinal atrophy may occur close to the disc. Clinical signs become apparent when blood levels have dropped to about 5 μg of vitamin A/ml, or 2 μg/g of liver. For diagnosis of vitamin A deficiency, liver levels are more reliable than blood levels.

Adult Cattle

1. Night blindness.
2. Papilledema.
3. Mottling of the tapetum.
4. Pallor of the nontapetal area.

Note: The 3rd and 4th items are both reversible with vitamin A therapy.

Pigs. The most common ophthalmic sign is birth of microphthalmic piglets to sows with vitamin A deficiency, although night blindness may occur later in the disease in adult pigs. In addition, affected adults show head tilt (otitis media), swaying gait (leading to hind limb paralysis), stiffness, and restlessness.

Sheep. Nyctalopia is the first sign of vitamin A deficiency.

Other reported signs—xerophthalmia, corneal edema, ulceration, photophobia, and corneal keratinization—are neither consistent, common, nor diagnostically useful and have resulted from extrapolation from the human disease. Vitamin A deficiency does cause keratinization of the conjunctive in tortoises and chickens.

Treatment and Prevention

The following regimen should be started for affected animals:

1. Vitamin A (water-soluble preparation), 440 IU/kg intramuscularly.

2. Provision of rations containing vitamin A, 65 IU/kg body weight/day.

Metabolic Disorders (Storage Disorders) (Table 17–14)

Inherited metabolic disorders of the nervous system occur in most domestic species and are models of comparable diseases in humans. All are progressive, degenerative disorders of the nervous system, usually of a recessive nature. The onset is usually some time after weaning. Signs represent diffuse involvement of the nervous system but often begin with pelvic limb ataxia and paresis. In the advanced stages of many of these diseases, blindness is common as the retina or visual pathways are affected. There is usually a lack of or severe deficiency of a specific degradative enzyme, which leads to abnormal accumulation of biochemical substrate normally metabolized by that enzyme. These metabolic disorders may be expressed in neurons by the accumulation of complex lipids in neuronal cytoplasm (lipodystrophy) or in the myelin by demyelination and accumulation of complex lipids in macrophages (leukodystrophy). Leukodystrophy involves abnormal metabolism of myelin and its subsequent degeneration, whereas lipodystrophy refers to abnormal neuronal metabolism associated with accumulations of complex lipids in neurons and their subsequent degeneration.

REFERENCES

Achesson GH (1938): The topographical anatomy of the smooth muscle of the cat's nictitating membrane. Anat Rec 71:297.

Aguirre GD, et al (1983): Feline mucopolysaccharidosis VI: General ocular and pigment epithelial pathology. Invest Ophthalmol Vis Sci 24:991.

Baird JD, Mackenzie CD (1974): Cerebellar hypoplasia and degeneration in part-Arab horses. Aust Vet J 50:25.

Baker HJ, et al (1971): Neuronal GM gangliosidosis in a Siamese cat with beta galactosidase deficiency. Science 174:838.

Barlow CM, Root WS (1949): The ocular sympathetic path between the superior cervical ganglion and the orbit in the cat. J Comp Neurol 91:195.

Barlow RM, et al (1981): Mannosidosis in Aberdeen Angus cattle in Britain. Vet Rec 109:441.

Barnett KC, Grimes TD (1974): Bilateral aplasia of the optic nerve in a cat. Br J Ophthalmol 57:663.

Barnett KC, et al (1970): Ocular changes associated with hypovitaminosis A in sheep. Br Vet J 126:561.

Bichsel P, et al (1988): Neurologic manifestations associated with hypothyroidism in four dogs. J Am Vet Med Assoc 192:1745.

Bistner S, et al (1970): Pharmacologic diagnosis of Horner's syndrome in the dog. J Am Vet Med Assoc 157:1220.

Blood DC, et al (1983): Veterinary Medicine, 5th ed. WB Saunders Co, Philadelphia.

Boysen BG et al (1974): Globoid cell leukodystrophy in the bluetick hound dog. 1. Clinical manifestations. Can Vet J 15(11):303.

Bromberg NM, Cabaniss LD (1988): Feline dysautonomia: A case report. J Am Anim Hosp Assoc 24:106.

Brouwer GJ (1987): Feline dysautonomia—Pharmacological studies. J Sm Anim Pract 28:350.

Canton DD, et al (1988): Dysautonomia in a cat. J Am Vet Med Assoc 192:1293.

Chrisp CE, et al (1970): Lipid storage disease in a Siamese cat. J Am Vet Med Assoc 156:616.

Christian RG, Tryphonas L (1971): Lead poisoning in cattle: Brain lesions and hematologic changes. Am J Vet Res 32:203.

Cogan DG (1956): Neurology of the Ocular Muscles, 2nd ed. Charles C Thomas. Springfield, IL.

Cowell KR, et al (1976): Mucopolysaccharidosis in a cat. J Am Vet Med Assoc 169:334.

Cummings JF, deLahunta A (1977): An adult case of canine neuronal ceroid-lipofuscinosis. Acta Neuropathol 39:43.

deLahunta A, Alexander JW (1976): Ischemic myelopathy secondary to presumed fibrocartilaginous embolism in nine dogs. J Am Anim Hosp Assoc 12:37.

Done JT (1976): Developmental disorders of the nervous system in animals. *In* Brandly CA, Jungherr EL (eds): Advances in Veterinary Science and Comparative Medicine, vol 20. Academic Press, New York.

Donnelly WJC, et al (1973): GM1 gangliosidosis in friesian calves. J Pathol 111:173.

Ernest JT (1976): Bilateral optic nerve hypoplasia in a pup. J Am Vet Med Assoc 168:125.

Everett CA, Jones GT (1972): Optic neuritis in dogs. J Am Vet Med Assoc, 160:68.

Fletcher TF, et al (1966): Globoid cell leukodystrophy (Krabbe type) in the dog. J Am Vet Med Assoc 149:165.

Fox JG, Gutnick MJ (1972): Horner's syndrome and brachial paralysis due to lymphosarcoma in a cat. J Am Vet Med Assoc 160:977.

Fraser DC, et al (1970): Myasthenia gravis in the dog. J Neurol Neurosurg Psychiatry 33:431.

Fraser H (1966): Two dissimilar types of cerebellar disorder in the horse. Vet Rec 78:608.

Gaskell CJ (1987): Feline dysautonomia—Introduction and background. J Am Anim Pract 28:337.

Gelatt KN, et al (1969): Bilateral optic nerve hypoplasia in a colt. J Am Vet Med Assoc 155:627.

Gelatt KN, et al (1971): Optic disc astrocytoma in a horse. Can Vet J 12:53.

Gerding PA, et al (1986): Pupillotonia in a dog. J Am Vet Med Assoc 189:1477.

Gilmore DR, deLahunta A (1987): Necrotizing myelopathy secondary to presumed or confirmed fibrocartilaginous embolism. J Am Anim Hosp Assoc 23:373.

Greene CE, Higgins RJ (1976): Fibrocartilaginous emboli as the cause of ischemic myelopathy in a dog. Cornell Vet 66:131.

Griffiths IR (1987): Feline dysautonomia—Pathology. J Am Anim Pract 28:347.

Griffiths IR, et al (1982): The Key-Gaskell syndrome: The current situation. Vet Rec 111:532.

Griffiths IR, et al (1985): Feline dysautonomia (the Key-Gaskell syndrome): An ultrastructural study of autonomic ganglia and nerves. Neuropathol Appl Neurobiol 11:17.

Guillery RW, Kaas JH (1971): A study of normal and congenitally abnormal retinogeniculate projections in cats. J Comp Neurol 143:73.

Guillery RW, Kaas JH (1973): Genetic abnormality of the visual pathways in a "white" tiger. Science 180:1287.

Harper PA, et al (1988): Neurovisceral ceroid-lipofucsinosis in blind Devon cattle. Acta Neuropathol 75:632.

Hartley WJ (1963): Polioencephalomalacia in dogs. Acta Neuropathol 2:271.

Hartley WJ, Blakemore WF (1973): Neurovisceral glucocerebroside storage (Gaucher's disease) in a dog. Vet Pathol 10:191.

Haskins ME, et al (1979): The pathology of arylsulfatase B deficient mucopolysaccharidosis. Am J Pathol 101:657.

Haskins ME, et al (1983): The pathology of the feline model of mucopolysaccharidosis I. Am J Pathol 112:27.

Hayes KC, et al (1968): Pathogenesis of the optic nerve lesion in vitamin A–deficient calves. Arch Ophthalmol 80:777.

Hegreberg GA, et al (1971): Morphologic changes in feline leuko-dystrophy. Fel Prod 30:341.

Hocking JD, et al (1972): Deficiency of alpha mannosidase in Angus cattle. Biochem J 128:69.

Hogan MJ, Zimmerman LE (1962): Ophthalmic Pathology, 2nd ed. WB Saunders Co, Philadelphia.

Hubel DH, Wiesel TN (1971): Aberrant visual projections in the Siamese cat. J Physiol 218:33.

Innes IJR, et al (1940): Familial cerebellar hypoplasia and degeneration in Hereford calves. J Path Bact 50:455.

Johnson G, et al (1975): Globoid cell leukodystrophy in a beagle. J Am Vet Med Assoc 167:380.

Johnson KH (1970): Globoid cell leukodystrophy in the cat. J Am Vet Med Assoc 157:2057.

Johnson RP, et al (1975): Myasthenia in springer spaniel littermates. J Sm Anim Pract 16:641.

Jolly RD, West DD (1976): Blindness in South Hampshire sheep: A neuronal ceroid-lipofuscinosis. New Zealand Vet J 24:123.

Jolly RD, et al (1987): Mannosidosis: Ocular lesions in the bovine model. Curr Eye Res 6:1073.

Kahrs RF (1968): Chronic mercurial poisoning in swine. A case report of an outbreak with some epidemiological characteristics of hog cholera. Cornell Vet 58:67.

Kalil RE, et al (1971): Anomalous retinal pathways in the Siamese cat. An inadequate substrate for normal binocular vision. Science 174:302.

Karbe E, Schiefer B (1967): Familial amaurotic idiocy in male German shorthair pointers. Pathol Vet 4:223.

Kay TJA, Gaskell CJ (1982): Puzzling syndrome in cats associated with pupillary dilation. Vet Rec 110:160.

Kern TJ, Erb N (1987): Facial neuropathy in dogs and cats: 95 cases (1975–1985). J Am Vet Med Assoc 191:1604.

Kern TJ, Riis RC (1981): Optic nerve hypoplasia in three miniature poodles. J Am Vet Med Assoc 178:49.

Kerr FWL, Hollowell OW (1964): Location of pupillomotor and accommodation fibres in the oculomotor nerve: experimental observations on paralytic mydriasis. J Neurol Neurosurg Psychiatry 27:473.

Koppang N (1970): Neuronal ceroid lipofuscinosis in English setters. Juvenile amaurotic familial idiocy in English setters. J Sm Anim Pract 10:639.

Koppang N (1973): Canine ceroid lipofuscinosis: A model for human neuronal ceroid lipofuscinosis and aging. Mech Ageing Dev 2:421.

Laws L, Saal JR (1968): Lipidosis of the hepatic reticuloendothelial cells in a sheep. Aust Vet J 44:416.

Leipold HW, Huston K (1968): Congenital syndrome with anophthalmia, microphthalmia and associated defects in cattle. Pathol Vet 5:407.

Leipold HW, et al (1971): Multiple ocular anomalies and hydrocephalus in grade beef shorthorn cattle. Am J Vet Res 32:1019.

Levy NS (1974): Editorial on recent advances: Functional implications of axoplasmic transport. Invest Ophthalmol 13:639.

Little PB, Sorenson DK (1969): Bovine polioencephalomalacia, infectious embolic meningoencephalitis and acute lead poisoning in feedlot cattle. J Am Vet Med Assoc 155:1892.

Lorenz MD, et al (1972): Neostigmine-responsive weakness in the dog similar to myasthenia gravis. J Am Vet Med Assoc 161:705.

Manktelow BW, Hartley WJ (1975): Generalized glycogen storage disease in sheep. J Comp Pathol 85:139.

Martin CL, et al (1986): Four cases of traumatic optic nerve blindness in the horse. Equine Vet J 18:133.

Mayhew IG, et al (1986): Ceroid-lipofucsinosis (Batten's disease): Pathogenesis of blindness in the ovine model. J Comp Pathol 254:543.

McConnon, JM, et al (1983): Pendular nystagmus in cattle. J Am Vet Med Assoc 182:812.

Meric SM (1988): Canine meningitis: A review. J Vet Int Med 2:26.

Miselbrook NG (1987): Peripheral neuropathy in a diabetic bitch. Vet Rec 121:287.

Murphy C (1987): Consider brain lesions with blindness. Assoc Avian Vet 1:11.

Nash AS, et al (1982): Key-Gaskell syndrome. Vet Rec 111:564.

Nash AS, et al (1982): The Key-Gaskell syndrome: An autonomic polyganglionopathy. Vet Rec 111:564.

Nash AS (1987): Feline dysautonomia—Clinical features and management. J Sm Anim Pract 28:339.

Owen RR (1974): Epistaxis prevented by ligation of the internal carotid artery in the gutteral pouch. Equine Vet J 6:143.

Palmer AC (1967): Cardiac arrest and cerebrocortical necrosis. Vet Rec 80:390.

Palmer AC (1970): Pathogenesis and pathology of the cerebellar vestibular syndrome. J Sm Anim Pract 11:167.

Palmer AC, Barker J (1974): Myasthenia in the dog. Vet Rec 95:452.

Palmer AC, et al (1972): Progressive ataxia of charolais cattle associated with a myelin disorder. Vet Rec 91:592.

Palmer AC, et al (1973): Cerebellar hypoplasia and degeneration in the young Arab horse: Clinical and neuropathological features. Vet Rec 93:62.

Palmer AC, et al (1973): Hereditary quadriplegia and amblyopia in the Irish setter. J Sm Anim Pract 14:343.

Palmer AC, et al (1974): Clinical signs including papilledema associated with brain tumors in twenty-one dogs. J Sm Anim Pract 15:359.

Parker AJ, et al (1973): Hemifacial spasms in a dog. Vet Rec 93:514.

Percy DH, Jortner BS (1971): Feline lipidosis. Arch Pathol 92:136.

Polin M, Sullivan M (1986): A canine dysautonomia resembling Kay-Gaskell syndrome. Vet Rec 118:402.

Rac R, Giesicke RR (1975): Lysosomal storage disease in Chihuahuas. Aust Vet J 51:403.

Read WK, Bridges CH (1968): Cerebrospinal lipodystrophy in swine. A new disease model in comparative pathology. Pathol Vet 5:67.

Read WK, Bridges CH (1969): Neuronal lipodystrophy—Occurrence in an inbred strain of cattle. Pathol Vet 6:235.

Richards RB, et al (1977): Bovine generalized glycogenosis. Neuropathol Appl Neurobiol 3:45.

Roberts SR, Vainisi SJ (1967): Hemifacial spasm in dogs. J Am Vet Med Assoc 150:381.

Robins GM (1976): Dropped jaw—Mandibular neuropraxia in the dog. J Sm Anim Pract 17:753.

Rochlitz I (1984): Feline dysautonomia (the Key-Gaskell or dilated pupil syndrome): A preliminary review. J Sm Anim Pract 25:587.

Rosen ES, et al (1970): Male fern retrobulbar neuropathy in cattle. J Sm Anim Pract 10:619.

Rosenblueth A, Bard P (1932): The innervation and function of the nictitating membrane in the cat. Am J Physiol 100:537.

Rubin LF (1974): Atlas of Veterinary Ophthalmoscopy. Lea & Febiger, Philadelphia.

Sandison AT, Anderson LJ (1970): Histiocytosis in two pigs and a cow. Conditions resembling lipid storage disorders in man. J Pathol 93:62.

Shull RM, et al (1982): Canine alpha-L-iduronidase deficiency, a model of mucopolysaccharidosis I. Am J Pathol 109:244.

Strain GM, et al (1987): Evoked potential and electroencephalographic assessment of central blindness due to brain abscesses in a steer. Cornell Vet 77:374.

Sweeney RW, Sweeney CR (1984): Transient Horner's syndrome following routine intravenous injections in two horses. J Am Vet Med Assoc 185:802.

Taylor RM, Farrow BR (1988): Ceroid-lipofucsinosis in border collie dogs. Acta Neuropathol 75:627.

Taylor RM, et al (1987): Canine fucosidosis: Clinical findings. J Sm Anim Pract 28:291.

van den Broek AHM (1987): Horner's syndrome in cats and dogs: A review. J Sm Anim Pract 28:929.

Vandevelde M, et al (1982): Hereditary neurovisceral mannosidosis associated with alpha mannosidase deficiency in a family of Persian cats. Acta Neuropathol (Berl) 58:64.

Vestre WA, et al (1982): Proliferative optic neuropathy in a horse. J Am Vet Med Assoc 181:490.

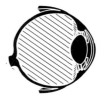

18

Orbit

ANATOMY	**ORBITAL DISEASES**	**OCULAR PROSTHESES**
PATHOLOGICAL MECHANISMS	**SURGICAL PROCEDURES**	**ORBITOTOMY**
DIAGNOSTIC METHODS		

ANATOMY

The orbit is the cavity that encloses the eye. In domestic animals there are two patterns:

1. Incomplete bony orbit—dog, cat (Figs. 18–1 to 18–3).

2. Complete bony orbit—horse, ox, sheep, pig (Figs. 18–4 and 18–5).

The orbit separates the eye from the cranial cavity, and the FORAMINA or FISSURES in its walls determine the path of blood vessels and nerves from the brain to the eye. The walls of the equine orbit are formed by the frontal, lacrimal, zygomatic, temporal, presphenoid, palatine, and maxillary bones and are similar in other species. In the dog and cat, the dorsolateral portion of the orbit is completed by the dense collagenous ORBITAL LIGAMENT, which passes from the zygomatic process of the frontal bone to the frontal process of the zygomatic bone. The basic foramina and fissures of the orbit are the orbital, rostral, and caudal alar, oval, supraorbital, ethmoidal, lacrimal, maxillary, sphenopalatine, round, and palatine. In cattle, the

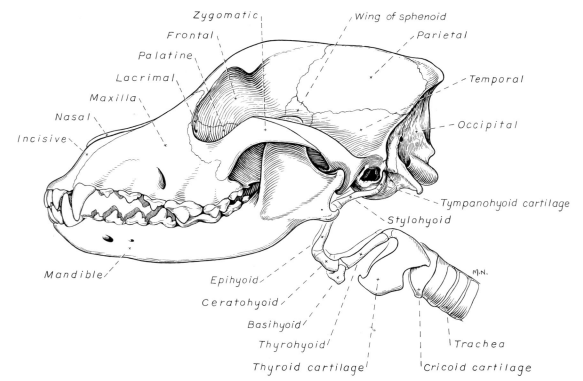

FIGURE 18–1. Bones of the skull, hyoid apparatus, and laryngeal cartilages. Lateral aspect. (From Evans HE, Christensen GC: Miller's Anatomy of the Dog, 2nd ed. WB Saunders Co, Philadelphia, 1979. © Cornell University 1964.)

478

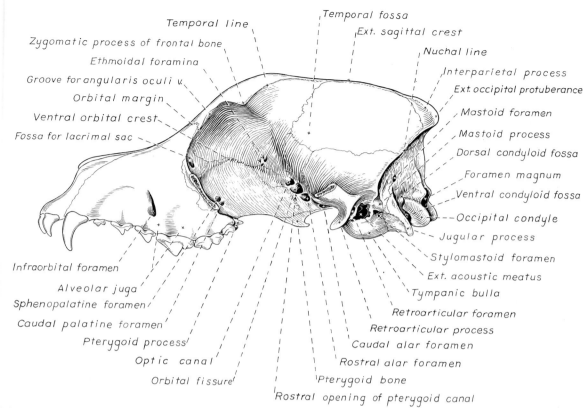

FIGURE 18–2. *Skull. Lateral aspect. (Zygomatic arch removed.) (From Evans HE, Christensen GC: Miller's Anatomy of the Dog, 2nd ed. WB Saunders Co, Philadelphia, 1979. © Cornell University, 1964.)*

Temporal line
Zygomatic process of frontal bone
Ethmoidal foramina
Groove for angularis oculi v.
Orbital margin
Ventral orbital crest
Fossa for lacrimal sac
Temporal fossa
Ext. sagittal crest
Nuchal line
Interparietal process
Ext. occipital protuberance
Mastoid foramen
Mastoid process
Dorsal condyloid fossa
Foramen magnum
Ventral condyloid fossa
Occipital condyle
Jugular process
Stylomastoid foramen
Ext. acoustic meatus
Tympanic bulla
Retroarticular foramen
Retroarticular process
Caudal alar foramen
Rostral alar foramen
Pterygoid bone
Rostral opening of pterygoid canal
Orbital fissure
Optic canal
Pterygoid process
Caudal palatine foramen
Sphenopalatine foramen
Alveolar juga
Infraorbital foramen

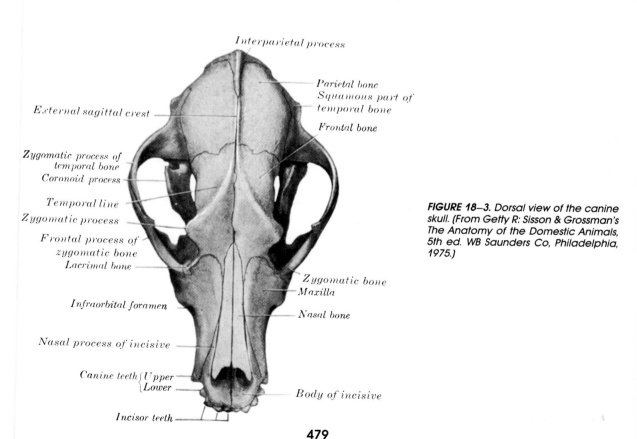

Interparietal process
Parietal bone
Squamous part of temporal bone
Frontal bone
External sagittal crest
Zygomatic process of temporal bone
Coronoid process
Temporal line
Zygomatic process
Frontal process of zygomatic bone
Lacrimal bone
Infraorbital foramen
Nasal process of incisive
Canine teeth { Upper
{ Lower
Incisor teeth
Zygomatic bone
Maxilla
Nasal bone
Body of incisive

FIGURE 18–3. *Dorsal view of the canine skull. (From Getty R: Sisson & Grossman's The Anatomy of the Domestic Animals, 5th ed. WB Saunders Co, Philadelphia, 1975.)*

479

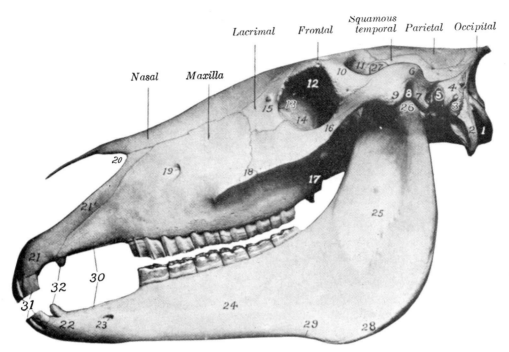

FIGURE 18–4. *Left lateral view of the equine skull. Note the enclosed dorsolateral surface of the orbit. (From Getty R: Sisson & Grossman's The Anatomy of the Domestic Animals, 5th ed. WB Saunders Co, Philadelphia, 1975.)*

orbital foramen and the foramen rotundum fuse to form the foramen orbitorotundum. The vessels and nerves that pass through these foramina and fissures in the dog are shown in Figures 1–11 to 1–15 and Figure 18–6.

The position of the orbit within the skull varies among species. In cattle, sheep, and horses, the eyes are situated laterally, giving panoramic vision, whereas in dogs and cats, the eyes are located anteriorly, allowing a greater degree of binocular vision and depth perception. The visual, orbital, and optic axes defined here do not coincide (Fig. 18–7).

VISUAL AXIS—line from the center of the most sensitive area of the retina to the object viewed.

ORBITAL AXIS—line from the apex of the orbit to the center of the external opening.

OPTIC AXIS—line from the center of the posterior pole of the eye through the center of the cornea.

The angle formed by the optic axes, a measure of binocularity, is shown in different species in Figures 18–8 and 18–9 (see also Figs. 1–3 and 1–4).

The relationships of the orbit to the *paranasal sinuses, teeth, zygomatic gland,* and the *ramus of the mandible* are important, as they affect incidence, diagnosis, and pathogenesis of clinical diseases of the eye and orbit.

1. *Infections of the sinuses or nasal cavity* may enter the orbit in all domestic species (Fig. 18–10). The junction of the frontal, lacrimal, and palatine bones in the medial wall of the canine orbit (see Fig. 18–1) is often thin and may be eroded by disease processes in the nasal cavity, which then enter the orbit. The bone is thicker in horses (Fig. 18–11).

2. *Fractures of walls of the sinuses* can cause emphysema, with gas visible beneath the conjunctiva or palpable under the skin.

3. *Infections of the roots of the molar teeth* can affect the orbit and periocular area in dogs and cats.

4. *Enlargement of the canine zygomatic salivary gland* can cause increased pressure within the orbit or protrusion of the gland into the ventral conjunctival fornix (Fig. 18–12).

On opening the mouth, especially in dogs and cats with greater mobility of the mandible, the ramus of the mandible moves forward, exerting pressure on the orbital contents (causing pain if inflammation is present).

The orbital contents are completely enclosed in a sheet of connective tissue—the PERIORBITA—which lies next to the bone in the bony parts of the orbital wall and is thicker laterally at the point at which the wall is incomplete (in carnivores). The periorbita is reflected over the extraocular muscles and forward over the globe to become TENON'S CAPSULE, lying beneath the conjunctiva (Fig. 18–13). The periorbita is continuous with the periosteum of the facial bones at the orbital rim, with the septum orbitale anteriorly, and with the dura mater of the optic nerve. The orbital fat pad lies between the periorbita and the orbital wall.

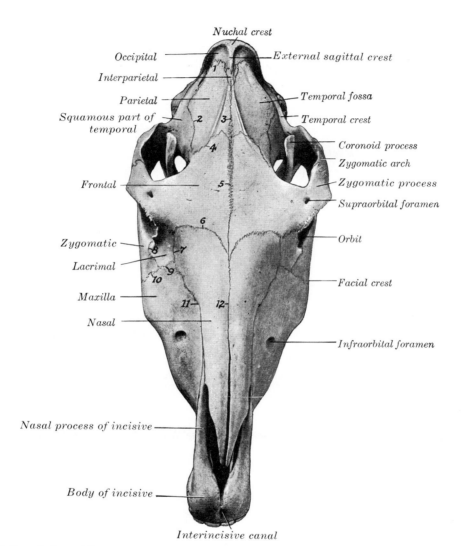

Nuchal crest

Occipital

Interparietal

Parietal

Squamous part of
temporal

Frontal

Zygomatic

Lacrimal

Maxilla

Nasal

External sagittal crest

Temporal fossa

Temporal crest

Coronoid process

Zygomatic arch

Zygomatic process

Supraorbital foramen

Orbit

Facial crest

Infraorbital foramen

Nasal process of incisive

Body of incisive

Interincisive canal

FIGURE 18–5. Dorsal view of the equine skull. (From Getty R: Sisson & Grossman's The Anatomy of the Domestic Animals, 5th ed. WB Saunders Co, Philadelphia, 1975.)

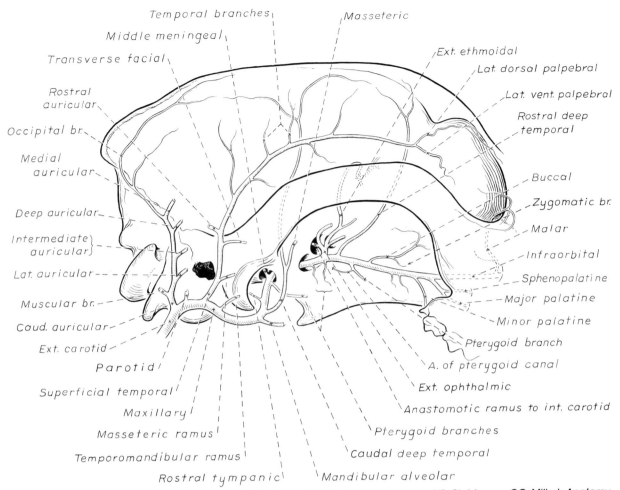

FIGURE 18–6. Arteries of the head in relation to lateral aspect of the skull. (From Evans HE, Christensen GC: Miller's Anatomy of the Dog, 2nd ed. WB Saunders Co, Philadelphia, 1979. © Cornell University 1964.)

FIGURE 18–7. The visual and optic axes of the eye. (From Getty R: Sisson & Grossman's The Anatomy of the Domestic Animals, 5th ed. WB Saunders Co, Philadelphia, 1975. Adapted from Walls GL: The Vertebrate Eye. Cranbrook Institute of Science. Bloomfield Hills, MI, 48013, 1942.)

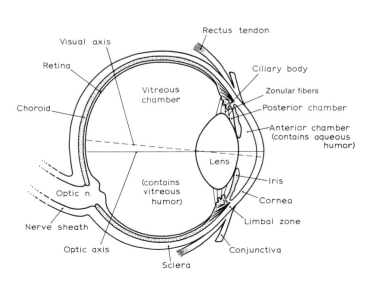

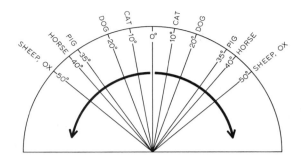

FIGURE 18–8. *Comparison of the angle formed by the optic axes of different species of domestic animals. (From Getty R: Sisson & Grossman's The Anatomy of the Domestic Animals, 5th ed. WB Saunders Co, Philadelphia, 1975.)*

Intraorbital fat lies between the muscles and fascial layers (Fig. 18–14). Orbital disease processes may thus be located in one of three planes:

1. Within the muscle cone
2. Outside the muscle cone but within the periorbita
3. Within the orbit but outside the periorbita (e.g., posterior to the periorbita laterally at the point at which there is no bony wall, as occurs in myositis of the temporal muscle)

The lacrimal gland lies beneath the orbital ligament on the dorsolateral surface of the globe (see Fig. 18–13). The base of the third eyelid and gland is held down by the **ORBITAL RETINACULUM**, poorly defined sheets of collagenous tissue continuous with the periorbita but containing smooth muscle with sympathetic innervation.

Extraocular Muscles

There are seven extraocular muscles and one levator muscle controlling movements of the globe and upper lid. The extraocular muscles arise from the annulus of Zinn, which circles the optic foramen and orbital fissure, and insert onto the globe. The general pattern of the extraocular muscles is shown in Figure 18–15. Functions of the muscles are summarized in Table 18–1. Neurological abnormalities in their function are discussed in Chapter 17.

For a discussion of orbital nerves, veins, and arteries, the reader is referred to standard anatomy texts.

PATHOLOGICAL MECHANISMS

Because the orbit forms a semiclosed space, increases and decreases in the volume of its contents affect the position of the eye in relation to the orbital rim and face and to the other eye. Space-occupying lesions (e.g., tumor, zygomatic mucocele, hydatid cyst, arteriovenous fistula, *Dirifilaria immitis,* and abscess) push the eye forward, causing **EXOPHTHALMOS** (Fig. 18–16); in dogs and cats, such lesions usually cause protrusion of the oral mucous membrane behind the last upper molar tooth, because this is an unrestricted portion of the orbital floor. With decreased volume of the orbital contents, for example, because of dehydration or atrophy of fat or muscle, the eye sinks further into the orbit—**ENOPHTHALMOS**—and the third eyelid protrudes.

Exophthalmos must be distinguished from apparent exophthalmos due to shallow orbits (in brachycephaly, hydrocephalus), euryblepharon, glaucoma, and facial paralysis.

The position of space-occupying lesions alters the direction of displacement of the globe and is used to determine the site of the offending mass (Fig. 18–17) and the desired route of surgical exploration.

Text continued on page 490

FIGURE 18–9. *Visual field of primate, showing a large binocular field, small uniocular areas, and a large blind area. (Reproduced by permission from Duke-Elder, Sir Stewart, editor: System of Ophthalmology. Vol I. The Eye in Evolution. St Louis, 1958, The CV Mosby Co.)*

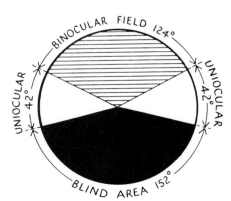

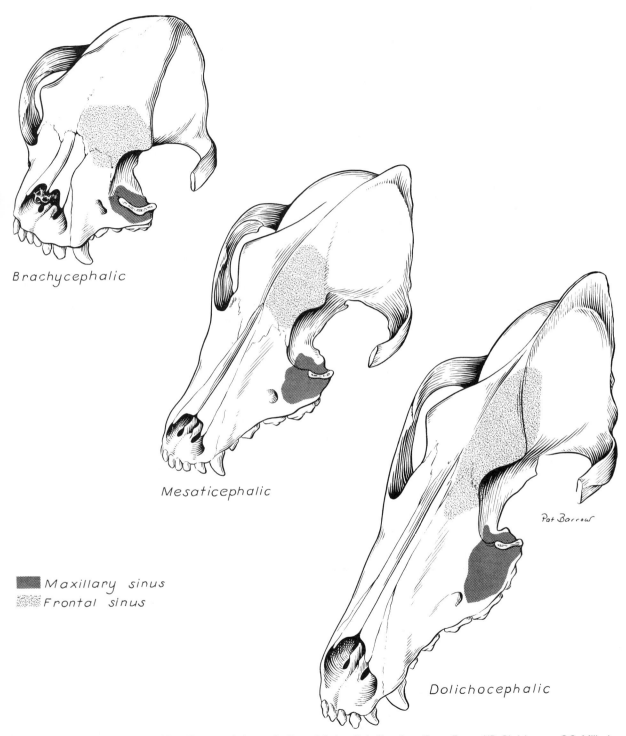

Brachycephalic

Mesaticephalic

Dolichocephalic

Pat Barrow

■ Maxillary sinus
▦ Frontal sinus

FIGURE 18–10. Relationship of the paranasal sinuses to the orbital walls in the dog. (From Evans HE, Christensen GC: Miller's Anatomy of the Dog, 2nd ed. WB Saunders Co, Philadelphia, 1979. © Cornell University 1964.)

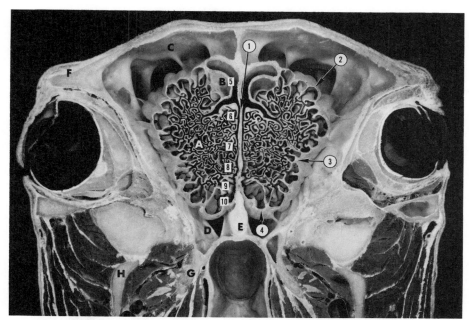

FIGURE 18–11. Transverse section through head of the horse at level of the orbital cavities; rostral surface of section. A = ethmoidal labyrinth; B = dorsal nasal conchal sinus; C = frontal sinus; D = sphenopalatine sinus; E = vomer bone; F = zygomatic process of frontal bone; G = palatine bone; H = mandible; 1 = perpendicular plate (lamina); 2 = tectorial plate; 3 = orbital plate; 4 = basal plate; 2, 3, 4 = papyraceous plate; 5 = dorsal nasal concha (endoturbinate I); 6 = middle nasal concha (endoturbinate II); 7–10 = endoturbinates II–VI, respectively. (From Getty R: Sisson & Grossman's The Anatomy of the Domestic Animals, 5th ed. WB Saunders Co, Philadelphia, 1975.)

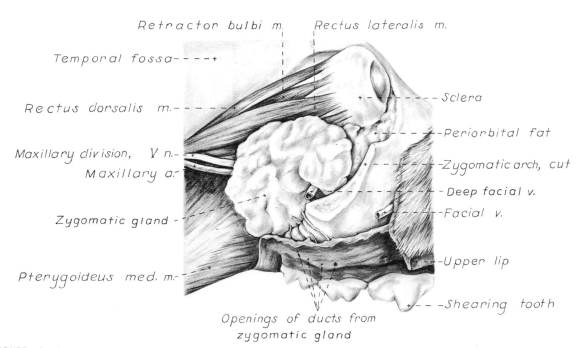

FIGURE 18–12. Lateral aspect of canine orbital contents and the zygomatic salivary gland. Note multiple ducts of the zygomatic gland entering the oral cavity. (From Miller ME, Christensen GC, Evans HE: Anatomy of the Dog, 1st ed. WB Saunders Co, Philadelphia, 1964. © Cornell University 1964.)

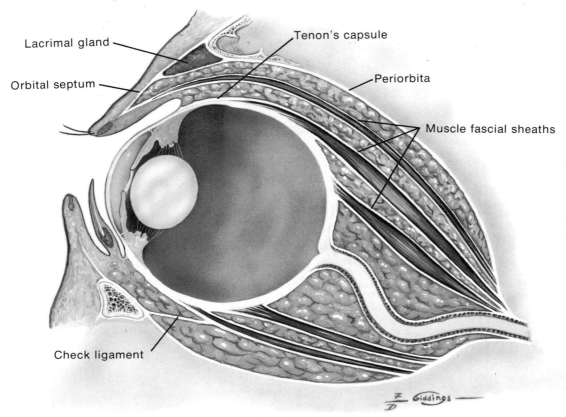

Lacrimal gland

Orbital septum

Tenon's capsule

Periorbita

Muscle fascial sheaths

Check ligament

FIGURE 18–13. Divisions of the periorbita.

FIGURE 18–14. Protrusion of intraorbital fat beneath the conjunctiva in a normal bovine eye.

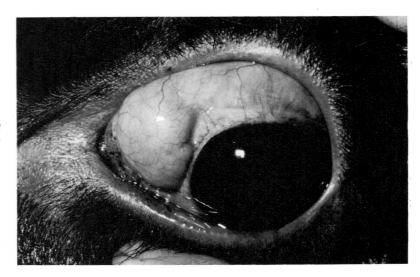

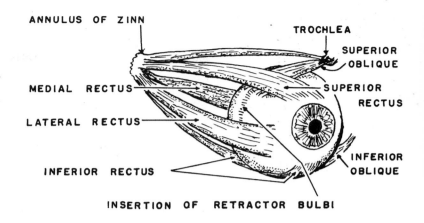

FIGURE 18-15. General arrangement of the orbital muscles. (Modified from Prince JH, et al: Anatomy and Histology of the Eye and Orbit in Domestic Animals. Courtesy of Charles C Thomas, Springfield, IL, 1960.)

TABLE 18-1. Extraocular Muscles

Muscle	Innervation	Action
Superior (dorsal) rectus m	Oculomotor III	Elevates globe
Inferior (ventral) rectus m	Oculomotor III	Depresses globe
Medial rectus m	Oculomotor III	Turns globe nasally
Lateral rectus m	Abducens VI	Turns globe temporally
Superior (dorsal) oblique m	Trochlear IV	Intorts globe (rotates 12 o'clock position nasally)
Inferior (ventral) oblique m	Oculomotor III	Extorts globe (rotates 12 o'clock position temporally)
M retractor bulbi	Abducens VI	Retracts globe
M levator superioris	Oculomotor III	Elevates upper lid

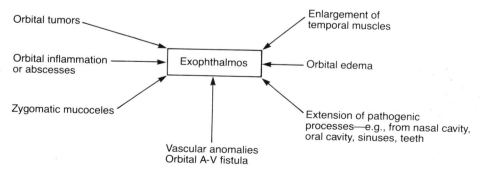

FIGURE 18-16. Mechanisms of exophthalmos.

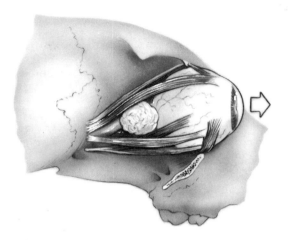

A WITHIN MUSCLE CONE

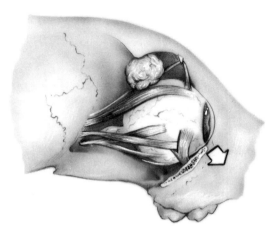

B DORSAL MASS

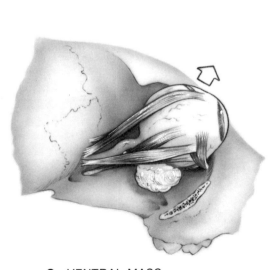

C VENTRAL MASS

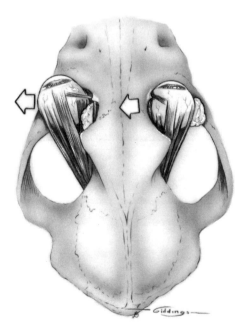

D NASAL AND TEMPORAL MASSES

FIGURE 18–17. Effects of position of space-occupying lesions on the direction of globe displacement.

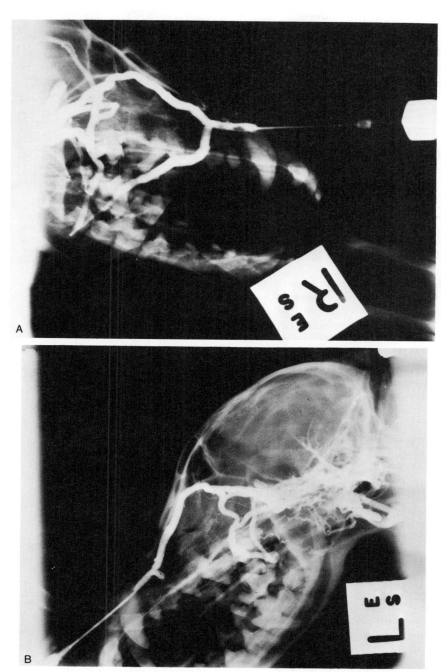

FIGURE 18–18. A, Normal lateral orbital venogram (right eye). B, Venogram of left orbit in a 5-year-old poodle with a lymphoid pseudotumor in the inferonasal orbit. The inferior ophthalmic vein is obliterated. (Courtesy of Dr. R. Dixon.)

Because the subconjunctival tissues and the orbit are connected, orbital diseases frequently cause *chemosis*. If the orbital lesion compresses the orbital veins, decreased posterior venous drainage occurs and chemosis is further increased. In horses, orbital swelling or inflammation frequently causes filling of the depression superior to the upper eyelid.

Exophthalmos frequently causes increased evaporation of the precorneal tear film and exposure keratitis.

Because of the many tissue types present, numerous kinds of neoplasms may affect the orbit.

DIAGNOSTIC METHODS

The diagnosis of orbital disorders requires special techniques in addition to a complete ophthalmic and fundus examination:

1. Orbital palpation. Careful orbital palpation along the rim and inside the orbit with the finger tip is useful in localizing lesions. The consistency and position of orbital contents can often be determined by placing pressure on the globe itself through the eyelids.

2. Determination of globe and optic axis displacement.

3. Aspiration of orbital contents for laboratory examination, that is, culture and cytological examination.

4. Contrast orbital venography (Fig. 18–18; see also Chap 5 and Figs. 5–37 and 5–38).

5. Contrast orbitography (Figs. 18–19 and 18–20; see also Chap 5).

6. Ultrasonography (see Chap 5, and Fig. 5–40A–C).

7. Orbital arteriography (Figs. 18–21 and 18–22).

8. Computerized axial tomography (CAT) (Fig. 18–23)—restricted to larger institutions. Nuclear magnetic resonance (NMR) studies, although potentially useful, are not readily available because of the high cost of equipment.

Localization of Foreign Bodies

Numerous sophisticated radiographic techniques have been devised for localization of orbital and ocular foreign bodies in humans. Because of the differences in orbital size and shape, such techniques are not transferable to animals. The most commonly used method in animals is to place a reference ring of wire at the limbus. Radiographs are taken at four different angles (lateral, ventrodorsal, oblique, frontal) to attempt to differentiate ocular and orbital foreign bodies and their location. Ultrasonography is also useful for localization (see Fig. 5–40A–C).

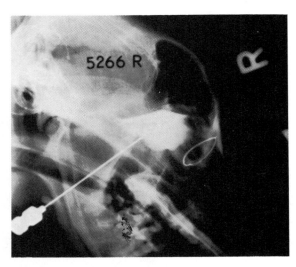

FIGURE 18–19. *Contrast orbitography. Lateral radiograph with the needle in position in the orbital cone after injection of 4 ml of contrast medium. The cone is well filled with leakage ventrally. A wire marker ring is present at the limbus. (From Munger RJ, Ackerman N: Retrobulbar injections in the dog: A comparison of three techniques. J Am Anim Hosp Assoc 14:490, 1978.)*

Orbital Arteriography

In orbital arteriography, a 21-gauge needle is passed into the infraorbital artery and 5 to 10 ml of contrast medium is forced in a retrograde direction up the artery to outline the arteries of the eye and orbit (see Figs. 18–22 and 18–23). Displacement, filling defects, and increased vascularity indicate the position of orbital lesions.

ORBITAL DISEASES

Orbital Cellulitis and Retrobulbar Abscess

Orbital cellulitis and retrobulbar abscess occur most commonly in dogs and cats.

ETIOLOGY

Although retrobulbar abscess is common, its cause is poorly understood and rarely confirmed. It is assumed to be bacterial in origin, the source being either hematogenous or by penetration from the oral cavity in association with a foreign body. Mixed flora and lack of growth are common findings on aerobic bacterial culture. *Aspergillus* spp and *Penicillium* spp have been isolated from orbital cellulitis in cats. The process begins as ORBITAL CELLULITIS, then localizes and an abscess usually forms. At the stage of cellulitis, the clinical signs are less extreme; for example, pain may

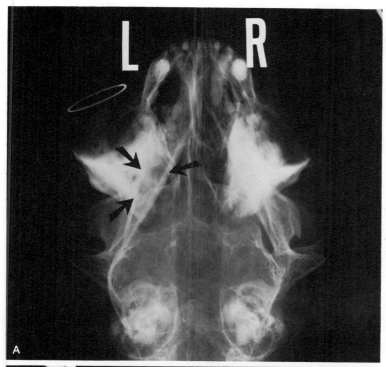

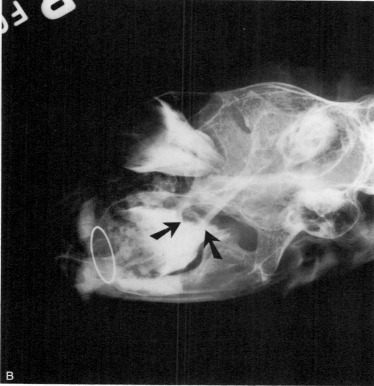

FIGURE 18–20. Contrast orbitography. A, Ventrodorsal radiograph of a cat after injection of contrast medium. The cat was blind and exhibited ophthalmoplegia and exophthalmos (orbital fissure syndrome). A filling defect (arrows) is present at the left orbital apex, owing to orbital extension of an intracranial lymphosarcoma involving the optic chiasm. B, A lateral oblique view of the skull, showing a filling defect (arrows) at the apex of the orbit. (Courtesy of Dr. R. Munger.)

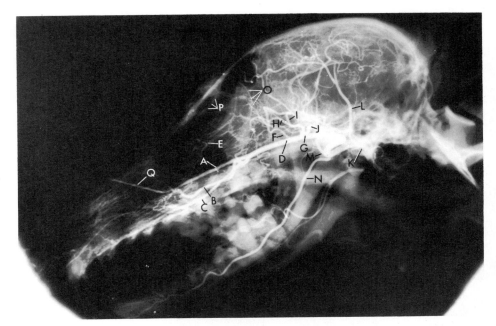

FIGURE 18–21. Lateral canine orbital arteriogram produced after a retrograde injection of contrast medium into the infraorbital artery. A = infraorbital artery; B = sphenopalatine artery; C = major palatine artery; D = maxillary artery; E = malar artery; F = anterior deep temporal artery; G = orbital artery; H = ventral muscular branch; I = external ethmoid artery; J = external ophthalmic artery; K = external carotid artery; L = superficial temporal artery; M = posterior deep temporal artery; N = mandibular alveolar artery; O = choroid; P = ciliary body; Q = cannula. (From Ticer JW: Radiographic Technique in Veterinary Practice, 2nd ed. WB Saunders Co, Philadelphia, 1984.)

FIGURE 18–22. Canine orbital arteriogram, open-mouth view, produced after a retrograde injection of contrast medium into the infraorbital artery. A = infraorbital artery; B = maxillary artery; C = major palatine artery; D = sphenopalatine artery; E = orbital artery; F = external ethmoid artery; G = external ophthalmic artery. (From Ticer JW: Radiographic Technique in Veterinary Practice, 2nd ed. WB Saunders Co, Philadelphia, 1984.)

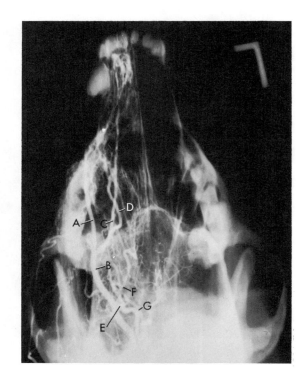

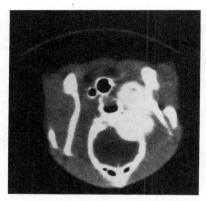

FIGURE 18–23. CAT scan of a multilobular ossifying fibroma (sarcoma) (chondroma rodens) originating from the right petrous temporal bone and extending rostrally to invade the orbit and nasal cavity and medially into the middle cerebral fossa via the frontal, temporal, and parietal bones. The eye was displaced anteriorly. The patient was a 12-year-old Brittany spaniel. (Courtesy of Dr. R. Bellhorn and the University of California.)

be less, oral signs may be nonexistent, and diagnosis may be more difficult.

CLINICAL SIGNS

1. Chemosis (unilateral) (Fig. 18–24).[1]
2. Pain on opening the mouth (often extreme).[1]
3. Fluctuating red swelling in oral mucous membrane behind last upper molar (Fig. 18–25).[1]
4. Protrusion of the third eyelid.
5. Exophthalmos (variable degree).
6. Periorbital swelling.
7. Pyrexia.
8. Anorexia.
9. Leukocytosis.
10. Onset is usually acute.

DIFFERENTIAL DIAGNOSIS

Retrobulbar abscess must be distinguished from orbital cellulitis (a generalized diffuse inflammation of orbital tissues), which has identical clinical signs. In orbital cellulitis, however, pain is less evident, pyrexia and anorexia are not as pronounced, and less exudate or no exudate is present on drainage. Orbital cellulitis may progress to retrobulbar abscess. Retrobulbar abscess may be distinguished from other causes of exophthalmos by its acute onset, pain, and pyrexia. Leukocytosis with neutrophilia is usually present. Retrobulbar abscess may be present with other ocular diseases (Fig. 18–26).

Clinical signs of retrobulbar abscess are often pathognomonic.

---

1. Most important signs.

TREATMENT

Orbital cellulitis and retrobulbar abscess are treated similarly, as follows:

1. Drainage via an incision behind the last upper molar (Fig. 18–27). A small incision is made in the mucous membrane, and a pair of curved Crile hemostats or a blunt probe (Fig. 18–28) is inserted and opened in small steps until the orbit is reached. This technique allows pockets of exudate to be drained while limiting damage to the orbit. Considerable amounts of exudate under pressure are often released, and dependent drainage to the oral cavity is established. Although exudate frequently is *not* obtained, drainage is an important *prerequisite* step in treatment. Failure to locate exudate indicates that the process is still at the cellulitis stage.

2. The orbit is flushed with sterile saline solution via the oral incision, and 2–3 ml of crystalline penicillin solution is instilled with a blunt needle or abscess cannula.

3. Systemic antibiotics (e.g., amoxicillin) are administered for 5–7 days.

4. Soft foods are fed during the recovery period.

Clinical improvement is usually rapid, occurring within 24 hours of treatment. In resistant cases, exploratory orbitotomy may be necessary.

Cystic Orbital and Periocular Lesions

Numerous lesions and tissues may cause cystic swellings, including dacryops (cyst of the lacrimal duct), zygomatic and lacrimal mucoceles, retained glandular tissue from the lacrimal or third eyelid gland after enucleation or trauma, transplanted parotid ducts, and mucosa of the nasal and frontal sinuses.

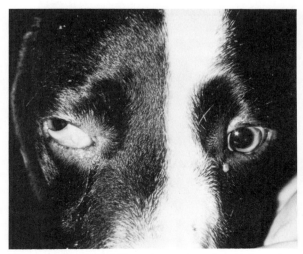

FIGURE 18–24. Retrobulbar abscess in a dog. Note periorbital swelling, protrusion of the third eyelid indicating orbital swelling, and epiphora.

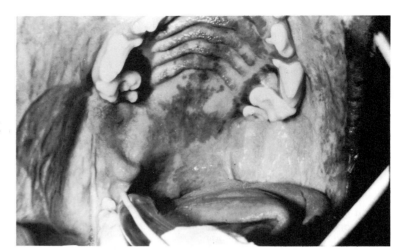

FIGURE 18–25. Fluctuating, reddened mucous membrane behind the last upper molar in the dog shown in Figure 18–24.

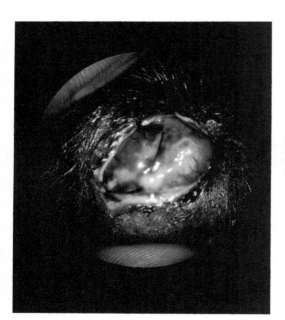

FIGURE 18–26. A poodle with unilateral retrobulbar abscess and keratoconjunctivitis sicca (KCS). KCS did not resolve spontaneously after treatment of the abscess, indicating permanent damage to the lacrimal gland.

FIGURE 18–27. Site of incision for drainage of retrobulbar abscess and orbital cellulitis.

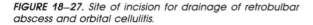

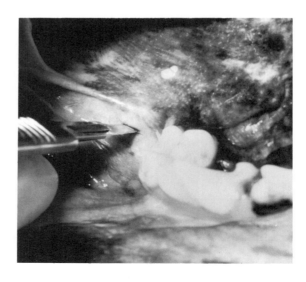

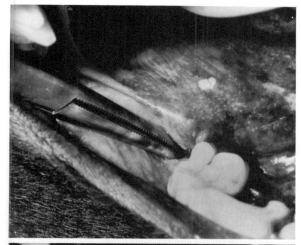

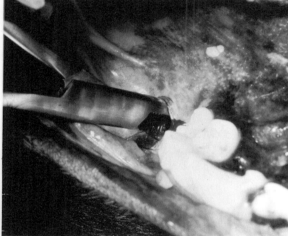

FIGURE 18–28. Progressive insertion of hemostats to establish drainage from the orbit to the oral cavity.

Neoplasms and Space-Occupying Lesions

Numerous orbital neoplasms have been described in domestic species, including meningioma, lymphosarcoma, adenocarcinoma, fibrosarcoma, osteosarcoma, glioma, myxoma, squamous cell carcinoma, rhabdomyosarcoma, and canine lymphoid pseudotumor. Retrobulbar neoplasms are not common. In the early stages, they present a diagnostic challenge. Correct diagnosis is essential to effective treatment.

CLINICAL SIGNS

1. Exophthalmos—usually unilateral, slowly progressive, and painless.
2. Deviation, displacement, or reduced motility of the globe (see Fig. 18–17).
3. Periocular swelling.
4. Prominent or protruding third eyelid.

5. Blindness in some cases, which is useful to differentiate from ocular enlargement caused by glaucoma, in which blindness is the rule.
6. Secondary exposure keratitis.
7. Retinal folds or detachment on ophthalmoscopic examination.
8. Dilated or eccentric pupil.
9. Papilledema.

TREATMENT

Thorough surgical removal is the treatment of choice. If specialized surgical assistance is available, an exploratory orbitotomy via zygomatic arch resection is recommended. This technique allows exploration and removal of the tumor mass, if possible, with retention of the globe. If the neoplasm is invasive, exenteration of the orbit and globe may be performed via the same approach. Orbitotomy allows removal of benign and non-neoplastic lesions without loss of the eye. If the lesion is small or well localized by diagnostic procedures, a transconjunctival approach or less radical orbitotomy is useful. Depending on tumor type, chemotherapy, immunotherapy, and radiation may be combined with surgery to control the neoplastic tissue, but these measures are ineffective alone. If radiation therapy is used, the ocular complications must be considered (see Chap 3).

Multilobular Osteoma

Synonyms: Chondroma rodens, calcifying aponeurotic fibroma

The multilobular osteoma occurs in dogs, cats, and horses and is discussed separately, as it arises from the flat bones of the skull and is not uncommon in the orbit. Exophthalmos is the most common sign in the orbit. Diagnosis is either by histopathological examination or from the radiographic signs—homogeneous stippling, evenly undulating well-demarcated borders, with a highly radiodense granular appearance. They are generally benign but are occasionally aggressive, and if localized they can be removed surgically. Growth is slow, metastasis is late, and local recurrence can be expected if removal is incomplete.

Zygomatic Mucocele

A mucocele is caused by leakage of saliva from a gland or duct, with consequent inflammation and fibrous tissue reaction to the saliva. The condition has been reported in dogs, both spontaneously and after head trauma. Zygomatic mucoceles are uncommon but must be considered in differential diagnosis of exophthalmos and space-occupying orbital lesions.

CLINICAL SIGNS

1. Orbital swelling
2. Exophthalmos
3. Protrusion of the third eyelid
4. Protrusion of the oral mucous membrane behind the last upper molar tooth
5. Protrusion of a mass beneath the conjunctiva in the inferior temporal or nasal conjunctival fornix

Position of the mucocele within the orbit is variable, with the clinical signs varying accordingly. Aspiration of fluid from within the sac may reveal tenacious, straw-colored, honeylike liquid. Zygomatic mucoceles are painless. A zygomatic sialogram may be used to outline the mucocele for planning surgical removal. Prior to removal, the gland may be outlined by injection of methylene blue up a zygomatic duct.

TREATMENT

Zygomatic mucoceles are best removed by localized orbitotomy, depending on the location of the mass:

1. For masses protruding beneath the conjunctiva behind the lower lid—transconjunctival approach via the inferior conjunctival cul de sac behind the lower eyelid.
2. For masses protruding beneath the conjunctiva laterally—an approach posterior to the orbital ligament and dorsal to the zygomatic arch. If necessary, the ligament may be transected and resutured.
3. If bulging of the oral mucous membrane is present, an oral approach behind the last upper molar tooth.

Periorbital Fractures

Periorbital contusions and fractures occur most commonly in horses and are caused by violent recovery from anesthesia, behavioral problems, and trauma. Diagnosis is more accurate by physical examination before and during surgical exploration rather than by radiography. Clinical signs include pain, crepitus, exophthalmos, periorbital swelling, abrasions, corneal ulceration, uveitis, blepharospasm, ocular entrapment, and facial asymmetry. Fracture of the supraorbital process with extension nasally to the supraorbital foramen and fractures of the lacrimal bone at the nasal canthus may damage the nasal mucosa, causing epistaxis. Bony fragments projecting into the orbit and causing pain, ocular entrapment, and exophthalmos have been observed in fractures in the area of the medial canthus. The nasolacrimal duct may also be damaged by manipulation of bone fragments in extensive fractures.

If fractures are demonstrated on oblique radiographs or by surgical exploration, small pieces of bone may be removed. The conjunctival fornices are palpated and any bony fragments palpable in the orbit are removed

or replaced surgically. Larger fragments may be wired in place, pinned, or treated conservatively by restricting the horse for 4–6 weeks. Early surgical treatment prevents fixation of fragments in abnormal positions by formation of fibrous tissue. Synthetic polymers may be used to restore facial contours for cosmesis. Associated ocular injuries, including corneal ulceration and traumatic uveitis, are frequent and should be looked for and treated. Contusions and associated edema are treated prophylactically with systemic penicillin and tetanus antiserum and are allowed to resolve spontaneously.

Early surgical intervention in equine periorbital fractures yields superior cosmetic results.

Eosinophilic Myositis

Eosinophilic myositis occurs most commonly in German shepherds and Weimaraners, but it is a rare disorder. *It is to be distinguished from orbital cellulitis and retrobulbar abscess.*

CLINICAL SIGNS[2]

1. Symmetrical swelling of masseter, temporal, and pterygoid muscles
2. Exophthalmos (variable in extent)
3. Eyelid edema
4. Protrusion of the third eyelid
5. Pain on opening the jaws fully

Some animals die during acute attacks; in others, the disease resolves, but recurrences are common. Attacks may last 10–21 days. Eosinophilia is not a constant sign. The disease may be diagnosed by clinical signs and temporal muscle biopsy. The cause of eosinophilic myositis is unknown. High doses of systemic steroids have been recommended for treatment. After recovery, temporal and masseter muscle atrophy may occur, together with atrophy of postorbital fat and enophthalmos. Affected animals often have difficulty opening the mouth because of scarring of the muscles of mastication.

Orbital Emphysema

Orbital emphysema occurs uncommonly in dogs and cats after trauma to the paranasal sinuses, with leakage of air into the orbit. The air is palpable as crepitus beneath the conjunctiva or periocular skin (Fig. 18–29).

---

2. From Magrane WG: Canine Ophthalmology, 3rd ed. Lea & Febiger, Philadelphia, 1977.

Orbital emphysema has been described in which the air may have entered the orbit via the nasolacrimal duct (Fig. 18–30) during labored respirations after a routine enucleation.

If emphysema is present, a radiographic study of the sinuses is indicated. The animal is placed on systemic antibiotics to prevent infection of the orbit via the paranasal sinuses. In reported cases, spontaneous resolution occurred. If the condition occurs after enucleation, the nasolacrimal duct may be ligated at its orbital exit.

Proptosis of the Globe

This condition constitutes an ocular emergency, and its treatment and prognosis are discussed in Chapter 20.

A summary of orbital diseases, classified by type, is given in Table 18–2.

SURGICAL PROCEDURES

The most common orbital procedures are those concerned with removal of all or part of the globe or orbital contents—ENUCLEATION, EXENTERATION, and EVISCERATION (Fig. 18–31):

Enucleation—removal of the globe, third eyelid, conjunctiva, and eyelids

Exenteration—removal of the globe, orbital contents, and eyelids

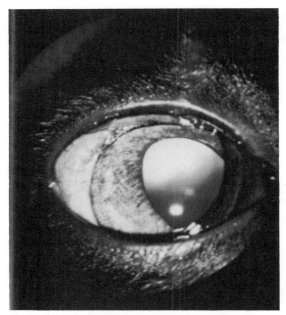

FIGURE 18–29. Subconjunctival emphysema following orbital trauma in a cat. Gas bubbles are visible beneath the conjunctiva laterally. (From Bryan GM: Subconjunctival emphysema in a cat. Vet Med Small Anim Clin 72:1087, 1977.)

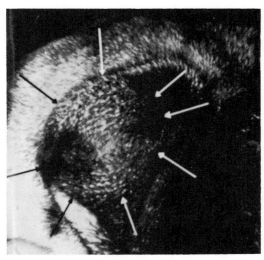

FIGURE 18–30. Orbital emphysema following enucleation in a pug. (From Martin CL: Orbital emphysema: A complication of ocular enucleation in the dog. Vet Med Small Anim Clin 66:986, 1971.)

Evisceration—removal of the intraocular contents, uvea, lens, retina, vitreous, and eyelids

Enucleation

INDICATIONS

1. Intraocular neoplasia.
2. Severe perforating ocular trauma with disruption and loss of ocular contents. An **intraocular** prosthesis can often be used instead to preserve cosmetic appearance.
3. Uncontrollable endophthalmitis or panophthalmitis.

Enucleation is an admission that therapeutic attempts to control a pathological process have failed. It is not used to replace a correct diagnosis.

After enucleation, an INTRAORBITAL prosthesis gives a far superior cosmetic result. Enucleation of a globe in a young animal results in a slower rate of growth of the orbit and a slower increase in orbital volume than in the contralateral normal orbit. This lower rate of growth is due to lack of orbital contents. Replacement of orbital volume with prosthetic materials after enucleation increases the growth rate toward normal.

There are numerous variations of enucleation techniques. The lateral subconjunctival and transpalpebral approaches are described here.

Text continued on page 502

TABLE 18–2. Summary of Orbital Diseases

Type of Disorder	Condition	Clinical Signs
Developmental abnormalities	1. Shallow orbit (brachycephalic breeds)	1. Exophthalmos, exposure keratitis, corneal ulceration, pigmentation
	2. Microphthalmia, anophthalmia	2. Small or no globe, nrrow palpebral fissure, prominent third eyelid, epiphora, blindness
	3. Hydrocephalus with orbital malformation	3. Exotropia, hypotropia, poor vision
	4. Euryblepharon	4. Long palpebral fissure resulting in apparent exophthalmos
	5. Orbital arteriovenous fistula	5. Exophthalmos, fremitus, pulse detectable ("exophthalmos pulsans")
Trauma	1. Hemorrhages	1. Subconjunctival and episcleral hemorrhages; retrobulbar hemorrhage with exophthalmos or proptosis
	2. Penetrating foreign bodies (grass awns, needles, and so on from mouth)	2. Discharging sinus fluid through the conjunctiva, periocular skin, buccal mucosa; pain on opening mouth (Figs. 18–24 and 18–26)
	3. Orbital fractures	3. Pain, crepitus, skin abrasions, displacement of globe
Infections	1. Bacteria, fungi	1. Ocular discharge usually secondary to penetrating foreign bodies from conjunctiva or oral cavity; sinusitis, rhinitis, or infections of roots of teeth
	2. Parasites (*Dirofilaria immitis; Pneumonyssus caninum*)	2. Granulomatous lesions due to wandering larvae, e.g., *Dirofilaria* (rare), or extension of infection from nasal cavity (*Pneumonyssus*)
Neoplasia	1. Primary orbital neoplasms—sarcoma, meningioma, adenocarcinoma from nasal cavity, lymphosarcoma in cattle	1. Exophthalmos, exposure keratitis, strabismus, displacement of globe (Fig. 18–17)
	2. Metastatic or invasive neoplasms	2. As for (1), plus nasal or neurological signs
Miscellaneous conditions	1. Zygomatic mucocele	1. Exophthalmos, strabismus, swelling in any part of orbit, or behind upper last molar tooth
	2. Infections of roots of teeth (especially carnassial)	2. Discharging fistula beneath eye in dogs
	3. Dehydration	3. Enophthalmos, passive protrusion of third eyelid
	4. Eosinophilic myositis	4. Exophthalmos, pain with dysphagia in acute stage; enophthalmos potentiated by opening mouth in chronic stage when temporal muscles have atrophied
	5. Horner's syndrome	5. Enophthalmos, miosis, ptosis, protrusion of third eyelid, ipsilateral sweating in horses, dermal vasodilation, and hyperthermia (see Figs. 17–9 and 17–10)
	6. Orbital emphysema	6. Crepitus beneath the conjunctiva (Fig. 18–29)

Modified from Smith JS: Diseases of the orbit. *In* Kirk RW (ed): Current Veterinary Therapy VI. WB Saunders Co, Philadelphia, 1977.

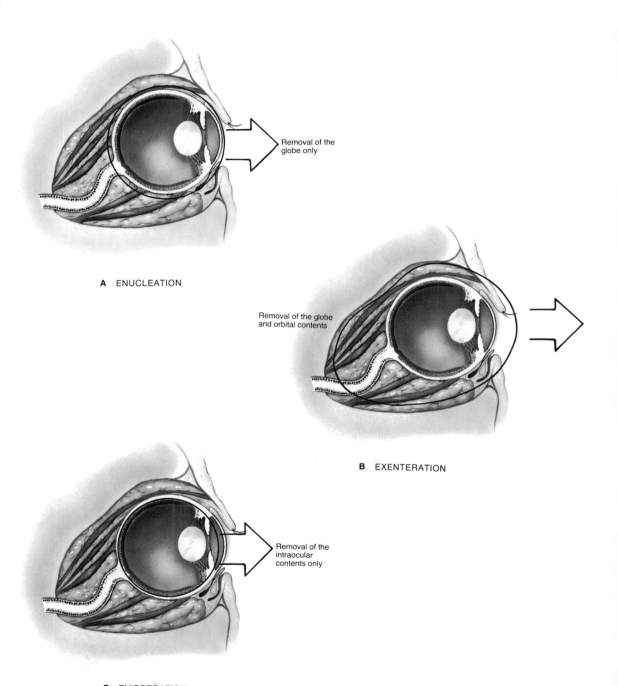

A   ENUCLEATION

Removal of the globe only

Removal of the globe and orbital contents

B   EXENTERATION

Removal of the intraocular contents only

C   EVISCERATION

FIGURE 18–31. *Diagrammatic representation of enucleation (A), exenteration (B), and evisceration (C).*

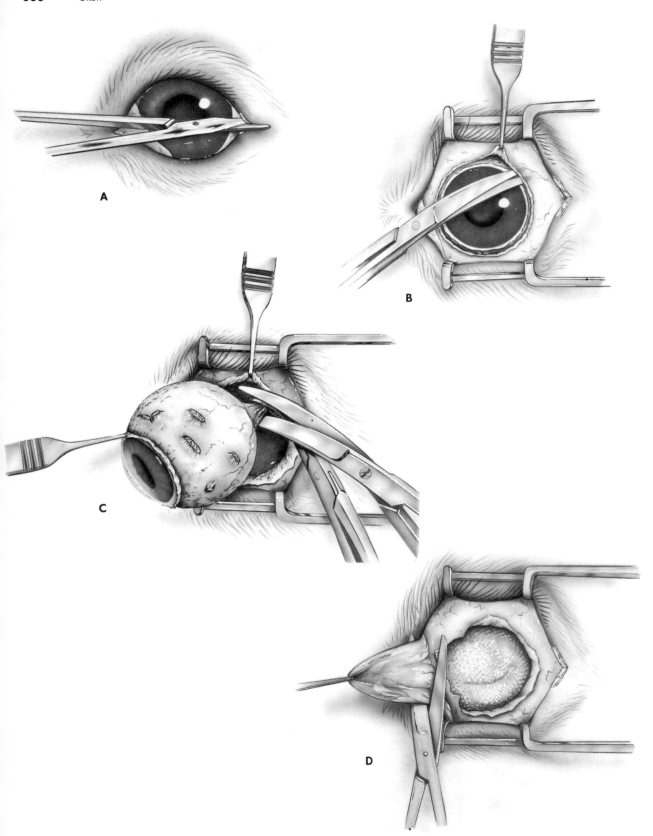

FIGURE 18–32 See legend on opposite page

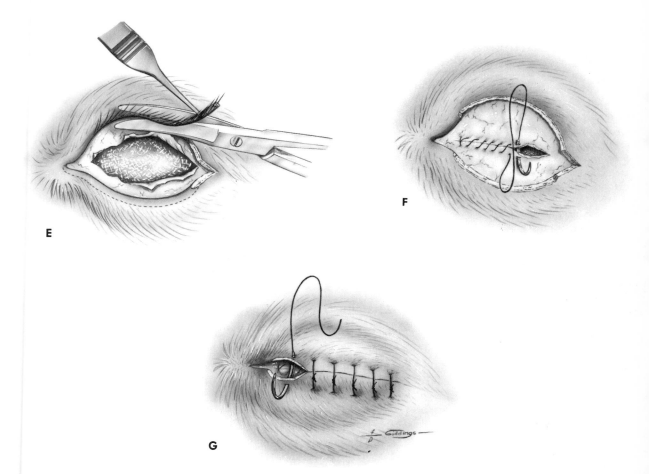

FIGURE 18–32. *Enucleation. A, A lateral canthotomy is performed. B, The globe is dissected free from the conjunctiva via a perilimbal incision. Extraocular muscle insertions and periorbita are dissected from the globe back to the optic nerve. C, The optic nerve is transected and the eye removed. D, The cavity is packed with sponges for temporary hemostasis, and the third eyelid is removed completely. E, The lid margins are removed. F, The sponges are removed, and the conjunctiva is sutured with 3/0 absorbable material. G, The lid incision is sutured right to the medial canthus with 4/0 nylon.*

LATERAL SUBCONJUNCTIVAL ENUCLEATION TECHNIQUE

This approach has the advantage of giving better exposure of the optic nerve and orbital vessels. It is used in dogs and cats.

1. A lateral canthotomy is performed for 1–2 cm in order to improve exposure (Fig. 18–32A).
2. The conjunctiva is grasped near the limbus with toothed forceps, and a 360° perilimbal incision is made beneath it (Fig. 18–32B).
3. The sclera is separated from the conjunctiva, Tenon's capsule, and extraocular muscles with curved Metzenbaum's or Mayo's scissors around to the optic nerve (Fig. 18–32B). The lacrimal gland beneath the orbital ligament is left attached to the globe, if possible.
4. The optic nerve may be severed with scissors or with an electrosurgical unit equipped with a tonsil snare (Fig. 18–32C). Excess traction *must not* be placed on the nerve, since damage to the optic chiasm may result, damaging vision in the remaining eye. A ligature may be placed around the nerve, encircling the associated short and long posterior ciliary vessels before entry to the sclera. The globe is removed and placed in fixative.
5. An attempt is made to control arterial and venous hemorrhage from the orbital cone with ligatures. If this is impossible, one or two surgical sponges are placed in the orbit (Fig. 18–32D).
6. The third eyelid and gland are carefully removed (Fig. 18–32D).
7. Two to 3 mm of the lid margins is removed from the lateral to the medial canthus (Fig. 18–32E).
8. Conjunctiva and Tenon's capsule are closed with a simple continuous suture of 3/0 absorbable material. After the conjunctiva has been almost closed, *the surgical sponges are removed* and closure is completed. This forms a seal to contain further hemorrhage (Fig. 18–32F).
9. The lid incisions are closed with simple interrupted sutures of 4/0 nylon (Fig. 18–32F).

Postoperative swelling is not unusual (especially if continuing hemorrhage occurs), but resolves within 3 or 4 days. As clots within the orbit break down, bloody fluid may appear at the nostril, via the nasolacrimal duct, on the 3rd–5th days, and owners should be advised accordingly.

The emotional resistance of owners to enucleation should not be underestimated.

All enucleated globes should be submitted for histopathological examination. Frequently, unsuspected disease processes are the cause of glaucoma or endophthalmitis (e.g., malignant melanoma, Fig. 18–33; lens capsule rupture). *Note:* Placement of foreign bodies in the orbit before closure, e.g., antibiotic powder, setons,

or irritating antiseptic solutions, is *unnecessary and undesirable.*

Insertion of an Intraorbital Prosthesis
(Fig. 18–34)

Shaped silicone orbital implants may be placed to prevent unsightly depressions in the orbit postoperatively. They should not be placed if the reason for enucleation was neoplasia outside the globe or infection inside the globe or if the patient has foci of possible hematogenous bacterial infection elsewhere—severe periodontal or gingival disease, pyoderma, prostatitis, chronic otitis externa.

The size of the implant is determined by the depth and diameter of the orbit—16–22 mm in dogs and cats, up to 35 mm in horses. The sphere is prepared by removing one third of the circumference with a clean horizontal slice and contouring the cut edges with a No. 10 scalpel blade. The prosthesis is inserted with the flat side uppermost. Crystalline penicillin (500,000 units) is placed around the prosthesis, which is secured *firmly* in place by suturing the periorbital fascia with a continuous absorbable 3/0 suture. A subcuticular suture layer and simple interrupted sutures close the incision. The success rate with orbital prostheses exceeds 95%. The cosmetic results with shaped silicone prostheses are superior to those obtained with methylmethacrylate spheres. A higher incidence of complications has been observed in cats with methylmethacrylate prostheses.

TRANSPALPEBRAL ENUCLEATION-EXENTERATION TECHNIQUE

This technique, which can be used in all species, differs from the lateral conjunctival approach in that dissection into the orbit is made *outside* the extraocular muscles, which are removed with the globe. It is preferable for removal of ocular neoplasms (e.g., bovine squamous cell carcinoma) that *have escaped from the globe*, as surrounding tissues are removed. It has the disadvantage, especially in small animals and horses, that a larger space is left in the orbit after the incision has healed. This is less acceptable cosmetically, and it leaves insufficient tissue to form a bed for an intraorbital prosthesis.

The transpalpebral approach is useful in the field for enucleation of bovine eyes with advanced squamous cell carcinoma. The cow is restrained in a head hail or crush, or against a strong railing fence, and tranquilized with xylazine (Fig. 5–8). Although a Pederson block can be used, the most consistent method is to infiltrate the upper and lower lids with 10 ml of lidocaine, 1 to 1.5 cm from the margin, and to place 5 to 10 ml into the orbit by retrobulbar injection with a 5- or 6-cm needle at each of four sites adjacent to the globe at the

Text continued on page 507

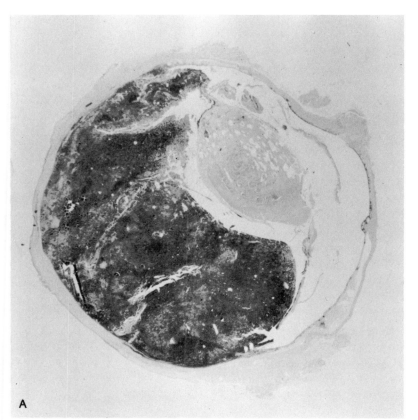

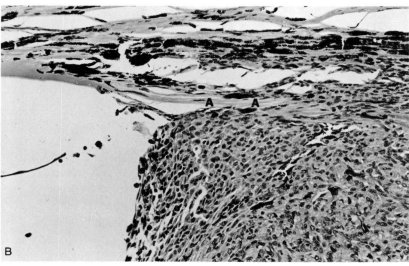

FIGURE 18–33. A, Intraocular melanoma in a dog, which presented as chronic glaucoma with buphthalmos. B, Neoplastic cells have infiltrated the drainage angle (A), which is collapsed. This is a primary indication for enucleation.

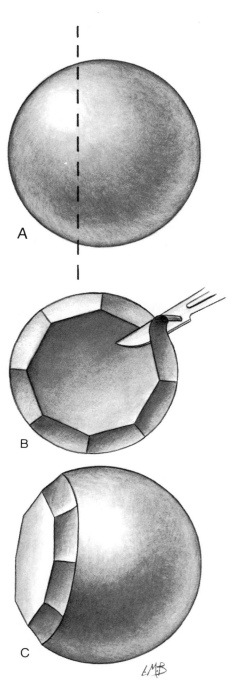

FIGURE 18–34. Preparation of the orbital prosthesis. A, One third of the silicone sphere is removed. B and C, The cut edge is contoured.

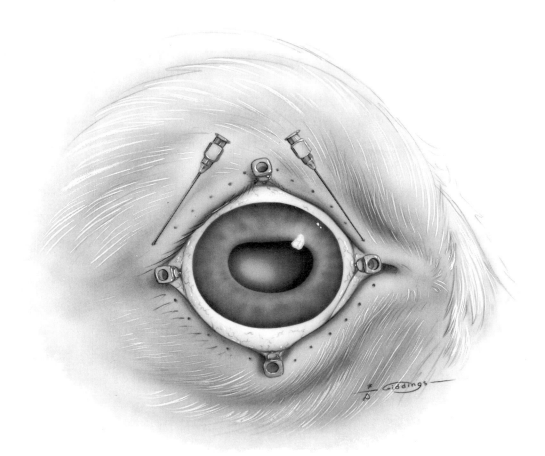

FIGURE 18–35. Injection sites for local anesthesia prior to transpalpebral enucleation in cattle. Five to 10 ml of lidocaine is injected at each site to produce anesthesia and proptosis.

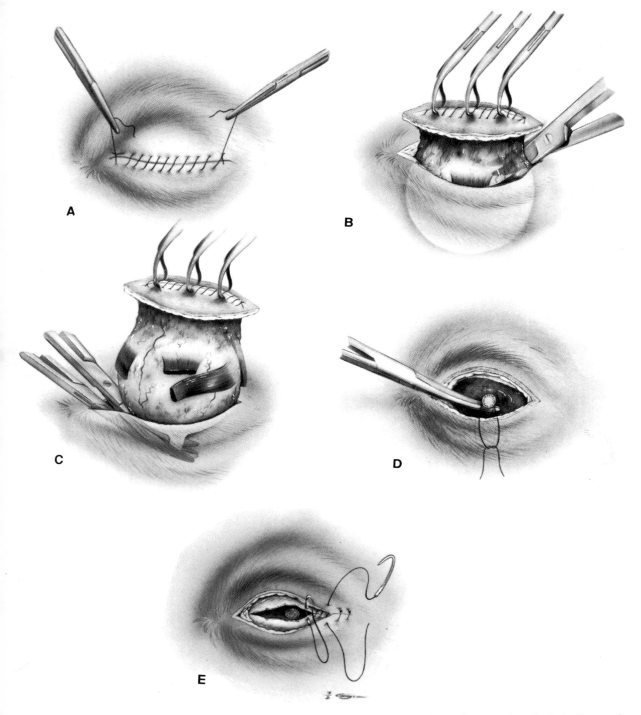

FIGURE 18–36. Transpalpebral enucleation. A, The eyelids are sutured with a simple continuous suture tied at either end and are held with hemostats. B, A periocular incision is made and dissection performed outside the extraocular muscles to the orbital apex. C and D, The optic nerve and associated vessels are clamped, ligated, and transected. E, Conjunctiva and Tenon's capsule are sutured with 3/0 absorbable suture, and the skin is closed with simple interrupted/nonabsorbable sutures appropriate for the size and environment of the patient (e.g., Supramid or Vetafil for horses and cattle; 4/0 silk or nylon for cats and dogs).

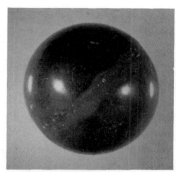

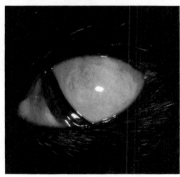

FIGURE 18–37. A, Silicone prosthesis. B, Postoperative appearance of an intraocular prosthesis. The cornea did not pigment postoperatively in this patient.

12, 3, 6, and 9 o'clock positions (Fig. 18–35). This produces anesthesia, akinesia, and exophthalmos, which aids in surgical exposure (Fig. 18–36). General anesthesia is used in dogs, cats, and horses. The plane of dissection in this technique may be extended to perform an exenteration.

Transpalpebral enucleation is suitable for ocular neoplasia. The lateral subconjunctival approach is preferable in most other instances.

Exenteration

Exenteration refers to removal of the globe and as much of the ocular contents as possible. It is performed in cases of orbital neoplasia or ocular neoplasia that has extended beyond the globe. For orbital neoplasms, far better exposure is gained for exenteration by lateral orbitotomy. For ocular neoplasms, an extension of the transpalpebral approach is used, with wider removal of orbital tissues.

Evisceration

Evisceration (Fig. 18–31) consists of removal of the contents of the sclera and is appropriate for insertion of

an intraocular prosthesis in dogs and cats and occasionally horses (see further on).

OCULAR PROSTHESES

Ocular prostheses are of three types:

1. Intraocular—used in the treatment of chronic glaucoma and to prevent phthisis bulbi in the early stages following severe trauma.

2. Extrascleral—a porcelain shell placed on the surface of the globe for cosmetic purposes.

3. Intraorbital—used to replace an enucleated globe.

Intraocular Prosthesis

In the past, intrascleral prostheses in dogs and cats were associated with persistent infection and extrusion. Use of a silicone ball and careful technique has removed these difficulties. This prosthesis is particularly useful in chronic glaucoma and is indicated when buphthalmos has begun and the condition cannot be controlled with cyclocryotherapy. It is also used after severe ocular trauma, when no infection or severe contamination is present, to prevent phthisis bulbi. The diameter of the prosthesis is equal to the horizontal corneal diameter of the contralateral normal eye, *plus* 1 mm.

The prosthesis (Fig. 18–37) is placed in the sclera and cornea after thorough removal of the remaining intraocular contents by evisceration. After insertion into buphthalmic eyes, the sclera and cornea contract to the size of the prosthesis, the time for contraction depending on the original size of the eye. In very large eyes, contraction may take up to 6 weeks.

The cornea sometimes remains clear but may also

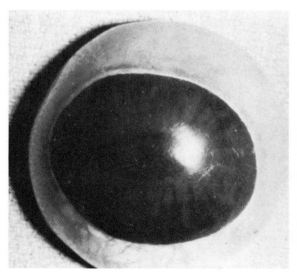

FIGURE 18–38. A porcelain shell prosthesis with an eye painted on the anterior surface. (Courtesy of Dr. G. A. Severin.)

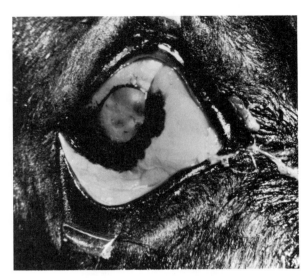

FIGURE 18–39. A horse with phthisis bulbi prior to prosthesis insertion. (Courtesy of Dr. G. A. Severin.)

vascularize in the 2–3 weeks after insertion of the prosthesis. This vascularization resolves over the first postoperative 6 weeks but may alarm owners and is explained to them in advance. After insertion, the cornea frequently becomes pigmented, but the degree of pigmentation is unpredictable. The complication rate with this procedure is also very low when performed in correctly chosen cases.

Extrascleral (Shell) Prosthesis

The extrascleral prosthesis is a porcelain shell, inserted into the conjunctival sac over a disfigured cornea or phthitic globe. An eye (i.e., conjunctiva, cornea, and iris) is painted onto the external surface of the shell (Fig. 18–38). Shell prostheses are used mainly in horses but are also available for dogs. The manufacture and insertion of a shell prosthesis is a time-consuming and expensive procedure but one that gives gratifying results for those clients prepared to bear the cost (Figs. 18–39 and 18–40). Each shell is individually cast to fit the affected eye, fitted over a period of several weeks, then painted to match the remaining eye. After insertion it must be removed daily and washed by the owner (a relatively simple procedure in a tractable horse). Shell prostheses are made and painted to special order by manufacturers of human prostheses).

Intraorbital Prosthesis

See page 502.

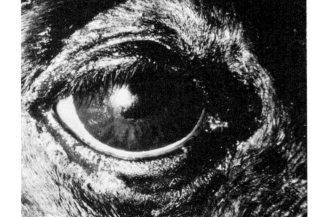

FIGURE 18–40. Same patient as in Figure 18–39 after insertion of the prosthesis. (Courtesy of Dr. G. A. Severin.)

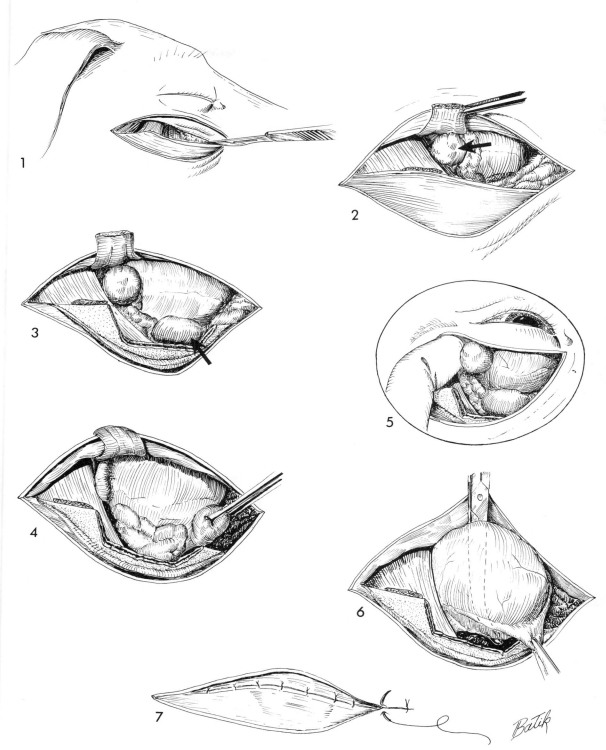

FIGURE 18–41. Exposure of the inferior lateral orbit by limited orbitotomy. The globe, zygomatic salivary gland, and transected orbital ligament are visible. (From Bistner SI, et al: Atlas of Veterinary Ophthalmic Surgery. WB Saunders Co, Philadelphia, 1977.)

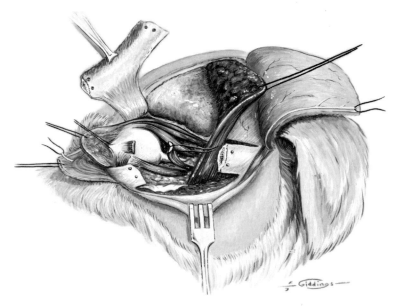

FIGURE 18–42. Exposure of deep orbital tissues by orbitotomy with zygomatic arch resection.

ORBITOTOMY[3]

A detailed discussion of orbitotomy techniques is beyond the scope of this text, as the procedure is almost always performed by veterinary ophthalmologists or specialist veterinary surgeons on an elective basis. The choice of approach to the orbit depends on the size and position of the lesion being excised:

1. Superior, medial, and lateral transconjunctival approaches are used for small lesions anterior to the equator.

2. Limited orbitotomy involving transection of the orbital ligament is used when limited exposure to the orbit is required (Fig. 18–41), for example, for removal of a well-delineated zygomatic mucocele.

3. Orbitotomy with zygomatic arch resection is used to completely expose the orbit, for example, for cases of neoplasia (Fig. 18–42).

REFERENCES

Adams WA, et al (1987): Radiotherapy of malignant nasal tumors in 67 dogs. J Am Vet Med Assoc 191:311.

Barnett KC, Grimes TD (1972): Retrobulbar tumor and retinal detachment in a dog. J Sm Anim Pract 13:315.

Barnett KC, et al (1988): Retrobulbar hydatid cyst in the horse. Equine Vet J 20:136.

Bedford PGC (1979): Orbital pneumatosis as an unusual complication to enucleation. J Sm Anim Pract 20:551.

Bellhorn RW (1972): Enucleation technique. A lateral approach. J Am Anim Hosp Assoc 8:59.

Brightman AH, et al (1977): Intraocular prosthesis in the dog. J Am Anim Hosp Assoc 13:481.

Bryan GM (1977): Subconjunctival emphysema in a cat. Vet Med Small Anim Clin 72:1087.

Buyukmihci N (1977): Orbital meningioma with intraocular invasion in a dog. Vet Pathol 14:521.

Buyukmihci N, et al (1975): Exophthalmos secondary to zygomatic adenocarcinoma in a dog. J Am Vet Med Assoc 167:162.

Caron JP, et al (1986): Periorbital skull fractures in five horses. J Am Vet Med Assoc 188:280.

Diesem C (1975): Organ of vision. In Getty R (ed): Sisson and Grossman's Anatomy of the Domestic Animals, 5th ed. WB Saunders Co, Philadelphia.

Duke-Elder S (1958): System of Ophthalmology, vol 1, The Eye in Evolution. H Kimpton, London.

Evans HE, Christensen GC (1979): Miller's Anatomy of the Dog, 2nd ed. WB Saunders Co, Philadelphia.

Harvey CE, et al (1968): Orbital cyst with conjunctival fistula in a dog. J Am Vet Med Assoc 153:1432.

Hayden DW (1976): Squamous cell carcinoma in a cat with intraocular and orbital metastases. Vet Pathol 13:332.

Knecht CD, et al (1969): Zygomatic salivary cyst in a dog. J Am Vet Med Assoc 155:625.

Koch SA (1969): The differential diagnosis of exophthalmos in the dog. J Am Anim Hosp Assoc 14:490.

Koch SA, Buel BE (1970): Medial orbital abscess in a collie. J Am Vet Med Assoc 156:1905.

Koch SA, et al (1980): Orbital surgery on two horses. Vet Surg 9:61.

Langhan RF, et al (1971): Primary retrobulbar meningioma of the optic nerve of a dog. J Am Vet Med Assoc 159:175.

Lavach JD, Severin GA (1977): Neoplasia of the equine eye, adnexa and orbit: A review of 68 cases. J Am Vet Med Assoc 170:202.

LeCouteur RA, et al (1982): Computed tomography of orbital tumors in the dog. J Am Vet Med Assoc 180:910.

Magrane WG (1965): Tumors of the eye and orbit in the dog. J Sm Anim Pract 6:165.

Martin CL (1971): Orbital emphysema: A complication of ocular enucleation in the dog. Vet Med Small Anim Clin 66:986.

Martin CL (1971): Orbital mucocele in a dog. Vet Med Small Anim Clin 66:36.

Martin CL, et al (1987): Cystic lesions of the periorbital region. Comp Cont Ed 9:1022.

Meek LA (1988): Intraocular prosthesis in a horse. J Am Vet Med Assoc 13:343.

---

3. For further details see Slatter DH, Chambers ED: Orbit. In Slatter DH (ed): Textbook of Small Animal Surgery, vol 2. WB Saunders Co, Philadelphia, 1985.

Munger RJ, Ackerman N (1978): Retrobulbar injections in the dog: A comparison of three techniques. J Am Anim Hosp Assoc 14: 490.

Nasisse MP, et al (1988): Use of methylmethacrylate orbital prostheses in dogs and cats: 78 cases (1980–1986). J Am Vet Med Assoc 192:539.

Pletcher JM, et al (1979): Orbital chondroma rodens in a dog. J Am Vet Med Assoc 175:187.

Prechter TK, Sarnat BG (1973): Comparison of direct and indirect determinations. Acta Morphol Neerl Scand 11:151.

Prince JH, et al (1960): Anatomy and Histology of the Eye and Orbit in Domestic Animals. Charles C Thomas, Springfield, IL.

Rebhun WC, Edwards NJ (1977): Two cases of orbital adenocarcinoma of probable lacrimal gland origin. J Am Anim Hosp Assoc 13:691.

Richardson DW, Acland H (1983): Multilobular osteoma (chondroma rodens) in a horse. J Am Vet Med Assoc 182:289.

Roberts SM, et al (1987): Ophthalmic complications following megavoltage irradiation of the nasal and paranasal cavities in dogs. J Am Vet Med Assoc 190:43.

Sarnat BG, Shanedling PD (1965): Postnatal growth of the orbit and upper face in rabbits. Arch Ophthalmol 73:829.

Sarnat BG, Shanedling PD (1970): Orbital volume following evisceration, enucleation, and exenteration in rabbits. Am J Ophthalmol 70:1970.

Schmidt GM, Betts CW (1978): Zygomatic salivary mucoceles in the dog. J Am Vet Med Assoc 172:940.

Siebold HR (1974): Juvenile alveolar rhabdomyosarcoma in a dog. Vet Pathol 11:558.

Slatter DH (1979): Lateral orbitotomy by zygomatic arch resection. J Am Vet Med Assoc 175:1179.

Slatter DH, Chambers ED (1985): Orbit. In Slatter DH (ed): Textbook of Small Animal Surgery. WB Saunders Co, Philadelphia.

Ticer JW (1984): Radiographic Technique in Veterinary Practice, 2nd ed. WB Saunders Co, Philadelphia.

Turner AS (1979): Surgical management of depressed fractures of the equine skull. Vet Surg 8:29.

Wilkinson GT, et al (1982): Aspergillus spp infection associated with orbital cellulitis and sinusitis in a cat. J Sm Anim Pract 23:127.

Williams JO, et al (1961): Glioma of the optic nerve of a dog. J Am Vet Med Assoc 138:377.

Valde H, Rook JS (1981): Use of fluorocarbon polymer and carbon fiber for restoration of facial contour in a horse. J Am Vet Med Assoc 188:249.

Wolf D (1988): Personal communication.

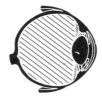

19

Systemic Diseases

In collaboration with Dr. Elizabeth Chambers

DOGS	SHEEP AND CATTLE	PIGS
CATS	HORSES	

Systemic diseases commonly have associated ocular lesions and signs in all domestic species, including chickens, turkeys, and laboratory animals. A knowledge of ocular signs assists both ocular and systemic diagnosis, as the eye can be examined readily. This allows earlier and more accurate diagnosis of systemic disorders and more effective evaluation of treatment. Many ocular signs of less common systemic diseases are poorly documented. Although it is impossible to cover all diseases with ocular manifestations here, common disorders are discussed.

Ocular examination is an essential part of a complete physical examination.

DOGS

Infectious diseases common to dogs and cats are discussed in the section on dogs (Table 19–1). Specific feline conditions can be found in the section on feline disorders.

Bacterial Disorders

BRUCELLOSIS

Brucella canis infection has been associated with uveitis, glaucoma, and endophthalmitis locally, and uveitis when it occurs remote from the eye.

TETANUS

Ocular and facial signs of tetanus include protrusion of the third eyelid, slight enophthalmos, spasm of the facial and auricular muscles, causing a grinning expression, and erect ears. Hypertrophy of lymphoid follicles has been observed on the bulbar and palpebral surfaces of the third eyelid.

NONSPECIFIC BACTEREMIAS

Severe gingivitis, abscessed teeth, prostatitis, and pyometra may cause uveitis and panophthalmitis.

Viral Disorders

CANINE DISTEMPER

Bilateral mucoid conjunctivitis is an early sign of canine distemper. It appears within the first week of exposure to the virus. As the exudate becomes mucopurulent, the cytological response proceeds from mononuclear to polymorphonuclear (Fig. 19–1).

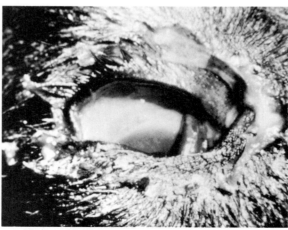

FIGURE 19–1. Mucopurulent conjunctivitis in canine distemper. (Courtesy of Dr. G. A. Severin.)

TABLE 19–1. Systemic Canine Diseases with Ocular Signs

Infectious	Endocrine	Neoplastic	Hematological and Circulatory	Miscellaneous
Bacterial	Diabetes mellitus	Lymphosarcoma	Hypertension	Hyperlipoproteinemia
Brucellosis	Hyperadrenocorticism	Metastases	Polycythemia	Allergic inhalant
Tetanus	Hyperparathyroidism		Arteriovenous fistula	dermatitis syndrome
Viral	Hypoparathyroidism		Anemia	Sjögren's syndrome
Distemper	Hypothyroidism		Monoclonal gammopathy	Autoimmune-mediated
Infectious canine hepatitis				skin diseases
Infectious tracheobronchitis				Myasthenia gravis
Yeasts and Fungi				Hydrocephalus
Blastomycosis				Cyclic hematopoiesis
Coccidioidomycosis				Ehlers-Danlos syndrome
Cryptococcosis				Deafness
Histoplasmosis				
Dermatomycoses				
Protozoal Disorders				
Babesiosis				
Leishmaniasis				
Toxoplasmosis				
Algae				
Protot(h)ecosis				
Geotrichosis				
Miscellaneous				
Ehrlichiosis				
Parasitic Disorders				
Dirofilaria spp				
Thelazia spp				
Toxocara canis				

Cytoplasmic inclusion bodies are present in conjunctival epithelial cells after about 6 days but are not easily demonstrated. Immunofluorescent methods are used on conjunctival epithelium, serum, macrophages, and footpads. The conjunctivitis usually responds well to broad-spectrum antibiotics, regular cleaning, and artificial tears. Artificial tears are used because distemper virus causes adenitis of the lacrimal gland, decreasing tear production. This acute and short-lived keratitis sicca is seen in most dogs with distemper. Severe central corneal ulcers may develop and become refractory to treatment.

Acute isolated or multifocal chorioretinitis occurs frequently in affected animals. The appearance of the acute and chronic retinal lesions (Figs. 19–2 and 19–3) is similar to that in retinitis of other causes (see Chap. 16). Retinal lesions may be small and have little

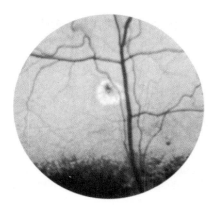

FIGURE 19–2. *Area of retinal atrophy with hyperreflectivity and pigmentation in a dog surviving distemper. (From Rubin LF: Atlas of Veterinary Ophthalmoscopy. Lea & Febiger, Philadelphia, 1974.)*

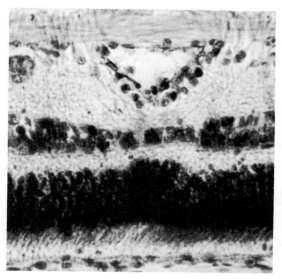

FIGURE 19–3. *Acute retinitis in a dog with perivascular cuffing by mononuclear cells in the ganglion cell layer. (From Saunders LZ, Rubin LF: Ophthalmic Pathology of Animals. S Karger AG, Basel, 1974.)*

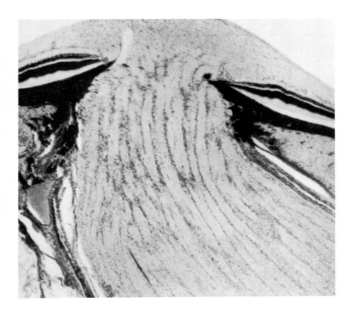

FIGURE 19–4. Optic neuritis, papilledema, and glial proliferation in acute canine distemper. (From Saunders LZ, Rubin LF: Ophthalmic Pathology of Animals. S Karger AG, Basel, 1974.)

effect on vision or may be widespread and cause blindness. Lesions also occur to a variable degree in the optic nerve (Fig. 19–4) and optic tracts and may cause blindness with minimal or no retinal lesions.

INFECTIOUS CANINE HEPATITIS

The ocular lesions of primary and postvaccinal infectious canine hepatitis (ICH) are discussed in Chapter 11 because the first observed clinical signs are seen in the cornea.

INFECTIOUS TRACHEOBRONCHITIS

Synonym: "Kennel cough"

Infectious tracheobronchitis causes conjunctivitis and a variable mucopurulent discharge in a manner very similar to that in canine distemper. Nervous and retinal signs are lacking, and the condition is distinguished by history of exposure, a hacking cough, and upper respiratory signs. Serological evidence of canine distemper virus infection is lacking.

Yeasts and Fungi

Yeast and fungal infections are characterized by a granulomatous histological response, which causes similar clinical signs in both dogs and cats. Features of granulomatous diseases caused by *Cryptococcus* spp (Fig. 19–5), *Blastomyces* spp, *Coccidioides* spp, *Histoplasma* spp, *Prototheca* spp, *Toxoplasma* spp,[1] and *Mycobacterium bovis* are summarized in Table 19–2. Secondary glaucoma is

---

1. A newly recognized, fatal protozoan disease of dogs caused by *Neosporum caninum* has been found responsible for some cases previously diagnosed as *Toxoplasma gondii* infection. The clinical significance is unknown.

a frequent result of the panophthalmitis and rubeosis iridis caused by these organisms.

In dogs living in the central United States east of the Mississippi River, blastomycosis should be included in the differential diagnosis when uveitis is present, especially when lesions of lung, lymph node, skin, bone, or testicle are present. Dogs diagnosed early may be successfully treated. Similarly, dogs in Arizona, Nevada, and the central valley region of California with uveitis and systemic lesions should have samples taken to eliminate coccidioidomycosis.

Primary toxoplasmosis is a rare cause of ocular disease in dogs. Dermatomycoses affecting the lids and periocular area are discussed in Chapter 7. The prognosis for treatment of disseminated canine cryptococcosis is poor, but it is more favorable in cats provided that treatment with ketaconazole is continued. If diagnosed early, the prognosis for treatment of canine blastomycosis with ketaconazole is good.

Protozoal and Miscellaneous Diseases (Table 19–3)

Protozoal diseases with ocular manifestations are uncommon in dogs and cats.

Algae

Algae are uncommon causes of ocular disease. *Geotrichium* and *Prototheca* are discussed in Table 19–2.

Miscellaneous Infectious Agents

EHRLICHIOSIS (See Table 19–3)

Synonym: Topical canine pancytopenia

Ehrlichia canis infection has been reported widely in California, Florida, Maryland, New Jersey, Pennsylva-

TABLE 19–2. Systemic and Ocular Granulomatous Diseases of Dogs and Cats

Disease	Ocular Signs	Systemic Signs	Diagnostic Aids	Treatment
Cryptococcosis (*Cryptococcus neoformans*) (Worldwide distribution)	Retinitis (Fig. 19–5), choroiditis, papilledema, hyphema, anterior uveitis	Meningitis, encephalitis, rhinitis (cats)	1. Histopathology 2. Cytology of exudates 3. Culture 4. Grayish gelatinous exudate in cultures Note association of eye and central nervous system signs	Ketaconazole Dog, 10–20 mg/kg once daily or divided twice daily Cat, 10–20 mg/kg twice daily every other day or 50 mg/kg once daily OR 5-Fluorocytosine* 200 mg/kg/day per os in 4 divided doses
Blastomycosis (*Blastomyces dermatitidis*) (North America)	Uveitis, glaucoma, blindness, retinal detachment, optic neuritis, corneal edema	Pulmonary, hepatic, bone, lymph node, and skin involvement; chronic cough, phasic pyrexia, wasting	1. Skin tests 2. Serology (variable reliability) 3. Culture 4. Histopathology	Ketaconazole Dog, 10–20 mg/kg once daily or divided twice daily Cat, 10–20 mg/kg twice daily every other day or 50 mg/kg once daily OR Amphotericin B† 0.5–1.0 mg/kg in 10 ml of 5% dextrose, 3 times per week (Caution!)
Coccidioidomycosis (*Coccidioides immitis*) (Southwest United States)	Anterior uveitis, deep keratitis, hypopyon	Pulmonary and bone lesions, cough, dyspnea, pyrexia, chronic wasting	1. Skin tests 2. Complement-fixing antibodies 3. Thoracic radiographs	Ketaconazole Dog, 10–20 mg/kg once daily or divided twice daily Cat, 10–20 mg/kg twice daily every other day or 50 mg/kg once daily OR Amphotericin B (as above)
Histoplasmosis (*Histoplasma capsulatum*)	Uveitis (uncommon)	A. *Respiratory form*— pneumonia with coughing, pyrexia, depression, and wasting B. *Intestinal form*— intractable enterocolitis, hepatosplenomegaly, jaundice, ascites, anemia C. *Lymphoid form*— lymphadenopathy, pyrexia, anemia	1. Thoracic radiographs (A) 2. Serology (variable reliability) 3. Skin tests (histoplasmin) 4. Histopathology 5. Culture	Ketaconazole Dog, 10–20 mg/kg once daily or divided twice daily Cat, 10–20 mg/kg twice daily every other day or 50 mg/kg once daily OR Amphotericin B (as above)
Protothecosis (*Prototheca* spp)	Uveitis, retinitis	—	Histopathology	—
Geotrichosis (*Geotrichium candidum*)	Uveitis, retinitis (rare)	—	Histopathology	Rare; human treatment with *oral* potassium iodide and gentian violet recorded
Toxoplasmosis (*Toxoplasma gondii*)	*Dog:* Mydriasis, anisocoria, congestion of retinal vessels, anterior uveitis *Cat:* Exudative anterior uveitis, retinochoroiditis, myositis of extraocular muscles	*Dog:* Pneumonia, hepatitis, encephalitis *Cat:* Pyrexia, bilirubinemia, dyspnea, pneumonia, leukopenia, anemia, encephalitis	1. Paired serum tests a. Sabin-Feldman dye test b. Indirect fluorescent antibody test 2. Fecal exam for oocysts in cats (often negative at this stage)	Sulfadiazine, 60 mg/kg/day in 4–6 divided doses, alone or in combination with pyrimethamine‡ 0.5–1.0 mg/kg/day§

Table continued on following page

TABLE 19–2. Systemic and Ocular Granulomatous Diseases of Dogs and Cats (*Continued*)

Tuberculosis (*Mycobacterium bovis*)	Conjunctivitis, keratitis, uveitis, chorioretinitis (cats more susceptible than dogs)	Variable, depending on primary focus *Dog*—thoracic form *Cat*—intestinal form	1. Culture of exudates and lesions 2. Histopathology	1. Isoniazid 2. Streptomycin 3. Bacille Calmette-Guérin vaccination (Euthanasia *may* be desirable for public health reasons) *Note:* tuberculosis in dogs and cats often comes from *human* infection

*Ancobon—Roche Laboratories, Nutley, NJ.
†Fungizone—Squibb, Princeton, NJ.
‡Daraprim—Burroughs Wellcome, Research Triangle Park, NC.
§From Frenkel JK: Toxoplasmosis. *In* Kirk RW (ed): Current Veterinary Therapy VI. WB Saunders Co, Philadelphia, 1977.

nia, Texas, the Philippines, Australia, and Thailand. It is not restricted to tropical areas. Ocular signs include hyphema, conjunctival hemorrhages, retinal vascular engorgement, retinal atrophy, and anterior uveitis. Systemic signs include anemia, leukopenia, thrombocytopenia, and epistaxis. Hypergammaglobulinemia may be demonstrated by high serum globulin levels and by electrophoresis. A positive indirect fluorescent antibody titer ($\geqq$ 1:20) is the most reliable method of diagnosis. Treatment is with tetracycline, 66 mg/kg daily for 14–21 days. Doxycycline and minocycline (5 mg/kg) have also been recommended.

TABLE 19–3. Ocular Signs of Protozoal Disorders

Disease	Etiological Agent	Ocular Signs	Systemic Signs	Treatment
Ehrlichiosis (tropical canine pancytopenia)	*Ehrlichia canis*	Hyphema, conjunctival hemorrhages, retinal vascular engorgement, retinal atrophy	Anemia, leukopenia, thrombocytopenia, epistaxis	1. Tetracycline, 66 mg/kg daily for 14 days 2. Blood transfusions
Leishmaniasis (kala-azar) (Europe, Africa, Asia, South America)	*Leishmania donovani*	Keratitis, conjunctivitis, anterior uveitis, scleritis, blepharitis	Anorexia, emesis, diarrhea, epistaxis, ataxia	1. Good diet 2. Sodium stibogluconare (Pentostam)
Babesiosis	*Babesia canis, Babesia gibsoni*	Jaundice, iris hemorrhages, anemia	Pyrexia, splenomegaly, jaundice, anorexia, anemia, hemoglobinuria	1. Removal of vectors 2. Phenamidine 0.3 ml/kg; Acaprin 0.25 mg/kg; Diminazene aceturate (Berenil) 7 mg/kg
Toxoplasmosis*	*Toxoplasma gondii*	Chorioretinitis, anterior uveitis (both granulomatous and nongranulomatous signs are reported), myositis of extraocular muscles Diagnosis: serological or histological examination	Pyrexia, debilitation; cachexia, multisystem signs	1. Sulfadiazine 60 mg/kg/day in 4–6 divided doses 2. Pyrimethamine 0.5–1.0 mg/kg/day 3. Folic acid
Trypanosomiasis†	*Trypanosoma brucei Trypanosoma congolense*	Limbal corneal edema, hypopyon, hyphema	Severe anemia, pyrexia, splenomegaly, lymph adenopathy, muscular pain, subcutaneous edema, orchitis, neurological changes, convulsions, death	

*Primary ocular infection with *Toxoplasma* is probably much less common than previously believed.
†Severe signs of trypanosomiasis may occur in dogs introduced into endemic areas.

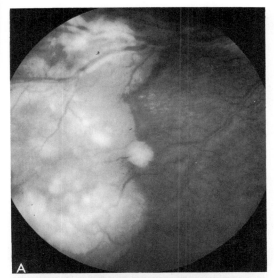

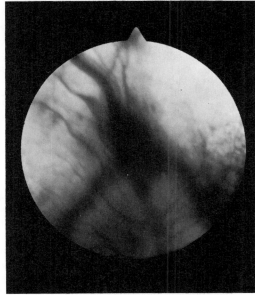

FIGURE 19–5. *Ocular manifestations of cryptococcosis. A, Temporal quadrant of a canine fundus, showing areas of granulomatous retinitis associated with cryptococcal infection. (From Roberts SR, Bistner SI: Ocular diseases. In Ettinger SJ [ed]: Textbook of Veterinary Internal Medicine, Vol 1. WB Saunders Co, Philadelphia, 1975.) B, Retinal hemorrhages and optic neuritis in a 6-year-old Weimaraner with ocular and nervous signs due to cryptococcus.*

Dogs with ehrlichiosis may also have a monoclonal gammopathy,[2] and must be differentiated from dogs with primary multiple myeloma. Similarities include older dogs, lameness, weight loss, ocular lesions, neurological dysfunction, polyuria, susceptibility to infections, anemia, leukopenia, renal insufficiency, hyperproteinemia, hyperviscosity, monoclonal spike on serum

and urine electrophoresis, and plasmacytosis on bone marrow examination. Differentiating features in myeloma include hypercalcemia, Bence-Jones proteinuria, and osteolytic lesions, and a differentiating feature in ehrlichiosis includes positive *Ehrlichia canis* titers. Thrombocytopenia may occur in either but is more common in ehrlichiosis.

Parasitic Diseases

Dirofilaria immitis is frequently reported in the canine eye. It causes uveitis, physical damage to the corneal endothelium with opacity, and retinitis. Parasites in the anterior chamber can be successfully removed surgically, with visual results depending on the degree of previous damage.

Thelazia spp are seen in the conjunctival sac in endemic areas and cause conjunctivitis, blepharospasm, and mild keratitis. The worms are removed under local anesthesia and can also be destroyed with echothiophate iodide (0.25%) drops.

Toxocara canis larvae cause focal areas of retinitis followed by atrophy and proliferation of pigment epithelium in the center of the atrophic areas. Massive infestation and migration are thought to cause much more severe retinal lesions in sheepdogs in Australia and New Zealand (see Chap 16). The retinal lesions caused by *Toxocara* spp rarely cause clinical signs but are important because of their dramatic appearance on ophthalmoscopic examination.

Endocrine Disorders

DIABETES MELLITUS[3]

Diabetes mellitus causes lesions in the lens and retina in dogs. Diabetic cataracts develop rapidly in affected animals. This may be the first sign observed by the owner, and maturity may occur in as little as 1 week from onset. The incidence of cataracts in spontaneous diabetes may reach 55% (up to 84% has been reported in experimental diabetes). Cataracts are, for practical purposes, the only lesions of clinical significance in diabetic dogs. Glucose levels may be elevated in canine tears in diabetic patients. This is a useful screening test if results are positive, but false-negative results are frequent.

Diabetic retinopathy is of comparative interest because of the high incidence of human diabetes mellitus and resultant blindness from diabetic retinopathy. It is primarily a disease of the retinal vessels with loss of pericytes from the vessel wall and the formation of microaneurysms and small hemorrhages. These lesions occur in diabetic dogs only after long-term maintenance on insulin or in poorly controlled diabetes.

All dogs with sudden onset of cataracts should be

2. Breitschwerdt EB, et al: Monoclonal gammopathy associated with naturally occurring canine ehrlichiosis. J Vet Int Med 1:2, 1987.

3. See also Chap 14.

evaluated for diabetes mellitus. Lenses with *sudden onset* of diabetic cataract are also susceptible to occasional, severe, lens-induced uveitis, and if cataract extraction is planned, topical dexamethasone therapy is recommended after the initial diagnosis. The patient with diabetes has a good prognosis for cataract extraction.

Dogs with diabetic cataract should have the diabetes controlled before cataract extraction and should be placed on topical dexamethasone to prevent lens-induced uveitis.

HYPERADRENOCORTICISM

Synonym: Cushing's disease

Ocular signs in up to 20% of affected dogs include corneal ulceration and neovascularization, with secondary bacterial conjunctivitis. Less frequent associations include keratoconjunctivitis sicca and hypercholesterolemia, hypertriglyceridemia, diabetes mellitus, and hypothyroidism. Corneal ulcerations are slow to heal. In a large epidemiological study, 21.4% of dogs with hyperadrenocorticism had pituitary tumors. Boxers had a higher risk of pituitary tumors causing hyperadrenocorticism, poodles had a higher risk for idiopathic hyperadrenocorticism, and dachsunds had a higher risk for hyperadrenocorticism caused by an adrenocortical tumor.

HYPERPARATHYROIDISM

Increased serum calcium levels have been associated with dystrophic calcification of the cornea. Similar calcification is also seen in senile canine keratopathy when hypercalcemia is not present.

HYPOPARATHYROIDISM

Ocular signs of hypoparathyroidism include punctate or linear lens opacities outlining the lens fibers (Fig. 19–6). The lesions may be associated with the hypocalcemia present in the disease and with other diseases causing chronic hypocalcemia.

HYPOTHYROIDISM

Ocular signs include ptosis, seborrhea with blepharitis, secondary lipid keratopathy and lipemia retinalis in severe cases, keratoconjunctivitis sicca, and facial paralysis (see Chap 17). (See also Hyperlipoproteinemias further on.)

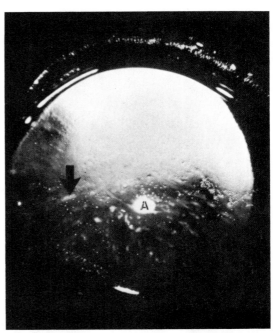

FIGURE 19–6. *Canine lens viewed by retroillumination. Note the short white linea opacities (arrows), located in the subcapsular anterior and posterior cortical regions. A = strobe artifact. (From Kornegay J, et al: Idiopathic hypocalcemia in four dogs. J Am Anim Hosp Assoc 16:727, 1980.)*

Neoplastic Disorders

LYMPHOSARCOMA

Clinical Signs

The presence and type of ocular signs in lymphosarcoma can assist in differential diagnosis initially and can give valuable information for grading and prognosis in relation to treatment. About 35% of dogs with lymphosarcoma exhibit some ocular signs, although they may not be the reason for presentation. Patients with ocular signs are more likely to have severe hematological abnormalities (anemia, thrombocytopenia, and leukemic lymphoma) and have a shorter survival time than those without ocular signs (Krohne et al, 1987).

The clinical staging is as follows:

I   Involvement of a single lymph node or organ
II   Involvement of many lymph nodes in a region
III   Generalized lymph node involvement
IV   Internal organ involvement (liver and spleen)
V   Manifestation in the blood and bone marrow or other organ systems, or both

Uveitis and intraocular hemorrhage are correlated with bone marrow involvement. Patients with these signs are graded as Class V.

General Ocular Signs

1. Secondary glaucoma
2. Blindness
3. Intraocular hemorrhage

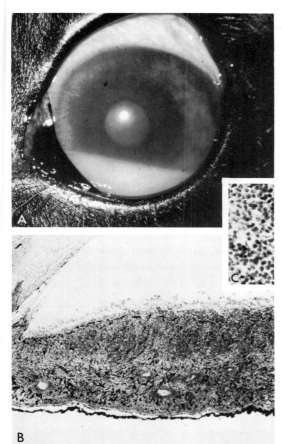

FIGURE 19–7. Ocular manifestations of lymphosarcoma. A, Ocular manifestations of lymphosarcoma in a dog, with infiltration of the anterior uvea with neoplastic cells and hypopyon. B, Infiltration of iris and trabecular meshwork with immature lymphocytes. C, Higher-power magnification of cell type in iris. (From Roberts SR, Bistner SI: Ocular diseases. In Ettinger SJ [ed.]: Textbook of Veterinary Internal Medicine, Vol 1. WB Saunders Co, Philadelphia, 1975.)

Uvea

1. Anterior uveitis with flare and cells in the anterior chamber (Fig. 19–7A)
2. Miosis
3. Swollen iris (Fig. 19–7C)
4. Hypotony
5. Keratic precipitates

Cornea

1. Keratitis with vascularization
2. Corneal edema
3. Keratic precipitates
4. Intrastromal corneal hemorrhage
5. Centrally migrating white band
6. Corneal ulceration in chronic cases

Fundus

1. Tortuous or dilated veins
2. Superficial and deep retinal hemorrhages
3. Perivascular sheathing
4. Retinal detachment

Interested readers should refer to standard surgery, oncology, or internal medicine texts for details of chemotherapy of lymphosarcoma.

MULTIPLE MYELOMA

In multiple myeloma, similar ocular signs have been reported when increased amounts of immunoglobulins are produced. Initial presentation may be for these ocular signs: aqueous flare, retinal detachment and hemorrhages, corneal edema, and "cattle truck" appearance of retinal vessels associated with hyperviscosity syndrome. This syndrome with ocular signs has been reported with myelomata producing IgA, IgG, and IgM. In cats, retinopathy may also be due to coexistent anemia.

Diagnostic Aids

Radiographic examination for characteristic radiolucent areas, especially in the spine

Laboratory examination for anemia, azotemia, leukopenia, hypercalcemia, hypoalbuminemia and hyperglobulinemia, and thrombocytopenia

Urinalysis for proteinuria and Bence-Jones proteins

Serum electrophoresis for immunoglobulin gammopathies

METASTASES

Metastases from distant sites are commonly seen in the eye and include those from malignant mammary tumors, osteosarcoma, thyroid carcinoma, pancreatic adenocarcinoma, pulmonary squamous cell carcinoma,

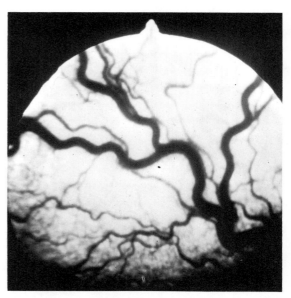

FIGURE 19–8. Fundus photograph of retinal vascular congestion in a dog with congestive heart failure and mitral insufficiency. (From Roberts SR, Bistner SI: Ocular diseases. In Ettinger SJ [ed]: Textbook of Veterinary Internal Medicine, Vol 1. WB Saunders Co, Philadelphia, 1975.)

TABLE 19–4. Ocular Signs of Hematological Disorders in Dogs and Cats

Disorder	Ocular Signs
Monoclonal gammopathy and hyperviscosity	Retinal hemorrhages (small or large), dilated tortuous retinal veins with irregular filling ("cattle truck" appearance), conjunctival hemorrhages, massive intraocular hemorrhages (rare)
Thrombocytopenia and thrombasthenia	Subconjunctival hemorrhages, retinal and anterior uveal hemorrhages, hyphema
Severe anemia	Retinal and vitreous hemorrhages (Fig. 19–9), secondary retinal detachment
von Willebrand's disease	Retinal hemorrhages, retinal detachment, conjunctival petechiae

seminoma, renal carcinoma, rhabdomyosarcoma, and hemangiosarcoma. Neoplasia remote from the eye is frequently associated with uveitis that is refractory to treatment or recurs after treatment.

Hematological and Circulatory Disorders

HYPERTENSION (See discussion under Cats, p 528)

Polycythemia rubra vera (Packed Cell Volume > 60)

In congenital cardiac diseases associated with polycythemia, retinal vessels may appear engorged and tortuous. In Figure 19–8, an arteriovenous fistula has caused pulsating exophthalmos in a dog. Some of the ocular signs of more common blood dyscrasias are summarized in Table 19–4.

Miscellaneous Disorders

HYPERLIPOPROTEINEMIAS

Hyperlipoproteinemias (HLPEs) are not uncommon. Primary HLPE occurs as a distinct entity in the miniature schnauzer. HLPE occurs in the following disorders:

1. Spontaneous hyperlipoproteinemia (types I–V)
2. Diabetes mellitus
3. Pancreatitis
4. Hypothyroidism
5. Postprandial plasma lipid elevations

It occurs less commonly in hyperadrenocorticism, liver disease, pregnancy, drug toxicosis, obesity, nephrotic syndrome, and gram-negative sepsis.

Laboratory determinations of serum lipid levels in dogs should be made after a 12–24-hour fast.

Ocular lesions and signs associated with hyperlipoproteinemia in dogs include:

1. *Lipemia retinalis*—retinal vessels appear creamy white owing to increased serum lipid levels.

2. *Lipid keratopathy*—the presence of central and peripheral corneal opacities that have a crystalline appearance (Fig. 19–10). Lipid deposits in the corneal stroma are more extensive if the cornea is vascularized, for example, in a corneal ulcer (Fig. 19–11). Animals with lipid keratopathy frequently do not have elevated lipid levels.

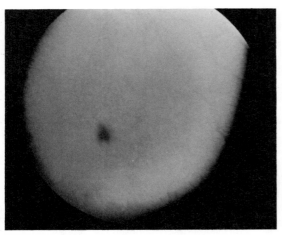

FIGURE 19–9. Deep retinal hemorrhages in a cat with severe anemia. (Courtesy of Dr. G. Bryan.)

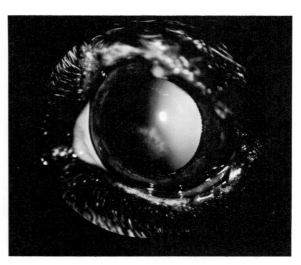

FIGURE 19–10. Unilateral central lipid keratopathy in a 3-year-old Samoyed (fasting serum cholesterol: 365 mg/dl).

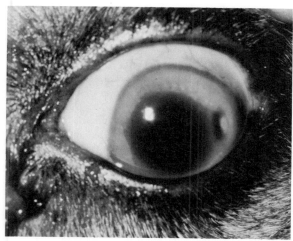

FIGURE 19–11. *Extensive lipid keratopathy in a 1-year-old beagle with ulcerative keratitis next to the limbus and hyperlipoproteinemia (fasting serum cholesterol: 1000 mg/dl).*

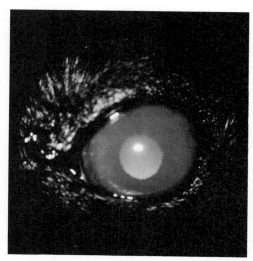

FIGURE 19–13. *Anterior chamber lipemia in a 5-year-old poodle with hyperlipoproteinemia (serum cholesterol: 600 mg/dl). Hyperlipoproteinemia responded to a low-fat diet within 4 weeks. Aqueous lipid disappeared within 24 hours of therapy for uveitis.*

These animals should receive a lipid evaluation (see Fig. 19–12), which is usually available from human laboratories, in which such tests are used routinely in the study of atherosclerosis and ischemic heart disease. An association between corneal lipid deposits and hypothyroidism in dogs has been noted experimentally and clinically.

3. *Anterior chamber lipemia*—lipoproteins do not normally cross the blood-aqueous barrier, but in uveitis, they may enter the aqueous when the barrier is broken down, causing a cloudy appearance and interfering with vision (Fig. 19–13). Thus, both hyperlipoproteinemia and uveitis are necessary for lipids to be present in the aqueous. If the uveitis is treated (and sometimes even if it is not), the lipids disappear from the anterior chamber in 48–72 hours and vision is restored. Animals with anterior chamber lipemia should be thoroughly evaluated to determine the cause of their hyperlipemia.

Hyperlipoproteinemia should not be confused with either systemic hypertension or atherosclerosis. The three conditions are separate, although each results in eye lesions in dogs, and any combination of the three may occur.

Treatment of HLPE

Underlying causes of HLPE should be treated, for example, hypothyroidism.

SERUM LIPID PROFILE

Serum cholesterol   Lipoprotein
Serum triglyceride   electrophoresis*
Serum total lipid   Serum cholesterol esters*
T4   Serum phospholipids*

FIGURE 19–12. *Serum lipid profile. (*Optional.)*

Dietary Therapy. Spontaneous HLPE often responds to a low-cholesterol, low-triglyceride diet:
1. All vegetable diets
2. Prescription Diet R/D[4]
3. Low-cholesterol human diets.
4. Medium-chain triglycerides[5] (MCTs) (0.5 ml/kg/day) provide calories without causing chylomicron and triglyceride synthesis by the small intestine but must be supplemented with vegetable oil daily for essential fatty acids. Portagen (Mead Johnson) containing MCT and corn oil can also be used.

Drug Therapy. Clofibrate, gemfibrozil, and niacin are used to reduce triglycerides and cholesterol in humans. Their use is insufficiently tested to be recommended in animals as yet.

CANINE ALLERGIC INHALANT DERMATITIS

Synonyms: Atopy, atopic dermatitis, allergic dermatitis, allergic eczema

Canine allergic inhalant dermatitis (CAID) is discussed in relation to conjunctival disorders (see Chap 8). In CAID, IgE antibodies and clinical allergy to inhaled antigens develop. It is one of the most common allergic skin diseases in dogs, accounting for 2–10% of all skin diseases. Onset is usually between 1 and 3 years, but it is rare after 6 years of age.

Clinical Signs

The clinical signs of CAID are shown in Table 19–5. The signs are initially seasonal (spring, summer,

---

4. Hill's Pet Products, Topeka, KS.
5. MCT Oil, Mead Johnson, Evansville, IN.

TABLE 19–5. Clinical Signs of Canine Allergic Inhalant Dermatitis

Nonocular Signs	Ocular Signs
Face rubbing	Allergic conjunctivitis (frequently
Feet licking	responsive to topical and
Armpit scratching	systemic corticosteroids)
Staining of coat in these areas	Epiphora
Xerosis of the skin	Periocular erythema and alopecia
Lichenification of axillary,	Rubbing of the eyes
inguinal, perioral,	Slight overflow of tears around
periorbital, and distal limb	the entire lid margins
regions	Keratitis
Hyperhidrosis	Cataracts
Seborrhea	
Pyoderma	
Otitis externa	
Rhinitis	
Lower urinary tract infections	
Infertility	
Irregular estrus cycles	
Pseudocyesis	

autumn) but eventually may occur throughout the year with chronicity of the disease. Some animals may exhibit the disease during specific climatic conditions, for example, when Santa Ana winds blow in southern California and allergens are blown from the desert. Whether the condition dissipates or becomes established thereafter is variable. Affected animals are usually 1–3 years old.

Breeds commonly affected include Lhasa apso, Dalmatian, wire-haired fox terrier, West Highland white terrier, golden retriever, beagle, Irish setter, Cairn terrier, miniature schnauzer, Scottish terrier, pug, Boston terrier, and English bulldog.

Secondary bacterial conjunctivitis, keratoconjunctivitis sicca, and staphylococcal keratoconjunctivitis and blepharitis may follow in susceptible animals.

Diagnosis

Diagnosis is by history and clinical signs. Intradermal testing is rarely necessary when ocular signs are correctly interpreted.

Treatment

Treatment consists of
1. Treatment of established bacterial infections
2. Removal of the offending allergen if possible
3. Intermittent very low dose oral corticosteroid therapy, preferably with a drug having high glucocorticoid and low mineralocorticoid activity, for example, dexamethasone
4. Topical low-potency corticosteroids, for example, hydrocortisone drops, 0.5%, 2–3 times daily
5. Hyposensitization if possible (Scott, 1978)

SJÖGREN'S-LIKE SYNDROME

In Sjögren's syndrome (named after the human disorder), mucus production from the lacrimal glands, salivary glands, and vaginal mucous membrane is decreased. It is thought to be due to an autoimmune-mediated destruction of exocrine glands. Reduced IgA in the mucus causes chronic bacterial infections on the membrane surfaces. Ocular signs and treatment are as for keratoconjunctivitis sicca. The presence of Sjögren's syndrome is important in evaluation of potential candidates for parotid duct transposition, because if the parotid gland is affected the procedure will be unsuccessful. Parotid secretion can be evaluated by placing a drop of ophthalmic atropine in the dog's mouth and observing for saliva production. The syndrome is seen more frequently in the miniature schnauzer. Most dogs with keratoconjunctivitis sicca *do not have* Sjögren's syndrome.

AUTOIMMUNE-MEDIATED SKIN DISEASES

Pemphigus and pemphigoid-type disorders frequently involve the eyelids (see Chap 8).

MYASTHENIA GRAVIS

Congenital and acquired myasthenia gravis occur in dogs and cats. The major ocular signs of myasthenia gravis are ptosis and palpebral areflexia. Other signs include muscle tremors, a short, choppy gait, megaesophagus, ventroflexion of the neck, a change in the voice, and regurgitation.

It can be diagnosed by:
1. A positive response to anticholinesterase–edrophonium hydrochloride,[6] 0.25–0.5 mg intravenously in cats—which resolves the weakness within 60 seconds and persists for 3–5 minutes
2. Demonstration of serum autoantibodies to cholinesterase

Myasthenia gravis can be treated in cats with pyridostigmine bromide syrup, 1.5 mg orally every 12 hours.

Cyclic Hematopoiesis (Gray Collie Syndrome)

Cyclic hematopoiesis is widespread in collies and is inherited as an autosomal recessive trait. Affected animals are gray. Changes may occur soon after weaning and include bilateral keratitis, lethargy, anorexia, fever, arthritis, respiratory infections, and gastrointestinal disorders. Most dogs die within 6 months. Affected animals may be treated with antibiotics, fluid therapy, and lithium—150 to 300 mg by mouth daily.

EHLERS-DANLOS SYNDROME

The Ehlers-Danlos syndrome is an inherited disorder of connective tissue. Lens luxation, cataract, and hyperelasticity of the palpebral skin, tearing of the skin, and excessive joint laxity occur.

---

6. Tensilon—Roche Laboratories, Nutley, NJ.

DEAFNESS AND OCULAR DEFECTS[7]

A predisposition to deafness has been noted in the Dalmatian, Australian cattle dog, English setter, Australian shepherd, Boston terrier, Old English sheepdog, and English bulldog. With the exception of the English setter, these breeds are affected with the merle gene, and associated ocular defects reported include blindness (cause unspecified), microphthalmia, persistent pupillary membrane, coloboma, retinal detachment, heterochromia iridis, and ectropion.

HYDROCEPHALUS

See Chapter 17.

CATS

Infectious diseases that are common to cats are shown in Table 19–6.

Bacteria

SALMONELLOSIS

Salmonella spp infection has been reported to cause conjunctivitis and protrusion of the third eyelids in association with dehydration.

7. Hayes HM, et al: Canine congenital deafness: Epidemiologic study of 272 cases. J Am Anim Hosp Assoc 17:473, 1981.

TUBERCULOSIS (See Table 19–12)

Mycobacterium bovis causes enophthalmitis in cats. The usual source of infection is contaminated milk or infected humans in the cat's household.

Viruses

UPPER RESPIRATORY INFECTIONS

Calicivirus, feline herpesvirus, reovirus, *Chlamydia* spp, and *Mycoplasma* are compared and described in Table 8–6.

FELINE INFECTIOUS PERITONITIS

Feline infectious peritonitis (FIP) is a chronic viral disorder characterized by fibrinous pleuritis and peritonitis with pyogranulomatous lesions in many organs. It has been widely reported throughout the world. About 20% of affected cats show eye lesions.

Ocular Signs of FIP

Cats with FIP are frequently presented because of ocular signs.
  Anterior Uveitis (Fig. 19–14B–D)
  Aqueous flare
  Cells in the anterior chamber
  Keratic precipitates
  Hemorrhage

TABLE 19–6. Systemic Feline Diseases with Ocular Signs

Infectious	Endocrine	Neoplasia	Hematological and Circulatory	Miscellaneous

Bacteria
  Salmonellosis
  Tuberculosis
	Hyperthyroidism	Myeloproliferative disease
		Lymphosarcoma
		Metastases
		Post-traumatic sarcoma
			Hypertension
			Anemia
				Taurine deficiency
				Thiamine deficiency
				Waardenburg's syndrome
				Chediak-Higashi syndrome
				Chronic renal disease

Viruses
  Calicivirus infection
  Feline infectious
    peritonitis
  Feline leukemia
  Feline rhinotracheitis
  Panleukopenia
  Reovirus infection
  Pleuropneumonia-
    like organisms
  Chlamydia spp				

Yeasts and Fungi
  Aspergillosis
  Blastomycosis
  Coccidioidomycosis
  Cryptococcosis
  Dermatomycoses
  Histoplasmosis				

Protozoal Disorders
  Hemobartonella
  Leishmaniasis
  Toxoplasmosis				

Parasitic Disorders *Toxocara canis*				

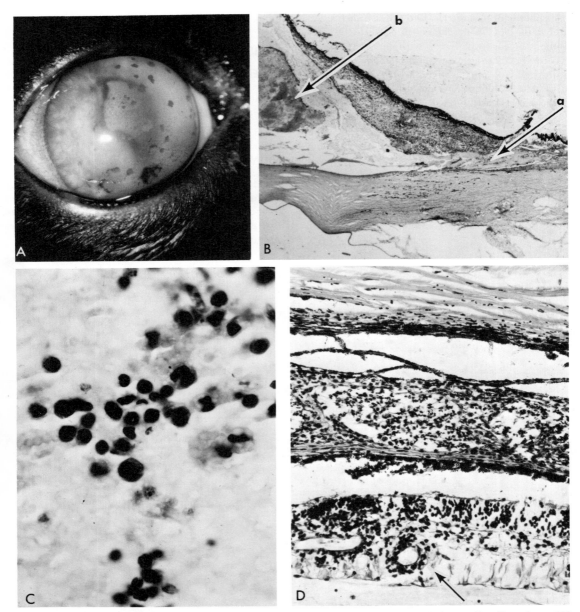

FIGURE 19–14. *Ocular manifestations of FIP. A, Ocular manifestations of FIP with acute anterior uveitis with cells and "flare" in the anterior chamber. There are numerous large and small keratitic precipitates present on the corneal endothelium and extensive posterior synechia. B, Photomicrograph of iris and anterior drainage angle from a case of FIP. Note the exudate and cells present in the anterior drainage angle (a) and in the anterior chamber (b), and the infiltration of the iris by inflammatory cells. C, Photomicrograph. Higher magnification than B to demonstrate inflammatory cell type that is predominantly mononuclear. D, Photomicrograph. Retinitis from same case as B and C. Both perivascular cutting and diffuse infiltration of the retina and choroid are present. There is a secondary degeneration of photoreceptor elements. (From Roberts SR, Bistner SI: Ocular disease. In Ettinger SJ [ed]: Textbook of Veterinary Internal Medicine, Vol 1. WB Saunders Co, Philadelphia, 1975.)*

Miosis

Iris edema

Occlusion of the pupil

Synechiae

Hypotony

Keratitis

Corneal edema (Fig. 19–14*A*)

Vascularization

Retinitis

Superficial and deep retinal and preretinal hemorrhages (keel-shaped) (Fig. 19–15)

Retinal edema

Engorged retinal vessels

Serous retinal detachments

Areas of tapetal and nontapetal retinitis

Although the diagnosis is confirmed histologically, the associated nervous signs and fluid accumulations in the thorax or abdomen are useful in differentiating FIP from other granulomatous disorders with similar ocular signs (see Table 19–1).

Cats with FIP are frequently presented because of ocular signs.

Pathogenesis

In *effusive* FIP, large amounts of fluid accumulate in the abdominal and thoracic cavities. A *noneffusive* form exists in which other organ systems may be affected. The disease is progressive (most affected animals die in 2–3 months) and is characterized by numerous superficial lesions on the peritoneal and pleural surfaces, although marked variation occurs in the extent and variety of organs involved. Extraserosal lesions restricted

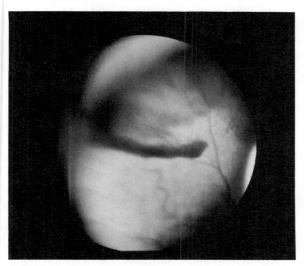

FIGURE 19–15. *Preretinal hemorrhages in a cat with FIP. (Courtesy of Dr. W. Yakely.)*

to specific organ systems (e.g., eye, kidney, central nervous system [CNS]) may be reflected by specific organ signs:

Liver	Subcapsular infiltration of plasma cells and lymphocytes, multiple subcapsular foci of hepatic cell necrosis
CNS	Leptomeningitis, focal spinal meningitis, and CNS lesions usually restricted to meninges, choroid plexuses, and ependyma, with little involvement of the brain parenchyma
Genital	Periorchitis in males
Eye	Necrotizing uveitis and panophthalmitis
Kidney	Most frequently affected secondary organ system; granulomatous lesions

FIP is characterized by multifocal necrotizing pyogranulomatous lesions with a predilection for necrotizing vasculitis. Feline leukemia virus (FeLV) infection predisposes cats to FIP.

EFFUSIVE FIP

Effusive FIP causes chronic weight loss, depression, and abdominal distention. In about 20% of affected cats, dyspnea and weight loss are the presenting signs. Fever is variable, and terminal signs of liver failure are frequent. Ocular or CNS signs, or both, may be associated with this form of FIP. In a study of 41 cases of effusive FIP, Pedersen and coworkers (1974) observed clinical signs referable to various organ systems in the distribution shown in Table 19–7.

Diagnosis

1. *Serological evidence* of FIP infection. False-positive results occur because of cross reactions with other coronaviruses.
2. *Analysis of pleural and peritoneal exudates.* The exudate is characteristically high in protein and contains 1600–50,000 while blood cells/cu mm (mostly neutrophils). It is usually sterile and contains fibrin and clots.
3. *Complete blood count*
   a. Leukocytosis with absolute neutrophilia and lymphopenia with a low-grade anemia.
   b. Total proteins—greater than 7.8 g/dl in 54% of

TABLE 19–7. Organ Systems Affected by Effusive Feline Infectious Peritonitis

Organ Systems	Number of Cases
Peritoneal cavity	25
Peritoneal and pleural cavities	6
Pleural cavity	3
Peritoneal cavity and eyes	2
Peritoneal cavity and CNS	2
Peritoneal and pleural cavities and CNS	1
Peritoneal and pleural cavities, CNS, and eyes	1
Pleural cavity and CNS	1

cases to absolute increase in beta and gamma globulins. Albumin/globulin decreased.

   c. Plasma fibrinogen—elevated (greater than 400 mg/dl in 20% of cases).

   d. Icterus index—7.5 in terminal stages.

4. *Radiological findings*

   a. Abdominal effusion.

   b. Pleural effusion and pleuritis.

   c. Liver, kidney, and spleen enlarged in some cases.

Differential Diagnosis of Effusive and Noneffusive FIP (Based on Systemic Signs)

   1. Lymphosarcoma

   2. Myeloproliferative disease (including reticuloendotheliosis)

   3. *Hemobartonella felis* infection

   4. Toxoplasmosis

   5. Pyothorax

   6. Steatitis

   7. Congestive heart failure

   8. Liver disease

   9. Hypoproteinemia

   10. Cryptococcosis

NONEFFUSIVE FIP

Lack of specific fluid accumulations make this form of FIP more difficult to diagnose. The disease may be present in many organ systems, but the presenting clinical signs are usually referable to one or two. Pedersen and coworkers (1974), studying 28 cases of noneffusive FIP, found the distribution of clinical signs shown in Table 19–8.

Chronic weight loss, fever, and debilitation are the most common signs. The kidneys are often enlarged and irregular with elevated levels of blood urea nitrogen (BUN) and proteinuria. Lymphosarcoma is often suspected because of renal involvement. Ocular lesions are *more common in effusive FIP.*

Diagnosis

1. Complete blood count

   a. Variable leukocytosis, neutrophilia, and lymphopenia

   b. Total plasma proteins—7.8% in 71% of cases

   c. Fibrinogen—greater than 400 mg/dl in 20% of cases

2. *Cerebrospinal fluid (CSF) analysis* in neurological cases

   a. Elevated CSF proteins—90–2000 mg/dl

   b. Elevated white blood cells—from 90 to 8250 white blood cells/cu mm

3. *Ocular lesions*

   a. Retinal and uveal lesions

   b. Aqueous cytological features—neutrophils and macrophages

TABLE 19–8. Organ Systems Affected by Noneffusive Feline Infectious Peritonitis

Organ System	Number of Cases
Peritoneal cavity	12
Ocular	7
Peritoneal cavity and eyes	2
CNS	5
CNS and eyes	2

Differential Diagnosis of Eye Lesions

Other causes of uveitis and chorioretinitis are:

   1. Toxoplasmosis

   2. Cryptococcosis

   3. Blastomycosis

   4. Histoplasmosis

   5. Malignant lymphoma and associated diseases

   6. Tuberculosis

Treatment

All patients die eventually (most within 2–3 months). Palliative treatment may include:

   1. Drainage of fluid from thorax and abdomen

   2. Fluid therapy for dehydration

   3. Steroids to reduce fever

   4. Broad-spectrum antibiotics (tylosin, 50 mg/kg/day has been suggested, but it has no special advantage over other agents)

FeLV

FeLV infection can cause a uveitis similar in appearance to uveitis caused by FeLV-negative lymphosarcoma. The clinical signs are nonspecific and are similar to uveitis caused by many organisms in cats—*Cryptococcus, Blastomyces, Histoplasma,* and *Toxoplasma* spp, and to ocular involvement with lymphosarcoma and myeloproliferative disorders. The frequency of this uveitis is controversial. In our experience, FeLV-positive titers are uncommon in cats with uveitis, but serological evaluation is justified, as for other infectious agents. Cats may also be afflicted with systemic infectious diseases because of immune status compromised by FeLV.

FELINE PANLEUKOPENIA

Panleukopenia virus causes cerebellar hypoplasia, retinal dysplasia, retinal degeneration, and immunosuppression in the kittens of queens infected during pregnancy (Figs. 19–16 to 19–18). (Panleukopenia virus shares this pathogenic ability with the viruses of bluetongue and mucosal disease–viral diarrhea.) There are no ocular manifestations of the disease in adults except enophthalmos and prominent third eyelids resulting from dehydration.

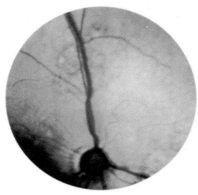

FIGURE 19–16. Mottled hyperreflective area surrounding the superior arteriole and venule in a 10-week-old kitten with cerebellar hypoplasia due to panleukopenia virus. (From Rubin LF: Atlas of Veterinary Ophthalmoscopy. Lea & Febiger, Philadelphia, 1974.)

Bacteria-Like Organisms

Chlamydia psittaci (See Table 8–2 and Chap 8)

Chlamydia spp cause a severe, chronic, and often unilateral conjunctivitis, often associated with upper respiratory signs. It may cause severe chemosis in the early stages and must be distinguished from feline herpesvirus infection and toxic insults, which it resembles because of its acute and severe onset.

Yeasts and Fungi

DERMATOMYCOSES (See Chap 7)

ASPERGILLOSIS (See Table 19–2)

Aspergillosis (*Aspergillus flavus*) is the second most frequently recognized fungal infection in cats and is often associated with panleukopenia, upper respiratory infection, and chronic sinusitis. Immunosuppression may play a role in the establishment of this disease.

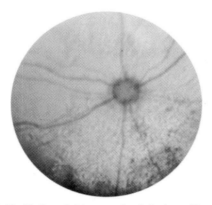

FIGURE 19–17. Tapetal hyperreflectivity in a littermate of the cat illustrated in FIGURE 19–16. (From Rubin LF: Atlas of Veterinary Ophthalmoscopy. Lea & Febiger, Philadelphia, 1974.)

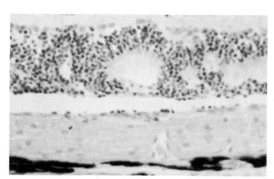

FIGURE 19–18. Section of a retina from a kitten affected with panleukopenia virus. There is severe disorganization of the inner and outer nuclear layers. (From Rubin LF: Atlas of Veterinary Ophthalmoscopy. Lea & Febiger, Philadelphia, 1974.)

Affected cats often have a history of treatment with cyclophosphamide and corticosteroids before aspergillosis appears. Ocular signs include orbital cellulitis and ocular proptosis.

CRYPTOCOCCOSIS (See Table 19–2)

Cats are frequently affected by *Cryptococcosis neoformans*. The combination of respiratory or central nervous signs with an apparently granulomatous ocular disease indicates investigation and advice to the owner on hygiene because of the zoonotic potential of *Cryptococcosis* spp.

Prolonged treatment with ketaconazole (see Table 19–2) is required and may result in return of vision. Patients are frequently anorexic because of their systemic disease and require hand feeding. Progression of the disease can be monitored by serum antigen and antibody titers. If treatment is successful, antigen titers fall and often, after *months*, antibody titers rise. Free antibody titer alone is an unreliable indication of response.

BLASTOMYCOSIS, COCCIDIOIDOMYCOSIS, HISTOPLASMOSIS, TOXOPLASMOSIS

Each of these conditions can cause uveitis in the cat. The clinical signs are similar. For differences in systemic signs, diagnosis, and treatment see Table 19–2. The results of treatment of blastomycosis in cats is uniformly poor. Coccidioidomycosis can be present even though latex particle agglutination, agar gel immunodiffusion, and complement fixation test results are negative.

Protozoal Disorders

HEMOBARTONELLOSIS

Synonym: Feline infectious anemia

The ocular signs of *Hemobartonella felis* infection are pale conjunctivae and, in severe cases, retinal hemorrhages associated with the anemia rather than the organism per se.

LEISHMANIASIS (See Table 19–3)

Parasites

TOXOCARA CANIS

Toxocara canis larvae cause retinal lesions in cats that are similar to those described in the dog.

Endocrine Disorders

HYPERTHYROIDISM

Retinal vessel engorgement may be observed in addition to secondary hypertension. Exophthalmos and the orbital signs of hyperthyroidism (Graves's disease) seen in humans are *not* observed in animals.

Hematological and Circulatory Disorders (See also Table 19–4)

HYPERTENSION

Hypertension occurs in both dogs and cats and causes hypertensive retinopathy. Hypertension may be primary or it may be secondary to renal disease, hyperthyroidism, hyperlipidemia, pheochromocytoma, and probably other unrecorded disorders.

Clinical Signs (Fig. 19–19)

1. Sudden loss of vision
2. Loss or suppression of direct pupillary reflex
3. Retinal hemorrhages
4. Retinal detachment, often bilateral
5. Iris hemorrhages
6. Vitreous hemorrhages

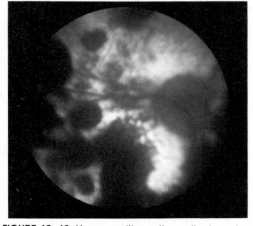

FIGURE 19–19. *Hypersensitive retinopathy in a dog.*

TABLE 19–9. Normal Blood Pressure Values (mmHg)

	Cat*	Dog†
Systolic	171 ± 22	148 ± 16
Diastolic	123 ± 17	87 ± 8

*From Gordon DB, Goldblatt H: Direct percutaneous determination of systemic blood pressure and production of renal hypertension in the cat. Proc Soc Exp Biol Med 125:177, 1967.
†From Cowgill LCD, Kallet AJ: Systemic hypertension. *In* Kirk RW (ed): Current Veterinary Therapy IX. WB Saunders Co, Philadelphia, 1986.

7. Hyphema
8. Glaucoma
9. Rubeosis iridis (neovascularization of the surface of the iris, possibly associated with chronic retinal detachment rather than the hypertension per se)

Diagnosis

1. Clinical signs
2. Blood pressure measurement (Table 19–9). Indirect measurement is more practical and can be performed in most conscious patients. It should be performed in all patients with unexplained retinal detachments or retinal, vitreous, or iris hemorrhages or hyphema. Ultrasonic measurement gives similar values. Pressures in anesthetized patients are 10–15 mmHg lower. Restrained or excited cats may show higher values.
3. Serum chemistry profile with evaluations of platelet count and thyroid, adrenal, diabetic, and lipid status as indicated. Primary hyperlipidemia does not cause hypertension in dogs but may be associated with other factors that do.

Treatment

The aims of treatment are to reattach the retina (see Chap 16) and control the systemic condition. Significant return and improvement of vision can often be achieved in cats if treatment is instituted *early*. In dogs with hypertension secondary to renal disease, reported results of treatment have been poor.

Patients with acute retinal detachment should be referred early for evaluation and therapy by a veterinary ophthalmologist if vision is to be saved.

ANEMIAS

Nonspecific signs of anemias include conjunctival pallor and, in severe anemia, retinal hemorrhages.

Neoplasia

MYELOPROLIFERATIVE DISORDERS AND LYMPHOSARCOMA

Myeloproliferative disorders are subclassified into *myelodysplastic syndromes* and *acute myelogenous leukemias* (Table 19–10). Infiltration of ocular tissues with malignant cells can be observed in either of these disorders and in lymphosarcoma. The clinical signs are similar to those of chronic granulomatous uveitis (see Table 19–1). The ocular signs may respond to topical dexamethasone, subconjunctival depot betamethasone injection, and systemic chemotherapy.

METASTASES

Metastases to the feline eye may occur from numerous types of tumor (see section on metastases in dog section).

POST-TRAUMATIC SARCOMA

Feline eyes subjected to trauma may develop sarcoma years later. For this reason, nonfunctional eyes severely damaged by trauma should be removed (and replaced with an orbital prosthesis if the best cosmetic appearance is desired). Post-traumatic sarcoma has the potential to produce bone in the eye and become osteosarcoma.

TABLE 19–10. Signs of Feline Myeloproliferative Disorders

Sign	Myelodysplastic Disorders (%)	Acute Myelogenous Leukemia (%)
*Clinical Signs**		
Retinal hemorrhages	14.3	12.8
Unresponsive fever	19.0	0.0
Dyspnea	14.3	23.1
Hepatomegaly and/or splenomegaly	0.0	33.3
Pica	14.3	5.1
Icterus	4.8	5.1
Ecchymoses	4.8	2.5
Gingival hemorrhages	4.8	2.5
Melena	4.8	2.5
Laboratory Parameters		
Severe anemia		
PVC <10%	23.8	55.3
Macrocytic	47.6	55.3
Leukopenia	42.9	28.9
Leukocytosis	4.8	36.8
Neutropenia	42.9	44.7
Thrombocytopenia	66.7	92.1
Myeloblastosis	0.0	68.4
FeLV positive	71.4	89.5
Serum iron increased	80.0	85.7

From Blue JT, et al: Nonlymphoid hematopoietic neoplasia in cats: A retrospective study of 60 cases. Cornell Vet 78:21, 1988.
*Most cats had anorexia, weight loss, pallor, and lethargy.

Miscellaneous Disorders

Taurine Deficiency

Taurine deficiency is discussed in Chapter 16 because of the retinal lesions it causes. Taurine deficiency also causes a reversible cardiomyopathy in affected cats, and feline cardiac patients should receive an ophthalmoscopic examination to help confirm taurine deficiency by the presence of retinal lesions.

THIAMINE DEFICIENCY

Clinical signs include:
Stage 1
1. Anorexia and salivation
2. Weight loss
3. Vomiting
4. Ataxia of the hindquarters
Stage 2 (Critical Stage)
Sudden onset of neurological disturbances:
1. Rapid series of short tonic convulsions with ventroflexion of the head and neck
2. Impaired righting and vestibulocular reflexes
3. Spasticity
4. Mydriasis with a depressed direct light reflex
5. Circling
6. Dysmetria
7. Spinal hypersensitivity
8. Retinal hemorrhages
9. Papilledema
Stage 3 (Semicoma)
1. Continuous crying
2. Opisthotonus
3. Extensor rigidity
4. Death within 1–2 days

Diagnosis

1. Clinical signs
2. Rapid response to thiamine or B-complex vitamins

Treatment

Thiamine, 1 mg intramuscularly or 5 mg orally, causes signs to disappear within a day if given at stage 2.

WAARDENBURG'S SYNDROME

Waardenburg's syndrome consists of:
1. Deafness
2. Heterochromia iridis
3. White coat color
Although this hereditary syndrome occurs most commonly in white, blue-eyed cats, it also occurs in dogs (especially the Australian cattle dog, the Great Dane, and the Dalmatian), mice, and humans. Not all white,

blue-eyed cats are affected. In cats, it is inherited as a dominant trait with complete penetrance for the white coat and incomplete penetrance for deafness and blue irides. Not all white blue-eyed cats are deaf.

CHEDIAK-HIGASHI SYNDROME

The Chediak-Higashi syndrome has been reported in Persian cats. Abnormal granulation of neutrophils and melanocytes occurs, with immune deficiency. Ocular signs include light yellow-green irides, photophobia, a "basket-weave" pattern to the iris surface, spontaneous nystagmus, decreased fundic pigmentation, tapetal degeneration, and cataracts.

CHRONIC RENAL DISEASE

Cats with chronic renal disease may have ocular signs associated with anemia and hypertension, but in addition retinal detachment and atrophy have been reported (Table 19–11).

SHEEP AND CATTLE

Infectious diseases common to sheep and cattle are given in Table 19–12.

Bacteria

ACTINOMYCOSIS AND NECROBACILLOSIS

Actinomycosis in cattle *may* cause exophthalmos by invasion of the soft tissues of the orbit and pterygopalatine fossa by *Actinomyces bovis*. Similar signs may be seen in necrobacillosis (*Sphaerophorus necrophorus*) (*Fusobacterium necrophorum*) in calves.

LISTERIOSIS

Listeriosis is a bacterial disease of the brain caused by *Listeria monocytogenes*. The organisms have a predilection for the brain stem, producing foci of necrosis and inflammation. Multiple neurological signs are produced, including unilateral facial paresis or paralysis, abducent paralysis, trigeminal motor paralysis, and pharyngeal paralysis. Signs of disturbance to consciousness, as well as circling and paresis or paralysis of the limbs, indicate that the lesion is confined to the CNS. Vestibular signs often accompany the lesion because of the involvement of vestibular nuclei in the medulla. CSF is often abnormal, with changes characteristic of nonsuppurative disease (despite the fact that this is a bacterial disease).

There are no ocular signs in listerial abortion. Lis-

TABLE 19–11. Findings in Chronic Feline Renal Disease

Feature	Percentage	Feature	Percentage
Clinical Findings		*Laboratory Findings*	
Retinal detachment	4.4	Increased serum	96.9
Retinal atrophy	1.5	creatinine	95.8
Lethargy	93.0	Uremia	72.5
Weight loss	79.1	Hypercholesterolemia	58.3
Dehydration	61.8	Hyperphosphatemia	61.6
Emaciation	44.1	Hyperproteinemia	69.5
Polyuria, polydyspia	35.6	Proteinuria	56.8
Vomiting	27.4	Isosthenuria	56.9
Diarrhea	5.5	Lymphopenia	41.1
Irregular kidneys	25.0	Nonregenerative anemia	27.4
Enlarged kidneys	25.0	Leukocytosis	4.1
Oral ulcers	10.3	Leukopenia	2.7
Pale mucous membranes	7.3	Hypoproteinemia	29.7
Nephrotic syndrome	1.4	Hypokalemia	29.7
Ascites	1.4	Hyponatremia	23.5
Fever	6.9	Hyperglycemia	18.6
Hypothermia	15.5	Increased anion gap	11.5
		Hypercalcemia	14.8
Radiographic Findings		Hypocalcemia	11.1
Small kidneys	41.5	Hyperalbuminuria	11.1
Large kidneys	31.7	Hypoalbuminemia	7.8
Osteoporosis	9.8	Hypernatremia	6.2
Nephrocalcinosis	7.3	Hyperkalemia	4.8
		Hypochloremia	3.2
Autopsy Findings		Hyperchloremia	20.0
Chronic tubulointerstitial nephritis	52.7	Glucosuria	47.7
Renal lymphosarcoma	16.2	Cylindruria	12.5
Renal amyloidosis	9.5	Pyuria	12.5
Chronic pyelonephritis	9.5	Hematuria	
Chronic glomerulonephritis	8.1		
Polycystic renal disease	2.7		
Pyogranulomatous nephritis (FIP)	1.35		

From DiBartola SP, et al: Clinicopathologic findings associated with chronic renal disease in cats: 74 cases (1973–1984). J Am Vet Med Assoc 190:1196, 1987.

TABLE 19–12. Systemic Diseases of Cattle and Sheep with Ocular Signs

Infectious	Neoplasia	Hematological and Circulatory	Metabolic
Bacteria	Lymphosarcoma	Anemia	Polio encephalomalacia
Actinomycosis			Pregnancy toxemia
Listeriosis			
Necrobacillosis			
Ovine chlamydial polyarthritis			
Thromboembolic meningoencephalitis			
Viruses			
Arthrogryposis-hydrancephaly			
Bluetongue			
Infectious bovine rhinotracheitis			
Malignant catarrhal fever			
Mucosal disease–viral diarrhea			
Protozoal Disorders			
Babesiosis			
Parasitic			
Elaeophorosis			
Gedoelstiasis			

teriosis must be distinguished from other diseases that cause blindness and nervous signs in sheep and cattle (see Chap 21). The differential diagnosis for bovine listeriosis includes middle ear infections, polioencephalomalacia, thromboembolic meningoencephalitis (TEM), and rabies. Cattle with ear infections may show head tilt, ataxia, circling, and facial nerve dysfunction, but they are alert, responsive, and strong, as distinct from cattle with listeriosis, and they have no other neurological defects. Animals with polioencephalomalacia have severe depression and blindness, with intact pupillary reflexes, and lack signs of cranial nerve dysfunction except for dorsal esotropia caused by trochlear ear nerve involvement. TEM can be differentiated by acute, diffuse onset of neurological signs, short course, and recumbency within 48–72 hours. Cranial nerve deficits can be present, but the predominant signs are fever, depression, chorioretinitis and retinal hemorrhages, and neutrophilia and increased protein in the CSF (Table 19–13).

OVINE CHLAMYDIAL POLYARTHRITIS

Chlamydia psittaci causes epiphora, conjunctival hyperemia and follicular hyperplasia, keratitis with edema, and neovascularization in association with lameness and swollen joints in lambs. Elementary bodies in smears and the presence of joint signs allow differentiation from infectious ovine keratoconjunctivitis. The disease is usually self-limiting. It may be a different manifestation of chlamydial infection rather than a separate entity.

TEM

TEM in cattle is caused by *Hemophilus agni* infection and occurs in feedlot situations in North America, especially during cold weather. The mortality rate is high (95%), with death occurring within 6 hours after signs first occur.

Clinical Signs

1. Pyrexia
2. Head held up and forward
3. Stupor
4. Opisthotonis
5. Ataxia
6. Weakness
7. Paralysis
8. Retinal hemorrhages and retinitis (Fig. 19–20)

Variable Signs

1. Circling
2. Nystagmus
3. Strabismus
4. Blindness

TEM may be diagnosed ophthalmoscopically.

TABLE 19–13. Signs of Listeriosis in Cattle and Sheep

Meningoencephalitic Form	Septicemic Form (Mostly in Young Animals)
Dummy syndrome	Keratitis
Head pressing	Panophthalmitis
Unilateral facial paralysis	Hypopyon
Deviation of head (no rotation)	Nystagmus
	Dyspnea
Circling	Opisthotonus
Panophthalmitis	Early death
Hypopyon	

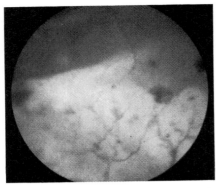

FIGURE 19–20. *Retinitis and retinal hemorrhages in bovine TEM. (Courtesy Dr. G. A. Severin.)*

Viruses

ARTHROGRYPOSIS-HYDRANENCEPHALY

Arthrogryposis-hydranencephaly is believed to be caused by a virus (Akabane virus). Calves born to affected cows show arthrogryposis (permanent joint contracture) and hydranencephaly (replacement of missing cerebral tissue). This condition frequently causes dystocia. Surviving calves are blind and mentally deranged. Ocular lesions include optic atrophy, vascular attenuation, tapetal hyperreflectivity, and pigmentation. Diagnosis is confirmed by a rising serum titer to the virus.

BLUETONGUE

Vaccination of pregnant ewes with attenuated bluetongue virus in the first half of pregnancy causes necrotizing retinopathy and CNS malformations in the offspring. During the last half of pregnancy the fetus is resistant.

Ewes should not be vaccinated for bluetongue in the first half of pregnancy.

INFECTIOUS BOVINE RHINOTRACHEITIS

Synonym: Rednose

Infectious bovine rhinotracheitis (IBR) occurs in two forms—the *conjunctival form,* in which no other signs are present, and the more common *respiratory form,* in which conjunctivitis is sometimes lacking. In both, conjunctivitis is acute, erythematous, and serous, with profuse lacrimation. White plaques may be present on the conjunctiva. Chemosis is sometimes present, but corneal lesions are rare. In the respiratory form, anorexia, fever, hyperemia of the nasal mucosa, nasal

discharge, and salivation occur. In the early acute stages, ocular lesions of IBR are distinguished from those of infectious bovine keratoconjunctivitis by *lack of corneal involvement.*

IBR is distinguished from infectious bovine keratoconjunctivitis (IBK) by lack of corneal involvement.

Vaccination with modified live IBR virus exacerbates outbreaks of IBK.

MALIGNANT CATARRHAL FEVER

Synonym: Bovine malignant catarrh

Malignant catarrhal fever (MCF) is a highly fatal viral disease of cattle. The catarrhal inflammation of upper respiratory and alimentary mucous membranes aids in differentiating the disease from other fulminating bovine viral diseases. Keratoconjunctival exanthema and lymph node enlargement also occur. Ocular lesions distinguish MCF from mucosal disease, rinderpest, muzzle disease, and infectious stomatitis. The corneal lesions of MCF start at the limbus and progress toward the center of the cornea, distinguishing them from IBK, which usually begins in the center of the cornea.

MUCOSAL DISEASE–BOVINE VIRAL DIARRHEA

Mucosal disease–bovine viral diarrhea (MD–BVD) is a widespread contagious viral disease of cattle occurring in *mild, acute,* and *chronic* forms. The clinical signs of each form are listed in Table 19–14. In addition to corneal opacity in adults, exposure of the fetus to the virus causes cataract, retinal atrophy, optic neuritis, microphthalmia with retinal dysplasia, and cerebellar hypoplasia. The retinal lesions are characterized by a gray optic disc, vascular attenuation, tapetal hyperreflectivity, and multifocal depigmentation of the nontapetal fundus.

Protozoal Diseases

BABESIOSIS

Babesiosis (*Babesia* spp) causes conjunctival injection and icterus in affected cattle.

Parasitic Diseases

COENUROSIS

Synonyms: Gid, sturdy

Coenurosis is invasion of the ovine brain by intermediate stages of *Taenia multiceps* and *T. serialis.*

TABLE 19–14. Clinical Forms of Mucosal Disease—Bovine Viral Diarrhea

Mild Form	Acute Form	Chronic Form
Fever	Fever	Laminitis with elongated, distorted hooves
Seromucoid nasal discharge	Obvious respiratory distress	Arched back
Rapid breathing	Leukopenia	Stools are pasty consistency, unformed, and abnormal in color
Nonproductive cough	Hyperemia and ulcers of oral mucosa	
Leukopenia	Weight loss	Rough haircoat, failure to shed
Decreased lactation	Dehydration	Slow weight gain
Variable appetite	Drying and peeling of muzzle	
Transient diarrhea		
Slow weight gain	Epiphora	
	Corneal opacity (in up to 10% of cases)	
	Anorexia	
	Acute laminitis	
	Diarrhea	

Modified from Rosner SF, Bittle JL: *In* Bovine Medicine and Surgery. American Veterinary Publications, Wheaton, IL, 1970.

ELAEOPHOROSIS

The adult worms of *Elaeophora schneideri* live in the carotid arteries and their branches in sheep, deer, and elk in the western United States, causing retinal necrosis, corneal opacity, uveitis, cataract, optic atrophy, retinal edema, and chorioretinal atrophy. Ophthalmoscopy aids diagnosis.

GEDOELSTIASIS

The migrating larvae of *Gedoelstia hassleri* (nasal botfly) in South Africa cause conjunctivitis, keratitis, exophthalmos, and panophthalmitis in sheep, cattle, goats, and horses in endemic areas.

Neoplasia

LYMPHOSARCOMA

Exophthalmos is seen in about 10% of cattle with lymphosarcoma, owing to infiltration of orbital tissues. Systemic involvement should be suspected in cattle with exophthalmos. Unilateral involvement is most common. Without the presence of other enlarged lymph nodes or other areas of lymphocytic infiltration, differential diagnoses include orbital cellulitis, orbital trauma, retrobulbar hemorrhage, and chronic sinusitis with orbital extension. The cornea on the affected side can be expected to undergo rapid dessication and ulceration. Affected animals are sent to slaughter.

Hematological Disorders

ANEMIA

Profound anemias in numerous intestinal parasitisms in sheep and cattle are first indicated by the pale appearance of the mucous membranes, especially the conjunctiva, for example, in *Haemonchus contortus* infection in sheep and ostertagiasis in cattle.

Metabolic Diseases

POLIOENCEPHALOMALACIA

Synonym: Cerebrocortical necrosis

Polioencephalomalacia occurs in pigs, sheep, and cattle and may be related to thiamine deficiency. Lambs between 2 and 4 months and calves about 6 months are most commonly affected. Polioencephalomalacia occurs at pasture and in feedlots.

Clinical Signs

Sheep
1. Blindness*
2. Trochlear paralysis (eye extorts and points medially) (see Fig. 17–6)*
3. Aimless wandering or motionless standing
4. Head pressing
These initial signs progress to:
5. Recumbency
6. Opisthotonus
7. Hyperesthesia
8. Nystagmus*
9. Tonic-clonic convulsions
Cattle
1. Blindness*
2. Muscle tremor (head especially)
3. Salivation
4. Opisthotonus
5. Convulsions
6. Head pressing
These signs are followed by:
7. Recumbency
8. Nystagmus*
9. Papilledema*
After progression to these last three signs, the animal either dies or recovers.

_____

*Ocular signs.

Differential Diagnosis

Sheep

Enterotoxemia *(Clostridium perfringens type D)* (glycosuria), focal symmetrical encephalomalacia, pregnancy toxemia

Cattle

Acute lead poisoning, enterotoxemia, hypomagnesemic tetany, hypovitaminosis A, arsenic and mercury toxicity, ketosis

PREGNANCY TOXEMIA AND ACETONEMIA

Pregnancy toxemia in sheep and acetonemia in cattle occur when animals are subjected to heavier demands on their resources of glucose and glycogen than can be met by their digestive and metabolic activity (Blood et al, 1979).

Conditions of Occurrence

Sheep and Goats

1. Ewes late in pregnancy
2. Ewes with twins or a large lamb
3. Falling plane of nutrition or short period of starvation
4. Cold weather

Cattle

1. High-producing, heavily fed dairy cows
2. Cattle at pasture or those inadequately fed
3. Cattle with specific nutritional deficiency

Clinical Signs

Sheep and Goats

Separation from flock
Blindness*
Grinding of teeth
Standing still
More severe nervous signs
Tremors and convulsions
Head pressing

Cattle

Nervous Form

Blindness*
Erratic behavior
Hyperesthesia
Tremor or tetany
Signs last 1–2 hours and recur at 8- to 12-hour intervals.

Wasting Form

Anorexia
Depressed milk yield
Loss of weight
Depression
Partial blindness and staggering (rare and transient)*

----

*Ocular signs.

TABLE 19–15. Systemic Equine Diseases with Ocular Signs

Disease	Ocular Signs or Lesions
Influenza/parainfluenza	Serous conjunctivitis, conjunctival erythema
Leukoencephalomalacia	Visual disturbance, dementia, circling, lethargy, pharyngeal paralysis
Leptospirosis	Conjunctival injection, jaundice; recurrent equine uveitis 1–2 years later
Equine viral arteritis	Chemosis, conjunctival hemorrhage, erythema, palpebral edema, epiphora, keratitis
Purpura hemorrhagica	Petechial conjunctival hemorrhages, orbital edema
Tetanus	Prominent third eyelid
Strangles	Chorioretinitis
Toxoplasmosis	Optic atrophy and focal retinal atrophy

Clinical Signs

1. Frenzy
2. Convulsions
3. Salivation

These initial signs are followed by:

4. Dullness
5. Head pressing
6. Ataxia
7. Blindness
8. Papilledema
9. Head deviation
10. Circling

HORSES

Ocular signs of systemic diseases are less common in horses than in other species and are summarized in Table 19–15.

TABLE 19–16. Systemic Porcine Diseases with Ocular Signs

Disease	Ocular Signs or Lesions
Hog cholera (swine fever)	Retinitis, uveitis
African swine fever	Keratitis, phthisis bulbi, blindness
Edema disease	Severe eyelid edema, exophthalmos
Mulberry heart disease	Severe eyelid edema, exophthalmos
Swine pox	Conjunctivitis, blepharitis, keratitis
Hypovitaminosis A	Microphthalmia (piglets), night blindness (late)
Teschen's disease (encephalomyelitis)	Retinitis

PIGS

Ocular signs of systemic diseases in pigs are summarized in Table 19–16.

Toxoplasmosis in Wallabies

Severe ocular lesions of *Toxoplasma* infection have been recorded in captive wallabies, resulting in cataracts and endophthalmitis (Ashton, 1979). Differential diagnosis of the cataracts should include nutritional causes.

REFERENCES

Abdelbaki YA, Davis RN (1972): Ophthalmoscopic findings in elaeophorosis of domestic sheep. Vet Med 67:69.

Adcock J, Hibler CP (1969): Vascular and neuroophthalmic pathology of elaeophorosis in elk. Path Vet 6:185.

Albert RA (1970): Lesions of the ocular fundus associated with systemic disease. J Am Vet Med Assoc 157:1635.

Angell JA, et al (1985): Ocular coccidioidomycosis in a cat. J Am Vet Med Assoc 187:167.

Angell JA, et al (1987): Ocular lesions associated with coccidioidomycosis in dogs: 35 cases (1980–1985). J Am Vet Med Assoc 190:1319.

Ashton N (1979): Ocular toxoplasmosis in wallabies *(Macropus rufogriseus)*. Am J Ophthalmol 88:322.

Barnett KC, Cottrell BD (1987): Ehlers-Danlos syndrome in a dog: Ocular, cutaneous and articular abnormalities. J Sm Anim Pract 28:941.

Bertoy RW, et al (1988): Intraocular melanoma with multiple metastases in a cat. J Am Vet Med Assoc 192:87.

Bistner SI, et al (1970): The ocular lesions of bovine viral diarrhea—mucosal disease. Pathol Vet 7:275.

Blood DC, et al (1983): Veterinary Medicine, 5th ed. Bailliere, Tindal & Cassell, London.

Breitschwerdt EB, et al (1987): Monoclonal gammopathy associated with naturally occurring canine ehrlichiosis. J Vet Int Med 1:2.

Brieder MA, et al (1988): Blastomycosis in cats: Five cases (1979–1986). J Am Vet Med Assoc 193:570.

Brooks, D, et al (1984): Ophthalmomyiasis interna in two cats. J Am Anim Hosp Assoc 20:157.

Bussanich MN, Rootman J (1983): Intraocular nematode in a cat. Feline Pract 13:24.

Buyukmihci N (1982): Ocular lesions of blastomycosis in the dog. J Am Vet Med Assoc 180:426.

Buyukmihci NC, Moore PF (1987): Microscopic lesions of spontaneous ocular blastomycosis in dogs. J Comp Pathol 97:321.

Campbell HB, et al (1984): Pulmonary squamous cell carcinoma with intraocular metastasis in a cat. J Am Vet Med Assoc 185:307.

Carlton WW (1976): Intraocular lymphosarcoma: Two cases in Siamese cats. J Am Anim Hosp Assoc 12:83.

Carter JD, et al (1971): Ocular and clinical features of canine thrombocytopenic purpura. Vet Med 66:125.

Cello RM (1960): Ocular manifestations of coccidioidomycosis in a dog. Arch Ophthalmol 64:897.

Cello RM, Hutcherson B (1962): Ocular changes in malignant lymphoma of dogs. Cornell Vet 52:492.

Center SA, Smith JF (1982): Ocular lesions in a dog with serum hyperviscosity syndrome secondary to an IgA myeloma. J Am Vet Med Assoc 181:811.

Clinkenbeard KD, et al (1987): Disseminated histoplasmosis in cats: 12 cases (1981–1986). J Am Vet Med Assoc 190:1445.

Collier LC, et al (1979): Ocular manifestations of the Chediak-Higashi syndrome in four species of animals. J Am Vet Med Assoc 175:587.

Collier LC, et al (1985): Tapetal degeneration in cats with Chediak Higashi syndrome. Curr Eye Res 4:767.

Cotter SM (1973): Multiple cases of feline leukemia and feline infectious peritonitis in a household. J Am Vet Med Assoc 162:1054.

Crispin SM, Barnett KC (1978): Arcus lipoides corneae secondary to hypothyroidism in the Alsatian. J Sm Anim Pract 19:127.

Doherty MJ (1971): Ocular manifestations of feline infectious peritonitis. J Am Vet Med Assoc 159:417.

Dubey JP, et al (1988): Newly recognized fatal protozoan disease of dogs. J Am Vet Med Assoc 12:1269.

Dubielzig RR (1984): Ocular sarcoma following trauma in three cats. J Am Vet Med Assoc 184:578.

Dunbar M, et al (1983): Treatment of canine blastomycosis with ketaconazole. J Am Vet Med Assoc 182:156.

Engerman RL, Bloodworth JMB (1965): Experimental diabetic retinopathy in dogs. Arch Ophthalmol 73:204.

Feldman ED, Nelson RW (1987): Canine and Feline Endocrinology and Reproduction. WB Saunders Co, Philadelphia.

Fischer CA (1970): Retinopathy in anemic cats. J Am Vet Med Assoc 156:1415.

Fischer CA (1971): Retinal and retinochoroidal lesions in early neuropathic canine distemper. J Am Vet Med Assoc 158:740.

French TW, et al (1987): A bleeding disorder (von Willebrand's disease) in a Himalayan cat. J Am Vet Med Assoc 190:437.

Frenkel JK (1977): Toxoplasmosis. *In* Kirk RW (ed): Current Veterinary Therapy VI. WB Saunders Co, Philadelphia.

Freundlich JJ, et al (1972): Indirect blood pressure determination by the ultrasonic Doppler technique in dogs. Curr Ther Res 14:73.

Garner HE, et al (1975): Indirect blood pressure measurements in the dog. Lab Anim Sci 25:197.

George L, et al (1988): Enhancement of infectious bovine keratoconjunctivitis by modified live infectious bovine rhinotracheitis virus vaccine. Am J Vet Res 49:1800.

Guildford WG, et al (1987): Primary immunodeficiency diseases of dogs and cats. Comp Cont Ed 9:641.

Gwin RM, et al (1978): Hypertensive retinopathy associated with hypothyroidism, hypercholesterolemia and renal failure in a dog. J Am Anim Hosp Assoc 14:200.

Gwin RM, et al (1980): Ocular lesions associated with *Brucella canis* infection in a dog. J Am Anim Hosp Assoc 16:607.

Hamilton HB, et al (1984): Pulmonary squamous cell carcinoma with intraocular metastasis in a cat. J Am Vet Med Assoc 185:307.

Hancock WK, Coats G (1911): Tubercle of the choroid in the cat. Vet Rec 23:533.

Hayes HM, et al (1981): Canine congenital deafness: Epidemiologic study of 272 cases. J Am Anim Hosp Assoc 17:473.

Hoganesch H, et al (1987): Seminoma with metastases in the eyes and the brain in a dog. Vet Pathol 24:278.

Holzworth J (1987): Mycotic diseases. *In* Holzworth J (ed): Diseases of the Cat. WB Saunders Co, Philadelphia.

Hribernik TN, et al (1982): Serum hyperviscosity syndrome associated with IgG myeloma in a cat. J Am Vet Med Assoc 170:169.

Hurvitz AI, et al (1970): Macroglobulinemia with hyperviscosity syndrome in a dog. J Am Vet Med Assoc 157:455.

Joseph RJ, et al (1988): Myasthenia gravis in the cat. J Vet Int Med 2:75.

Kilham L, et al (1967): Congenital infections of cats and ferret feline panleukopenia virus, manifested by cerebellar hypoplasia. Lab Invest 17:465.

Kilman L, et al (1971): Cerebellar ataxia and its congenital transmission in cats by feline panleukopenia. J Am Vet Med Assoc 158:888.

Kirschner SE, et al (1988): Blindness in a dog with IgA-forming myeloma. J Am Vet Med Assoc 193:349.

Kornegay J, et al (1980): Idiopathic hypocalcemia in four dogs. J Am Anim Hosp Assoc 16:723.

Krohne SDG, et al (1987): Ocular involvement in canine lymphosarcoma—A retrospective study of 94 cases. Proc Am Coll Vet Ophthalmol, Fort Worth, TX.

Kurtz HJ, Finca DR (1970): Granulomatous chorioretinitis caused by *Cryptococcus neoformans* in a dog. J Am Vet Med Assoc 157:934.

Lawford JB, Neane H (1923): Biocular choroidal tuberculosis with detachment of the retina in two kittens. Br J Ophthalmol 7:305.

Legendre AM, et al (1981): Canine blastomycosis: A review of 47 clinical cases. J Am Vet Med Assoc 178:1163.

Littman MP, et al (1988): Spontaneous systemic hypertension in dogs: Five cases (1981–1983). J Am Vet Med Assoc 193:486.

McConnell EE, et al (1970): Visceral leishmaniasis with ocular involvement in a dog. J Am Vet Med Assoc 156:197.

Miller WW, Boosinger TR (1987): Intraocular osteosarcoma in a cat. J Am Anim Hosp Assoc 23:320.

Montali RJ, Strandberg JD (1972): Extraperitoneal lesions in feline infectious peritonitis. Vet Pathol 9:109.

Morrison WI (1981): The pathogenesis of experimental *Trypanosoma brucei* infection in the dog. I. Tissue and organ damage. Am J Pathol 102:168.

Mushi EZ, et al (1980): Isolation of bovine malignant catarrhal fever virus from ocular and nasal secretions of wildebeest calves. Res Vet Sci 29:168.

Neer TM (1988): Disseminated aspergillosis. Comp Cont Ed 10:465.

O'Donnell JA, Hayes KC (1987): Nutrition and nutritional disorders. *In* Holzworth J (ed): Diseases of the Cat. WB Saunders Co, Philadelphia.

Olin DD, et al (1976): Lipid-laden aqueous humor associated with anterior uveitis and concurrent hyperlipemia in two dogs. J Am Vet Med Assoc 168:861.

Pedersen NC (1987): Basic and clinical immunology. *In* Holzworth J (ed): Diseases of the Cat. WB Saunders Co, Philadelphia.

Piper RC, et al (1970): Natural and experimental ocular toxoplasmosis in animals. Am J Ophthalmol 69:662.

Rebhun WC (1982): Orbital lymphosarcoma in cattle. J Am Vet Med Assoc 180:149.

Rebhun WC (1986): Diseases of the bovine orbit and globe. J Am Vet Med Assoc 190:171.

Rebhun WC, deLahunta A (1982): Diagnosis and treatment of bovine listeriosis. J Am Vet Med Assoc 180:395.

Rhodes KH, et al (1987): Comparative aspects of canine and human atopic dermatitis. Semin Vet Med Surg 2:166.

Roberts SR, Bistner SI (1974): Ocular diseases. *In* Ettinger SJ (ed): Textbook of Veterinary Internal Medicine. WB Saunders Co, Philadelphia.

Roeder PL, et al (1986): Pestivirus fetopathogenicity in cattle: Changing sequelae with fetal maturation. Vet Rec 118:44.

Rubin LF (1974): Atlas of Veterinary Ophthalmoscopy. Lea & Febiger, Philadelphia.

Saunders LZ, Rubin LF (1974): Ophthalmic Pathology of Animals. S Karger, Basel.

Scott DW (1978): Immunologic skin disorders in the dog and cat. Vet Clin North Am 8:641.

Shively JM, Whiteman CE (1970): Ocular lesions in disseminated coccidioidomycosis in two dogs. Path Vet 7:1.

Silverstein AM, et al (1971): An experimental virus-induced retinal dysplasia in the fetal lamb. Am J Ophthalmol 72:22.

Slatter DH, et al (1973): Ocular manifestations of myeloproliferative disease. Aust Vet J 50:164.

Slatter DH, et al (1979): Effects of experimental hyperlipoproteinemia on the canine eye. Exp Eye Res 29:437.

Slauson DO, Finn PJ (1972): Meningoencephalitis and panophthalmitis in feline infectious peritonitis. J Am Vet Med Assoc 160:729.

Stephens LR, et al (1981): Infectious thromboembolic meningoencephalitis in cattle: A review. J Am Vet Med Assoc 178:378.

Vainisi SJ, Campbell LH (1969): Ocular toxoplasmosis in cats. J Am Vet Med Assoc 154:141.

van den Broek AHM (1987): Horner's syndrome in cats and dogs: A review. J Sm Anim Pract 28:929.

Waddle JR, Littman MR (1988): A retrospective study of 27 cases of naturally occurring canine ehrlichiosis. J Am Anim Hosp Assoc 24:615.

Whiteley HE, et al (1985): Ocular lesions of bovine malignant catarrhal fever. Vet Pathol 22:219.

Willeberg P, Priester WA (1982): Epidemiological aspects of clinical hyperadrenocorticism in dogs (canine Cushing's syndrome). J Am Anim Hosp Assoc 18:717.

Williams LW, et al (1981): Ophthalmic neoplasms in the cat. J Am Anim Hosp Assoc 17:999.

Woog J, et al (1983): Osteosarcoma in a phthisical feline eye. Vet Pathol 20:209.

Yang S (1987): Gray collie syndrome—Letter to the editor. J Am Vet Med Assoc 191:390.

Zerbe C (1986): Canine hyperlipemias. *In* Kirk RW (ed): Current Veterinary Therapy IX. WB Saunders Co, Philadelphia.

20

Ocular Emergencies

MATERIALS REQUIRED	SEVERE OCULAR AND ADNEXAL	HYPHEMA
PROPTOSIS OF THE GLOBE	CONTUSIONS AND	ACUTE ANTERIOR UVEITIS
GLAUCOMA	CONCUSSION	SEVERE CORNEAL ULCERATION
CORNEAL LACERATION	PENETRATING INJURIES	SUDDEN BLINDNESS
LID LACERATIONS	DESCEMETOCELE AND IRIS	
	PROLAPSE	

The conditions discussed in this chapter are the most important disorders in which early action is necessary to prevent severe or permanent damage to the eye. Emergency treatment is outlined separately for ready clinical reference, followed by further discussion for those conditions not covered elsewhere in the text.

MATERIALS REQUIRED

Basic Diagnostic Instruments and Supplies

Magnifying loupe 2× to 4× magnification
Direct ophthalmoscope and Finnoff's transilluminator
Lid retractors—handheld
Sterile eye wash
Fluorescein strips
"Weck cell" cellulose sponges
Schiøtz tonometer
Culture swabs and media

Surgical Instruments

Needle holders (Derf's or Castroviejo's)
Tenotomy scissors
Lacrimal cannula
Irrigating bulb
Fixation forceps
No. 15 scalpel blade
Foreign body spud
Lid retractors (Castroviejo's or Vierheller's)

Medications

Topical anesthetic
Tropicamide (Mydriacyl), 1%

Atropine, 1%, drops and ointment
Mannitol, 20%, parenteral
Chilled glycerin
Diamox, 500-mg vial, intravenous (IV) preparation
Pilocarpine, 2%, drops
Neosporin drops
Chloromycetin drops and ointment
Tear replacement solution

Before manipulating the eye, always perform a thorough clinical examination.

PROPTOSIS OF THE GLOBE
(Fig. 20–1)

Emergency Treatment for Proptosis of the Globe[1]

1. Anesthetize the patient.
2. Replace the globe as soon as possible to prevent severe corneal damage. If first aid is to be administered by a client in a distant location prior to transport, advise keeping the eye moist with wet cotton or whatever is available and to avoid additional trauma from movement.
3. Flush the conjunctival sac free of extraneous debris with sterile saline solution and lubricate the cornea with tear replacement solution and antibiotic drops.
4. Using fine Vetafil or 4/0 nylon, place three or four simple, interrupted sutures as shown in Figure 20–2A and B. If possible, sutures

---

1. Modified from Severin GA: Veterinary Ophthalmology Notes, 2nd ed. Fort Collins, CO, 1976.

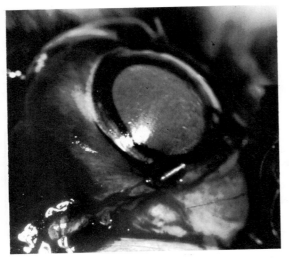

FIGURE 20–1. A prolapsed globe in a Pekingese. (Courtesy of Dr. R. Cooper.)

should emerge on the lid margin rather than on the conjunctival surface to prevent corneal abrasion after replacement of the globe.

5. Apply a suitable antibiotic ointment (e.g., chloramphenicol) to the eye.

6. Place a scalpel handle across the cornea, beneath the sutures, and draw up on each of the sutures simultaneously, as shown in Figure 20–1C and D. This pulls the lids forward to protect the cornea and replaces the globe within the orbit.

7. The sutures are tied (Fig. 20–1E). If necessary, that is, if pressure is extensive, additional intermarginal lid sutures may be placed between the original traction sutures.

8. Using the dorsal rim of the orbit as a landmark, inject 10–20 mg of triamcinolone 2–3 cm by retrobulbar injection.

9. Apply atropine ointment (1%) and chloromycetin ointment to the conjunctival sac between the sutures.

10. Give an IV injection of dexamethasone (10–15 mg), and flunixin meglumine (1 mg/kg) to limit and control secondary uveitis. (For maintenance therapy, see further on.)

Prognosis

The sooner the eye is replaced, the better the prognosis, both for saving the eye and for shortening the convalescent period. Unfortunately, some eyes are inevitably lost despite early and vigorous treatment. The following features are useful prognostic indicators.

AVULSION OF EXTRAOCULAR MUSCLES

The medial and inferior (ventral) recti and inferior (ventral) oblique muscles rupture first. Because branches of the ciliary artery to the anterior segment enter the globe with the extraocular muscles, complete avulsion of all muscles indicates a grave prognosis. In eyes with only a few of the muscles ruptured, temporary postoperative deviations of the visual axis occur.

HYPHEMA

Marked hyphema is an unfavorable sign, as it is usually associated with severe damage to the ciliary body, leading to hypotension and phthisis bulbi.

PUPIL SIZE

1. *Miotic pupil*—favorable prognosis as this is the normal response to trauma.

2. *Mydriatic pupil*—indicates damages to oculomotor or optic nerves or ciliary ganglion. Prognosis is guarded to unfavorable for vision.

Note: Complete transection of the optic nerve may result in a pupil of nearly normal size if associated with disruption of both sympathetic and parasympathetic innervation.

PUPILLARY REFLEXES

A consensual reflex to the unaffected eye is a favorable sign. Loss of reflexes in the injured eye is of little prognostic significance, but if the reflexes have not returned within a week it is likely that there is permanent ocular damage. According to Severin, the most favorable set of prognostic indicators is the following:

1. Lack of hyphema
2. Partial prolapse only (the globe is held tightly against the lids)
3. Minimal damage to extraocular muscles (only one or two affected)
4. Pinpoint miotic pupil

Maintenance Therapy

1. Continued systemic antibiotics for 7 days.

2. Continued application of antibiotic and 1% atropine ointment through the medial canthus twice daily by the owner (*note:* only if the patient is easily handled).

3. Initial sutures are left in place for 3 weeks. If the lids do not meet (lagophthalmos), the sutures should be replaced for 2–3 weeks longer to allow residual orbital swelling to regress and to prevent corneal desiccation and ulceration.

4. During resolution, deep corneal vascularization proceeds from the limbus to the center of the cornea. It should *not* be inhibited by corticosteroids. The cornea

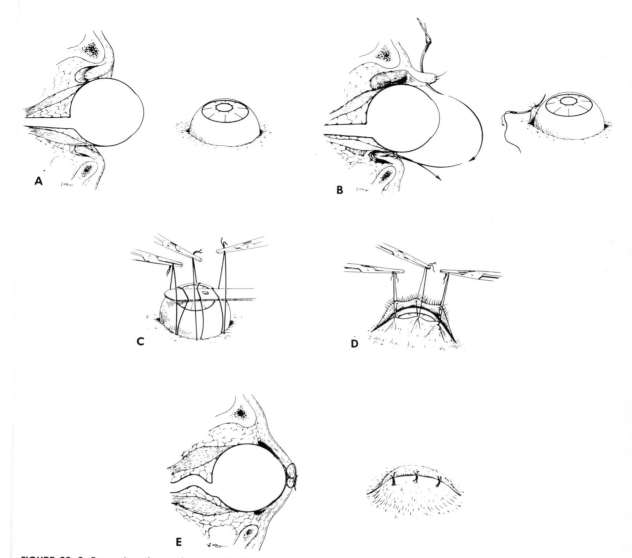

FIGURE 20–2. *Procedure for replacement of prolapsed globe. A, Prolapsed globe. B, Placement of simple interrupted traction sutures of 4/0 nylon or fine Vetafil. C, Placement of scalpel handle. D, Traction on the sutures and replacement of the globe. E, Completion of the sutures. (Courtesy of Dr. G.A. Severin.)*

gradually clears from the limbus to the center, and at this final stage, topical steroids may be used. The course may run as long as 4–6 weeks in severely damaged corneas.

5. Traumatic strabismus is a frequent complication of prolapse of the globe. The visual axis is usually deviated dorsally and laterally (see Fig. 20–1) resulting from rupture of the inferior oblique and medial rectus muscles. Although such deviation may appear unsightly (Fig. 20–3) and can be corrected surgically, most cases resolve spontaneously in 6–9 months. If deviation is noted at the time of replacement, it may be repaired at that time by attempting to resuture the ends of the damaged muscle (usually the medial rectus). With

time, the ends of the muscle retract, making accurate reapposition more difficult.

6. Prolapse occurs most frequently in brachycephalic breeds with shallow orbits (e.g., Pekingese, Boston terrier, pug). It is extremely important that excessive pressure around the neck of these breeds be avoided, especially after prolapse.

7. If continued lagophthalmos occurs (and lid innervation is intact) after suture removal, a temporary tarsorrhaphy is performed and left in place for 3–6 months. In some patients, long-term partial exophthalmos remains, probably because of scar tissue in the orbit, or lid retraction, causing partial drying of the cornea. Medial and sometimes lateral reconstructive

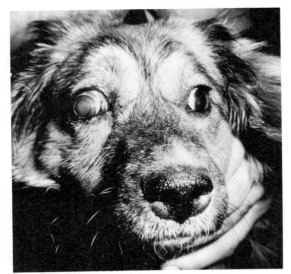

FIGURE 20–3. *Postprolapse deviation (exotropia). (Courtesy of Dr. G.A. Severin.)*

blepharoplasty and artificial tear supplementation are indicated to decrease precorneal tear film evaporation and to protect the cornea in such patients.

With severely damaged eyes, it is preferable to replace the globe and wait several days before resorting to enucleation, unless rupture has occurred. Most prolapsed eyes can be salvaged.

GLAUCOMA

The steps outlined in the box are for emergency treatment only.

Emergency Treatment of Glaucoma

1. IV mannitol, 1.5 g/kg (7.5 ml/kg of 20% solution) over 5–10 minutes.

2. IV acetazolamide (Diamox), 5–10 mg/kg—*caution is necessary if the patient has been previously medicated with oral carbonic anhydrase inhibitors.*

3. Oral glycerin, 0.2 ml/kg, fed chilled and in three divided doses daily. This method is especially useful for owners.

4. Pilocarpine drops, 2%, administered every 5 minutes for 30 minutes, then every 3 hours. Monitor for bradycardia and other side effects of parasympathetic stimulation during this time.

Paracentesis is contraindicated in the emergency treatment of glaucoma.

Interim Therapy

After initial lowering of pressure, interim therapy is often required to prevent pressure elevation before the veterinary ophthalmologist is consulted for further diagnostic procedures and maintenance therapy. If pupillary block is not present, the following maintenance regimen can be used until final diagnosis is made and treatment is begun.

1. Oral glycerin, 2 ml/kg, fed chilled and divided into three doses daily.

2. Carbonic anhydrase inhibitors, for example, dichlorphenamide, 2 mg/kg, 3 times daily by mouth, or ethoxyzolamide, 5 mg/kg, 2 or 3 times daily by mouth.

3. Pilocarpine (2%) drops, 3 times daily.

Definitive diagnosis and therapy should be commenced as soon as possible.

CORNEAL LACERATION

Emergency Treatment of Corneal Laceration

1. Carefully examine the eye, and if laceration is suspected place the patient under general anesthesia to prevent further damage and allow a closer examination.

2. Avoid pressure on the globe. Stain the eye with fluorescein and examine the anterior chamber with a focal light source to determine if the cornea has been perforated.

3. Place a third eyelid flap over the affected eye (see p 137).

4. Institute systemic antibiotic therapy and topical antibiotic drops (*not* ointment).

5. Administer 1% atropine drops 3 times daily.

6. Administer flunixin meglumine, 1 mg/kg, IV (or appropriate equine dosage).

7. If penetration has occurred, give systemic corticosteroids (e.g., dexamethasone, 1 mg/kg, intramuscularly [IM]) to limit uveitis and fibrin exudation into the anterior chamber.

8. If the laceration is superficial, treat as described in Chapter 11. Penetrating or doubtful lacerations should be treated by a veterinary ophthalmologist after full ophthalmic examination to determine the extent of ocular injuries.

LID LACERATIONS[2]

Treatment

Three factors determine the treatment of lid lacerations:

1. Time since injury, which affects degree of bacterial contamination.

2. Involvement of lid margin and especially lacrimal puncta and canaliculi.

3. Extent of lesion (plastic reconstruction may be necessary).

Emergency Treatment of Lid Lacerations

1. Determine the time since injury, and proceed accordingly; that is:

a. Four hours or less—immediate repair.

b. Four to 24 hours—immediate or delayed repair, depending on evaluation of injury.

c. After 24 hours—treat as an open wound until gross infection is controlled, then repair as an elective procedure.

2. Induce general anesthesia.

3. Administer systemic antibiotics—gentamicin, 4 mg/kg IV and 4 mg/kg IM or cefazolin 20 mg/kg IV and 20 mg/kg IM.

4. If the lid margins are involved, accurate reapposition and suturing is performed, using 5/0 or 6/0 silk, to prevent "notching," postoperative scarring, ectropion, and epiphora and to generally improve the cosmetic appearance (see Chap. 7, Fig. 7–34).

5. If lid margins are not involved, treat as a simple skin laceration, avoiding tension on the lid margins.

6. If the wound is extensive, requires plastic repair, or involves the lacrimal canaliculi, initial first aid procedures are completed, and the wound is protected against further damage (e.g., by use of bandage, Elizabethan collar, and systemic antibiotics) before the animal is transported to a referral center for final evaluation and treatment.

Important Facts

1. Débridement is minimized in repair of lid lacerations.

2. Because of the excellent blood supply to the eyelids, lid lacerations usually heal well, even if contaminated.

3. Because lid lacerations are often irritating during

---

the healing phase, the following measures may be taken if necessary to prevent self-mutilation:

a. Elizabethan collar.

b. Taping of dewclaws.

c. Sedation.

SEVERE OCULAR AND ADNEXAL CONTUSIONS AND CONCUSSION

A *contusion* is damage due to direct contact with the globe by an object. *Concussion* is damage due to trauma adjacent to the eye when forces are transmitted to the eye.

Two important points should be kept in mind when treating contusions or concussions involving the eye:

1. External trauma may cause severe intraocular injuries even if the globe is not penetrated.

2. Post-traumatic uveitis is frequent and must be controlled.

Common Clinical Signs Associated with Ocular Trauma

1. Hyphema
2. Chemosis
3. Subconjunctival hemorrhages
4. Corneal desiccation
5. Proptosis of the globe (Fig. 20–2)
6. Swollen lids
7. Paralysis of lids
8. Lack of pupillary light reflexes
9. Pain on palpation
10. Fibrin in the anterior chamber
11. Miosis or anisocoria (difference in the size of pupils)
12. Corneal edema
13. Lens luxation or subluxation
14. Retinal detachment and hemorrhages
15. Decreased motility or deviation of the globe
16. Blindness or visual field defects
17. Associated signs of central nervous system (CNS) damage—for example, coma, nystagmus

---

Emergency Treatment of Ocular Contusions and Concussions
(Fig. 20–4)

1. After a general physical examination and treatment of life-threatening disorders, examine the eye and adnexa and record findings. If necessary, anesthetize the patient. Palpate the orbital rim and facial bones and, if necessary, radiograph the area.

2. Examine direct and consensual pupillary light reflexes.

3. Carefully examine the cornea with a mag-

---

2. See also Chap. 7.

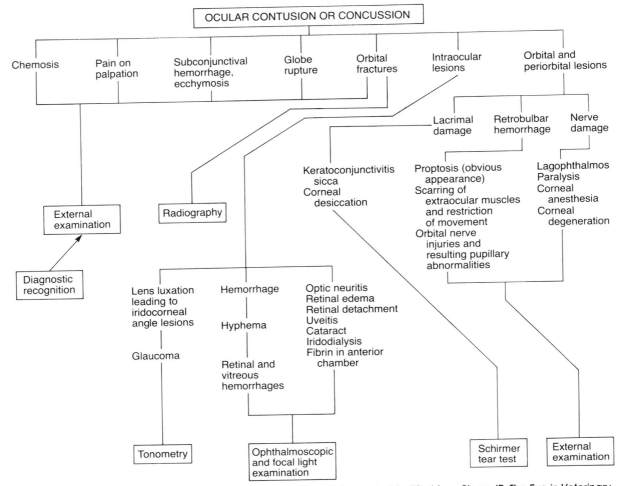

FIGURE 20—4. Ocular contusions and concussions—sequelae and diagnosis. (Modified from Blogg JR: The Eye in Veterinary Practice. VS Supplies, North Melbourne, Victoria, Australia, 1975.)

nifying loupe and, if necessary, stain with fluorescein.

4. Perform an ophthalmoscopic examination and check for the position of the lens, hemorrhages in the vitreous or retina, retinal detachment, and fibrin in the anterior chamber.

5. Administer the following:

   a. Systemic corticosteroids (dexamethasone, IM or IV).

   b. Flunixin meglumine (1 mg/kg IV or appropriate equine dosage).

   c. Systemic antibiotics (chloramphenicol, 25 mg/kg).

   d. Atropine, 1% drops, twice daily.

   e. Tear replacement solutions as necessary.

6. Institute cage rest or stable confinement immediately, and examine the eye frequently (at least every 4 hours) thereafter.

7. If complications develop or severe intraocular lesions are suspected, refer for specialist treatment.

PENETRATING INJURIES

Emergency Treatment of Penetrating Injuries

Initial attempts are directed at preventing further injury.

1. Administer tranquilizers or analgesics as necessary to prevent self-trauma.

2. Avoid all pressure on the eye and periorbital area.

3. Carefully examine the eye to evaluate the extent of injuries.

4. Administer systemic antibiotics to prevent infection. High doses of Na^+ or K^+ penicillin (25,000–50,000 units/kg) are useful, as the blood-eye barrier is permeable after trauma. Administer topical antibiotics (drops) frequently, but avoid gentamicin, which is toxic intraocularly.

5. Administer systemic corticosteroids (e.g., dexamethasone, 2–5 mg IM in an average-sized dog) to limit uveitis after antibiotics have been administered.

6. Administer flunixin meglumine (1 mg/kg) IV to reduce uveitis.

7. Obtain a thorough history of the cause of the trauma and how it occurred. This is important so that preventive measures to avoid further complications may be taken if necessary; for example, in the case of vegetable foreign bodies, which are sources of saprophytic fungal infections.

8. Protect the eye from further trauma by the following means, as necessary:

    a. Third eyelid flap or intermarginal tarsorrhaphy.

    b. Elizabethan collar.

    c. Taping of dewclaws.

    d. Tranquilizers and analgesics.

    e. Cross-tying or neck brace in horses.

9. Maintain antibiotic and steroid cover until specialist assistance can be obtained (all penetrating or severe ocular injuries should be treated by a veterinary ophthalmologist, if possible).

DESCEMETOCELE AND IRIS PROLAPSE

Once the diagnosis has been confirmed, immediate steps are undertaken to prevent rupture of the cornea or further displacement of the iris and to stabilize and support the cornea until definitive surgical treatment can be performed.

Emergency Treatment of Descemetocele and Iris Prolapse

1. Anesthetize or tranquilize the patient.

2. Administer 25 mg/kg acetazolamide IV and begin a drip with 20% mannitol, 1 g/kg, to reduce intraocular pressure.

3. Begin anticollagenase therapy (Chap 3) and topical antibiotics.

4. In descemetocele, a third eyelid or 360° conjunctival flap may be used if surgical correction is to be delayed, for example, by direct suturing, corneoscleral transposition, or temporary supportive keratoplasty.

5. In iris prolapse, the protruding piece of iris (usually a grayish color) may be excised, the cornea sutured, and the anterior chamber reconstituted with an air bubble (Fig. 20–5). Such

treatment should be attempted by experienced persons only.

HYPHEMA

Hyphema is the presence of blood in the anterior chamber. It most commonly results from hemorrhage in the iris and ciliary body. Less frequently, blood originates from the posterior uveal tract or retina, for example, in the scleral ectasia syndrome.

Emergency Treatment of Hyphema[3]

1. Prevent further ocular trauma and confine the patient as soon as possible after injury.

2. Administer corticosteroid drops (dexamethasone, 0.1%, prednisolone, 1%, 3 or 4 times daily.

3. If the hyphema is mild, administer pilocarpine (1%) drops 3 times daily, and every 2nd day dilate the pupil with phenylephrine, 10%, to prevent posterior synechia formation.

4. If the hyphema is severe, administer 1% atropine drops 3 times daily to control the presumed uveitis present, and monitor intraocular pressure daily as the blood resorbs. Rebleeding occasionally occurs within the first 5 days.

5. If the color of the hyphema changes from bright red to bluish black ("eight-ball hemorrhage") 5–7 days after onset, and intraocular pressure increases, surgical intervention may be indicated.

6. If recurring hyphema occurs, begin laboratory examination 2nd work-up including complete blood count, platelets, toenail bleeding time, and clotting parameters.

7. The use of vitamins C and K, calcium, and estrogens has not been beneficial in the treatment of hyphema.

Note: Although uveitis is often present with hyphema, use of prostaglandin inhibitors is not advised because many of them also prolong blood clotting through their effect on platelets.

ACUTE ANTERIOR UVEITIS

This condition requires urgent treatment because
1. It can be extremely painful.

---

3. Prostaglandin inhibitors, which affect platelets and clotting, are contraindicated in hyphema.

The use of atropine and pilocarpine in hyphema is controversial, with conflicting experimental and human clinical data used to support significantly differing regimens.

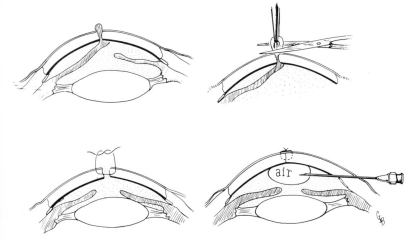

FIGURE 20–5. Technique for removal of incarcerated iris tissue in a corneal wound. Sutures in the cornea lie deep in the middle third of the corneal stroma and do not enter the anterior chamber. The anterior chamber can be re-formed by an air bubble delivered through a needle entering the eye at the limbus. Adequately closed corneal wounds are airtight, permitting the anterior chamber to maintain its depth. (From Bistner SI, Aguirre GD: Management of ocular emergencies. Vet Clin North Am 2:359, 1972.)

2. Life-threatening systemic disorders may be associated with it.

3. Permanent structural lesions may result in undesirable sequelae—for example, secondary glaucoma, iris bombé, cataract.

Emergency Treatment of Acute Anterior Uveitis

After diagnosis, the following treatment is instituted:

1. Topical atropine, 1%, 3 times daily.
2. Broad-spectrum systemic antibiotics.
3. Topical antibiotics, for example, chloramphenicol, 4 times daily.
4. Subconjunctival *nonrepository* corticosteroids, for example, 1 mg dexamethasone.[4]
5. Topical and systemic corticosteroids.[4]
6. Systemic therapy with prostaglandin inhibitors, for example, flunixin meglumine, aspirin. (See Chaps 3 and 12.)
7. Full ophthalmic and physical examination and laboratory studies to find the cause of the uveitis. This search may be unrewarding.

SEVERE CORNEAL ULCERATION

A thorough eye examination is performed, with special attention to the eyelids, third eyelid, and anterior chamber.

Emergency Treatment of Corneal Ulceration

1. A Schirmer tear test is performed.
2. A moistened bacterial swab and scraping

---

are taken from the margins of the ulcer for culture, cytological examination, and Gram's staining.

3. The ulcer is stained with fluorescein and accurately drawn, as a reference to determine the efficacy of future treatment.

4. A subconjunctival injection of an appropriate antibiotic is given—for example, 10 mg gentamicin, tobramycin, or amikacin, 40 mg chloramphenicol, 1 million units Na$^+$ penicillin with 0.1 ml epinephrine (1:1000).

5. Atropine (1%) drops 2 times daily if keratoconjunctivitis sicca is not present.

6. If ulceration is especially severe, a third eyelid flap (p 137) or conjunctival flap is applied, and compound ulcer medication is used (for formula see Chap 11).

Further diagnostic attempts and maintenance therapy (e.g., subpalpebral lavage) may be commenced.

In all corneal ulcers, inspect beneath the third eyelid for foreign bodies.

SUDDEN BLINDNESS

A complete history and eye examination is necessary to diagnose the cause of sudden loss of vision. Differential diagnosis in dogs includes:

1. Acute glaucoma
2. Retinal detachment
3. Acute uveitis with retinal detachment, optic neuritis, for example, a Vogt-Koyanagi-Harada–like syndrome.
4. Retinal or vitreous hemorrhages, for example, feline hypertensive retinopathy, rodenticide poisoning.

---

4. Use with caution or not at all if an infectious cause is suspected.

5. Sudden acquired retinal degeneration (canine).

6. After epileptic seizures.

7. Various toxicities, for example, owner administered marijuana in small animals, *Stypandra imbricata* toxicity in sheep.

8. End-stage progressive retinal degenerations.

9. Acute onset of cataract, for example, in diabetes mellitus.

10. Inflammatory disorders of the central visual pathways, for example, postdistemper encephalitis, reticulosis.

Refer to detailed discussion of the responsible condition for appropriate therapy, and algorithms in Chapter 21.

REFERENCES

Bistner SI, Aguirre GD (1972): Management of ocular emergencies. Vet Clin North Am 2:359.

Paton D, Goldberg MF (1976): Management of Ocular Injuries. WB Saunders Co, Philadelphia.

Rosin E (1989): In press. Am J Vet Res

Severin GA (1976): Veterinary Ophthalmology Notes. 2nd ed. Fort Collins, CO, 1976.

21

Differential Diagnosis of Common Ocular Diseases and Syndromes

---

COMMON OCULAR DISEASES
THE RED EYE
EPIPHORA
THE DISCOLORED EYE
CORNEAL ULCERATION
THE PAINFUL EYE
PROMINENT THIRD EYELID
COMMON NEONATAL OCULAR DISORDERS
NEONATAL OCULAR DISORDERS IN FOALS
PERIOCULAR ALOPECIA OR DERMATITIS

CHRONIC CONJUNCTIVITIS IN DOGS
FELINE CONJUNCTIVITIS
BLINDNESS IN SHEEP
BLINDNESS AND NERVOUS DYSFUNCTION IN CATTLE
COMMON BOVINE OCULAR DISORDERS

SUDDEN ACQUIRED BLINDNESS
SUDDEN BLINDNESS, RETINAL DETACHMENTS, HEMORRHAGES, AND UVEITIS
ANISOCORIA
OCULAR DISEASES OF CAGED BIRDS
OCULAR CONDITIONS OF FISH
OCULAR DISEASE IN POULTRY
OCULAR DISEASE IN RABBITS, RODENTS, AND REPTILES

In considering common ocular syndromes, it is important to be familiar with the major disease problems in a breed (see Appendix II), species, or age group. This assists the veterinarian in general practice in making a reasonable differential diagnosis and not overlooking common disorders. It also helps prevent the "zebra diagnosis."[1]

In this chapter, common groups of clinical signs are presented graphically for clinical reference. Detailed consideration of specific conditions is omitted. For further details refer to relevant text chapters.

---

1. If hoofbeats are heard outside the barn, they are more likely to belong to a horse than to a zebra.

COMMON OCULAR DISORDERS

THE RED EYE

GLAUCOMA

1. Elevated intraocular pressure
2. Pain
3. Corneal edema
4. Mydriasis
5. Breed predisposition
6. Lens luxation
7. Blindness
8. Corneal edema over the site of endothelial touch by the luxated lens
9. Episcleral vascularization
10. Optic disc cupping

CORNEAL ULCERATION

1. Fluorescein-positive
2. Ulcer visible
3. Blepharospasm
4. Photophobia
5. Hypopyon
6. Concurrent conjunctivitis and uveitis
7. Pain

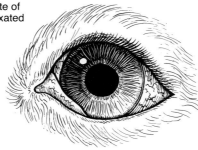

CONJUNCTIVITIS

1. Mucopurulent discharge
2. Superficial vascular engorgement
3. Neutrophils on scrapings
4. Positive bacteria, fungal culture
5. Occasional chemosis
6. Few visual consequences
7. Normal pressure
8. Normal pupil size and reflexes

UVEITIS

1. Miosis
2. Aqueous flare
3. Hyphema
4. Fibrin clots
5. Vitreous haze
6. Blepharospasm
7. Photophobia
8. Hypopyon
9. Pain
10. Ciliary flush
11. Decreased intraocular pressure

EPIPHORA

SHEEP
1. Painful corneal lesion
2. Entropion (lambs)
3. Infectious ovine keratoconjunctivitis

HORSES
1. Painful corneal lesion
2. *Habronema* conjunctivitis
3. Nasolacrimal obstruction
4. Influenza and parainfluenza

CATTLE
1. Painful corneal lesion
2. Infectious bovine keratoconjunctivitis

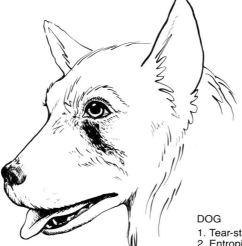

CAT
1. Tear-staining (Persians)
2. Lacrimal punctal atresia
3. Dacryocystitis
4. Entropion
5. Painful corneal lesions
6. Punctal scarring after conjunctivitis
7. Feline corneal necrosis syndrome

DOG
1. Tear-staining syndrome
2. Entropion
3. Lacrimal punctal atresia
4. Dacryocystitis
5. Painful corneal lesions
6. Distichiasis
7. Ectopic cilia
8. Allergic inhalant dermatitis (atopy)

THE DISCOLORED EYE

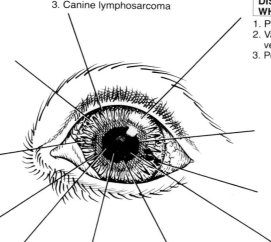

CORNEAL EDEMA

BLUISH WHITE
1. Hazy blue
2. Vascularization if chronic
3. Intraocular pressure—
   normal or increased
   (glaucoma may be present)
4. Stain with fluorescein
5. Onset—acute or chronic

VASCULARIZATION

RED OR BLUE
1. Ciliary or corneal
2. Deep or superficial
3. Signs of uveitis

HYPHEMA

RED OR RED/BLACK
1. Trauma
2. Blood dyscrasias
3. Diffuse or clotted
4. Intraocular pressure—
   normal, decreased, or
   elevated
5. Pupil size

CORNEAL STROMAL HEMORRHAGE

RED
1. Usually near limbus
2. Trauma
3. Canine lymphosarcoma

AQUEOUS LIPEMIA

WHITE
1. Miosis
2. Signs of uveitis
3. Serum lipemia
4. Visual deficit
5. Distinguish from
   corneal edema by a
   clear cornea
6. Early resolution

HYPOPYON

YELLOW
1. Diffuse or ventral
2. Corneal lesions
3. Systemic bacteremia
   or signs
4. Signs of uveitis

FIBRIN

YELLOW-BROWN
1. Signs of uveitis
2. Systemic signs
3. Trauma
4. Intraocular pressure
   depressed

CORNEAL SCAR

**DISORGANIZED, BLUISH-
WHITE COLLAGEN**
1. Previous corneal injury
2. Vascularization or ghost
   vessels
3. Possible pigmentation

DILATED PUPIL

**APPEARS GREEN OR
YELLOW, THE COLOR OF
THE TAPETUM**
1. Increased tapetal reflectivity
2. Breed susceptibility

PIGMENTATION

BLACK OR BROWN
1. Usually chronic
2. Vascularization usually
   present
3. Brachycephalic patient

LENS OPACITY

MILKY WHITE
1. Lens visible
2. Progressive or stationary
3. Visual deficit
4. Purkinje's images
5. Breed susceptibility
6. Fundus visible (distinguish
   sclerosis)

CORNEAL ULCERATION

SUGGESTIVE SIGNS

1. Fluorescein-positive
2. Ulcer visible
3. Blepharospasm
4. Epiphora
5. Photophobia

LID ABNORMALITIES

1. Entropion
2. Distichiasis
3. Ectopic cilia
4. Nasal fold trichiasis
5. Facial paralysis
6. Euryblepharon

ACUTE ONSET

1. Check third eyelid for foreign body
2. Trauma

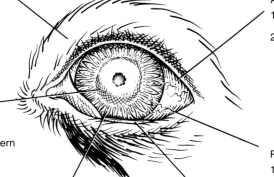

RECURRENT ULCERATION

1. Check lids
2. Check Schirmer test
3. Dendritic or geographical pattern (herpes—cats)
4. Deep or superficial
5. Breed susceptibility (boxer or corgi)
6. Neurotrophic keratitis

POSITION OF GLOBE

1. Exophthalmos— abnormal or normal for breed
2. Exposure keratitis

INFECTIOUS CAUSES

1. Culture sensitivity
2. Gram's and Giemsa's staining on scraping
3. Rapidly progressing (producing collagenase)
4. Previous steroid therapy
5. Species susceptibility:*
   Cattle—IBK, MCF
   Sheep—IOK
   Goats—ICK

SCHIRMER TEAR TEST

1. 0–5 mm/min—KCS[†]
2. 5–9 mm/min—equivocal
3. 7–10 mm/min—normal
4. Check for iatrogenic removal of nictitans gland

---

*IBK = infectious bovine keratoconjunctivitis; MCF = malignant catarrhal fever; IOK = infectious ovine keratoconjunctivitis; ICK = infectious caprine keratoconjunctivitis.

[†]KCS = keratoconjunctivitis sicca.

THE PAINFUL EYE

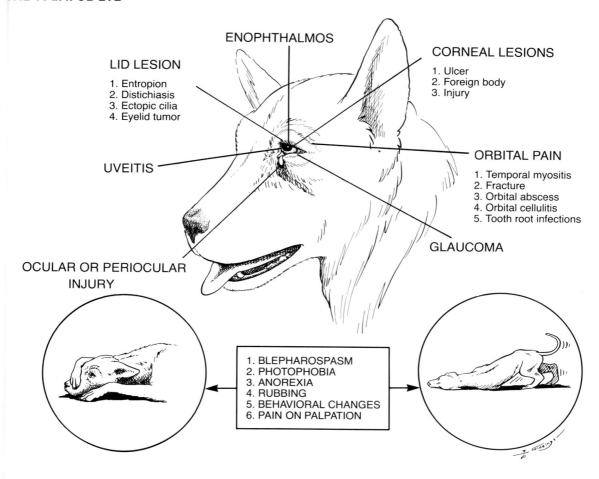

ENOPHTHALMOS

LID LESION

1. Entropion
2. Distichiasis
3. Ectopic cilia
4. Eyelid tumor

CORNEAL LESIONS

1. Ulcer
2. Foreign body
3. Injury

UVEITIS

ORBITAL PAIN

1. Temporal myositis
2. Fracture
3. Orbital abscess
4. Orbital cellulitis
5. Tooth root infections

GLAUCOMA

OCULAR OR PERIOCULAR
INJURY

1. BLEPHAROSPASM
2. PHOTOPHOBIA
3. ANOREXIA
4. RUBBING
5. BEHAVIORAL CHANGES
6. PAIN ON PALPATION

PROMINENT THIRD EYELID

DOG

1. Horner's syndrome
2. Tetany
3. Tranquilization
4. Ocular pain (see previous figure,
   The Painful Eye)
5. Excision of cartilage of third eyelid
6. Excision of nictitans gland
7. Loss of orbital fat

CAT

1. Horner's syndrome
2. Dehydration
3. Tranquilization
4. Ocular pain
5. Excision of nictitans gland
6. Loss of orbital fat

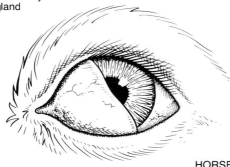

CATTLE AND SHEEP

1. Horner's syndrome
2. Tetany
3. Ocular pain—IBK, IOK, MCF*
4. Encephalitis

HORSES

1. Horner's syndrome
2. Tetany
3. Ocular pain—recurrent equine
   uveitis, foreign body, trauma

---

*IBK = infectious bovine keratoconjunctivitis; IOK = infectious ovine keratoconjunctivitis; MCF = malignant catarrhal fever.

COMMON NEONATAL OCULAR DISORDERS

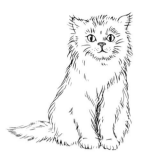

KITTEN

1. Ophthalmia neonatorum
2. Eyelid agenesis
3. Lacrimal atresia
4. Congenital open eyelids
5. Viral upper respiratory tract infections
6. Bilateral esotropia

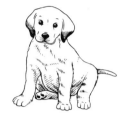

PUPPY

 1. Entropion
 2. Ophthalmia neonatorum
 3. Lacrimal atresia
 4. Congenital open eyelids
 5. Retinal dysplasia
 6. Scleral ectasia syndrome
 7. Distichiasis
 8. Dermoid
 9. Persistent pupillary membranes
10. Cataracts
11. Optic nerve hypoplasia

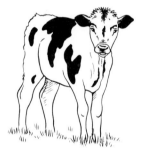

CALF

1. Subconjunctival hemorrhages
2. Coloboma (charolais)
3. Dermoid

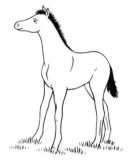

FOAL

1. Entropion
2. Subconjunctival and retinal hemorrhages
3. Jaundice (neonatal isoerythrolysis)
4. Corneal ulceration and birth trauma

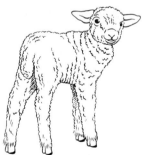

LAMB

1. Entropion
2. Foreign bodies

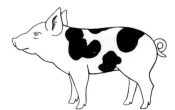

PIGLET

1. Ophthalmia neonatorum
2. Anophthalmia-microphthalmia (vitamin A deficiency)
3. Cataracts
4. Eyelid edema and chemosis (edema disease)

Note: Uncommon developmental disorders have been omitted.

NEONATAL OCULAR DISORDERS IN FOALS

TABLE BY DRS. R. G. STANLEY AND J. R. BLOGG

Disorder	Breeds	Etiology	Essential Features and Management
Microphthalmia May be associated with other ocular defects, e.g., multiple ocular defect syndrome cataracts, retinal detachments.	All breeds. Thoroughbreds have higher incidence.	Not established; most cases are idiopathic, some due to toxic, infectious, or nutritional episodes	Small eyes, prominent third eyelid. No treatment; lid surgery for secondary entropion.
Strabismus	Appaloosa.		Rare. Strabismus usually convergent; some patients have compensatory head deviation. Surgery to straighten eyes has been described.
Eyelid Coloboma May be associated with multiple occular anomalies.			Defects in eyelid margin. Surgery, depending on extent of other problems.
Ankyloblepharon Congenita			Partial fusion of upper and lower lids. Surgery.
Entropion Primary. Secondary.		Some patients have oversized palpebral fissures. Prematurity or illness.	Inturned eyelids, epiphora, corneal ulceration. Manual eversion of the eyelids, palpebral injections or horizontal mattress sutures or surgery to turn out the eyelids. Treatment of underlying cause, then surgery.
Nasolacrimal Atresia of nasolacrimal meatus. Misplaced punctum. Atresia of punctum.			Absence of nasal opening. Watery eye; some patients have mucopurulent discharge. Dacrocystorhinography may aid in diagnosis. Surgery to create new opening. Surgery to enlarge punctum. Surgery to create new punctum.
Cornea Microcornea. May be associated with microphthalmia syndromes. Corneal melanosis. Dermoid. Probably most common congenital anomaly.		 Not known to be inherited.	Small cornea. No treatment. Superficial axial nonprogressive pigment. Superficial keratectomy. Lateral or ventral corneal conjunctival masses containing hair and sebaceous glands. Surgical removal.
Aniridia May be associated with cataracts.	Belgian draft horse.	Autosomal recessive.	Complete absence of iris tissue.
Uveal Cysts May be associated with heterochromia iridis.			Pigmented cysts in anterior chamber or pupillary edge. Can be transilluminated. Aspiration if large and vision obstructed.
Heterochromia Iridis	Many color-dilute breeds.	Pigment failure in one iris or part of one iris.	Tapatum may be absent, and iris can be hypoplastic.

TABLE BY DRS. R. G. STANLEY AND J. R. BLOGG *Continued*

Disorder	Breeds	Etiology	Essential Features and Management
Cataracts			
Some associated with microphthalmia syndromes.	Arabian; Belgian draft; Morgan; thoroughbred; Quarter horse.	May be inherited.	Spontaneous resorption can offer useful vision in stud animals. Consider surgery if the cataracts interfere with vision.
		Other cataracts can be due to trauma (prenatal and foaling) or poor nutrition, or metabolic or toxic causes.	*Note:* Need to differentiate from prominent posterior Y sutures, which are present in the majority of foals.
Persistent Pupillary Membranes (PPM)			
May be associated with other ocular anomalies.			Strands of iris tissue that can run to iris, cornea (opacity), or lens (cataracts). PPM may continue to atrophy during the 1st year of life.
Vitreous			
Remnants of hyaloid tissue.			Remnants of hyaloid tissues visible behind the lens. These are present in most foals and will atrophy by 6–9 months.
Persistent hyperplastic primary vitreous.			Uncommon. Fibrovascular membrane behind the lens.
Retina			
Retinal hemorrhages.		Mostly incidental. Difficult birth.	
Retinal dysplasia; may be associated with other defects.	Thoroughbred may have higher incidence.		Bilateral retinal disorganization; may also have retinal detachment.
Retinal detachment; may associate with dysplasia.			Complete retinal detachment.
Coloboma of the fundus.			Chorioretinal defect.
Retinal aplasia.		Possibly autosomal recessive.	Absence of the retina.
Stationary night blindness.	Appaloosa and other breeds.	Autosomal recessive defect in neuroretinal transmission.	No lesions visible on ophthalmoscopic examination. Some patients have microphthalmia or dorsal strabismus/nystagmus.
Optic Nerve			
Optic nerve hypoplasia (congenital optic atrophy); may be associated with other defects.			Small optic nerve heads either unilateral or bilateral. Slow or absent pupillary light reflex. Searching nystagmus.
Papilledema.		Maladjustment.	Swelling of optic nerve associated with cerebral edema.

PERIOCULAR ALOPECIA OR DERMATITIS

DOG

1. Demodectic mange
2. Sarcoptic mange
3. Dermatomycosis
4. Autoimmune skin disorder
5. Seborrhea
6. Allergic inhalant dermatitis (atopy)
7. Hypopigmentation
8. Solar dermatitis
9. Hypothyroidism
10. Self trauma

CAT

1. Dermatomycosis
2. Notoedric mange
3. Hypopigmentation

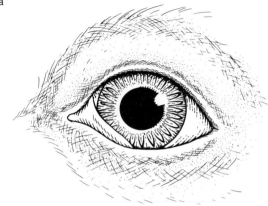

SHEEP

1. Photosensitization
2. Demodectic mange
3. Sarcoptic mange
4. Psoroptic mange

HORSE

1. Trauma
2. Dermatomycosis
3. Equine seborrhea
4. Demodectic mange
5. Sarcoptic mange
6. Psoroptic mange
7. Streptotrichosis

CATTLE

1. Dermatomycosis
2. Photosensitization
3. Sarcoptic mange
4. Psoroptic mange
5. Streptotrichosis

CHRONIC CONJUNCTIVITIS IN DOGS

DIFFERENTIATE FROM:
1. Glaucoma
2. Uveitis
3. Conjunctival injection due to sensitive vessel syndrome

LID ABNORMALITIES

1. Entropion
2. Ectropion
3. Distichiasis
4. Ectopic cilia
5. Seborrhea
6. Pyoderma
   (often generalized)

KERATOCONJUNCTIVITIS SICCA

1. Idiopathic
2. Sulfonamide administration
3. Phenazopyridine
4. Distemper
5. Hypoadrenocorticism
6. Nictitans gland removal
7. Hypothyroidism

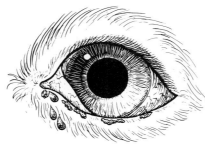

VIRUS INFECTION

Infectious tracheobronchitis

LACRIMAL ABNORMALITIES

1. Dacryocystitis
2. Lacrimal foreign bodies

IMMUNE-RELATED PHENOMENA

1. Allergic inhalant dermatitis
2. Autoimmune skin diseases
3. Bacterial allergy
   (e.g., *Staphylococcus aureus)*
4. Drug allergy (e.g., neomycin)
5. Immunodepressed states

OTHER INFECTIONS

1. Tarsal gland infection
2. Chronic staphylococcal infection (usually secondary)
3. Yeasts
4. Fungi
5. Thelaziasis

FELINE CONJUNCTIVITIS

RESPIRATORY TRACT INFECTIONS

FELINE HERPESVIRUS I
(feline viral rhinotracheitis)

1. Bilateral
2. Signs usually severe
3. Lacrimation; conjunctivitis
4. Chemosis, keratitis
5. Serous or mucopurulent discharge and sneezing
6. Occasional ulcers and vesicles in buccal epithelium
7. High morbidity
8. High kitten mortality
9. Intranuclear inclusions on early smears

CALICIVIRUS
(feline calicivirus infection)

1. Bilateral
2. Lacrimation
3. Mild to moderate signs
4. Occasional serous discharge
5. Sneezing
6. Frequent ulceration on dorsal margin of the tongue and hard palate (gingivitis)
7. High morbidity
8. Variable mortality

REOVIRUS
(feline reovirus infection)

1. Bilateral
2. Mild signs
3. Lacrimation
4. Rare nasal discharge
5. No oral lesions
6. 50% morbidity
7. Very low mortality

LACRIMAL ABNORMALITIES

1. Dacryocystitis
2. Keratoconjunctivitis sicca

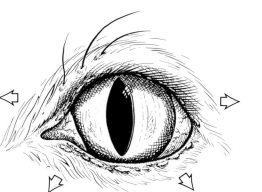

LID ABNORMALITIES

1. Entropion
2. Eyelid agenesis

A LESS EVIDENT RESPIRATORY TRACT INFECTION

CHLAMYDIA PSITTACI
(feline pneumonitis)

1. Often unilateral
2. Mild signs (acute may show chemosis)
3. Conjunctivitis
4. Nasal discharge rare
5. No oral lesions
6. Low morbidity
7. Very low mortality
8. Elementary bodies in smears

MISCELLANEOUS INFECTIONS
(*Mycoplasma* spp, *Staph. pyogenes, Strep. pyogenes, P. multicoda, B. bronchieseptica*)

1. Often unilateral
2. Mild signs
3. Conjunctivitis
4. No nasal signs
5. No oral lesions
6. Low morbidity
7. Very low mortality

BLINDNESS IN SHEEP

PREGNANCY TOXEMIA

1. Pregnancy
2. Adverse weather conditions
3. Declining plane of nutrition (usually)
4. Ketonuria

ORGANOPHOSPHATE POISONING

1. Miosis
2. Salivation
3. Blindness
4. Head pressing
5. History of exposure

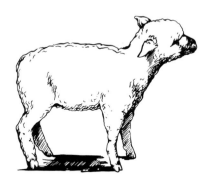

COENUROSIS

1. Circling
2. Endemic areas

POLIOENCEPHALOMALACIA

1. Trochlear nerve paralysis
2. Head pressing
3. No age distribution
4. Opisthotonus
5. Stubble or grain diet
6. Focal or symmetrical encephalomalacia
7. Less consistent muscle spasms
8. Younger sheep affected

PLANT TOXICITY

1. *Pteris aquilina* (United Kingdom)
2. *Stypandra imbricata* (Western Australia)
3. *Locoweed (Astragalus* and *Oxytropis* spp Western US)
4. *Swainsona galegifolia* (Australia)

BLINDNESS AND NERVOUS DYSFUNCTION IN CATTLE

POLIOENCEPHALOMALACIA
Autopsy findings

LISTERIOSIS

1. Sporadic
2. Circling
3. Facial paralysis
4. Some endophthalmitis
5. Head deviation (no rotation)
6. Dummy syndrome and convulsions

MALIGNANT CATARRHAL FEVER
(bovine malignant catarrh)

1. Endophthalmitis
2. Deep peripheral keratitis
3. Pyrexia
4. Necrosis of buccal and nasal mucosa
5. Nasal, oral, and ocular lesions
6. Nasal discharge and dyspnea

PLANT TOXICITY

Locoweed, rape,
and numerous
others

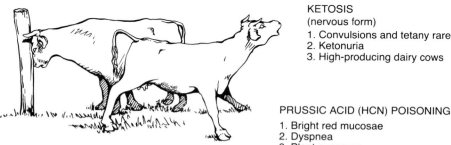

KETOSIS
(nervous form)

1. Convulsions and tetany rare
2. Ketonuria
3. High-producing dairy cows

LEAD POISONING

1. Mania
2. History of exposure
3. Kidney, liver, blood, and fecal analysis
4. Muscle tremors on head and neck
5. Mydriasis

PRUSSIC ACID (HCN) POISONING

1. Bright red mucosae
2. Dyspnea
3. Plant exposure
4. Numerous animals affected

HYPOMAGNESEMIA

1. Incoordination
2. Hyperesthesia
3. Tetany
4. Serum magnesium levels respond to therapy
5. Lactating animals affected first

RABIES

1. Ascending paralysis
2. Absence of tetany
3. Anesthesia
4. Bellowing
5. Salivation

THROMBOEMBOLIC MENINGOENCEPHALITIS

1. Early death
2. Retinal hemorrhages
3. Retinitis
4. Cold climates (e.g., North America)

HYPOVITAMINOSIS A
(calves)

1. Gait disturbances
2. Papilledema
3. Exophthalmos
4. Liver analysis

SPORADIC BOVINE ENCEPHALOMYELITIS

1. Pyrexia
2. Sporadic occurrence
3. Respiratory signs
4. Lameness, motor irritation (mild)

Note: Animals with any of these diseases may show blindness, nystagmus, strabismus, and prominent third eyelids, especially during convulsions.

Data from Blood DC, Henderson JA, Radostits O: Veterinary Medicine, 7th ed. Bailliére Tindall, London, 1989; Swan RA: Personal communication, 1979.

COMMON BOVINE OCULAR DISORDERS

> **COMMON FEATURES**
> Ocular discharge
> Corneal opacity
> Blepharospasm
> Epiphora
> Conjunctivitis

INFECTIOUS BOVINE KERATOCONJUNCTIVITIS

1. Unilateral or bilateral
2. Central corneal lesion
3. Most common in young
4. Resolves in 4–6 weeks
5. Herefords most susceptible but occurs in all breeds
6. Rare in *Bos indicus*

SQUAMOUS CELL CARCINOMA

1. Unilateral or bilateral
2. Painless until advanced
3. Affects:
   a. Limbus (80%)
   b. Lids (15%)
   c. Third eyelid (5%)
4. Usually affects animals over 3 years of age
5. Herefords most susceptible

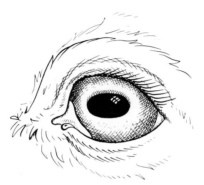

INFECTIOUS BOVINE RHINOTRACHEITIS

1. Bilateral
2. Occurs as outbreak
3. Profuse nasal discharge
4. Conjunctivitis (keratitis rare)
5. Pyrexia
6. Some outbreaks show chemosis and conjunctivitis as only symptoms
7. Most animals recover
8. High morbidity

MALIGNANT CATARRHAL FEVER
(bovine malignant catarrh)

1. Cattle often associated with sheep
2. Bilateral
3. Peripheral keratitis moving centrally (compare with IBK)
4. Sporadic
5. Hypopyon
6. Endophthalmitis
7. Most affected animals die
8. Pyrexia
9. Low morbidity (outbreaks have occurred)

SUDDEN ACQUIRED BLINDNESS

RED EYE ALGORITHM

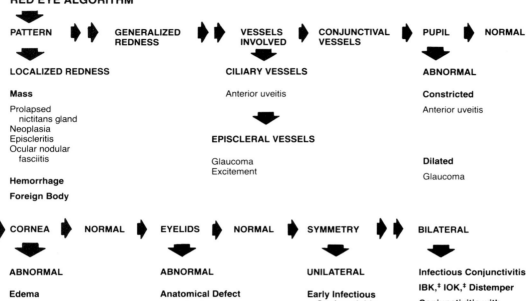

PATTERN ▶▶ **GENERALIZED REDNESS** ▶▶ **VESSELS INVOLVED** ▶ **CONJUNCTIVAL VESSELS** ▶ **PUPIL** ▶ **NORMAL**

LOCALIZED REDNESS

Mass

Prolapsed
   nictitans gland
Neoplasia
Episcleritis
Ocular nodular
   fasciitis

Hemorrhage

Foreign Body

CILIARY VESSELS

Anterior uveitis

EPISCLERAL VESSELS

Glaucoma
Excitement

ABNORMAL

Constricted

Anterior uveitis

Dilated

Glaucoma

▶ **CORNEA** ▶ **NORMAL** ▶ **EYELIDS** ▶ **NORMAL** ▶ **SYMMETRY** ▶▶ **BILATERAL**

ABNORMAL

Edema

Localized
• corneal ulcer
Generalized
• anterior uveitis
• glaucoma
• endophthalmitis

Keratitis

Localized
• Überreiter's
  syndrome
• exposure keratitis
• healing ulcer
• lid problem
• superficial corneal
  erosion

Generalized
• KCS*
• Überreiter's syndrome
• neurotrophic keratitis
• superficial punctate
  keratitis

ABNORMAL

Anatomical Defect
• entropion
• ectropion
• trichiasis
• distichiasis
• ectopic cilia
• neoplasia

Functional Defect

Lagophthalmos
• exophthalmos
• facial nerve
  paralysis
• orbital disease
• partial lid
  agenesis

Poor lid-corneal
   contact
• ectropion
• enophthalmos
• microphthalmos
• phthisis bulbi

Inflammatory Disease
• blepharitis
• meibomitis,
  chalazion

UNILATERAL

**Early Infectious
Conjunctivitis**
• herpes
• chlamydiae
• *Mycoplasma*
• *Moraxella*
• IBR†

Dacrocystitis

Trauma

Orbital Disease
• cellulitis
• proptosis
• retrobulbar
  mass
• retrobulbar
  abscess

Infectious Conjunctivitis

IBK,‡ IOK,‡ Distemper

**Conjunctivitis with
Systemic Disease**

Allergic Conjunctivitis

Follicular Conjunctivitis

Orbital Disease
• acute myositis

---

*KCS = keratoconjunctivitis sicca.
†IBR = infectious bovine rhinotracheitis.
‡IBK = infectious bovine keratoconjunctivitis; IOK = infectious ovine keratoconjunctivitis.

UVEITIS ALGORITHM*

  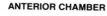   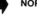

CORNEA → NORMAL → ANTERIOR CHAMBER → NORMAL → IRIS → NORMAL OR MIOTIC ONLY

ABNORMAL **ABNORMAL** **ABNORMAL**

EDEMA

Localized
- ulcerative keratitis
- perforating wound

Generalized

Severe—normal-sized eye
- ulcerative keratitis
- hepatitis-vaccination reaction
- endophthalmitis
- panophthalmitis

Severe—abnormal-sized eye
- phthisis bulbi
- glaucoma

Mild—nondiagnostic

Hemorrhage—Hyphema

Trauma
- perforating
- nonperforating

Clotting defect
- thrombocytopenia
- factor deficiency

Nondiagnostic

Fibrin Clot

Surgical trauma
Chronic hyphema
Nondiagnostic

Pus—Hypopyon

Infectious
- bacterial
- mycotic

Lipid
- hyperlipoproteinemia
- uveitis

Noninfectious—nondiagnostic

Diffuse Swelling

Edema—nondiagnostic
Neoplasia
Granulomatous inflammation

Localized Swelling

Neoplasia
Granuloma

Dyscoria

Synechiae
Lens luxation

Change in Color

Often darker after uveitis

FUNDIC REFLECTION OR PUPIL → NORMAL → FUNDUSCOPIC EXAM → NORMAL → SYSTEMIC DISEASE

ABNORMAL **ABNORMAL**

Leukocoria

Seclusion, occlusion of pupil
- chronic
- nondiagnostic
- iris bombé— glaucoma

Cataract
- lens-induced uveitis
- uveitis-induced cataract

Cyclitic membrane
- chronic, recurrent
- nondiagnostic

Retinal detachment
Vitreal exudate or haze

Hemorrhage

Trauma
Retinal detachment
Nondiagnostic

Exudative Detachment

Chorioretinitis
- active
- inactive

Optic Neuritis
- papillitis
- papilledema

Neurological

Gastrointestinal

Respiratory

Multisystem

Dermatological

Musculoskeletal

---

*Modified from Schmidt GM: Problem-oriented ophthalmology. Part 2. Anterior uveitis. Mod Vet Pract 57: 516–520, 1976.

SUDDEN BLINDNESS, RETINAL DETACHMENTS, HEMORRHAGES, AND UVEITIS

Minimum Data Base*

Complete Fundus and Physical Examination
  Serum chemistry profile and hematology
  Clotting panel
  Systolic blood pressure
  Serum titers

Dog	*Cat*
Toxoplasmosis	Toxoplasmosis
Blastomycosis	Blastomycosis
Histoplasmosis	Histoplasmosis
Coccidioidomycosis	Feline leukemia virus
Cryptococcosis	Cryptococcosis
Ehrlichiosis	Feline infectious peritonitis

  Coombs's Test
  Urinalysis
  Serum electrophoresis

*Because of financial constraints, the data base is usually accumulated in sequence until a diagnosis is made, depending on the most likely differential diagnoses based on the clinical examination and geographical locality.

ANISOCORIA

Pupillary Function and Vision Associated With Various Neurological Syndromes and a Left-Sided Lesion

Syndrome*	Resting Pupil Left	Resting Pupil Right	Vision Left	Vision Right	Pupillary Reflex in Left Eye Direct	Consensual (to Right Eye)	Pupillary Reflex in Right Eye Direct	Consensual (to Left Eye)
Cervicothoracic (Sympathetic)	Miotic	Normal	OK	OK	Yes	Yes	Yes	Yes
Cervical (Sympathetic)	Miotic	Normal	OK	OK	Yes	Yes	Yes	Yes
Vestibular (Sympathetic)	Miotic	Normal	OK	OK	Yes	Yes	Yes	Yes
Cerebellar (Unknown)	Miotic	Dilated	OK	OK	Yes	Yes	Yes	Yes
Midbrain (Parasympathetic)	Dilated	Miotic	OK†	OK†	No	Yes	Yes	No
Hypothalamic (Optic nerve or optic chiasm)	Dilated	Miotic	Poor	OK	No	No	Yes	Yes
	Dilated	Dilated	Poor	Poor	No	No	No	No
Cerebral (Optic tract)	Miotic	Normal/ Dilated	OK	Poor	Yes	Yes	Impaired	Impaired

From Braund KG: Anisocoria: Its relationship to neurologic syndromes. Vet Med 82:997, 1987.
*The abnormal pupillary reflex control mechanism is in parenthesis.
†Animals with this syndrome may be comatose.

OCULAR DISEASES OF CAGED BIRDS

TABLE BY DR. L. KARPINSKY

Disease or Condition	Species	Clinical Features	Treatment	Remarks
Parrot pox	Amazons, commonly; lovebirds; mild in young macaws	Proliferative lesions of eyelid borders; commissurae of beak; also feet of lovebirds; respiratory disease	Washing eyelid borders; topical dilute merbromin; vitamin A IM 10,000 to 25,000 IU per 300 g body weight once weekly	Results in distorted lid margins, lash loss, corneal crystals, epiphora
Mynah pox	Mynahs	Proliferative lesions of eyelid borders; commissurae of beak, wattles; ± keratitis, conjunctivitis	Topical antibiotics if keratitis present	Results in mild lid distortion; keratitis, chronic conjunctivitis
Cockatiel conjunctivitis	Cockatiels, especially white or albino mutations	Chemotic to proliferative conjunctivitis	Chlortetracycline in food	Recurrence common; transmitted to offspring
Lovebird eye disease	Lovebirds, especially peach-faced mutations	Blepharitis; serous ocular discharge; depression	Often fatal	Decrease stress
Chronic conjunctivitis in Amazons	Amazons	Edematous; inflamed to infiltrated conjunctiva	Topical corticosteroids or surgical removal	± Corneal ulcer
Periorbital abscess	Cockatiels, commonly; all species	Firm swelling in periorbital area	Drainage; appropriate antimicrobial	Follows sinusitis
Lacrimal sac abscess	All species	Swelling anteroventral to medial canthus	Flushing or removal of material in sac	Follows sinusitis
Sunken eyes and sinuses	Macaws, especially scarlet and green-winged	Globe sunken into orbit; collapse of orbital tissue	Flushing through nares with large volumes; systemic carbenicillin (100 mg/kg IM, BID or TID) and amikacin (40 mg/kg IM SID or BID)	Miniature macaws, Amazons, cockatoos respond poorly
Punctate keratitis in Amazons	Amazons	Punctate keratitis with blepharospasm	Topical vitamin A	Often chronic
Knemidokoptic mites (scaly face)	Budgerigars, commonly	Dry, flaking lesions of periorbital area and cere	Ivermectin IM (200 μg/kg)	
Oxyspirura nematodes	Cockatoos, commonly; mynahs	Worms in conjunctival sac and lacrimal duct; blepharitis, tearing	Manual removal; ivermectin IM (200 μg/kg)	

OCULAR CONDITIONS OF FISH

TABLE BY DR. R. C. RIIS

Fish Ophthalmic Pathology

Buphthalmos
Carotene deficiency
Endophthalmitis
N_2 gas accumulation

Exophthalmia
Aeromoniasis
Corynebacterial kidney disease
Flavobacteriosis
Fluke metacercaria
Ichthyosporidium
Infectious hemorrhagic necrosis
Infectious pancreatic necrosis
Pseudomoniasis
Trematode larvae
  Cryptocotyle lingua
  Nanophyetus salmincola
Tuberculosis
Vibriosis
Viral hemorrhagic septicemia

Cataracts
Asphyxia
Congenital
Inherent
N_2 gas accumulation
Nutritional
  Methionine deficiency
  Riboflavin deficiency
  Tryptophan deficiency
  Zinc deficiency
Parasitic
  Metacercaria and *Diplostomum* spp
Temperature shock
Toxicities: Acids/bases
  Chlorinated biphenols
  Cyanide
  Fungicides
  Heavy metals
  Herbicides
  Hydrocarbons
  Pesticides
  Soaps/detergents
  Thioacetamide
Trauma
Ultraviolet light

Retinal Degenerations
Dietary deficiency
  Methionine
  Cystine
  Vitamin A

Panophthalmitis
Septicemia
  Aeromonas
  Flavobacterium
  Pseudomonas
  Vibrio

Periocular Inflammation
Crustacean (*Artystone trysibia*)
Microsporidian (*Dermocystidium* sp)
Myxosporan
  (*Henneguya lagodon*)
  (*Myxosoma scleroperca*)
  (*Glugea pseudotumefaciens*)

Periocular Hemorrhage
Trauma
Viral hemorrhagic septicemia
Vitamin C deficiency

Intraocular Hemorrhage
N_2 gas
Septicemia
Trauma
Viral hemorrhagic septicemia

Ocular Manifestations of Systemic Disease
Ichthyophthirius multifiliis
Lymphocystis
Mycobacteriosis
Nocardiosis
Nutritional deficiency
Toxicities

Keratopathies
Bacterial opportunists
Fungal saprophytes (*Saprolegnia*)
Ichthyophthirius sp
Lymphocystis
Parasitic metacercaria
Riboflavin deficiency
Trauma
Water salinity/pH imbalances

TABLE BY DR. R. C. RIIS

Etiology of Ocular Lesions in Fish

Degenerations
Cataracts: Rule out—
  Nutritional causes
  Chemical toxicosis
  Ultraviolet light
  Infectious diseases
  Inherent
Exophthalmos/buphthalmos
  Infectious
  Nutritional deficiencies
  Hormonal imbalances
  Nitrogen gas accumulation
Retinal blindness
  Environmental etiologies
  Nutritional
  Inherent

Inflammation

Bacterial (Ocular Manifestations of Systemic Disease)
  Aeromonas
  Pseudomonas (necrosis and hemorrhage)
  Vibrio
  Flavobacteria (proliferative lesion)
  Tuberculosis (granulomatous lesion)

Viral (Ocular Manifestations of Systemic Disease)
  Infectious hematopoietic necrosis
  Infectious pancreatic necrosis
  Infectious hemorrhagic septicemia

Parasitic
  Protozoan
    Ichthyophthirius
    Microsporidian
    Myxosporan
  Crustacean
    Artystone trysibia
    Lernaeenicus sprattae
  Trematode
    Cryptocotyle lingua
    Strigeidae sp
    Nanophyetus salmincola
Fungi
  Ichthyosporidium
  Saprolegnia
  Others

Malformations
  Abnormal eye migration
  Anophthalmia/microphthalmia
  Cyclopia
  Trauma

Neoplasia/Hyperplasia
  Fibrosarcoma
  Hemangiosarcoma
  Melanosarcoma
  Lymphocystis (hypertrophy of fibroblasts)
  Medulloepithelioma
  Retinoblastoma

OCULAR DISEASE IN POULTRY

TABLE BY DRS. M. E. NAIRN AND K. A. NAIRN

Disease or Condition	Clinical Characteristics	Age	Differential Features	Diagnostic Methods and Samples	Key References
Nutritional					
Vitamin A deficiency	Watery discharge from eyes and nose	Usually growing birds	Raised white plaques on mucosal surface of esophagus and pharynx	Section of white plaques for histopathology (squamous metaplasia)	Hinshaw and Lloyd, 1934
Pantothenic acid deficiency	Encrustations on eyelids and commissurae of lips	Young chickens	Lesions confined to head	Analysis of diet	Gries and Scott, 1972
Biotin deficiency	Encrustations on eyelids, lips, and legs	Young chickens	Lesions on legs	Analysis of diet	Hofstad et al, 1978
Bacterial Infections					
Salmonellosis, including *S. pullorum* and *S. gallinarum*	Purulent panophthalmitis and opacity of cornea	Young chickens and turkey poults	May be other signs of infection, including brain lesions	Direct culture of eye lesions	Evans et al, 1955
Arizona infection (*Arizona hinshawii*)	Purulent panophthalmitis and corneal opacity	Young turkey poults	May be other signs of septicemia	Direct culture	Sato and Adler, 1966
Chronic cholera *Pasteurella multocida*	Caseous swelling of wattles, comb, sinuses, and eyelids	Adult fowl	Involvement of combs and wattles	Culture of lesions	Hofstad et al, 1978
Chronic respiratory disease (*Haemophilus gallinarum* infection)	Serous/mucoid inflammation of nasal sinuses and eyes	Young and adult chickens; Japanese quail	Inflammation confined to upper respiratory tract	Culture of section of trachea to eliminate infectious laryngotracheitis	Matsumoto and Yamamoto, 1971; Reece et al, 1981
Coliform infection (*Escherichia coli*)	Panophthalmitis and air sacculitis	Young chickens	Usually associated with mortality and severe air sacculitis	Culture lesion	Nakamura and Abe, 1987
Pseudomonas infection (*Pseudomonas aeruginosa*)	Keratitis	Young chickens	No other lesions	Culture	Niilo, 1959
Viral Infections					
Marek's disease (herpesvirus)	Iritis with "pearly" discoloration	Young and adult chickens	Central nervous system, peripheral nerve, and visceral lesions	Section of eye shows infiltration of lymphocytes	Hofstad et al, 1978
Infectious laryngotracheitis (herpesvirus)	Severe respiratory distress with watery conjunctivitis and caseous necrotic plaques in trachea	Chickens over 6 weeks of age	Presence of hemorrhagic necrotic plaques in trachea	Section of trachea taken for histopathology or virus isolation	Raggi and Armstrong, 1960
Avian influenza (orthomyxovirus)	Nonpurulent conjunctivitis	Adult turkeys and ducks	General depression and respiratory symptoms (nonspecific)	Virus isolation and serology	Hofstad et al, 1978
Avian adenovirus infection	Conjunctivitis	Quail and chickens (young and adult)	Nonspecific respiratory disease	Virus isolation	Aghakhan, 1974
Fowl pox (pox virus)	Severe proliferative lesions on face and eyelids with associated conjunctivitis	Adults	Lesions very proliferative	Histopathology of lesions	Hofstad et al, 1978

TABLE BY DRS. M. E. NAIRN AND K. A. NAIRN *Continued*

Disease or Condition	Clinical Characteristics	Age	Differential Features	Diagnostic Methods and Samples	Key References
Parasitic Diseases					
Oxyspirura mansoni and *O. petrouri*	Severe ophthalmitis and edema	Many species of fowl (adults)	Parasite in conjunctival sac and nasolacrimal duct	Direct examination of parasite	Mustaffa-Babjee, 1969
Philopthalmidae (3 genera and 12 species occur in birds)	Irritation and erosion of conjunctiva	Many species of birds (adults)	Parasite in conjunctival sac	Direct examination of parasite	Mustaffa-Babjee, 1969
Fungal Infections					
Aspergillosis (*Aspergillus fumigatus*)	Granulomatous panophthalmitis	Young chickens and turkey poults	Often associated with granulomatous lung lesions	Culture and histopathology	Moore, 1953
Moniliasis (*Candida albicans*)	Mild conjunctivitis with white opacity of third eyelids	Young ducks	May have crop lesions also	Culture	Crispen and Barnett, 1978
Other Infections					
Trichomoniasis (*Trichomonas gallinae*)	Caseous lesion in anterior chamber	Young chickens	Other organs usually involved, e.g., crop	Direct examination of wet preparation	Hofstad et al, 1978
Mycoplasma gallisepticum	Distention of sinuses and conjunctivitis	Adult turkeys	Mucoid discharge from sinuses	Culture	Hofstad et al, 1978
Plasmodium lophurae	Conjunctivitis	Adult turkeys	Confined to eye	Direct examination of stained smear	Becker et al, 1949
Ornithosis (*Chlamydia psittaci*)	Conjunctivitis, panophthalmitis, diarrhea, severe depression	Psittacine birds, ducks, and chickens (all ages)	Enlarged spleen	Direct examination of Giemsa-stained smears and egg inoculation	Hofstad et al, 1978; Barr et al, 1986
Miscellaneous					
Cataracts	Cataract	Adults	No other lesions	Histopathology	Keymer, 1977
Granulomatous chorioretinitis	Granulomatous inflammation of choroid and retina	Adults	No other lesions	Histopathology	Saunders and Moore, 1957
Formaldehyde irritation	Conjunctivitis and photophobia	Young chickens	No other lesions	History of access to agent	Hofstad et al, 1978
Ammonia burns	Keratoconjunctivitis and corneal opacity	Young chickens and turkey poults	No other lesions	History of access to ammonia fumes	Barber, 1947
Genetic blindness	Blind	Chickens	Feather amelanosis in some birds	Histopathology (agenosis of rods and cones)	Cheng et al, 1980
Light- and darkness-induced blindness	Buphthalmia and poor vision	Young chickens and turkeys	No other lesions	History of reduced or increased artificial light	

OCULAR DISEASE IN RABBITS, RODENTS, AND REPTILES

The eyes and adnexae of rabbits, rodents, and reptiles are subject to the same ophthalmic disease processes that affect higher vertebrates. The eye may be the primary site of disease or secondarily involved following systemic infection. The cause and clinical manifestations of these lesions are usually similar to those responsible for ophthalmic problems in other mammals and birds. Many diseases in rabbits, rodents, and reptiles result from inadequate knowledge of proper environmental and nutritional requirements. Correction of poor husbandry procedures is as much a part of the treatment as is any specific therapy aimed at ophthalmic diseases (Davidson, 1985). The table in this section correlates clinical signs, cause, and treatment of common ophthalmic problems in rabbits, rodents, and reptiles.

Rabbits

The optic nervehead is located approximately one disc diameter above the horizontal midline of the eye; the examiner must look upward into the rabbit eye in order to evaluate this structure. A prominent physiological cup in the optic nervehead is commonly present. The entire surface of the optic nervehead may be depressed and appear as cupping of the disc. This physiological cupping must be distinguished from cupping in hereditary glaucoma. In glaucoma, cupping of the disc is associated with a buphthalmic eye. Rabbits have an inferior nasolacrimal punctum only, located well below the eyelid margin; the superior punctum is absent. Since many rabbits possess the enzyme atropinase, tropicamide is generally more effective for mydriasis than is atropine.

Rodents

Because the rodent eye is small mydriasis is especially important for examination of the posterior segment.

The pupils of pigmented rodents are occasionally resistant to dilation because melanin granules in the iris bind the mydriatic and inhibit its action (Davidson, 1985). In such cases, 1% atropine solution mixed with equal parts of 10% phenylephrine solution and applied 3–4 times during a 15-minute period is effective (Bellhorn, 1981). The orbital lacrimal glands are large in most rodents. Problems with these glands are the basis for many ocular diseases in rodents.

Reptiles

SNAKES

The eyes of all snakes are covered anteriorly by a transparent spectacle, formed embryologically by a fusion of the eyelids. It is important to differentiate the subspectacular space from the anterior chamber (Millichamp et al, 1983). Topical treatment of the eye in snakes is usually ineffective because the keratinized spectacle is impervious to topically applied medications. The spectacle is normally shed with the rest of the skin during each molting cycle (ecdysis). Most ophthalmic problems in snakes are related to problems with the spectacle, especially when retention of the spectacle occurs (dysecdysis). Examination of the posterior segment and fundus with the aid of atropine or tropicamide is impossible in reptiles because of the striated muscle in the iris and ciliary body. Reptilian mydriasis is best accomplished under general anesthesia (Millichamp et al, 1983).

CHELONIANS (TURTLES AND TORTOISES)

Chelonians do not have a nasolacrimal duct. Tears are lost by evaporation, absorption across the conjunctiva, or spillage from the conjunctival sac. Therefore, any infection or excessive lacrimation results in severe epiphora. The orbital glands are large in most species, an important consideration in ocular manifestations of vitamin A deficiency.

Rabbits

TABLE BY DRS. J. M. A. DA SILVA CURIEL AND R. W. BELLHORN

Disease Process	Cause	Clinical Signs	Diagnostic Procedures	Treatment	References
Congenital glaucoma (buphthalmia).	Hereditary autosomal recessive trait in the New Zealand albino rabbit. Basic defect is an abnormal anterior chamber angle.	Increased intraocular pressure noted by 4–6 months of age. Cloudy cornea conjunctival injection, corneal diameter increases, eye becomes enlarged and more prominent, and vascular keratitis occurs. Later, intraocular pressure may return to normal owing to ciliary body degeneration. Globe remains enlarged, and exposure keratitis may develop. Optic nerve cupping occurs only later—distinguish from normal physiological cupping. Attenuation of retinal vessels and gray color of optic nerve head.	Measurement of intraocular pressures, gonioscopy.	Medications as for canine primary glaucoma are suitable for rabbits. Reductions in pressure are usually temporary. In chronic glaucoma, enucleation may be required if exposure keratitis occurs due to buphthalmia. Dipivyl epinephrine (Propine) (1 drop each eye every 12 hours).	Hanna et al, 1963
Conjunctivitis and ocular discharge.	1. Pasteurellosis (snuffles). Upper respiratory infection ("snuffles") caused by *Pasteurella multocida.*	Rhinitis, sneezing, nasal discharge, and chronic conjunctivitis. Most common—a white or yellow purulent discharge with epiphora. Loss of hair (medial canthus). Ocular signs can also occur in association with other diseases caused by *Pasteurella,* including rhinitis, pneumonia, otitis media, subcutaneous abscesses, septicemia, dacryocystitis, occlusion of the nasolacrimal duct, and anterior uveitis.	Culture and sensitivity of nasal discharge or material flushed from nasolacrimal duct.	Systemic antibiotics, plus topical chloramphenicol. Treatment does not eliminate the organism from the nasal passages; therefore, relapses may occur. Use systemic antibiotics with caution in order to prevent drug-induced diarrhea. In rabbits with blocked nasolacrimal ducts, the duct may be partially cannulated and the nasolacrimal sac flushed. Passage of a cannula or suture through the nasolacrimal duct into the nares is usually unsuccessful.	Fox et al, 1984; Harkness and Wagner, 1983; Raphael, 1981

Table continued on following page

Rabbits *Continued*

TABLE BY DRS. J. M. A. DA SILVA CURIEL AND R. W. BELLHORN *Continued*

				Improve husbandry, including providing adequate ventilation, isolating or culling affected animals, and eliminating environmental stress.	
	2. Noninfectious (irritant) conjunctivitis. Entropion, dust, trauma, and distichiasis have all been implicated.	Conjunctivitis and epiphora.	–	Eliminate source of ocular irritation	Fox et al, 1979, 1984; Hanna et al, 1963; Raphael, 1981
	3. Myxomatosis. Myxomatosis (poxvirus) is a viral disease that is enzootic in wild rabbits (*Sylvilagus*). In the United States, the disease only occurs in the coastal mountain ranges of Oregon and California. Transmitted to commercial and pet rabbits by mosquitos and fleas.	Blepharoconjunctivitis and thick mucoid ocular discharge. In chronic infections, gelatinous swelling of the face and urogenital area, and development of subcutaneous tumors. Mortality is 25–50%. A seasonal disease, seen in months when mosquito population is high.	Histological examination of conjunctival biopsies for intracytoplasmic inclusion bodies in epithelial cells.	No effective treatment. Destroy affected animals and dispose of by burning in order to prevent further spread of disease. Mosquito and flea control. Autogenous vaccines provide a 6- to 9-month immunity but must be given 1–2 months before mosquito season starts.	Brooks, 1986; Davidson, 1985; Patton and Holmes, 1977
Septicemic uveitis.	Septicemia is most commonly caused by *Pasteurella multocida* but also by staphylococcal infections (especially mastitis) and bacterial enteritis.	Anterior uveitis in association with other clinical symptoms referable to systemic infection. *P. multocida* can cause peracute deaths owing to septicemia in seemingly uncomplicated or minor cases of snuffles (see "Pasteurellosis" above).	—	Appropriate systemic antimicrobial therapy. Topical ophthalmic treatment with steroids and mydriatics.	Harkness and Wagner, 1983; Raphael, 1981

TABLE BY DRS. J. M. A. DA SILVA CURIEL AND R. W. BELLHORN *Continued*

Disease Process	Cause	Clinical Signs	Diagnostic Procedures	Treatment	References
Orbital cellulitis/ abscesses.	Penetrating wounds. Most commonly due to local or hematogenous spread of *Pasteurella* infections (especially from rhinitis).	Conjunctivitis, epiphora, blepharitis, and sometimes exophthalmos.	Culture and sensitivity.	Drain abscess, systemic antibiotic therapy. (See "Pasteurellosis" above).	
Colobomata.	Spontaneous.	Notch-like defects of optic nerve or adjacent retina, sclera, and choroid may occur. Occur frequently in rabbits with microphthalmic eyes. Focal retinal separations may be present. Coloboma of the lens also reported.	—	None required.	Bellhorn, 1973, 1981
Absence of nasolacrimal punctum.	Superior nasolacrimal punctum in rabbits is normally absent.	—	—	—	

Rodents

TABLE BY DRS. J. M. A. DA SILVA CURIEL AND R. W. BELLHORN

Disease Process	Cause	Clinical Signs	Diagnostic Procedures	Treatment	References
Rats and Mice Sialodacryoadenitis (SDA) complex.	Corona virus, infects nasopharynx, salivary glands, and harderian glands of rats. Salivary and lacrimal glands become inflamed.	Blinking and proptosis early signs—a result of inflammation and enlargement of glands. Epiphora and chromodacryorrhea (see below) are also early signs and are observed at about 6–8 weeks of age. Keratoconjunctivitis sicca may result from decreased tear formation, with subsequent keratitis. Iridocyclitis may develop, and synechia to the lens or peripheral cornea can occur. Endophthalmitis may occur, with secondary glaucoma or phthisis bulbi. Focal retinal atrophy (due to focal choroiditis from orbital gland inflammation) may occur unilaterally or bilaterally, and usually appears as a band of hyperreflectivity with sharply delineated borders. Gland swelling usually resolves in 10–14 days.	Clinical signs, histological lesions, and detection of serum-neutralizing and complement-fixing antibodies. Distinguish a chromodacryorrhea in SDA complex from that due to overgrown incisors. Unilateral focal or generalized retinal degeneration is more likely the result of SDA complex, whereas generalized bilateral retinal degeneration is more likely due to heredity or phototoxic retinopathy.	Treatment for secondary ophthalmic bacterial infections (most commonly *Pasteurella pneumotropica* and *Staphylococcus aureus*). In panophthalmitis, enucleation may be necessary. Disease confers long-lasting immunity against reinfection.	Bellhorn, 1973, 1981; Weisbroth and Peress, 1977
Chromodacryorrhea (bloody tears).	Secretion of pigmented tears is a normal physiological process in rats and mice. Pigment results from porphyrins synthesized in harderian gland and excreted with tears. Excessive pigment accumulation from epiphora (chromodacryorrhea) is abnormal. Overgrowth of lower incisor teeth can obstruct the nasolacrimal duct and cause epiphora.	Accumulation of red crusts on the medial canthus, nose, and forepaws. Distinguish from dried blood. Pigment fluoresces under ultraviolet light. Animals with dental malocclusion may drool.	—	Corrective dentistry if lower incisors are overgrown.	Harkness and Ridgway, 1980

TABLE BY DRS. J. M. A. DA SILVA CURIEL AND R. W. BELLHORN *Continued*

Disease Process	Cause	Clinical Signs	Diagnostic Procedures	Treatment	References
	Epiphora and pigment accumulation can also be due to infection of orbital and salivary tear glands with SDA virus (see above). Advanced chronic mycoplasma pneumonia, stress, and vitamin A and riboflavin deficiency have also been implicated.				
Light-induced (phototoxic) retinal degeneration.	High light levels are toxic to the retina and cause degenerative changes with blindness. Continuous light and higher temperatures enhance disease process.	Blindness or vision loss (usually not clinically significant in the rat or mouse). The albino rat is markedly susceptible owing to an absence of pigment. Older female rats are more susceptible.	Distinguish from heritable retinal degeneration (may be impossible to do) and from retinal lesions caused by SDA complex (see above). Fundic hyperreflectivity and retinal vessel narrowing are observed. Histopathological lesions can vary in severity from generalized thinning of the photoreceptor layer to complete loss of photoreceptors with proliferation and vascular invasion of retinal pigmented epithelium.	No treatment. Once the disease is established, it can continue even if nondamaging levels of light are reinstated. Preventative treatment—reduce intensity of light. Continuous lighting is harmful; ensure that cyclical light-dark lighting is available.	Bellhorn, 1980; Bellhorn et al, 1980; Everitt et al, 1987; Lai et al, 1978; Lanum, 1978
Environmental keratoconjunctivitis.	Ammonia build-up in bedding. Dust from bedding material.	Epiphora and sometimes keratitis and conjunctivitis due to irritating effects of ammonia vapor or dust.	—	Improve husbandry (regular cage-cleaning to prevent ammonia build-up). Use dust-free bedding materials.	
Pasteurella periorbital abscesses and keratoconjunctivitis of mice.	Disease of young weanling mice. A suppurative dacryoadenitis (involving primarily harderian gland) occurs and infects other orbital and ocular tissues by direct extension. *P. pneumotropica* and *P. hemolytica* var. *urea* have been cultured.	Conjunctivitis (frequently suppurative) usually accompanies periorbital abscesses and dacryoadenitis. Lesions appear between 12 and 21 days and are confined to the orbital region. Orbital abscesses are usually unilateral but can occur bilaterally.	Culture and sensitivity of purulent material from orbital abscesses or the conjunctiva.	Generally self-limiting without marked mortality in affected mice. Systemic antibiotics and topical ophthalmic antibiotic preparations may be used (based on results of culture and sensitivity).	Wagner et al, 1966
Cataracts.	1. Anesthetic-induced. Prolonged sedation or anesthesia. Lens	Spontaneous lens opacities occur	—	None required. The lens opacities are	Fraunfelder and Burns, 1966

Table continued on following page

Rodents *Continued*

TABLE BY DRS. J. M. A. DA SILVA CURIEL AND R. W. BELLHORN *Continued*

Disease Process	Cause	Clinical Signs	Diagnostic Procedures	Treatment	References
	opacities occur after prolonged periods of nonclosure of the eyelids. Anterior chamber is extremely shallow, and evaporation of fluids causes significant changes in aqueous, which affects the anterior lens transparency.	during periods of deep or prolonged anesthesia.		reversible and resolve on recovery.	
	2. Congenital.	—	—	—	
Corneal opacities (keratitis).	Sometimes associated with orbital gland inflammation. Due to the inflammation of the ducts and glands, and the close proximity of the cornea and iris, keratitis and focal iritis may develop.	Transient, unilateral or bilateral, nasal quadrant corneal opacities. In some, keratitis is associated with an underlying iris adhesion (adherent leukoma due to anterior synechia). Permanent corneal scarring.	Culture and sensitivity if suppurative conjunctivitis is involved. Serology and clinical signs for SDA virus.	Topical ophthalmic antibiotic solutions or ointments. Atropine. Systemic antibiotics if indicated.	
Congenital ocular disease.	Hereditary ocular diseases in rats include microphthalmia, cataracts, and retinopathy. Coloboma of the optic nervehead, is fairly common. Microphakia is also observed. Patent hyaloid vessels can be present in 80–90% of weanling rats, but usually disappear within 2–4 months.	—	—	—	Bellhorn, 1973, 1981

Guinea Pigs					
Cataracts.	Tryptophan deficiency (?).	—	—	—	
Conjunctivitis.	1. Inclusion (chlamydial) conjunctivitis. Naturally occurring ocular infection caused by *Chlamydia psittaci*. Also infects genital tract of guinea pigs, and offspring of infected animals can develop neonatal chlamydial conjunctivitis.	Conjunctivitis with follicle formation, slight chemosis, and serous ocular discharge.	—	—	Murray, 1964
	2. Bacterial conjunctivitis.				

TABLE BY DRS. J. M. A. DA SILVA CURIEL AND R. W. BELLHORN *Continued*

Disease Process	Cause	Clinical Signs	Diagnostic Procedures	Treatment	References
	Bordetella bronchiseptica and *Streptococcus pneumoniae* from enzootic respiratory infections.	Conjunctivitis and ocular discharge, ± signs of pneumonia. Active disease may occur in stressed carrier animals.	Culture and sensitivity of conjunctival discharge or tracheal exudate.	Prognosis for guinea pigs with *Bordetella bronchopneumonia* is poor. Systemic antibiotics or antibiotics in drinking water. Intranasal and intramuscular bacteria preparations have been used to prevent infection and eliminate carrier states.	Harkness and Wagner, 1983; Nakagawa et al, 1974; Shimizu, 1978
Gerbils					
Harderian gland hypersecretion.	Harderian gland secretion (containing porphyrins) is excreted in the nasolacrimal duct and mixes with nasal secretions, which gerbil combines with saliva and spreads over pelage. The build-up of gland secretions provokes scratching, with subsequent skin lesions, bleeding, formation of scabs, and loss of hair. May be hypersecretion of harderian gland material or failure of gerbil to spread material over pelage.	Lesions begin as reddened, scabby, hairless areas surrounding the external nares. Eventually, most of the dorsum of the head and forepaws become denuded, with bloody crusting. Does not respond to topical antibiotics or ectoparasite remedies. Usually worsens with time and is exacerbated by frequent scratching.	—	Remove gland, initiate grooming by raising environmental temperature, clear secretions from nose.	Theisen and Pendergrass, 1982
Chromodacryorrhea (bloody tears).	See "Chromodacryorrhea" (Rats and Mice) above.	—	—	—	
Hamsters					
Cataracts.	1. Anesthesia-induced cataracts (see "Cataracts, Anesthetic-induced" [Rats and Mice] above).	—	—	—	
	2. Diabetes-induced cataract. Cataract formation occurs in the Chinese hamster with hereditary diabetes mellitus.	—	Urine and blood glucose measurements.	Standard insulin therapy is possible.	
Retinal dysplasia.	Presumably congenital.	Dysplastic foci vary from retinal streaks to small, ovoid areas of cream-colored depigmentations. No visual deficits.	Fundic examination, histopathology.	—	Schiavo, 1980

Reptiles

TABLE BY DRS. J. M. A. DA SILVA CURIEL AND R. W. BELLHORN

Disease Process	Cause	Clinical Signs	Diagnostic Procedures	Treatment	References
Snakes					
Retention of spectacle.	1. Ectoparasites. Mites (most frequently *Ophionyssus*) and ticks. Scarring and accumulation of debris in periocular region interferes with molting of spectacle.	Retention of opaque spectacle after molting. See mites or ticks in recess between spectacle and periorbital scales.	Examine snake (especially periocular region) for ectoparasites.	Place dichlorvos-impregnated strip (Vapona Pest strip, Shell Chemical Corp, Atlanta, GA) in cage for 3 days. Follow with cage disinfection and repeat treatment in 10–14 days. Careful manual removal of ticks (taking care not to leave mouth parts behind).	Millichamp et al, 1983
	2. Dysecdysis (improper shedding). Failure of spectacle to be shed due to malnourishment, dehydration, lack of proper humidity in cage, chilling, systemic disease, or lack of scabrous substrate in cage.	Retention of spectacle (opaque) after snake molts. Spectacle may be retained after each molt such that several retained spectacles are present. Vision may be impaired.	—	Do not pull off old spectacle with forceps. Wait until next molt. Correct humidity to 50–60%, add bricks or logs to cage for snake to rub against. Correct ectoparasitism. Just before molting, spray snake and cage with water to raise humidity. If spectacles are not shed, soak snake in warm water (just enough to cover snake) overnight. Rub gently free with moistened cotton next day. Topical application of acetylcysteine may help loosen old spectacle.	Frye, 1981; Hanna et al, 1963; Jacobsen, 1977; Marcus, 1981; Millichamp and Jacobsen, 1986; Millichamp et al, 1983
Clouding of spectacle.	1. Normal. Normal shedding process	Skin and spectacle normally become dull with beginning of shedding. This cloudy/blue appearance fades in 7–10 days, and spectacle becomes transparent again just before outer skin is shed.	—	None required. Ensure that proper shedding occurs (see "Retention of spectacle" above).	

TABLE BY DRS. J. M. A. DA SILVA CURIEL AND R. W. BELLHORN *Continued*

Disease Process	Cause	Clinical Signs	Diagnostic Procedures	Treatment	References
	2. Distention of subspectacular space (see below).				
	3. Abscessation of subspectacular space (see below).				
Distention of subspectacular space.	1. Congenital Congenital absence or occlusion of nasolacrimal duct at its opening into mouth. Most congenital lesions in snakes are due to suboptimal incubation temperatures or conditions.	Distention of subspectacular space (may be unilateral or bilateral) with clear fluid.	Inject 10% sodium fluorescein dye into subspectacular space with a 30-gauge needle and observe roof of mouth (in area of vomeronasal organ) with a cobalt blue or ultraviolet light source for passage of dye.	Excision of a 30° wedge from ventral portion of spectacle temporarily relieves distention. Can create a new drainage route between mouth and subspectacular space by passing a 2/0 nylon suture or 0.0025-inch outer diameter Silastic tubing through a curved needle inserted between subspectacular space and roof of mouth. Leave in place for 4–8 weeks. Use concomitant prophylactic antibiotic therapy. Prognosis is guarded if secondary infection of space occurs.	
	2. Acquired. Occlusion usually occurs secondary to inflammatory conditions within mouth (especially ulcerative stomatitis). Ulcerative stomatitis usually due to *Aeromonas hydrophilia* infection (*Klebsiella* and *Pseudomonas* occasionally isolated). If bacterial colonization of harderian gland occurs, subspectacular abscessation may result.	Distention of subspectacular space (may be unilateral or bilateral) with clear or cloudy fluid.	Culture and sensitivity of subspectacular fluid. Culture and sensitivity of mouth if ulcerative stomatitis present. Identify and eliminate predisposing factors for stomatitis (malnutrition, vitamins C and A deficiency, force feeding, trauma from capture).	Treat stomatitis with 3% hydrogen peroxide mouthwashes, plus systemic antibiotic therapy. Clear obstruction in mouth. Wedge resection of ventral spectacle will temporarily relieve distention (usually resolves on its own, following successful treatment of ulcerative stomatitis). Flush subspectacular space with saline solution; instill a triple antibiotic ophthalmic solution into space. Disinfect cage.	Frye, 1981; Marcus, 1981; Millichamp et al, 1983; Wallach and Boever, 1983

Table continued on following page

Reptiles *Continued*

TABLE BY DRS. J. M. A. DA SILVA CURIEL AND R. W. BELLHORN *Continued*

Disease Process	Cause	Clinical Signs	Diagnostic Procedures	Treatment	References
Abscessation of subspectacular space.	1. Penetrating injury to eye. 2. Extension up nasolacrimal duct in ulcerative stomatitis. 3. Hematogenous extension from systemic disease. 4. Complication of dysecdysis or fluid distention of subspectacular space.	Ballooning of spectacle with white or yellow exudate beneath spectacle. In recovered animals, focal or diffuse deposits on inner surface of spectacle (must distinguish these deposits from keratic precipitates associated with uveitis on inner surface of cornea).	Culture and sensitivity of purulent material in subspectacular space. *Salmonella, Arizona, Proteus, Aeromonas,* and *Pseudomonas* are commonly cultured. Opportunistic fungal infections may occur (e.g., candidiasis). Biopsies of scales or smears of purulent material.	Treat mouth infections (see "Acquired distention of subspectacular space" above). Topical ophthalmic therapy is *not* effective. Excise a 30° wedge of spectacle ventrally; flush pus out of subspectacular space with physiological saline solution; infuse appropriate antibiotics if indicated. Local extension may result in panophthalmitis; enucleation in advanced cases. To prevent trauma and infection, live prey should be killed before feeding it to snake.	Fox et al, 1984; Frye, 1981; Marcus, 1981; Millichamp et al, 1983
Mycotic periocular dermatitis.	Poor husbandry. A continuously damp environment, unsanitary conditions, and suboptimal temperatures are predisposing factors. *Geotrichum, Fusarium, Trichoderma,* and *Penicillium* have all been isolated.	Necrotizing skin disease. Scales of head and spectacle often involved. Infection starts between scales and spreads to contiguous scales.	Culture and histopathology of biopsied scales. Fungus-stained sections have masses of hyphae and arthrospores, usually at bases of affected scales.	Correct environmental conditions. Topical application of tolnaftate, miconazole, or nystatin. Snake may be soaked in chlorhexidine (0.26 ml/L of water) for 1–2 hours daily, especially at time of shedding. Surgical removal of dermal granulomas.	Frye, 1981; Jacobsen, 1980, 1981; McKenzie and Green, 1976; Millichamp et al, 1983
Panophthalmitis.	Penetrating wounds, hematogenous spread from systemic infection, local invasion from subspectacular or orbital abscess, local trauma from ectoparasites.	Massively swollen and discolored eye(s) bulging from the orbit. Neovascular changes may be present in chronic cases.	Differentiate from subspectacular abscesses. Establish presence or absence of systemic disease. Culture and sensitivity.	Systemic antibiotic and supportive therapy. Panophthalmitis is extremely destructive and results in blind eye; therefore, surgical removal of affected eye is most effective treatment.	
Anterior uveitis/ hypopyon.	Penetrating wounds, manifestation of systemic disease; neoplastic invasion (especially lymphoreticular) of uveal tissue.	Unilateral or bilateral photophobia, cloudy corneas, iritis, aqueous flare, and miosis. Keratic precipitates may be present on the interior surface of the cornea. Hypopyon.	Establish presence of systemic disease (physical examination, complete blood count, and so on.) Differentiate hypopyon and keratic precipitates from subspectacular abscess.	Treat systemic disease with appropriate antimicrobial agent. Topical antibiotic or steroid therapy not effective in snakes due to impervious spectacle; therefore, these agents must be given	Frye, 1981

TABLE BY DRS. J. M. A. DA SILVA CURIEL AND R. W. BELLHORN *Continued*

Disease Process	Cause	Clinical Signs	Diagnostic Procedures	Treatment	References
				systemically or injected under spectacle. Atropine and tropicamide not effective for mydriasis. Intraocular injection of antimicrobials not recommended.	

Chelonians (Turtles and Tortoises)

Disease Process	Cause	Clinical Signs	Diagnostic Procedures	Treatment	References
Keratoconjunctivitis.	1. Termination of hibernation. Associated with end of hibernation.	Mucoid ocular discharge, excessive tearing or blepharospasm immediately after hibernation. May be an associated rhinitis.	—	Discharge and blepharospasm usually resolve with no treatment a few days after animal starts feeding. Keep periocular region clean until clinical signs disappear. Topical ophthalmic antibiotic.	Davidson, 1985
	2. Respiratory disease. *Klebsiella, Pasteurella,* or mycotic pneumonia.	Conjunctival hyperemia, ocular and nasal discharge, gaping of mouth, dyspnea, anorexia, listlessness, inability to maintain equilibrium (body is tilted) while swimming.	Culture and sensitivity of lung washings. Cytological examination of lung washings for hyphae.	Raise environmental temperature to at least 37°C. Antibiotics and supportive care for bacterial pneumonias. For mycotic pneumonias, treat with nystatin or potassium iodide solution. Dosages are empirical and are based on mammalian schedule, with longer intervals between doses.	Frye, 1981; Jacobsen, 1981
Hypovitaminosis A.	Vitamin A deficiency due to dietary deficiencies. Squamous metaplasia of orbital glands and ducts leads to eyelid and orbital edema. Secondary bacterial or fungal blepharitis or keratitis may occur.	Swollen eyelids on a young, growing turtle fed an all-meat diet.	Establish presence of inadequate diet.	Inject 1000–1500 units (depending on size) of vitamin A intramuscularly at weekly intervals (minimum of three treatments) until eyelid edema subsides. Topical ophthalmic antibiotic or antifungal preparation for eyes if secondary bacterial/fungal infection present. Correct diet to include vitamin A (feed commercial trout pellets); add small amounts of cod liver oil to diet.	Bellhorn, 1973; Millchamp et al, 1983

Table continued on following page

Reptiles *Continued*

TABLE BY DRS. J. M. A. DA SILVA CURIEL AND R. W. BELLHORN *Continued*

Disease Process	Cause	Clinical Signs	Diagnostic Procedures	Treatment	References
Epiphora.	May be normal (due to absence of nasolacrimal duct in chelonians), associated with hibernation (see above), or associated with keratoconjunctivitis resulting from other causes.	Excessive tearing.	—	Keep periocular area clean if discharge is excessive. Identify and treat corneal ulcers, and so on.	
Orbital abscesses.	Arthropod-borne bacterial infection. Extension from systemic infection. Penetrating wounds.	Abscessation may involve conjunctival, subconjunctival, retrobulbar, periorbital, and eyelid tissues. Infraorbital and periorbital spaces most frequently involved. Abscessation may extend behind globe and cause eye to bulge outward. Small localized abscesses may be found beneath the eyelids. Secondary septicemia may occur. Differential diagnosis is ear abscess.	Culture and sensitivity.	Evacuation of necrotic debris by lancing abscess, gentle evacuation using a blunt curette, flush cavity using a plastic catheter. Systemic antibiotics.	Frye, 1981

REFERENCES

Horses

Blogg JR (1980): The Eye in Veterinary Practice, vol 1, Extraocular Disease. WB Saunders Co, Philadelphia.

Blogg JR (1985): The Eye in Veterinary Practice, vol 2, Eye Examination of the Performance Horse. Chilcote Publishing, Melbourne, Australia.

Lavach JD (1987): The Handbook of Equine Ophthalmology. Giddings Studio Publishing, Ft Collins, CO.

Munroe GA, Barnett KC (1984): Congenital ocular disease in the foal. Vet Clin North Am 6:519.

Caged Birds

Bellhorn RW (1981): Laboratory animal ophthalmology. *In* Gelatt KN (ed): Veterinary Ophthalmology. Lea & Febiger, Philadelphia.

Clubb SL (1984): Therapeutics in avian medicine: Flock vs individual bird treatment regimens. Vet Clin North Am 14:345.

Karpinski LG, Clubb SL (1986): Clinical aspects of ophthalmology in caged birds, p 616. *In* Kirk RW, et al: Current Veterinary Therapy IX. WB Saunders Co, Philadelphia.

Karpinski LG, Clubb SL (1986): An outbreak of avian pox in imported mynahs. Proc Ann Mtg Assoc Avian Vet, p 35.

Murphy CJ (1984): Raptor ophthalmology. Proc Ann Mtg Assoc Avian Vet, p 43.

Murphy CJ, et al (1982): Ocular lesions in free-living raptors. J Am Vet Med Assoc 181:1302.

Slatter DH, et al (1983): Hereditary cataracts in canaries. J Am Vet Med Assoc 183:872.

Fish

Brandt TM, et al (1986): Corneal cloudiness in transported large-mouth bass. Prog Fish Cult 48:199.

Conroy DA, Herman RL (1970): Textbook of Fish Diseases. Jersey City, TFH Publications.

Dukes TW (1975): Ophthalmic pathology of fishes. *In* Ribelin WE, Migaki G (eds): *Pathology of Fishes*, p 383. University of Wisconsin Press, Madison.

Gaten E (1987): Aggregation of the eye fluke *Diplostomum spathecum* (Digenea: Diplostomatidae) in the lenses of various species of fish. J Fish Dis 10:69.

Hawkins WE, et al (1986): Intraocular neoplasms induced by methylazoxymethanol acetate in Japanese madaka. Jap N Cl 76:453.

Hoffert JR, Fromm PO: Biomicroscopic, gross, and microscopic observations of corneal lesions in the lake trout *Solvelinus namaycush*. J Fish Res Bd Can 22:761.

Noga EJ, et al (1981): Cataracts in cichlic fish. J Am Vet Med Assoc 179:1181.

Posten H, et al (1977): The effect of supplemental dietary amino acids, minerals, and vitamins on salmonids fed cataractog... diets. Cornell Vet 67:472.

Posten H, et al (1988): Nutritionally induced cataracts in salmonids fed purified diets. Marine Fisheries Rev 40:45.

Tumilson R, et al (1985): Multiple lenses in the eye of a large-mouth bass. Southwest Naturalist 30:147.

Wolfe MJ (1983): The morphogenesis of nutritional cataracts in rainbow trout. PhD Thesis, Cornell University, Ithaca, NY.

Yokote M (1974): Spontaneous diabetes in carp (Cyprinnus carpio). Spec Publ Japan Sea Fish Lab, p 67.

Poultry

Aghakhan SM (1974): Avian adenovirus. Vet Bull 44:531.

Barber CW (1947): Studies on the avian leucosis complex. I. The effects of rearing environment on the incidence of leucosis among white leghorn chickens. Cornell Vet 37:349.

Barr DA, et al (1986): Isolation of Chlamydia psitacci from commercial broiler chickens. Aust Vet J 63:377.

Becker ER, et al (1949): Eyelid lesion of chicks in acute dietary deficiency resulting from blood-induced Plasmodium lophurae infection. I. Description; role of pantothenic acid and biotin. J Infect Dis 85:230.

Cheng KM, et al (1980): An autosomal recessive blind mutant in the chicken. Poult Sci 59:2179.

Crispin SM, Barnett KC (1978): Ocular candidiasis in ornamental ducks. Avian Pathol 7:49.

Evans WM, et al (1955): Blindness in chicks associated with salmonellosis. Cornell Vet 45:239.

Gries CL, Scott ML (1972): The pathology of thiamin, riboflavin, pantothenic acid and niacin deficiencies in the chick. J Nutr 102:1269.

Hinshaw WR, Lloyd WE (1934): Hilgardia 8:281. Cited by Hofstad MS, et al (eds) (1978): Diseases of Poultry, 7th ed. Iowa State University Press, Ames.

Hofstad MW, et al (eds) (1978): Diseases of Poultry, 7th ed. Iowa State University Press, Ames.

Keymer IF (1977): Cataracts in birds. Avian Pathol 6:335.

Matsumoto M, Yamamoto R (1971): A broth bacterin against infectious coryza: Immunogenicity of various preparations. Avian Dis 15:109.

Moore EN (1953): Aspergillus fumigatus as a cause of ophthalmitis in turkeys. Poult Sci 32:796.

Mustaffa-Babjee A (1969): Specific and nonspecific conditions affecting avian eyes. Vet Bull 39:681.

Nakamura K, Abe F (1987): Ocular lesions in chickens inoculated with Escherichia coli. Can J Vet Res 51:528.

Niilo L (1959): Some observations on Pseudomonas infection in poultry. Can J Comp Med 23:329.

Olson LD (1981): Ophthalmia in turkeys infected with Pasteurella multocida. Avian Dis 25:423.

Raggi LG, Armstrong WH (1960): Conjunctivitis of chickens caused by a typical infectious laryngotracheitis virus. Avian Dis 4:272.

Reece RL, et al (1981): The isolation of Haemophilus paragallinarum from Japanese quail. Aust Vet J 57:350.

Sato G, Adler HE (1966): Experimental infection of adult turkeys with Arizona group organisms. Avian Dis 10:329.

Saunders LZ, Moore EN (1957): Blindness in turkeys due to granulomatous chorioretinitis. Avian Dis 1:27.

Rabbits, Rodents, and Reptiles

Bellhorn RW (1973): Ophthalmic disorders of exotic and laboratory animals. Vet Clin North Am 3:345.

Bellhorn RW (1980): Lighting in the animal environment. Lab Anim Sci 30:440.

Bellhorn RW (1981): Laboratory animal ophthalmology. In Gelatt KN (ed): Veterinary Ophthalmology, p 649. Lea & Febiger, Philadelphia.

Bellhorn RW, et al (1980): Retinal vessel abnormalities of phototoxic retinopathy in rats. Invest Ophthalmol Vis Sci 19:584.

Brooks DL (1986): Special medicine of rabbits, hares, and picas. In Fowler ME (ed): Zoo and Wild Animal Medicine, 2nd ed., p 711. WB Saunders Co, Philadelphia.

Davidson MG (1985): Ophthalmology of exotic pets. Compend Cont Ed Pract Vet 7:724.

Everitt JE, et al (1987): Diagnostic exercise: Eye lesions in rats. Lab Anim Sci 37:203.

Fox JG, et al (1979): Congenital entropion in a litter of rabbits. Lab Anim Sci 29:509.

Fox JG, et al (1984): Laboratory Animal Medicine, p 149. Academic Press, Orlando, FL.

Fraunfelder FT, Burns RP (1966): Effect of lid closure in drug-induced experimental cataracts. Arch Ophthalmol 76:559.

Frye FJ (1981): Biomedical and Surgical Aspects of Captive Reptile Husbandry, p 228. Veterinary Medical Publishing Co, Edwardsville, KS.

Hanna BL, et al (1963): Recessive buphthalmos in the rabbit. Genetics 47:519.

Harkness JE, Ridgway MD (1980): Chromodacryorrhea in laboratory rats (Rattus norvegicus): Etiologic considerations. Lab Anim Sci 30:841.

Harkness JE, Wagner JE (1983): The Biology and Medicine of Rabbits and Rodents, p 75. Lea & Febiger, Philadelphia.

Jacobsen ER (1977): Histology, endocrinology, and husbandry of ecdysis in snakes (a review). Vet Med Small Anim Clin 72:275.

Jacobsen ER (1980): Necrotizing mycotic dermatitis in snakes: Clinical and pathological features. J Am Vet Med Assoc 177:838.

Jacobsen ER (1981): Diseases of reptiles—Infectious diseases. Compend Cont Ed Pract Vet 3:195.

Lai YL, et al (1978): Age-related and light-associated retinal changes in Fischer rats. Invest Ophthalmol Vis Sci 17:634.

Lanum J (1978): The damaging effects of light on the retina. Empirical findings, theoretical and practical implications. Surv Ophthalmol 22:221.

Marcus LC (1981): Veterinary Biology and Medicine of Captive Reptile Husbandry, p 43. Lea & Febiger, Philadelphia.

McKenzie RA, Green PE (1976): Mycotic dermatitis in captive carpet snakes (Morelia spilotes variegata). J Wild Dis 12:405.

Millichamp NJ, Jacobsen ER (1986): Ophthalmic diseases of reptiles. In Kirk RW (ed): Current Veterinary Therapy IX, p 621. WB Saunders Co, Philadelphia.

Millichamp NJ, et al (1983): Diseases of the eye and ocular adnexa in reptiles. J Am Vet Med Assoc 183:1205.

Murray ES (1964): Guinea pig inclusion conjunctivitis virus. I. Isolation and identification as a member of the Psittacosis-Lymphogranuloma-Trachoma group. J Infect Dis 114:1.

Nakagawa M, et al (1974): Prophylaxis of Bordetella bronchiseptica infection in guinea pigs by vaccination. Jpn J Vet Sci 36:33.

Patton NM, Holmes HT (1977): Myxomatosis in domestic rabbits in Oregon. J Am Vet Med Assoc 171:560.

Raphael BL (1981): Pet rabbit medicine. Compent Cont Ed Pract Vet 3:60.

Schiavo DM (1980):Multifocal retinal dysplasia in the Syrian hamster: LVG (5 yr). J Environ Pathol and Toxicol 3:569.

Shimizu T (1978): Prophylaxis of Bordetella bronchiseptica infection in guinea pigs by intranasal vaccination with live strain ts-S43. Infect Immun 22:318.

Theisen DD, Pendergrass M (1982): Harderian gland involvement in facial lesions in the Mongolian gerbil. J Am Vet Med Assoc 181:1375.

Wagner JE, et al (1966): Spontaneous conjunctivitis and dacryoadenitis of mice. J Am Vet Med Assoc 155:1211.

Wallach JD, Boever WJ (1983): Diseases of Exotic Animals—Medical and Surgical Management, p 979. WB Saunders Co, Philadelphia.

Weisbroth SH, Peress N (1977): Ophthalmic lesions and dacryoadenitis: A naturally occurring aspect of sialodacryoadenitis virus infection of the laboratory rat. Lab Anim Sci 27:466.

APPENDIX I

Breed Predisposition to Eye Diseases[1]

This list provides an aid to diagnosis of the *more common* disorders and is not a complete account of all diseases recorded.

DOGS

Afghan Hound

Cataracts
Corneal dystrophy
Eversion of the cartilage of the third eyelid
Glaucoma (secondary to vaccination with canine adenovirus vaccines)
Mesodermal dysgenesis (goniodysgenesis) of the drainage angle
Persistent pupillary membranes
Progressive retinal degeneration (PRD) type I
Vogt-Koyanagi-Harada syndrome[2]

Airedale

Corneal dystrophy
Distichiasis
Entropion
PRD type I

Akita

Corneal dystrophy
Entropion
Eversion of the cartilage of the third eyelid
Multiple ocular anomalies (microphthalmia, congenital cataracts, posterior lenticonus, retinal dysplasia)
PRD type I
Vogt-Koyanagi-Harada syndrome

Alaskan Malamute

Corneal dystrophy
Hemeralopia (cone dysplasia)
Heterochromia iridis
PRD type I

American Cocker Spaniel

Cataract (juvenile and adult onset)
Corneal dystrophy
Distichiasis
Ectopic cilia
Ectropion
Entropion
Glaucoma (primary narrow-angle and secondary to lens luxation)
Hypoplasia of the optic nerve
Keratoconjunctivitis sicca (KCS)
Lacrimal punctal atresia
Lens luxation ($\pm$ secondary glaucoma)
Optic nerve colobomata
Optic nerve hypoplasia
Oversized palpebral fissure
Persistent pupillary membranes
PRD type I
Protrusion of the gland of the third eyelid

Redundant forehead skin
Retinal dysplasia
Staphylococcal blepharitis with hypersensitivity
Trichiasis

American Foxhound

Microphthalmia

American Staffordshire Terrier (Pit Bull)

Cataract
Persistent hyperplastic primary vitreous

Australian Cattle Dog ("Queensland Blue Heeler" [sic])

Chronic immune-mediated keratoconjunctivitis (Überreiter's syndrome, pannus, chronic superficial keratitis)
Heterochromia iridis
PRD type I

Australian Shepherd [sic]

Cataract
Colobomata
Corectopia, dyscoria
Heterochromia iridis
Microcornea
Microphthalmia with multiple congenital defects
Persistent pupillary membrane
PRD type I
Retinal detachment
Retinal dysplasia
Scleral ectasia syndrome

Vogt-Koyanagi-Harada
syndrome

Australian Terrier

Cataract
PRD type I

Basenji

Cataract
Coloboma of the optic disc
Corneal leukoma
Persistent pupillary membrane
Posterior segment colobomata
Progressive retinal atrophy
(PRA) type I

Basset Hound

Ectropion
Entropion
Lens luxation (± secondary
glaucoma)
Oversized palpebral fissure
PRA type I
Primary glaucoma (mesodermal
dysgenesis {goniodysgenesis})
Redundant forehead skin

Beagle

Cataract
Corneal dystrophy
Glaucoma (primary open-angle)
Globoid cell leukodystrophy
Optic nerve hypoplasia
Persistent pupillary membranes
PRD type I
Protrusion of the gland of the
third eyelid
Retinal dysplasia (±
microphthalmia and retinal
folds)

Bearded Collie

Cataracts
Persistent pupillary membranes
PRD type I

Bedlington Terrier

Atresia of lacrimal puncta or
canaliculi
Distichiasis
PRD type I

Retinal dysplasia

Black and Tan Coonhound

PRD type II

Blue Tick Hound

Globoid cell leukodystrophy

Bloodhound

Ectropion
Entropion
KCS
Redundant forehead skin

Border Collie

Ceroid lipofuscinosis
PRD type I
PRD type II (pigment epithelial
dystrophy)
Proliferative keratoconjunctivitis
Scleral ectasia syndrome (collie
eye anomaly)

Border Terrier

Cataract
PRD type I

Borzoi

Glaucoma (secondary to
vaccination with canine
adenovirus vaccines)
PRD type I
Retinal dysplasia

Boston Terrier

Cataracts
Corneal endothelial dystrophy
Distichiasis
KCS
Medical canthal entropion
PRD type I
Protrusion of the gland of the
third eyelid
Strabismus
Superficial corneal erosion
syndrome

Bouvier de Flandres

Cataracts
Ectropion
Entropion
Heterochromia iridis
Mesodermal dysgenesis

Boxer

Distichiasis
PRD type I
Superficial corneal erosion
syndrome

Briard

PRD type I
PRD type II

Brittany Spaniel

PRD type I
Retinal dysplasia

Brussels Griffon

Distichiasis

Bulldog (English)

See English Bulldog

Bullmastiff

Entropion
Eversion of the cartilage of the
third eyelid
Glaucoma
PRD type I

Bull Terrier

Blepharophimosis
(micropalpebral fissure)
Cataract (juvenile)
KCS
Persistent hyperplastic primary
vitreous
PRD type I

Cairn Terrier

Ectopic cilia
Globoid cell leukodystrophy
KCS

Lens luxation (± secondary
   glaucoma)
PRD type I

Cardigan Welsh Corgi

Lens luxation (± secondary
   glaucoma)
Persistent pupillary membrane
PRD type I
PRD type II
Superficial corneal erosion
   syndrome

Cavalier King Charles Spaniel

Cataracts
Corneal dystrophy (lipid)
Distichiasis
Posterior lenticonus, cataracts,
   and microphthalmia
PRD type I

Chesapeake Bay Retriever

Cataract (juvenile)
Distichiasis
Entropion
Eversion of the cartilage of the
   third eyelid
PRD type I
PRD type II

Chihuahua

Ceroid lipofuscinosis
Chronic immune-mediated
   keratoconjunctivitis syndrome
   (Überreiter's syndrome)
Corneal endothelial dystrophy
Iris atrophy
KCS
Lens luxation (± secondary
   glaucoma)
PRD type I
Trichiasis

Chow Chow

Anterior chamber cleavage
   syndrome
Blepharophimosis
   (micropalpebral fissure)
Displaced lacrimal puncta
Distichiasis

Entropion
Glaucoma
Oversized palpebral fissure
Persistent pupillary membrane
PRD type I
Redundant forehead skin

Cocker Spaniel

See American Cocker Spaniel,
   English Cocker Spaniel

Collie (Rough and Smooth)

Blepharophimosis
   (micropalpebral fissure)
Corneal dystrophy (lipid)
Distichiasis
Entropion
Hypoplasia of optic nerve
Microcornea
Microphthalmia
Optic nerve hypoplasia
Persistent pupillary membrane
PRD type I (rod-cone dysplasia)
PRD type II
Proliferative keratoconjunctivitis
Retinal dysplasia
Scleral ectasia syndrome (collie
   eye anomaly)

Corgi

See Cardigan Welsh Corgi,
   Pembroke Corgi

Curly-Coated Retriever

Cataracts
Distichiasis
Entropion
PRD type I

Dachshund

Atypical chronic keratitis
Ceroid lipofuscinosis
Corneal dystrophy (epithelial
   and endothelial)
Dermoid
Ectopic cilia
KCS
Microphthalmia
Optic nerve hypoplasia
Persistent pupillary membranes
PRD type I

Superficial corneal erosion
   syndrome

Dalmatian

Dermoid, conjunctiva
Entropion
Glaucoma
Heterochromia iridis
Neuronal ceroid lipofuscinosis

Dandie Dinmont Terrier

Goniodysgenesis
Persistent pupillary membrane

Doberman Pinscher

Anterior chamber cleavage syndrome
Cataract
Colobomata
Deep inferior conjunctival fornix
Enophthalmos
Entropion
Entropion secondary to enophthalmos
Eversion of the cartilage of the third eyel
Microphakia
Persistent hyperplastic primary vitreous
Persistent pupillary membrane
PRD type I

English Bulldog

Distichiasis
Ectopic cilia
Ectropion
Entropion
KCS
Nasal fold trichiasis
Oversized palpebral fissure
Persistent pupillary membrane
Redundant forehead skin

English Cocker Spaniel

Cataract
Distichiasis
Ectropion
Entropion
Fucosidosis
Glaucoma
Optic nerve colobomata
Persistent pupillary membrane
PRD type I
Retinal dysplasia

English Setter

Cataract
Ceroid lipofuscinosis
Ectropion
Entropion
KCS
Palpebral neoplasia
PRD type I

English Springer Spaniel

Cataract
Corneal dystrophy
    (subepithelial)
Distichiasis
Ectropion
Entropion
Glaucoma
Persistent pupillary membrane
PRD type I
PRD type II
Retinal dysplasia

Field Spaniel

PRD type I

Fox Terrier (Smooth)

Corneal dystrophy (epithelial)
Lens luxation ($\pm$ secondary
    glaucoma)
Trichiasis

Fox Terrier (Wire-Haired)

Cataract (juvenile)
Corneal dystrophy (epithelial
    and endothelial)
Distichiasis
Glaucoma (primary)
Lens luxation ($\pm$ secondary
    glaucoma)
PRD type I
Superficial corneal erosion
    syndrome

German Shepherd

Cataract
Chronic immune-mediated
    keratoconjunctivitis syndrome
    (Überreiter's syndrome,
    pannus)
Colobomata

Corneal dystrophy
Deep inferior conjunctival
    fornix
Dermoid
Euryblepharon (juvenile,
    transient)
Eversion of the cartilage of the
    third eyelid
Optic nerve hypoplasia
PRD type I
PRD type II (Europe)

German Short-Haired Pointer

Corneal dystrophy
Entropion
Eversion of the cartilage of the
    third eyelid
GM^2 gangliosidosis
Strabismus

Golden Retriever

Cataract
Cataract with microphthalmia
Distichiasis
Enophthalmos
Entropion
Persistent pupillary membrane
PRD type I
PRD type II
Retinal dysplasia
Vogt-Koyanagi-Harada
    syndrome

Gordon Setter

Entropion
PRD type I
Retinal dysplasia

Great Dane

Distichiasis
Ectropion
Enophthalmos
Entropion
Eversion of the cartilage of the
    third eyelid
Glaucoma
Mesodermal dysgenesis
Microphthalmia (merles)
Multiple iris cysts
Retinal dysplasia (harlequin
    coloring)
PRD type I

Great Pyrenees

Ectropion
Enophthalmos
Entropion
Persistent pupillary membrane

Greyhound

Cataracts
Chronic immune-mediated
    keratoconjunctivitis
    (Überreiter's syndrome,
    pannus)
Corneal dystrophy
Glaucoma (secondary to
    vaccination with canine
    adenovirus vaccines)
Persistent pupillary membrane
PRD type II
Retinal dystrophy

Irish Setter

Anterior chamber cleavage
    syndrome
Cataract
Corneal dystrophy
Deep inferior conjunctival
    fornix
Distichiasis
Enophthalmos
Entropion
Optic nerve hypoplasia
Persistent pupillary membrane
PRD type I (rod-cone dysplasia)
PRD type II
Vogt-Koyanagi-Harada
    syndrome

Italian Greyhound

Cataracts
Glaucoma (secondary to
    vaccination with canine
    adenovirus vaccines)
PRD type I
PRD type II

Jack Russell Terrier

Lens luxation ($\pm$ secondary
    glaucoma)

Keeshond

Ectopic cilia
Glaucoma

PRD type I
PRD type II

Kerry Blue Terrier

Blepharophimosis
Distichiasis
Entropion
KCS
PRD type I
Trichiasis

Labrador Retriever

Cataract
Distichiasis
Enophthalmos
Entropion
PRD type I
PRD type II
Retinal dysplasia ($\pm$ skeletal
abnormalities)

Lakeland Terrier

Distichiasis
Lens luxation ($\pm$ secondary
glaucoma)

Lapland

Glycogen storage disease type II
(Pompe's disease)

Large Munsterlander

Cataracts

Lhasa Apso

Cataracts
Chronic corneal exposure
syndrome
Distichiasis
Ectopic cilia
Entropion, medial lower lid
Euryblepharon
KCS
PRD type I
Retinal dysplasia

Maltese Terrier

Canine allergic inhalant
conjunctivitis (atopy)
Distichiasis
Ectopic cilia

PRD type I
Tear-staining syndrome

Manchester Terrier

Lens luxation ($\pm$ secondary
glaucoma)
PRD type I

Mastiff

Ectropion
Entropion
Persistent pupillary membrane

Miniature Bull Terrier

Lens luxation (recessive)

Miniature Pinscher

Entropion (medial)
KCS
PRD type I

Newfoundland

Ectropion
Entropion
Euryblepharon
Eversion of the cartilage of the
third eyelid

Norwegian Elkhound

Distichiasis
Glaucoma (primary open-angle)
PRD type I (rod dysplasia, early
retinal degeneration)

Nova Duck Tolling Retriever

PRD type I

Old English Sheepdog

Cataract (congenital and adult)
Distichiasis
Entropion
Glaucoma
Heterochromia iridis
Microphthalmia
PRD type I
Vogt-Koyanagi-Harada
syndrome

Papillon

Entropion

Pekingese

Atresia of lacrimal puncta and
canaliculi
Cataract
Chronic corneal exposure
syndrome
Corneal ulceration
Distichiasis
Ectopic cilia
Entropion (medial)
Euryblepharon
Exotropia
Microphthalmia
Nasal fold trichiasis
PRD type I
Traumatic proptosis
Trichiasis

Pembroke Corgi

Lens luxation ($\pm$ secondary
glaucoma)
Persistent pupillary membrane
PRD type I

Plott Hound

Mucopolysaccharidosis type I

Pointer

Cataract
Entropion
PRD type I

Pomeranian

Atresia of lacrimal puncta
Canine allergic inhalant
conjunctivitis (atopy)
Distichiasis
PRD type I
Tear-staining syndrome
Trichiasis

Poodle (Miniature and Toy)

Atresia of lacrimal puncta and
canaliculi
Canine allergic inhalant
conjunctivitis (atopy)

Cataract
Chronic immune-mediated
   keratitis
   (Überreiter's syndrome,
   pannus) (miniature poodle
   only)
Corneal dystrophy (epithelial
   and endothelial)
Distichiasis
Entropion (medial)
Glaucoma (primary open-angle,
   narrow-angle)
Hemeralopia (miniature poodle)
Iris atrophy
Microphthalmia
Optic nerve hypoplasia
PRD type I (rod-cone
   degeneration)
Superficial corneal erosion
   syndrome
Tear-staining syndrome
Trichiasis
Trichomegaly

Poodle (Standard)

Canine allergic inhalant
   conjunctivitis (atopy)
Cataract
Distichiasis
Optic nerve hypoplasia
Persistent pupillary membrane
PRD type I

Portugese Water Dog

Persistent pupillary membrane

Pug

Chronic corneal exposure
   syndrome
Corneal dystrophy
Distichiasis
Entropion (medial)
Euryblepharon
Nasal fold trichiasis
PRD type I
Trichiasis

Queensland Blue Heeler [*sic*]

See Australian Cattle Dog

Redbone Coonhound

PRD type II

Rottweiler

Cataract
Deep conjunctival fornix
Ectropion
Entropion
Euryblepharon
Microphthalmia
Oversized palpebral fissure
PRD type I
Retinal dysplasia

Saint Bernard

Dermoid
Distichiasis
Ectropion
Entropion
Eversion of the cartilage of the
   third eyelid
Microphthalmia with multiple
   congenital anomalies
Oversized palpebral fissure
Redundant facial skin
Vogt-Koyanagi-Harada
   syndrome

Saluki

Corneal dystrophy
Glaucoma (secondary to
   vaccination with canine
   adenovirus vaccines)
Mesodermal dysgenesis
   (goniodysgenesis)
Persistent pupillary membrane
PRD type I
Retinal detachment
Retinal dysplasia

Samoyed

Corneal dystrophy
Distichiasis
Mesodermal dysgenesis
   (goniodysgenesis)
Microphthalmos
Persistent pupillary membrane
Primary glaucoma
PRD type I
Retinal detachment, cataracts,
   and skeletal dwarfism
Retinal dysplasia
Vogt-Koyanagi-Harada
   syndrome

Schipperke

Distichiasis
Ectropion
Narrow palpebral fissure

Schnauzer (Giant)

PRD type I

Schnauzer (Miniature)

Atresia of lacrimal puncta and
   canaliculi
Cataract (congenital ±
   microphthalmia)
Cataract (juvenile)
Corneal dystrophy
Distichiasis
Entropion
KCS
Microcornea
Microphthalmia (± multiple
   congenital anomalies)
Optic nerve hypoplasia
Persistent hyperplastic primary
   vitreous
Persistent pupillary membrane
PRD type I (rod-cone dysplasia)

Schnauzer (Standard)

Persistent hyperplastic primary
   vitreous

Scottish Terrier

Persistent pupillary membrane
PRD type I

Sealyham Terrier

Atresia of the lacrimal puncta
   and canaliculi
Cataract
Lens luxation (± secondary
   glaucoma)
Retinal detachment
Retinal dysplasia

Shar Pei

Ectropion
Prolapse of the gland of the
   third eyelid
Redundant facial skin

Shetland Sheepdog

Atresia of the lacrimal puncta
    and canaliculi
Blepharophimosis
Cataract
Choroidal hypoplasia
Colobomata (optic disc)
Corneal dystrophy
Distichiasis
Ectopic cilia
Heterochromia iridis
Persistent pupillary membrane
PRD type I
PRD type II
Proliferative keratoconjunctivitis
    syndrome
Retinal dysplasia
Scleral ectasia syndrome (collie
    eye anomaly)
Vogt-Koyanagi-Harada
    syndrome

Shih-Tzu

Cataract
Chronic exposure keratitis
Corneal dystrophy (endothelial)
Deep corneal erosion
Entropion (medial)
Euryblepharon
KCS
PRD type I
Ulcerative keratitis

Siberian Husky

Cataract
Chronic immune-mediated
    keratoconjunctivitis syndrome
Corneal dystrophy (endothelial
    and epithelial)
Glaucoma
Heterochromia iridis
Palpebral neoplasia
Persistent pupillary membrane
PRD type I
Vogt-Koyanagi-Harada
    syndrome

Silky Terrier

Atopic conjunctivitis and
    blepharitis
Cataract
Neurovisceral glucocerebroside
    storage disease

Soft-Coated Wheaten Terrier

Cataract
PRD type I

Spitz

PRD type I

Staffordshire Bull Terrier

Cataract
Persistent hyperplastic primary
    vitreous

Tibetan Spaniel

PRD type I

Tibetan Terrier

Lens luxation (± secondary
    glaucoma)
Persistent pupillary membrane
PRD type I (nyctalopia 1–3
    years, and congenital)

Toy Havanese

PRD type I

Toy Terrier

Lens luxation (± secondary
    glaucoma)

Vizsla

PRD type I

Weimaraner

Distichiasis
Entropion
Eversion of the cartilage of the
    third eyelid

Welsh Springer Spaniel

Cataract
Glaucoma (dominant)
PRD type I

Welsh Terrier

Lens luxation (± secondary
    glaucoma)

West Highland White Terrier

Atopic conjunctivitis and
    blepharitis
Cataract
Globoid cell leukodystrophy
KCS

Whippet

Glaucoma (secondary to
    vaccination with canine
    adenovirus vaccines)
PRD type I

Yorkshire Terrier

Atopic conjunctivitis and
    blepharitis
Cataract
Distichiasis
KCS
Retinal dysplasia

CATS

Albinotic Felidae

Esotropia

Burmese

Eyelid hypoplasia ("coloboma")
PRD type I

Domestic Short Hair

Mucopolysaccharidosis type I

Himalayan

Cataracts

Persian

Atresia of the lacrimal puncta
    and canaliculi
Chediak-Higashi syndrome
Entropion
Feline corneal necrosis
Retinal degeneration

Siamese

Esotropia
Feline corneal necrosis

Globoid cell leukodystrophy
Glycogen storage disease type II
  (Pompe's disease)
GM$_1$ gangliosidosis
Herpetic keratitis
Iris atrophy
Mucopolysaccharidosis type VI
PRD type I
Sphingomyelin lipidosis
  (Niemann-Pick disease)
Tapetal degeneration
  (hereditary)

CATTLE

Aberdeen Angus

Mannsidosis

Ayrshire

Heterochromia iridis
Pendular nystagmus

Beef Master

Neuronal lipodystrophy

Brown Swiss

Extra lacrimal drainage
  openings
Multiple ocular anomalies
  (including cataracts)

Charolais

Colobomata (posterior pole)

Devon

Ceroid lipofuscinosis

Friesan (Holstein)

Cataracts (recessive)
  GM$_1$ gangliosidosis
Heterochromia iridis
Pendular nystagmus

German Spotted Cattle

Squamous cell carcinoma

Guernsey

Heterochromia iridis
Multiple ocular anomalies
Pendular nystagmus

Hereford

Cataracts (recessive)
Chediak-Higashi syndrome
Coloboma (associated with
  incomplete albinism)
Dermoids (hereditary)
Infectious bovine
  keratoconjunctivitis
Multiple ocular anomalies
Squamous cell carcinoma

Jersey

Cataracts (recessive)
Corneal opacity
Esotropia
Pendular nystagmus

Shorthorn

Esotropia
Exophthalmos
Glycogen storage disease type II
Multiple ocular anomalies
Susceptibility to infectious
  bovine keratoconjunctivitis
Susceptibility to squamous cell
  carcinoma

SHEEP

Corriedale

Glucocerebroside storage disease
  type II
Glycogen storage disease type II

South Hampshire

Ceroid lipofuscinosis

HORSES

Appaloosa

Congenital night blindness

Morgan Horse

Cataracts (congenital, dominant)

GOATS

Angora

Squamous cell carcinoma

PIGS

Yorkshire

Cerebrospinal lipodystrophy
Glucocerebroside storage disease

REFERENCES

Bistner SI, et al (1977): Atlas of Veterinary Ophthalmic Surgery. WB Saunders Co, Philadelphia.
Blogg JR (1980): The Eye in Veterinary Practice, vol 1. WB Saunders Co, Philadelphia.
Clark RD, Stainer JR (1983): Medical and Genetic Aspects of Purebred Dogs. Veterinary Medicine Publishing Co, Edwardsville, KS.
Kirk RW (ed) (1986): Current Veterinary Therapy IX. WB Saunders Co, Philadelphia.
Magrane WG (1977): Canine Ophthalmology, 3rd ed. Lea & Febiger, Philadelphia.
Rubin LF (1989): Inherited Eye Diseases in Purebred Dogs. Williams & Wilkins, Baltimore.
Severin GA, Lavach JD (1977): Congenital and hereditary disease of the canine and feline eye. In Kirk RW (ed): Current Veterinary Therapy VI. WB Saunders Co, Philadelphia.
Whitley RD (1988): Focusing on eye disorders among purebred dogs. Vet Med 83:50.

APPENDIX II

Ophthalmic Equipment and Supplies for General Practice

SUPPLIES

1% tropicamide (mydriatic)
Proparacaine hydrochloride (Ophthetic) (topical anesthetic)
Fluorescein strips
Schirmer tear test
Balanced salt solution (irrigating fluid) extraocular
Tear replacement solution

EMERGENCY SUPPLIES

20% Mannitol
Parenteral acetazolamide (Diamox)
Chloramphenicol drops
Sterile balanced salt solution (intraocular)
Chilled glycerin
Atropine (1%) drops

SUTURE MATERIALS

4/0 silk (cutting needle)
6/0 polyglactin 910 (Vicryl) (cutting needle)
4/0 nylon (cutting needle)
6/0 silk (corneal needle)

EQUIPMENT

Direct ophthalmoscope
20-D lens (for indirect ophthalmoscopy)
Focal light source (penlight or Finnoff trans-illuminator)
Magnifying loupe (magnification × 2)
Lacrimal cannula
Conjunctival fixation forceps
Schiøtz tonometer and calibration table

BASIC SURGICAL INSTRUMENTS

Derf needle holders
Castroviejo lid retractors
Conjunctival forceps
Corneal forceps
Strabismus scissors
No. 3 scalpel handle
No. 11 scalpel blades (Bard-Parker)
No. 15 scalpel blades (Bard-Parker)

SUPPLEMENTARY INSTRUMENTS

Castroviejo needle holders (with lock)
Cilia forceps
Corneal scissors
Additional conjunctival fixation forceps
Foreign body spud

Glossary

abiotrophy—premature degeneration of a tissue after it has reached maturity. A term once applied to progressive retinal degeneration type I.

accommodation—the adjustment of the eye for seeing at different distances, usually accomplished by changes in the shape of the lens through action of the ciliary muscle, which result in focusing a clear image on the retina. In some species (e.g., horses), the mechanism is different.

acuity—visual ability to distinguish shapes; applies to central vision.

adnexa—orbit, orbital contents, lids, lacrimal system, conjunctiva, third eyelid.

agenesis—failure of development of an organ.

albinism—inherited absence or deficiency of tyrosinase, characterized by an absence or decrease of melanin in the skin, hair, and eyes.

amaurosis—nearly obsolete term indicating loss of vision.

amblyopia—reduced vision in an eye that appears normal at examination.

ancoria—lack of a pupil.

angle-closure glaucoma (narrow-angle glaucoma)—ocular abnormality in which the intraocular pressure increases, often quickly, because the anterior aqueous is mechanically prevented from reaching the trabecular meshwork.

angstrom (Å)—unit of wavelength equal to 10^{-10} meter (nanometer now preferred [10^{-9} meter]).

aniridia—absence of iris, usually incomplete, with iris root present.

aniseikonia—optical condition in which the retinal images in the two eyes are of different sizes.

anisocoria—condition in which the pupils of the two eyes are of unequal size.

ankyloblepharon—condition in which the margins of the eyelids are fused together.

anophthalmos—absence of the eye.

anterior chamber—space filled with aqueous, bounded anteriorly by the cornea and posteriorly by the iris and lens.

anterior chamber angle—see *iridocorneal angle.*

aphakia—absence of the lens.

aphakic crescent—when a ventrally subluxated lens is seen through a dilated pupil, the "new moon" area between the pupil and the lens equator is called an aphakic crescent

aqueous—the clear, watery fluid that fills the anterior and posterior chambers within the front part of the eye.

aqueous flare—Tyndall beam observed with a biomicroscope when excessive protein is present in the anterior aqueous.

aqueous, secondary (plasmoid)—aqueous

produced when the blood-aqueous barrier is disturbed.

asteroid hyalosis—fixed opacities composed of a calcium lipid complex that occur in an otherwise normal vitreous body; there are no symptoms.

astigmatism—optical condition in which the refractive power is not uniform in all meridians; when regular, there are two main meridians of refractive power; when irregular, there are a number of meridians of refractive power.

bedewing of cornea—subepithelial corneal edema, often associated with sudden, prolonged increase in intraocular pressure or wearing of contact lenses for an excessively long period.

Bergmeister's papilla—small mass of glial cells that surrounds the hyaloid artery in the center of the optic disc; on occasion it persists and obliterates the physiological cup of the optic disc.

binocular vision—the ability to use the two eyes simultaneously to focus on the same object and to fuse the two images into a single image.

biomicroscope—microscope for examining the eye, consisting essentially of a dissecting microscope combined with a light source that projects a rectangular light beam that can be changed in size and focus.

blepharitis—inflammation of the upper or lower eyelids.

blepharochalasis—relaxation of the eyelid skin (may indicate redundancy).

blepharoclonus—exaggerated reflex blinking.

blepharophimosis—inability to open the eye to the normal extent.

blepharoplasty—plastic surgery of the eyelids.

blepharoptosis—drooping of the upper lid due to paralysis of the oculomotor nerve (cranial nerve III) or the sympathetic nerves or to excessive weight of the upper eyelids.

blepharospasm—tonic spasm of the orbicularis oculi muscle.

blindness—inability to see.
  cortical b.—caused by a lesion in the cortical visual center.
  night b.—inefficient dark adaptation, so the vision is markedly reduced in reduced illumination.
  snow b.—inability to open eyes to see; secondary to ultraviolet keratitis.

blood-aqueous barrier—functional barrier between the vasculr system and the aqueous.

bulla—a large vesicle or blister.

bullous keratopathy—disease of the cornea associated with bullae.

buphthalmos—enlargement of the eye due to glaucoma.

canaliculus—small tear drainage tube at the inner aspect of the upper and lower lids, leading from the punctum to the common canaliculus and then to the tear sac.

canthoplasty—a plastic operation on the canthus.

canthorrhaphy—suturing of the canthus.

canthotomy—incision of the canthus.

canthus—the angle at either end of the eye aperture; specified as nasal (medial) or temporal (lateral).

caruncle—a small piece of skin at the medial canthus from which hairs often protrude.

cataract—opacity of the lens or its capsule or both.

central progressive retinal atrophy—progressive retinal degeneration type II.

cerebellar nystagmus—a pathological tremor of the globes due to damage to the deep nuclei of the cerebellum. If the flocculonodular lobe is involved, the nystagmus will be associated with loss of equilibrium.

chalazion—chronic lipogranuloma of a tarsal gland.

chalcosis—retention of copper (or its alloys of brass or bronze) in the eye.

chemosis—edema of the conjunctiva.

chloroid—part of the uveal tract immediately external to the retina; responsible for nutrition of the outer retinal layers.

choroiditis—inflammation of the choroid.

chronic superficial keratitis—see *syndrome, Überreiter's.*

ciliary body—part of the uveal tract between the iris and the choroid; consists of ciliary processes that produce aqueous and the ciliary muscle.

ciliary injection—hyperemia of the subconjunctival (ciliary) vessels ("ciliary vessels" does *not* refer to the lids).

cilium—eyelash.

closed-angle glaucoma—see *glaucoma.*

collie eye anomaly—scleral ectasia syndrome.

collyrium—eyewash.

coloboma—a gap, hole, or fissure in ocular tissue (e.g., the iris, choroid, or optic disc).
  typical c.—a defect lying in or near the fetal ocular cleft (a line from the center of the optic disc to the pupil, slightly nasal to the center of the lower border of the pupil)
  atypical c.—a defect lying in an area other than the fetal ocular cleft.

cone—cells responsible for vision in bright light and for fine visual acuity.

conjugate ocular movements—similar ocular movements of both eyes, such as eyes right, eyes left, eyes up, eyes down (version).

conjunctiva—mucous membrane lining the posterior aspect of the eyelids and covering the anterior sclera.

conjunctival follicles—see *follicles, conjunctival.*

conjunctivorhinostomy—surgical creation of a communication between the conjunctiva and the nasal cavity.

consensual light reflex—constriction of the pupil in the contralateral eye when the retina is stimulated by light.

contact lens—thin plastic lens that fits directly on the cornea under the eyelids.

contralateral—situated on or pertaining to the opposite side.

corectopia—displacement of the pupil from its normal position.

corneal erosion—see *erosion, corneal.*

corneal graft—operation to restore vision by replacing a section of opaque cornea with transparent cornea.

corneal ulcer—see *ulcer, corneal.*

corpora nigra—irregular oval bodies on the dorsal and occasionally the ventral pupillary edges of the iris in herbivora.

cotton wool spots—a microinfarct causing acute edema of the nerve fiber layer of the retina (cytoid body).

couching—an ancient surgical procedure of dislocating the lens from its optical axis.

cryotherapy—localized tissue destruction by freezing.

cul de sac—fornix; the area where the conjunctival layers covering the lower lid and the globe meet.

cyclitic membrane—organized exudate seen as a transverse membrane behind the lens as a result of uveitis.

cyclitis—inflammation of the ciliary body.

cyclocryotherapy—localized destruction of parts of the ciliary body by freezing.

cyclodialysis—surgical procedure for glaucoma to establish a communication between the anterior chamber and the suprachoroidal space.

cyclodiathermy—destruction of a portion of the ciliary body by diathermy to reduce the quantity of aqueous produced in glaucoma.

cycloplegia—paralysis of the ciliary muscle giving rise to paralysis of accommodation.

dacryoadenitis—inflammation of the lacrimal or gland of the third eyelid.

dacryocystitis—inflammation and infection of the lacrimal sac.

dacryostenosis—atresia of the lacrimal duct.

dark adaptation—biochemical and neurological process by which the eye becomes more sensitive to light.

decussation—referring to the crossing of nerve fibers or tracts from one side of the nervous system to the opposite side. The optic chiasm is the crossing of some fibers of the optic nerve to the opposite side of the brain.

denervation supersensitivity—sensitivity to neural effector substance that follows postganglionic interruption of the nerve supply of organs innervated by the autonomic nervous system.

dermoid—a congenital tumor consisting of skin and its appendages.

descemetocele—herniation of the basement membrane of the corneal endothelium.

detachment, retinal—separation of the sensory retina from the retinal pigment epithelium.

dialysis of retina—separation at the ora ciliaris retinae of the sensory retina from the retinal pigment epithelium.

diopter—unit of measurement of the refractive power of lenses, equal to the reciprocal of the focal length of lens expressed in meters.

diplopia—the perception of one object as two images ("double vision").

disinsertion of retina—retinal dialysis at the ora ciliaris retinae in which the sensory retina is separated from the retinal pigment epithelium.

dislocation (luxation) of lens—condition in which the crystalline lens is completely unsupported by the zonular fibers, so that the lens is free, either in the vitreous body or in the anterior chamber.

distichiasis—supernumerary row of eyelashes.

drainage angle—see *iridocorneal angle.*

dyscoria—abnormally shaped pupil.

dystrophy—noninflammatory, developmental, nutritional, or metabolic abnormality.

ectasia—dilatation or distention; may be toward the observer (e.g., corneal ectasia) or away from the observer (e.g., posterior scleral ectasia).

ectopia—displacement or malposition, especially congenital.

ectropion—eversion or turning out of the eyelid.

electroretinogram—a graphic record of the action potential that follows stimulation of the retina by light.

emmetropia—refractive condition in which no refractive error is present with accommodation at rest.

endophthalmitis—inflammation of the intraocular contents.

enophthalmos—abnormal recession of the eye within the orbit.

entropion—turning inward of the eyelid.

enucleation—removal of the eye.

epilation—removal of hair, especially cilia.

epiphora—faulty drainage of tears, permitting overflow and tearing.

episcleritis—localized inflammation of the superficial tissues of the sclera.

erosion, corneal—recurrent loss of corneal epithelium.

esotropia—inward deviation that occurs with both eyes open.

evisceration—surgical removal of the intraocular contents, with retention of the cornea (sometimes) and the sclera.

exenteration, orbital—removal of all the orbital tissues, including the eye and its nervous, vascular, and muscular connections.

exodeviation—turning outward of the eyes.

exophthalmos—abnormal protrusion of the eye.

ophthalmoplegic e.—inability to move the eye because of exophthalmos.

pulsating e. (exophthalmos pulsans)—associated with an arteriovenous fistula of the orbit.

exotropia—outward deviation of the eyes.

feline keratitis nigrum—see *sequestration.*

field, visual—see *visual field.*

filtration angle—see *iridocorneal angle.*

fluorescein angiography—serial photography of the ocular fundus following intravenous administration of fluorescein solution.

fluorescence—reradiation of energy with increase of wavelength by an absorbing substance.

focus—point of convergence of light rays.

follicles, conjunctival—lymphatic hypertrophy in response to conjunctival inflammation.

fornix—the reflection of the conjunctiva from the eyelid or third eyelid to the globe.

fundus—the posterior portion of the eye visible through an ophthalmoscope.

glands of Moll—apocrine glands of the upper and lower eyelid margins.

glands of Zeis—sebaceous glands of the upper and lower eyelid margins.

glaucoma—increase in intraocular pressure.

narrow-angle or closed-angle g.—glaucoma arising because of apposition of the iris to the peripheral cornea.

gonioscope—a special instrument for studying the iridocorneal angle of the anterior chamber of the eye.

gonioscopy—examination of the iridocorneal angle using a corneal contact lens, (goniolens), magnifying device, and light source.

guttate—drop-shaped.

haws—a lay term indicating protrusion of the third eyelid.

hemeralopia—day blindness; defective vision in a bright light.

hemianopia—blindness of one half of the visual field.

heterochromia iridis—condition in which the irises of the two eyes are not of uniform color.

heterotropia—condition in which the eyes deviate; strabismus.

hippus—spasmodic dilatation and contraction of the pupil independent of stimulation with light.

hordeolum—stye; a localized, purulent, inflammatory infection of one or more sebaceous glands of the eyelid.

external h.—infection of the glands of Moll or Zeis

internal h.—infection of the tarsal glands.

Horner's syndrome—see *syndrome, Horner's.*

hyaloid—pertaining to the vitreous.

hydrophthalmos—buphthalmos or the distended eye that occurs in infantile glaucoma.

hyperopia (hypermetropia)—refractive state of the eye in which the parallel rays of light would come to focus behind the retina if not intercepted by it.

hypertropia—deviation of the eyes in which one eye is higher than the other.

hyphema—blood in the anterior chamber.

hypopyon—pus in the anterior chamber.

hypotony—diminished ocular pressure.

image—the visual impression of an object formed by a lens or mirror.

Purkinje's i.—image reflected from the surface of the cornea, the anterior surface of the lens, and the posterior surface of the lens.

real i.—in optics, the inverted image in which refracted rays pass through the image point.

virtual i.—in optics, the erect image in which the refracted rays do not pass through the image point but appear to come from it.

infrared radiation—part of the electromagnetic spectrum that has a wavelength of more than 700 nm and less than 10,000 nm.

intumescent lens—a swollen or enlarged lens.

iridectomy—removal of a part of the iris.

peripheral (basal) i.—removal of a portion of the peripheral iris.

sector i.—removal of an entire sector of the iris, extending usually from the pupillary margin to the root of the iris.

iridencleisis—surgical procedure for glaucoma in which an incision is made at the limbus, and the iris is incarcerated in the wound to create a filtering wick between the anterior chamber and the subconjunctival space.

iridocorneal angle (filtration, anterior chamber, or drainage angle)—the angle between the iris and the cornea through which aqueous leaves the eye.

iridocyclitis—inflammation of the iris and ciliary body.

iridodialysis—separation of the base of the iris from the ciliary body; main cause is blunt trauma to the eye.

iridodonesis—tremulousness of the iris occurring after loss of support due to luxation or removal of the lens.

iridoplegia—paralysis of the sphincter pupillae of the iris.

iris bombé—adherence of the pupil to the lens, so that aqueous accumulates in the posterior chamber; the iris tends to balloon forward peripherally and may close the angle, causing secondary glaucoma.

iris prolapse—protrusion of the iris through a perforated corneal or corneoscleral wound.

iritis—inflammation of the iris.

keratectomy—excision of the cornea.

keratic precipitates (KPs)—clumps of leukocytes adhering to the corneal endothelium in uveal tract inflammation; customarily classified as either mutton fat precipitates (macrophages), which occur in granulomatous inflammations, or punctate precipitates (lymphocytes), which occur in nongranulomatous inflammations.

keratitis—inflammation of the cornea.

keratoconjunctivitis—simultaneous inflammation of the cornea and conjunctiva.

keratoconus—conical protrusion of the cornea.

keratoglobus—enlargement of the cornea in which the cornea is protruded and globular in shape.

keratomycosis—keratitis caused by fungi.

keratoplasty—transplantation of a portion of the cornea.

lamellar k.—replacement of superficial layers.

penetrating k. (deep)—replacement of the entire thickness of a portion of the cornea.

lacrimation—section of the precorneal tear film (tears).

lagophthalmos—condition in which the globe is not entirely covered when the eyelids are closed.

lens—glass or other transparent material used to optically modify the path of light.

lenticonus—abnormality of the lens, characterized by a conical prominence on the anterior or posterior lens surface.

lentiglobus—exaggerated curvature of the lens, producing a spherical bulging on its surface.

leukoma—a corneal opacity; a less marked type is called a macula, and a minor type of opacity is a nebula.

adherent l.—corneal opacity to which the iris is adherent.

limbus—circular boundary between the cornea and the sclera.

luxation—complete displacement of the lens from the hyaloid fossa. See also *subluxation of lens.*

lysozyme (muramidase)—an antibacterial enzyme found in tears, leukocytes, egg albumin, and plants; mainly effective against nonpathogenic bacteria and found in low levels in the normal eyes of domestic animals.

macula—a moderate corneal scar; a cone-rich area in the posterior retina that is devoid of blood vessels.

microphakia—abnormally small lens.

microphthalmia—abnormally small globe.

miosis—constriction of the pupil.

miotic—pertaining to or characterized by constriction of the pupil or to a drug that causes pupillary constriction.

Mittendorf's dot—opacity of the posterior lens capsule marking the site of hyaloid artery attachment.

morgagnian cataract—a hypermature cataract in which the cortex is liquefied, permitting the lens nucleus to float or sink within the capsule.

mummification—see *sequestration.*

mydriasis—dilatation of the pupil.

mydriatic—a drug that causes pupillary dilatation.

myopia—optical condition in which parallel rays of light come to focus in front of the retina.

axial m.—myopia caused by abnormal length of the anteroposteior diameter of the eye.

nanometer (nm)—unit of wavelength equal to 10^{-9} of a meter; formerly called millimicron (mμ).

narrow-angle glaucoma—see *glaucoma.*

nebula—minor corneal opacity.

neurotrophic keratitis—keratitis caused by anesthesia of the cornea.

nyctalopia—night blindness.

nystagmus—oscillatory movement of the eye.

jerk n.—nystagmus having a fast and a slow phase.

labyrinthine n.—nystagmus occurring when the labyrinths are irritated or diseased (synonym: vestibular nystagmus).

optokinetic n.—nystagmus in normal individuals (especially humans) that occurs when a succession of moving objects traverse the field of vision, as when one gazes out of a window of a moving vehicle at a succession of stationary objects.

pendulous n.—nystagmus occurring in individuals in whom vision in both eyes has been defective since birth.

rotatory n.—nystagmus in which the eye partially rotates around the visual axis.

occlusion of the pupil—see *pupil, occluded.*

O.D.—oculum dexter, the right eye.

open-angle glaucoma—that form of increased intraocular pressure in which the aqueous humor has access to the trabecular meshwork.

ophthalmia neonatorum—conjunctivitis in the newborn.

ophthalmoplegia—paralysis of the ocular muscles.

o. externa—paralysis of the external ocular muscles.

o. interna—paralysis of the muscles of the iris and the ciliary body.

total o.—combination of both intrinsic and extrinsic paralysis.

ophthalmoscope—an instrument with a special illumination system for viewing the inner eye, particularly the retina and associated structures.

optic atrophy—atrophy of the optic nerve.

optic disc—ophthalmoscopically visible portion of the optic nerve in the globe.

O.S.—oculum sinister, the left eye.

pannus—newly formed vascular tissue involving the cornea.

panophthalmitis—inflammation of all ocular tissues, including the corneoscleral envelope, Tenon's capsule, and often orbital tissue as well.

papilla (optic papilla)—the optic disc.

papilledema—passive edema of the optic disc.

papillitis—inflammation of the optic disc, or optic neuritis.

peripheral anterior synechiae (PAS)—adhesion of peripheral iris to the cornea (seen by gonioscopy).

persistent pupillary membrane—web-like strands stretching across the pupil from the region of the collarette.

photophobia—ocular discomfort induced by bright light.

photopic—pertaining to vision in the light; an eye that has become light-adapted.

photoreceptor—a nerve and organ sensitive to light; classified as a rod or a cone.

phthisis bulbi—degenerative shrinkage of the eye.

polycoria—occurrence of more than one pupil in the iris; classified as true polycoria if surrounded by sphincter muscle, and pseudopolycoria if not.

posterior chamber—space between the back of the iris and the front of the lens; filled with aqueous.

presbyopia—refractive condition in which there is a diminished power of accommodation, arising from impaired elasticity of the crystalline lens, as occurs with aging.

progressive retinal atrophy (PRA)—progressive retinal degeneration (PRD).

prolapse of the iris—protrusion of the iris through a perforated cornea or corneoscleral wound.

proliferative keratoconjunctivitis—a disease complex seen largely in rough collies and characterized by cholesterol crystals in superficial corneal stroma, inflammatory infiltration of the cornea from the lateral limbus, and inflammatory infiltration of the third eyelid.

proptosis—forward displacement of the globe; exophthalmos.

pseudoenophthalmos—apparent recession of the globe, such as in the animal with swollen lids, microphthalmia, or phthisis bulbi.

pseudoproptosis—apparent exophthalmos, such as that suggested when lid retraction is seen.

ptosis—drooping of the upper eyelid.

pupil—the round hole in the center of the iris that corresponds to the lens aperture in a camera.

   occluded p.—opaque fibrous tissue covering the pupil.

   secluded p.—adhesion of the whole pupillary circumference to the lens capsule; leads to iris bombé.

pupillary block—blockage of the passage of aqueous through the pupil between the posterior and the anterior chambers.

pupillary membrane—anomaly of the iris, usually minor, in which there is failure of the fetal pupillary membrane to atrophy; often a persistent strand extends between the iris collarette and the anterior lens capsule.

Purkinje's shift—luminosity curve of dark-adapted individual peaks at 500 nm, whereas the luminosity curve of light-adapted individuals peaks at 550 nm; indicates two types of retinal photoreceptors.

red eye—lay term applied to any condition with dilatation of conjunctival or ciliary body vessels.

reflex—involuntary, invariable, adaptive response to a stimulus.

   conjunctival (lid) r.—closure of the eyelids induced by touching the conjunctiva (also called corneal reflex).

   consensual light (crossed) r.—constriction of the pupil when the opposite retina is stimulated with light.

   direct light r.—contraction of the sphincter pupillae induced by stimulation of retina with light (also called pupillary reflex)

   lacrimal r.—secretion of tears induced by irritation of the cornea and conjunctiva.

   oculocardiac (eye compression) r.—decrease of heartbeat caused by pressure on the eye.

retina—the innermost tunic of the eyeball, containing the neural elements for reception and transmission of visual stimuli.

   disinsertion of—see *disinsertion of retina.*

retinal atrophy, progressive—see *progressive retinal atrophy (PRA).*

retinal detachment—see *detachment, retinal.*

retinal dysplasia—abnormal differentiation of retinal layers.

retinitis—inflammation of the retina.

retinopathy—any disease condition of the retina.

retinoschisis—a congenital cleft of the retina; a cleavage of retinal layers.

retrobulbar neuritis—inflammation of the optic nerve occurring without involvement of the optic disc.

retrolental fibroplasia—a condition characterized by the presence of gliotic tissue behind the lens, associated with detachment of the retina and arrest of growth of the eye, due to excessively high concentrations of oxygen in the care of the prematurely born (hence, the synonymous term retinopathy of prematurity).

rod—part of the outer retina responsible for vision in dim light. The animal retina is a rod-rich retina, in contrast to the cone-rich human retina.

rubeosis iridis—neovascularization of the iris.

Schirmer test—test for tear formation in which absorbent paper is folded over the lid margin for 1 minute and the amount of wetting measured.

scleritis—inflammation of the sclera.

scotopic—pertaining to vision in the dark; refers to an eye that has become dark-adapted.

seclusion of pupil—see *pupil, secluded.*

sequestration (mummification; also known as feline keratitis nigrum)—the partial separation of black necrotic cornea following severe keratitis in the cat.

slit lamp—see *biomicroscope.*

spherophakia—spherically shaped lens.

squint—see *strabismus.*

staphyloma—ectasia of the wall of the eye, lined with uveal tract.

strabismus—condition in which the eyes are not simultaneously directed to the same object.

   comitant s.—deviation of the eye in which there is no ocular muscle paralysis, and the degree of crossing is the same in all directions of gaze.

   noncomitant s.—deviation of the eyes from parallelism in which a muscle is paretic or paralytic.

stye—purulent inflammation of a gland of Zeis or Moll, or of a tarsal gland. See also *hordeolum.*

subhyaloid hemorrhage—hemorrhage between the neural retina and the vitreous body; a meniscus level is often present.

subluxation of lens—condition of the lens when a portion of the supporting zonule is absent and the lens lacks support in one or more quadrants, resulting in partial displacement from the hyaloid fossa.

symblepharon—adhesion between palpebral and bulbar conjunctiva.

synchysis scintillans—cholesterol crystals in liquefied vitreous.

*****syndrome**—a group of symptoms and signs that occur together; a disease or definite morbid process having a characteristic sequence of symptoms; may affect the whole body or any of its parts.

   Chediak-Higashi—recessive albinism with leukocytic inclusions.

   chiasma—optic atrophy and bitemporal hemianopia.

   Ehlers-Danlos—a widespread systemic disorder with overextensibility of joints, hyperplasticity and fragility of the skin, and pseudotumors following trauma; there may be epicanthal folds, esotropia, blue sclera, glaucoma, ectopic lenses, proliferating retinopathy, and acanthocytosis.

   Horner's—sympathetic nerve paralysis with miosis, blepharoptosis, enophthalmos, and protrusion of the third eyelid.

   Kennedy's (Foster Kennedy)—ipsilateral optic atrophy and contralateral papilledema in frontal lobe tumors, aneurysms, or abscesses.

   Niemann-Pick—heredofamilial lipid disorder.

   Peters's anomaly—adherent corneal leukoma with absence of Descemet's membrane and endothelium.

   Tay-Sachs disease—infantile amaurotic familial idiocy; a sphingolipidosis.

   Überreiter's—a specific corneal disease affecting the dog.

---

*Many of these eponymous terms refer to human diseases but are used to describe analogous conditions in animals.

synechiae—adhesion between the iris and the adjacent structures.

anterior s.—synechiae between the iris and the cornea.

peripheral anterior s.—occurs with unrelieved attacks of angle-closure glaucoma when the iris remains in contact with the cornea or following surgery when the anterior chamber does not form.

posterior s.—adhesion between the iris and the lens, as occurs commonly in uveitis.

tapetum—fluorescent layer in the choroid in the dorsal third of the fundus; triangular in shape.

tarsorrhaphy—operation in which the lids are sutured together, as in treatment of lagophthalmos.

tear film BUT—tear film break-up time.

Tenon's capsule—fascia bulbi, a connective tissue sheath encircling the globe, posterior to the limbus.

Tenon's space—episcleral space between Tenon's capsule and the globe.

tonography—test to determine the amount of fluid forced from the eye by a constant pressure during a constant period.

tonometer—instrument for measuring ocular tension.

applanation t.—instrument used to measure intraocular pressure in which the globe is not indented.

Schiøtz t.—indentation type of instrument.

TRIC agents—acronym derived from *tra*choma and *i*nclusion *c*onjunctivitis, members of the psittacosis–lymphogranuloma venereum–trachoma (*Chlamydia* or *Bedsoniae*) group of microorganisms.

trichiasis—condition in which there are supernumerary eyelashes.

tumor—a swelling or enlargement of varying size that may involve any structure; usually but not always neoplastic.

ulcer, corneal—a break in continuity of corneal epithelium with or without loss of stroma; often slow to heal.

uvea (uveal tract)—entire vascular coat of the globe: iris, ciliary body and choroid, including the tapetum.

anterior u.—iris and ciliary body.

posterior u.—choroid.

uveitis—inflammation of the iris, ciliary body, or choroid, or a combination of these.

endogenous u.—inflammation of the uveal tract, arising from causes within the body.

exogenous u.—inflammation of the uveal tract, arising from causes outside the body, as in injuries.

vision—faculty of seeing; sight.

binocular v.—faculty of using both eyes synchronously.

color v.—ability to distinguish subjectively a large variety of wavelengths of light in the visible spectrum.

photopic v.—vision in bright illumination.

scotopic v.—vision in dim illumination or vision following the biochemical or neurological changes occurring in dark adaptation.

visual field—locus of objects or points in space that can be perceived when the head and eyes are kept fixed; the field may be monocular or binocular.

vitreous flare—vitreous opacity associated with uveitis.

vitreous veils—faint, curtain-like opacities seen by focal light through a dilated pupil in the normal eye; the veils move gently in the vitreous when the eye moves.

Wood's light—electromagnetic energy with a wavelength of about 3650 Å; an apparatus equipped with a nickel oxide filter that produces ultraviolet light of that quality.

xerophthalmia—conjunctivitis with atrophy, producing a dry eye.

xerosis—abnormal dryness of the eye or skin.

zonulus—the numerous fine tissue strands (ligaments) that stretch from the ciliary process to the lens equator (360°) and hold the lens in place.

zonulysis—dissolution of the zonules, as with chymotrypsin, to facilitate removal of the lens in cataract surgery.

Index

Note: Page numbers in *italics* refer to illustrations; those followed by a (t) indicate tables. Color plates are indicated by the word plate followed by the appropriate roman numeral.